THE ACOUSTICS OF SPEECH COMMUNICATION

FUNDAMENTALS, SPEECH PERCEPTION THEORY, AND TECHNOLOGY

J. M. PICKETT

Professor Emeritus, Gallaudet University
Proprietor, Windy Hill Lab, Surry, Maine

ALLYN AND BACON

Boston   London   Toronto   Sydney   Tokyo   Singapore

Executive Editor: Stephen D. Dragin
Editorial-Production Administrator: Joe Sweeney
Editorial-Production Service: Walsh & Associates, Inc.
Composition Buyer: Linda Cox
Manufacturing Buyer: Julie McNeill
Cover Administrator: Jennifer Hart

Copyright © 1999 by Allyn & Bacon
A Viacom Company
160 Gould Street
Needham Heights, MA 02494
www.abacon.com

Library of Congress Cataloging-in-Publication Data
Pickett, J. M. (James M.)
     The acoustics of speech communication : fundamentals, speech
perception theory, and technology / J. M. Pickett.
       p.   cm.
     Includes bibliographical references and index.
     ISBN 0-205-19887-2
     1. Speech perception.   2. Speech—Physiological aspects.
3. Psychoacoustics.   4. Phonetics.   5. Auditory perception.
I. Title.
BF463.S64P5   1998
153.7′5—dc21   98-38945
                                                            CIP

Printed in the United States of America

Dedicated to the memory of Dennis Klatt

1970—An instructive dialogue with Dennis:
Author J.M. Pickett: "How do you see the future of speech technology?"
Dennis: "Speech tech will be very, very big! ! !"
1998—Bill Gates quoted by Business Week, *February 23:*
"Speech is not just the future of Windows, but the future of computing itself"

CONTENTS

PREFACE

DEVOTED TO SPEECH SOUNDS

Story of a Speech Book

School debate tournaments got me into a lifetime study of speech acoustics. My mentors were the debating coach, engineering instructors in WWII, and the phonetician/psychologist R.H. Stetson. He inspired me to go for the forefront of knowledge about speech because, even in his retirement career, he had developed a unique electronic laboratory for the study of speech movements and speech sound analysis.

I went from zero to zealous about speech sounds, from 1939 to 1952, when I started work in acoustic speech research for the U.S. Air Force. Thanks to the developing new technology of speech, it was possible to offer that introductory experience in the 1980 book, condensed into a one-semester course of study (Pickett, 1980).

A Revised Book

My basic aim, similar to my 1980 book, is to teach the technical acoustics of speech and its perception to the nontechnical student. We go deeply enough into these subjects to provide a strong background for reading the literature and beginning research. The first part, Chapters One through Ten, develops the basic concepts used in sound analysis and applies them to the speech sound distinctions employed in English. It is intended to be a thorough introduction to acoustic phonetics. Here I have used much of the 1980 book, edited, updated, and supplemented with computer-generated illustrations and phonological notes. The rest, Chapters Eleven through Seventeen, present some of the major findings of acoustic research on speech perception and current theoretical explanations, including how this knowledge may be employed in speech technology and understanding speech for people with hearing impairments. This part is almost totally new, written primarily by my coauthors.

Help from Colleagues

Gunnar Fant's basic theory and interests figured heavily in the 1980 book because of his generous welcoming of guest researchers to work in his Department at the Swedish Royal Institute of Technology. As before, I'm grateful for the many comments of my students at Gallaudet University and the intense speech interests of many Gallaudet associates, especially Sally Revoile, Ingo Titze, Tim Bunnell, and Lynne Bernstein. Tim unknowingly contributed to this revision via his development of easy-to-use analysis programs in his Edwav suite; Sally wrote a new chapter. Ingo sent me computer-generated vocal folds.

Enthusiastic users of the 1980 book offered comments from an astonishing variety of laboratories and departments. Those I especially remember are Adrian Fourcin and Evelyn Abberton, Sarah Hawkins, John Gilbert, Don Jamieson, Björn Lindblom, George Allen, Nina Thorsen, Arthur Abramson, and Yael Frank. Thanks also to reviewers Ray Daniloff, University of North Texas, and Susan Nittrouer, Boys Town National Research Hospital.

Dennis Klatt is especially remembered. He was always ready for an advisory visit, even when I brought along my research dean. We often talked about the book, about research strategies, about aids for the speech-handicapped, and even about the industrial future of speech technology. Everyone in our field will remember how, late in his shortened life, he still gave an effective lecture with only half a voice.

Recently, my personal motivations, after I retired from the major concerns of Gallaudet University, remained strongly stimulated by people in the Speech Communication Group of the Research Laboratory of Electronics at Massachusetts Institute of Technology, particularly when I talked with Kenneth Stevens and Corine Bickley, in discussions of their development work with Robert Berkovitz, President of Sensimetrics Corporation. I can never thank that Sensimetrics crew enough for providing SpeechStation, for their enthusiastic encouragement, for critical comments on the book, and for considerable contributions toward the revision. We devised a CD-ROM course in speech production and perception, an activity that synergized with the book at important points.

Coauthors who stuck it out despite teaching commitments and responsibilities for the survival of their research programs were: Sarah Hawkins, Winifred Strange, Sally Revoile, Corine Bickley, Ann Syrdal, Juergen Schroeter, and Diane Kewley-Port.

We should all thank the Gods of Phonetics for colleagues like these.

Finally, though she's not a phonetician, I thank my wife, Dr. Betty H. Pickett, a companion scientist who supported both books and our research sojourn in Sweden. Kathy Whittier of Walsh & Associates was invaluable in the final assembly of this book from diverse files of our authors.

PART ONE

ACOUSTIC PHONETICS: SPEECH ENCODING FROM ARTICULATION TO SOUND STREAM

People usually communicate by talking. It is convenient: Your talking instrument is always with you. It is fast: You can talk almost as fast as you can think of what to say. Your speed is afforded by a remarkably efficient code that uses two human activities: (1) your vocal organs encode what you want to say into a stream of speech sounds and, (2) your listener's hearing decodes what your message is (Liberman, 1996). You encode the phonemes (vowels and consonants) of your message into a flowing stream of sound, and speech perception by the listener decodes your speech stream back into the phonemes of your message.

This book is a detailed tutorial on how this speech code operates. Part One of our study, Acoustic Phonetics, describes phonemes and how speech articulation encodes them, via vowel and consonant shaping of acoustic voice sources, into a flowing stream of complex acoustic patterns. In Part Two we study how listeners decode the stream of acoustic patterns back to phonemes and the theories proposed to explain the decoding. Then we describe some applications to hearing-impaired decoding and coding/decoding by computers.

CHAPTER ONE

LANGUAGE, PHONETICS, AND SPEECH PRODUCTION

INTRODUCTION: LANGUAGE AND SCIENCE

Each of us enjoys language in many personal ways: getting information, asking questions, telling things, instructing, arguing, persuading, cheering, singing, amusing, joking; is there any limit to our uses? A language scientist wonders how language does these things and wants to satisfy that curiosity by building formal schemes to explain what language can achieve.

When I talk, I launch some sounds from my mouth, confident they will mean something to another speaker of my language. How can this happen? Obviously my sounds must be coded or patterned in certain ways to be detected, deciphered, and recognized by my listener. Companion speakers understand what I say by decoding my speech patterns. Speech sound patterning is what phoneticians want to know all about; they ask how the sounds are formed, what their essential code patterns are, and how language employs the patterns to convey meaning.

What do our sounds look like? I asked a neighbor family to record Son, Mother, and Father bedtime reading and then made some sound landscapes of their greetings on the tape, as seen in Figure 1-1. The first soundscape in the top row is Mother saying "Hi Mac" and next is her 9-year-old son repeating her; Father's soundscape is on the right. We can see there are two groups of ridges running from left to right, one group for "Hi" and another for "Mac," separated by a gap above the [m]-sound of "Mac." The ridges are far apart vertically in the "Hi's" and closer for the "Mac's." These ridges, spaced upward from the bottom of the plot toward the top, are closer

for Mother than for Son and even closer for Father.

Despite these differences, Mother's, Son's, and Father's words sound like exactly the same words: "Hi Mac." How could this be? Examine the bottom-to-top spacing of the ridges. Within each word the Son's first, second, and third ridges are more widely spaced apart, but the proportions of Son's spacing are about the same as Mother's and Father's. Father's words have ridges that are closer together than Mother's and even closer than Son's. In other words, it looks like the proportions of the spacing are what defines the words. It is the proportions that form the words, not just the distances between the ridges.

In the bottom row of soundscapes, where the family is saying "Hi Sam," the two word-ranges are separated by a bank of bumpy "clouds" higher up the scale in each soundscape. The cloud-banks represent the S-sound of "Sam." Their bumpiness is due to the chaotic turbulence of the S-sound. Each cloud is tallest in the area marked "S-ridge" for each person. For Mother the location of the tall S-ridge tends to be at a middle place going up the cloud, but it is farther up for Son and lower for Father. Thus, the S-frequencies of the family members, in relation to each other, are similar in proportions to the ridges in the words, but higher up vertically in the soundscape.

Similarities and differences like these are what our study of acoustic phonetics is all about. The speech landscapes were plotted by a computer system that presented acoustical analyses of the "Hi Mac" and "Hi Sam" sound waves plotted in

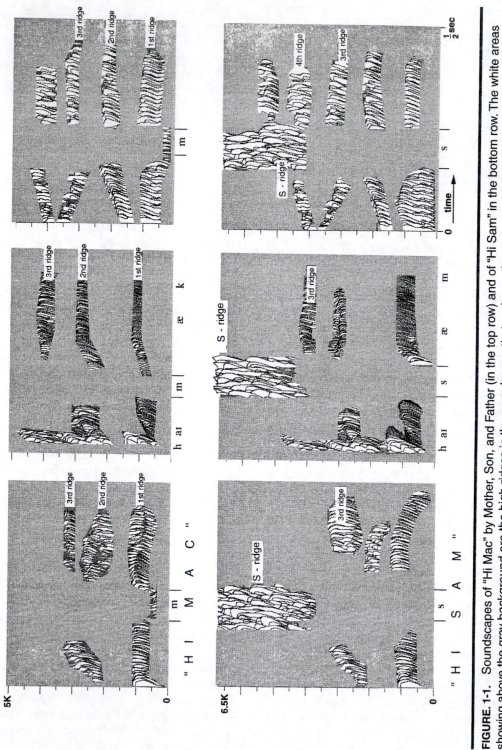

FIGURE. 1-1. Soundscapes of "Hi Mac" by Mother, Son, and Father (in the top row) and of "Hi Sam" in the bottom row. The white areas showing above the gray background are the high ridges in the soundscape that make up the coded acoustic information of those greetings. (Soundscapes were derived and plotted, retouched, as energy patterns in frequency [vertically] and time [horizontally] by the Perspectrogram program in SpeechStation2 from Sensimetrics Corporation)

4

time, left-to-right, in *frequency*, bottom-to-top, and in *intensity*, height of ridges. We will explain all the features of speech sounds in that way, by means of frequency and intensity of sound as they change over time.

HOW SIGNIFICANT IS ACOUSTIC PHONETICS?

Speech is coded to form words and sentences in a language. The code of speech resides in its sounds. Thus a scientific understanding of speech communication depends on knowing the sound patterns of the speech code. The scientific study of speech sounds is acoustic phonetics, which focuses especially on the sound patterns that function in language. In other words, acoustic phonetics is the language science dealing with the sound code of speech. Acoustic phonetics is a part of the general field of speech science, or experimental phonetics, which also includes physiological phonetics. Physiological phonetics describes how the nervous system, muscles, and other organs operate in speech. Acoustic phonetics describes the speech sounds themselves and how they are formed acoustically. Acoustic and physiological phonetics are closely related, as we will often see in our study.

Speech science is basic to the understanding of a very broad range of challenging problems, including speech perception and hearing, child language acquisition, teaching of language and speech, pathologic speech and language, speech communication technology and speech processing, synthetic speech, automatic recognition of spoken messages, speech communication aids for handicapped people, personal voice characteristics and voice identification, dialects, phonetic comparison of languages, and linguistics in general. Acoustic phonetics contributes to each of these.

Our first aim in this book is to present the facts and theories of acoustic phonetics and speech perception, as a background for further study in the many fields related to speech science and linguistics. Later we apply acoustic phonetics to speech technology and speech audibility for hearing-impaired people.

To begin our study of speech, some linguistic units are defined and the production of speech sounds is described generally.

LINGUISTICS, PHONETICS, AND PHONOLOGY

Linguists have found that the code of every spoken language consists of units arranged in a hierarchy of small units embedded within larger units. The smallest units are the individual sounds, that is, the vowels and consonants, the *phonemes* in linguistics. The sounds form syllables, which contain one or more phonemes. The syllables form words of one or more syllables. Words form sentences of one or more words, to express a thought.

Speech events that encode words are called *phonemes*. Consider, for example, the spoken words *man*, *ban*, and *pan*, each of which consists of a sequence of three sounds. These words differ only in their beginnings. Other sets of words are differentiated in the same way, such as *mean*, *bean*, and *peen*. In *mam* and *map*, the difference is in events at the end; in *bean* and *ban*, the difference is in the middle sound. These are all examples for defining the phonemes /m, b, p, i/ and /ae/ of spoken English. By convention the phonemes are written within slashes, using symbols of the International Phonetic Alphabet. The phonemes of General American English are listed in Table 1-1; for each phoneme key words are given containing the phoneme in different positions.

The phonemes of a language are determined by linguists, who make comparisons among many utterances in each language they study; they construct long lists of example words and phrases to define each phoneme; the word lists are much longer but essentially like the three-word lists we gave in the previous paragraph; over time they revise these phoneme lists to reach a consensus. The linguist's ear and knowledge of the language are the main tools for this type of study. A linguist who is not a native speaker of the language uses native speakers to pronounce sentences and words

TABLE 1-1. The phonemes of General American English. Each phoneme is given by its symbol in the International Phonetic Alphabet followed by examples of words containing the phoneme.

CONSONANTS	VOWELS AND DIPHTHONGS
/ m / *me*, *aim*, *smile*, *ramp*	/ i / *heed*
/ w / *wet*, *swoop*	/ ɪ / *hid*
/ ʌ / *whet*	/ ɛ / *head*
/ b / *be*, *mob*	/ æ / *had*
/ v / *van*, *give*	/ ɑ / *odd*
/ p / *pan*, *map*, *spill*, *apt*	/ ɔ / *awed*
/ f / *fan*, *wife*, *soft*	/ o / *tote*
/ ð / *that*, *bathe*	/ ʊ / *hood*
/ θ / *thing*, *bath*	/ u / *who*
/ n / *no*, *pan*, *snap*, *bend*	/ ʌ / *ton*
/ l / *lawn*, *pole*, *slap*, *belt*	/ ə / *a ton*
/ d / *dawn*, *good*	/ ɚ / *earth*
/ z / *zip*, *ways*	/ aɪ / *hide*
/ t / *tan*, *bat*, *still*, *cats*	/ ɔɪ / *coin*
/ s / *sip*, *face*, *fast*, *cats*	/ aʊ / *out*
/ tʃ / *chop*, *each*	/ eɪ / *pain*
/ ʤ / *joke*, *age*	/ oʊ / *code*
/ j / *you*	/ ɪu / *few*
/ r / *ran*, *press*, *hard*	
/ ʒ / *azure*, *garage*	
/ ʃ / *show*, *fresh*	
/ ŋ / *sing*, *thin*	**REGIONAL VOWELS**
/ g / *give*, *bag*	/ a / Bostonian "*hard*"
/ k / *key*, *sick*, *skip*, *picked*	/ ʌ / New York Manhattan "*better*"; "*her*"
/ h / *had*	/ ø / Northeastern "*earth*"

for comparison and listing. Some cultures play games with words that reveal phonemes and syllables to the linguist (Campbell, 1986). A real-life description of how linguists work appeared in the newsletter of the Acoustical Society of America (Ladefoged, 1995).

We should note that phonemes are determined by linguists according to their function in differentiating words. Thus, although the sequence of phonemes in a word may be perceived as a sequence of sound patterns, phonemes are not defined acoustically by their sound characteristics, but by their function in a language system. Speech scientists sometimes speak of a *phone*, for example, the phone [s], which means a sound pattern having some acoustic features that are

strongly similar to other sounds that could be called examples of the phoneme /s/. So, spoken examples of a particular phoneme usually have some acoustic features in common, as we shall see, but they also vary in important ways depending on the adjacent events in the stream of speech. We must think of a phoneme as a sort of group or class of sound-events; usually the group has some common pattern of articulation. Any spoken instance of a given phoneme is actually a variation on an "average" or representative configuration of events, a variant of a typical pattern.

A definable, systematic variant of a phoneme is called an *allophone*. Let us see what we mean here by "definable, systematic variant." Consider some variant examples of the phoneme /s/: In the words *sill*, *still*, and *spill*, each [s] is slightly different because it is spoken as tied into a different following sound, and the same differences occur between the [s]'s in the words *seed*, *steed*, and *speed*. You can hear these differences by pronouncing those words. Even better, you can feel those different [s]'s by speaking the words silently (Catford, 1988, Exercise 58). The [s] of *speed* has a lower pitch than it does in *steed* where it is lower in pitch than in *seed*. The reason for the differences in pitch is the overlap, with the s-formation, of gestures toward the following different sounds, /p, t, i/. The very same sort of differences occur between *spill*, *still*, and *sill*. There is a systematic variation. All such systematic variants of /s/, its allophones, comprise the phoneme /s/. Each phoneme thus actually designates a large class of sounds. For example, the phoneme /s/ consists of more than 100 allophones.

Linguists often call phonemes the "segmental" units of language because they are the smallest units whose sequences differentiate words. Acoustically speaking, the phonemes of an utterance are not always separable or segmentable from each other by their sound patterns in the flow of speech. So, in acoustic phonetics, using the word "segment" for "phoneme" can be misleading. To be sure, there are sequential sound changes in a spoken word that correspond to the phoneme sequence of the word; for example, in the word "mass" we hear that a murmur-like [m]-sound is followed by an [æ]-sound and then a hissy [s]-sound. We hear a phoneme sequence but, as we shall see later, the sound-cues we use to perceive each phoneme can be much intertwined with the sounds of its neighboring phonemes, without sound-boundaries that are very clear. In linguistics, on the other hand, the term "segmental" is pertinent to the phonemes' sequentiality and permutability to form the words of a language: The phoneme segments of "mass" can be rearranged to make the word "Sam" or even as the first part of "smash." The permutability of our language's phonemes as segments, to form almost an infinity of words, allows us to generate all the thousands of words that we know and use.

In our acoustic studies of speech we usually describe only the most general or common features of a phonemic sound and are not concerned with all of its allophones. For example, an acoustic characteristic of /s/-allophones is their sharply hiss-like quality produced by the breath rushing over the tongue-tip and against the teeth. However, the exact tone of the hiss will depend on whether the following phoneme is /i/, /t/, or /p/. You heard this in pronouncing the words *seed*, *steed*, and *speed*. Any one of these allophones is called a *speech sound* or *phone*, not a phoneme. To label such a sound, the same symbols as in Table 1-1 are used with brackets instead of slashes, as you may have noticed above when we were talking about the term *phone*; thus [s], for example, refers to a sound pattern produced like other [s] sounds that may be classed as, or serve as examples of, the phoneme /s/.

Phonemes are the basic sequential units or segments of speech and thus the features of phonemes are sometimes called *segmental features*. However, as we said above, this term is largely a linguistic one. In the acoustic stream of speech, phoneme-correlated features are subject to intermixing and so may not be very clearly demarcated, because speech production is a rapid, flowing activity, with a lot of overlap of the acoustic features of one phoneme on others. The basic unitary aspect of the phoneme resides not in acoustic demarcation, but in linguistic evidence that the phoneme is the smallest interchangeable element in a language. In addition, perceptual and behavioral evidence prove the phoneme to be a basic unit. For example, in "slips of the tongue" phonemes usually interchange as units (Fromkin, 1972).

The *syllable* is the next larger unit of speech after the phoneme. Phonemes are always embedded in syllables. A syllable typically consists of a vowel and one or more consonants. The vowel functions as the "carrier" of the syllable, with the consonants riding on the beginning and end. For this reason the vowel is sometimes called the *syllable nucleus*. Some syllables consist of a single vowel, or of a single voiced consonant, such as /n/

or /l/, forming the second syllable of words like *garden* /gardn/ and *ladle* /leidl/.

Syllables, like phonemes, are linguistic units, not acoustic units. Some linguists view the syllable as the basic building block of spoken language, citing evidence from the organization of speech production, how speech sounds are perceived, and slips of the tongue (Fry, 1964; Kozhevnikov & Chistovich, 1965).

Sounds may be described in very many ways, so speech scientists have benefited from applying linguistic concepts to guide their explorations. The concept of the *phoneme* tells the phonetician approximately where to look sequentially in a stream of speech sounds, say in a word, for acoustic events that are essential to differentiate it from other words. This has led to a body of knowledge of the sound differences used by many languages. Often the sounds used in a language can be described in a universal feature system called *distinctive feature theory*. A feature theory connects the phonemes of a language to the words on the one hand and the sound differences on the other. The whole, feature systems and rules for combining the features into phonemes and for forming words, is called the *phonology* of that language.

So we might guess that a good theory of the distinctive features of languages would depend on collaboration between a phonologist and an acoustic scientist. Our acoustic studies in Part One are primarily acoustic. A prominent version of the theory is given us in an advanced tutorial article by two distinguished scientists at MIT: the phonologist, Morris Halle, and the acoustic scientist, Kenneth Stevens (Halle & Stevens, 1991). Students who are deeply interested in acoustic feature theories should read this article, but only after study of the first nine chapters of our book or a similar text.

Not so broadly phonological, our study will concentrate primarily on General American English. Still, we like to note ties between phonetics and phonology, particular connections between acoustic features and their phonological function in languages in general. These "Phonology Notes" will give findings by some of the experimental linguists who have advanced our knowledge to encompass the phonetics of all languages, beyond the most intensively studied languages, French, German, Italian, Russian, Spanish, Swedish, and our own study-language, English. Our phonology notes come mostly from studies at the University of California (Los Angeles) Phonetics Laboratory of their Phonological Segment Inventory Database (UPSID) by Maddieson (1984); pages there will be cited after "Madd:". UPSID describes all the different phonemes of each of 317 representatives, scoping the major and minor families of the world's spoken languages. Maddieson discovers many interesting phonological relationships and provides several indexes according to language families, phoneme types, and articulatory features. UPSID is thus a base for detailed analyses to try to find further phonological principles used by languages in constructing their basic communication codes (see also Ladefoged & Maddieson, 1995).

GENERAL CONDITIONS OF SPEECH PRODUCTION

Before we begin a detailed study of speech sounds, we need a general knowledge of how speech is produced. Only an overall picture of the breathing movements, the speech articulatory movements, and the basic mechanisms of speech sound production is given in this chapter. Later each of these topics is studied in more detail.

We will usually proceed from articulatory shapes and movements to the sound patterns. This is because articulations can be seen and felt, but sounds have to be described with special acoustic concepts. Once you have learned the acoustic concepts and have used them to describe the relations between articulations and speech sounds, you will find sounds are as easy to understand as articulations.

Speaking is a motor skill and, like other skills, it consists of coordinated movements acting upon an object. In speaking, the object acted upon is the air contained in the respiratory passages, that is, the air in the lungs, trachea, larynx, pharynx, nose, and mouth. When we speak, we perform movements that act on these air spaces. The movements occur in consistent gestural patterns to produce the speech sounds.

The gestures of speech are performed primarily by the organs of the upper alimentary tract: glottis, tongue, lips, jaw, and velum. These gestures are coordinated with movements by the respiratory system to fashion sound patterns from the basic airflow as a power source. When referring to speech the term *vocal tract* is used to include the passages of the larynx, mouth, and nose. The organs and passages involved are diagrammed in Figure 1-2.

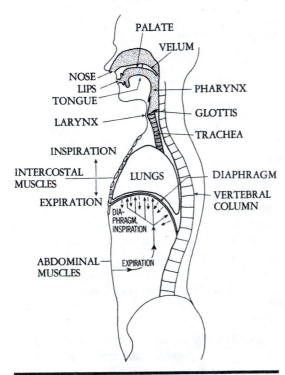

FIGURE 1-2. Diagram of the organs used in speech production. In breathing and in speaking, the expiratory muscles act to move air from the lungs through the trachea and onward toward the outside. The expiratory muscles are the internal intercostals, which lower the rib cage when they contract, thus compressing the lungs, and the abdominal muscles, which push the viscera and diaphragm upward. The airstream moving outward (breath stream) is modified by movements of the glottis and the other downstream organs to produce speech sounds.

Respiration for Speech

In the production of speech the air in the lungs is pressed upon by the chest and lung tissues, resulting in a flow of air from the lungs toward the outside; we call this flow the *breath stream*. If the vocal tract is open, the breath stream is unimpeded and the air flows out the nose or mouth, as in ordinary breathing. During speech, however, some part of the vocal tract is constricted to a degree that impedes the outward airflow and then the pressure of the tracheal air rises. This tracheal air pressure is the fundamental basis of speech sounds; in fact, the sounds originate in variations in the flow of air from the trachea powered by the tracheal air pressure.

Let us examine the control of the breath stream in more detail, referring to Figure 1-2. Breathing is controlled by two opposed sets of forces on the lungs: forces of inspiration and forces of expiration. The *inspiratory forces* expand the lung volume by raising the rib cage and lowering the floor of the lung cavity. The major inspiratory muscles are the diaphragm and external layer of the intercostal muscles between the ribs. The diaphragm forms the floor of the chest cavity. Contraction of these muscles expands the chest, air flows in, and the lungs expand.

The *expiratory forces* contract the lung volume by lowering the rib cage and pushing the floor of the chest cavity upward. Major expiratory muscles are the abdominal muscles—which pull the abdominal wall inward, thereby pressing on the viscera and pushing the floor of the chest upward—and other abdominal muscles that pull downward on the rib cage. The intercostal muscles also exert a contracting force on the rib cage. Another expiratory force is provided by the elastic recoil of the lung tissues and those other chest tissues, stretched by the increased volume of the chest after an inspiration of air. The expiratory forces push air out of the lungs causing air to flow outward through the respiratory passages.

How are these breathing muscles used in speech? Here is a brief summary.[1]

[1]Based on research studies by Draper, Ladefoged, and Whitteridge (1959), Ladefoged (1963, 1967), and Hixon (1987).

The chest movements for conversational speech are light, easy movements that are not noticeably effortful. The lungs are only slightly distended; thus the elastic recoil force is low, and the internal intercostal muscles between the bony parts of the ribs probably provide the main expiratory force. This force, on the average, is very moderate, producing a pressure in the trachea, under vocal tract constriction for speech, that is only slightly above atmospheric pressure. Atmospheric pressure is 1055 cm of water and the tracheal pressure in speech is about 10 cm above atmospheric pressure, with small variations up and down because of the speech rhythm or stress pattern. Thus the tracheal air pressure, constituting the energy source of speech, averages only about 1% above the ambient atmospheric pressure.

The average outward flow of air during speech is also rather low on the order of 100 to 300 cc of air per second, which is less than 1/2 pint per second. During certain speech sounds the flow is much lower or is even completely blocked momentarily, as in stop consonants like [p, t, k]. For other sounds the airflow can be much higher than average. For example, during fricatives like [s] and [ʃ] and in the release of stop consonants like [t] in the word *tea*, the airflow briefly reaches rates equivalent to about 1000 to 2000 cc of air per second.

The chest movements of shouting and of very low vocal effort can be radically different from those of normal conversation. In shouting, the pressures and flow rates may be higher; with very low effort they are lower. However, adequate volume of voice is primarily a matter of the voice action of the glottis in the larynx and the resonances of the vocal tract, not of strong pressure by the chest.

Long streams of speech, uninterrupted by air intakes, require a very large air reservoir at the beginning, and thus the elastic recoil force may be too high for the voice level desired; in this case the inspiratory muscles contract in order to oppose the recoil and hold the tracheal pressure to the desired low level. Then, as air is expended in speaking and the lung tissues become less dis-tended, the recoil force decreases and the opposing inspiratory contractions disappear. When the air reservoir reaches normal and lower levels, the expiratory muscles come into play to maintain the tracheal pressure.

The expiratory muscles also contract in increased amount to produce increases in tracheal air pressure at places in the stream of speech where stress or emphasis is required. These pressure pulses for stress may also be produced by sudden relaxations of the inspiratory opposition to the elastic recoil. The vocal mechanisms for stress are described in Chapter Five in more detail.

Articulation of Speech

At first glance speaking seems like a very complicated activity: The respiratory movements and the articulations of glottis, pharynx, velum, jaw, tongue, and lips must all be well coordinated to produce intelligible speech. These coordinations involve rapid movements resulting from very complex patterns of muscular contractions. Still, to most people speaking seems to be very easy and natural. Perhaps speaking, like walking, is basically a simple act despite the diversity and complexity of the muscles involved. Another indication of the simplicity of speaking is its easy acquisition by children, very early in life, naturally, without any formal training; this has suggested to some researchers that speech coordinations may be largely innate (Lenneberg, 1967).

Speaking is like other rhythmic body movements where a postural adjustment serves as a base on which smaller, rapid movements are superimposed. In tapping a rhythm by hand, for example, the shoulders and arms provide a postural base for the rapid tapping movements of the hand. In speech the postural base is the adjustment of the breathing muscles to provide the outward airflow of the breath stream, and the articulatory movements of the tongue, lips, and jaw are small, rapid movements rhythmically superimposed on the breath stream. Thus, speaking is basically like making any simple rhythm.

General Time Features of Speech

The time pattern of syllables determines many of the time features of speech sounds. Therefore, it is important to know the typical character of syllable timing; later we use this to describe the time patterns of vowels and consonants.

The syllables of speech occur at an average rate of two to five syllables per second, depending on the style of speaking. The slow rate of two syllables per second is typical of careful, exaggerated enunciation; the fast rate of five syllables per second would be for very rapid, fluent conversation that is still clearly articulated.

Let us examine the time sequence of a very simple sequence of articulations. Consonant articulations constrict the vocal tract more than vowel articulations. Typically, there are no gaps between the phonemes or the syllables. Thus, for a fluent sequence of syllables we can think of the utterance simply as an alternation over time between a constricted articulation and an open articulation.

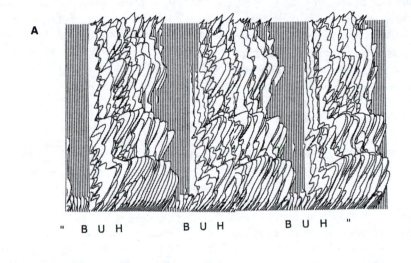

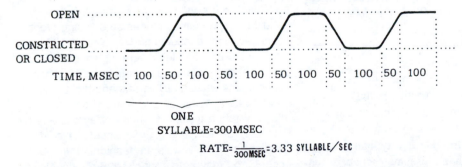

FIGURE 1-3. (A) Soundscape of an utterance "buh,buh,buh," timed like the schematic articulatory movements below. (B) Schematic representation of the consonant and vowel articulatory movements for the "buh,buh,buh." The durations of the movement phases are idealized, average durations, typical of those found in speech at a moderate rate of utterance. Further explanation in text.

(Perspectrogram soundscape from SpeechStation2 from Sensimetrics Corporation)

We begin with a very regular oscillation in constriction, producing a sequence of syllables much like babies make in "babbling" their first speech-like vocalizations (Davis & MacNeilage, 1995). Our example utterance is an adult babbling. In Figure 1-3 the top part shows a speech soundscape of a series of three syllables: "BUH,BUH, BUH." The bottom part shows schematic motions of the vocal tract, alternating between the B-constrictions and the UH-vowels. The open states produce the vowel sounds; the constricted states produce the consonant sounds.

For the medium rate of speaking used for the soundscape utterance we can assign typical time durations, based on average measurements, of the constricting and opening movements. For simplicity let us assume that the constricting and opening cycles succeed each other at exactly equal intervals of time; this is not actually true, because usually some syllables are stressed or emphasized more than others and these differences are highly important in language, as shown later in Chapter 5, but at this stage of our study we need some simple, easily remembered durations for typical speech events. Events for a succession of equal syllables are sketched in Figure 1-3; these events are very rapid, so it is customary to use a time unit of 1/1000 second, or a millisecond (ms). The constricted period (consonant) is about 100 ms, the opening transition between constricted and open takes about 50 ms, the open period (vowel) is about 100 ms, and the closing transition from open to constricted takes about 50 ms. The total time for one consonant-vowel syllable, from constricted to open and back to the beginning of the consonant constriction in the next syllable, would be the sum of these periods. The sum is 300 ms, which corresponds to a rate of 3.33 syllables per second. This rate is a typical average rate for careful speech falling somewhere between slow, exaggerated enunciation and rapid but clear conversation. This is only an average syllable rate. In real speech at this rate syllables of about 300 ms are common, but the shortest syllables may be as little as 100 ms in duration and the longest syllables as long as 500 ms.

Phonology Note: Consonants versus Vowels

All languages articulate primarily by alternating between constricted and open states of the vocal tract, between consonant and vowel. Consonants, as phonemes, appear to carry more information than vowels. In fact, our alphabet originated with consonants alone because the vowels played only minor roles in identifying words in Semitic languages. Ancient Semitic people, in commerce in eastern Mediterranean areas, were among the first to write phonetically. For these traders, words were made of the "strong bones of consonants with the vowels floating above like invisible spirits" (Burgess, 1992). Those "bones" were so singular that a Hebrew scribe, Ben Kamtzar of Talmudic/ Midrash legend, could write a word of four consonants (and four syllables) with one flourish of his hand, using four pens wedged between his fingers (Braude, 1992:164). Ancient Greeks added vowels to the alphabet they adopted from Semitic writing, because Greek employed stable vowel phonemes (Stetson, 1951, Appx III, pp. 155–157 in Kelso & Munhall, 1988; Gaur, 1992).

Languages often employ more than one consonant between successive vowels. To put a number on the consonant/vowel ratio I consulted the UPSID phoneme lists; the typical language of that "population" employs 2.8 different consonant phonemes to every different vowel phoneme. If a language employs more than the typical number of different phonemes it does so by using proportionately more consonants (Maddieson, 1984). In the UPSID list of all the different phonemes found over all the languages, I counted 548 different consonants versus 120 vowels and diphthongs, a ratio of 4.6 to 1. It seems no matter how you count them, within a typical language or across a large number of languages, consonants are more important than vowels in fashioning language codes. You may note, though, that my counts did not take account of how often each of the phonemes is used in its language, either in generating words or by speakers in using them. Still it seems plausible that consonants would dominate communication.

SPEECH SOUND SOURCES

The gestures of speech produce sounds by modulating the airflow from the trachea (breath stream). These essential modulations or fluctuations in the breath stream, being the basic signal material of speech, are called *source* sounds. There are three distinctly different types of sound source: *voiced*, *turbulent*, and *transient*. We consider here, in just a general way, how each of these three "raw materials" of speech is generated by the vocal tract. Later these sound types are described in more detail.

Voiced Sound Source

The majority of speech sounds are formed on the "voiced source," a type of modulation of the breath stream that produces periodic sounds. Voiced sounds are based on a periodic modulation of the breath stream by the action of the glottis. This action to produce the voiced source is a repeated opening and closing of the glottal slit between the vocal folds in the larynx. Voicing action occurs more or less automatically when the vocal folds are adjusted for "voicing" and supplied with tracheal air pressure. The action produces periodic pulses of airflow by repeatedly passing and shutting off the breath stream. The airflow pulses succeed each other at a very rapid rate, about 125 pulses per second for adult male talkers and about 200 per second or higher for women and children. This pulsing sound has a buzz-like quality. It propagates up through the vocal tract to the air outside the speaker. Examples of speech sounds produced with the voiced sound source are the vowels, the nasal consonants [m, n, ŋ], and glide consonants like [w].

Turbulent Sound Source

The second type of modulation of the breath stream is produced when it passes through a narrow constriction and the flow of air through the constriction becomes turbulent. The turbulence produces a sound having a hissing quality; the turbulent breath stream does not pulse periodically as

---

Phonology Note: Transients in Languages

The three types of sound source, voiced, turbulent, and transient, are the ones employed in English and many other languages of the world. Transient-producing stops (plosives) are probably the primary articulations of the world's languages (Henton, Ladefoged, & Maddieson, 1992; Maddieson, 1984:25), but there are several other types of transient sound sources. A few languages employ "clicks" formed by sucking actions released by the lips or tongue, and some languages employ glottal ejections or an inspiratory breath stream to make "ejective" or "implosive" sounds (Maddieson, 1984:98–110). English speakers use clicks and inspiratory sounds as expressive interjections, like "tsk, tsk," but not as phonemic distinctions. For examples of phonemic clicks and implosives, see Ladefoged (1993, pp. 130-138) where he tells how to make them.

---

for the voiced sounds, but has random variations in airflow. This type of sound is called *aperiodic*. Aperiodic sound is the basic type of sound source that is further modified to produce speech sounds like the fricatives, [s, ʃ, θ], and [f].

Transient Sound Source

Sudden, step-like increases in the airflow occur whenever there is a sudden release of the air pressure built up behind a constriction in the vocal tract. This occurs upon the release of the complete constriction of consonants like [p], [t], and [k]. Later we see how these transients generate sound.

SUMMARY

Thus far we have seen that speech consists of linguistic units of sound sequences, the phonemes and syllables, which form words and sentences in a language. Speech production is based on movements of the breathing mechanism, which produce a flow of air through the vocal tract. This airflow is modified by articulatory movements to produce sequences of syllables consisting of a rapid alternation between constricted articulation for consonant phonemes and open articulation for vowel phonemes. Three basic types of airflow modulation provide the sound sources of speech: (1) a periodic or voiced sound source, (2) a turbulent, hissing sound source, and (3) a transient, step-like sound source. In addition to modulated breath flow, some languages employ sounds made with airflow initiated by glottal or oral movements.

In our study of acoustic phonetics we concentrate first on acoustic patterns that serve to differentiate the vowel phonemes. Then vowel features of stress, emphasis, and expression are studied in Chapter Five. Further chapters describe the features of consonant phonemes. Finally, some of the acoustic effects seen in phoneme interaction are studied.

The next chapter explains how speech sounds are analyzed into their acoustic components; we look for the components of the [b]-portion in one of the "buh" syllables in Figure 1-3.

CHAPTER TWO

SOUNDS, RESONANCE, AND SPECTRUM ANALYSIS

Like most sounds, vowels and consonants are complex in form. Fortunately, though, we have relatively simple concepts and terms to give us a concise description of any sound. We simplify complex sounds by analysis into components. Figure 2-1 (bottom) shows the sound wave of a [b] and how I took it from the beginning of the second "buh" in the speech soundscape of Figure 1-3. At the start of the wave, the form of fluctuation of the sound amplitude is very regular. We shall see later that it is very similar to a sine wave; however, toward the end on the right another smaller fluctuation is coming in, making the wave look more complicated. We will find simple ways to represent these complexities, via sound analysis.

This chapter introduces the basic principles of sound analysis, important concepts we will apply later in our study of all the sounds of speech. First I describe how sound waves are produced and propagated. Then the sine wave, a wave resulting from simple harmonic motion, is described. Sine waves are the simple waves used as components to describe complex sounds. The sine wave components represent the spectrum of a sound, and the spectrum is the concise description that we need.

Resonances in sound-producing devices allow us to identify them by ear. That is how we perceive speech, so we need to know how resonances are formed in the vocal tract and how to find them in speech sounds. Actually, we have already found one in Figure 2-1, because the beginning simple sinuous wave of the [b] originates in the resonance of the mouth cavity behind the closed lips. Later, I explain how resonance occurs in the vocal tract and how resonant sound waves are analyzed into sine waves to represent the spectrum of resonant sounds. First, we look at how soundwaves are produced.

SOUND PRODUCTION AND PROPAGATION

Sound originates as a disturbance of the positions of particles within a substance. The initial disturbance also moves all the neighboring particles, these in turn move their neighbors, and in this way the sound is propagated outward through all parts of the substance. The disturbance propagates as a momentary change in position, forth and back, of each particle. Usually air is the substance that propagates sound to us from its place of origin. Airborne sounds generated at one place reach us at another place because the disturbances of the air particles at the original location are faithfully relayed through the intervening air.

In speech the vocal organs produce sound by causing a local disturbance in positions of the air particles at some point in the vocal tract. The disturbance causes successive motions of the particles, to and fro, at each adjacent point in the vocal tract, thus propagating the vocal sound outward to the outside air and onward to distant points. For example, during a vowel sound the disturbances initiating the sound are pulses of air emitted by the glottis. Each pulse is propagated upward from the glottis to the lips and to the outside air. In the production of a fricative consonant, the breath stream is forced through a constriction in the vocal tract, causing a turbulent disturbance that is propagated away from the constriction to the lips and the outside air.

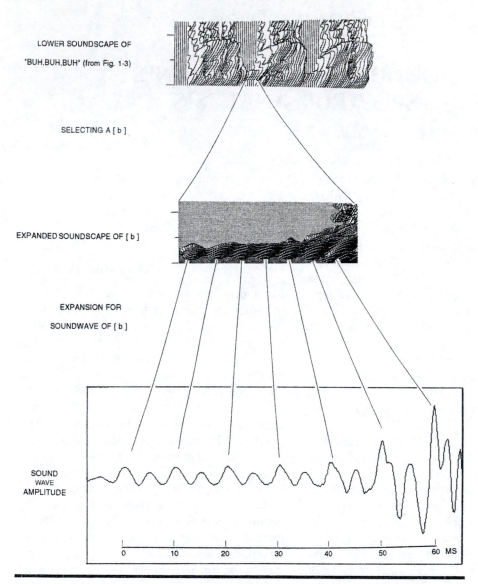

LOWER SOUNDSCAPE OF
"BUH,BUH,BUH" (from Fig. 1-3)

SELECTING A [b]

EXPANDED SOUNDSCAPE OF [b]

EXPANSION FOR

SOUNDWAVE OF [b]

SOUND
WAVE
AMPLITUDE

0   10   20   30   40   50   60   MS

FIGURE 2-1. The expanded wave of sound at the beginning part of a [b] in the soundscape of "buh,buh,buh" in the top of the previous Figure 1-3. The first part of the wave is like a sine wave (compare with Figure 2-4) but an additional fluctuation comes in as the [b]-wave continues.

(Wave plotted by Bunnell Edwav, Gallaudet University)

The propagation speed of sound in air is about 1129 feet per second. This is a very high speed compared with the rate of flow of the breath stream, which moves only about 1 foot per second. Thus, although disturbances in the breath stream are the initiating sources of speech sounds, the sounds themselves are propagated through the vocal tract air at a much higher speed than the breath. The speech sounds, traveling at the speed of sound, or about 770 miles per hour, can be thought of as riding on the very slow wind of the breath stream, which is moving outward at less than 1 mile per hour.

SIMPLE HARMONIC MOTION

The air motions of speech sounds are complex in form. However, complex motions can be described concisely by considering them to be made up of simple oscillations. This is done by breaking down the complex motions into a set of simple vibrations called *simple harmonic motions*. Simple harmonic motion is a basis for describing all forms of motion no matter how complex.

A familiar example of simple harmonic motion is the swing of a pendulum. An ideal pendulum, one with no friction, moves back and forth in simple harmonic motion. The pendulum motion is very regular in time, but still it involves many different speeds and positions. Fortunately, this motion can be represented very simply by relating it to uniform motion on a circle. Let us see how this happens.

Imagine the situation illustrated in Figure 2-2. In the figure we view together, and from the side, the motions of a pendulum and of a peg moving on a turntable. When we adjust the turntable speed so the time per oscillation of the pendulum and revolution of the turntable are the same, then the motions of the peg and bob are found to be in perfect synchrony at every moment. In other words, the simple harmonic motion of an ideal pendulum is the same as a constant circular motion viewed from the side looking along the plane of the circle. In terms of geometry, simple harmonic motion can be represented by circular motion projected on a line in the plane of rotation. This affords a very simple description of the pendulum motion because the circular motion can be described just by specifying two values, one giving the rate of motion and another giving the size of the motion. If we find other types of motion produced by the same type of force mechanism as in the pendulum, we can describe them too in terms of projected circular motion.

What is the force mechanism of the pendulum motion? The motion is produced by a restoring

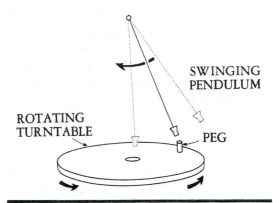

FIGURE 2-2 Demonstration showing how the back-and-forth motion of a pendulum can be represented by uniform motion in a circle viewed from the side. When the turntable speed is adjusted to one revolution for each swing of the pendulum, the peg and pendulum will be seen always to be at the same horizontal position, the peg exactly under the swinging bob, even though the peg moves continuously in a circle and the bob moves along a line between two momentary stops.

(Adapted from Benade, 1960)

force that is proportional to the distance of the pendulum bob from its resting position, the location where it remained still until disturbed. There are many other types of motion produced by forces proportional to the distance from a resting position; all such motions have a form related to simple harmonic motion. Examples of harmonic motions that produce sound are the vibrations of the prongs of a tuning fork, the main vibration of a plucked guitar string, and the vibration of the sides of a wine glass when tapped. Because all these motions are like simple harmonic motion, each can be described using the two aspects that describe a uniform circular motion: (1) the time, or period, for one complete revolution, and (2) the size of the motion, which is determined by the distance from the center of rotation to the moving point. In sound vibrations, these two aspects are: (1) the period for one complete cycle, to and fro, of air particle vibration, and (2) the extent or amplitude of the particle motion.

A plot in time of the motion of the ideal pendulum gives a wave like the one shown in Figure 2-3. This wave is called a *sine wave*; its sinuous form is the form in time for all simple harmonic motions. The form of this wave is called *sinusoidal*.

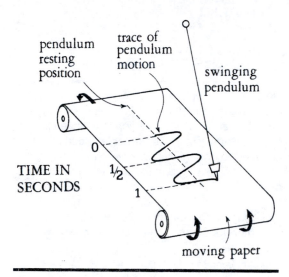

FIGURE 2-3. The motion of the pendulum traces a path in time that is a sine wave. The *period*, i.e., the time for one complete cycle of oscillation, is 1/2 second and the *frequency* of oscillation is 2 Hz, for the pendulum shown.
(Adapted from Benade, 1960)

The sine wave contains various types of curvatures, nearly straight lines, turns, and reversals, so we might expect it to be useful for representing the curves of other waves or even of random waves. This is true in actuality, and sine waves are used in combinations to duplicate any sound wave. Conversely, any sound wave can be analyzed into its sine wave components.

DEFINITIONS OF SINE WAVE CHARACTERISTICS

The *period* of a sine wave is the time for one complete cycle; this aspect, related to the rate of oscillation, is often given as the *frequency of repetition* of the cycle in a unit of time. This *frequency* is simply the reciprocal of the period. The *frequency* is given in cycles per second or Hertz (Hz). For example, in Figure 2-3, the period of the pendulum motion is 1/2 second and the frequency is 2 cycles per second or 2 Hz.

The distance or amount of sine wave motion is called the *amplitude*. It corresponds to the extent of the oscillation from the original resting position. This is illustrated in Figure 2-4 where a sine wave of 1 Hz frequency is traced by a point projected from a uniform circular motion that is being translated horizontally in time.

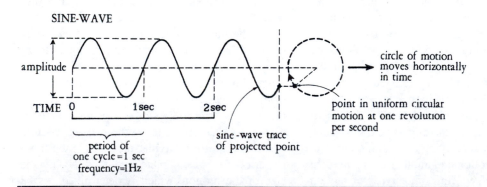

FIGURE 2-4. The *amplitude*, *period*, and *frequency* of a sine wave generated by a point rotating at one revolution per second and moving horizontally. For example, the sine wave would be the path traced by the vertical position of the peg on a turntable that is held on its side facing us and moving horizontally at a constant speed.

The frequencies of sound vibrations are usually much higher than 1 or 2 Hz; for example, notes of the guitar go up to about 2000 Hz. The range of the frequencies found in speech is from about 50 Hz to over 10,000 Hz, covering almost the entire range of hearing. Figure 2-5 shows some sine waves having frequencies and amplitudes like those in speech. Here there is a time scale in 1/1000 of a second (milliseconds or ms) instead of the seconds involved in our slow-swinging pendulum.

In sound vibrations the air particles move back and forth. If the original disturbance is a simple harmonic motion, the resulting air particle motions will also be simple harmonic in form, and the frequency and amplitude of their movement will follow perfectly the sine wave form of the original disturbance. For any sound wave the extent or amplitude of the motion and its form describe the sound completely, in physical terms. When a sound is received by ear, the extent of air particle motion determines the loudness of the sound heard; the form of the motion determines the timbre or quality of the sound heard. The

heard quality and loudness of sound are very important to us and these are very neatly represented by means of the frequency and amplitude of simple harmonic motions. Consider the form of the sound from tapping a wine glass. After the tap, which displaces the glass particles from their resting position, the sides of the glass continue to move in and out in a form similar to simple harmonic motion. The moving sides of the vibrating glass move the adjacent air particles; that motion is propagated through the air to our ears, and we hear the beautiful ringing tone of the wine glass. The "pure" tonal quality of this sound is caused by a sinusoidal motion of air particles at our ears. Sinusoidal sounds are called *pure tones*. The sensation of a pure tone is hard to describe but the sound wave producing it can be described exactly just by noting that it is sinusoidal in form and has a given frequency and amplitude of motion. If the amplitude were to remain constant and not die out, the vibration would be pure simple harmonic motion and the wave of motion in time would be a sine wave, like that traced in time by an ideal pendulum.

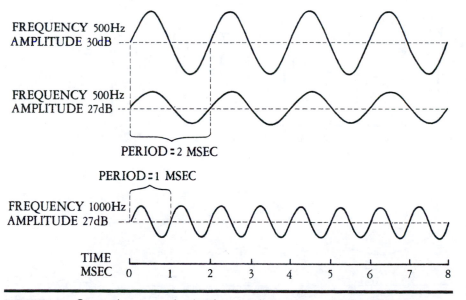

FIGURE 2-5.   Some sine waves having frequencies and intensities (amplitudes in dB) found in components of speech.

Vibrations of actual objects are always affected by "damping" forces affecting the amplitude of motion. These cause a regular decrease in amplitude of oscillation, as in the gradual dying away of the tone from a ringing wine glass. The same thing happens to the vibration of a guitar string and to the swing of a real pendulum: The vibrations die out gradually in time. The causes of damping are air friction and the internal resistance to bending of the wine glass and the guitar string. The resulting waves are called damped oscillations. A *damped oscillation* will be sinusoidal in form if it is produced by restoring forces proportional to the displacement from resting position, but a sinusoidal damped oscillation is not a sine wave because it is not constant in amplitude. Still, as we will soon see (Figures 2-8 and 2-9), damped sinusoids can be analyzed into a set of sine waves.

RESONANCE

An oscillating object, like the swinging pendulum or the ringing wine glass, vibrates at just one frequency, called its *natural* or *resonant frequency*. Another example is air resonance in a bottle. The air in a bottle has a natural, resonant frequency of vibration; if we displace the air particles at the mouth of a bottle by pulling out a cork or by blowing across the open mouth, the bottle produces a resonant, tonal sound. This type of resonance plays a very important role in speech.

Let us now see exactly what makes a bottle give a resonant "pop" when the cork is pulled and then we will apply it to speech. In essence, pulling the cork produces a pulse of airflow that results in a damped sinusoidal oscillation of the air particles in the bottle. First, let us see why the oscillation is sinusoidal in form.

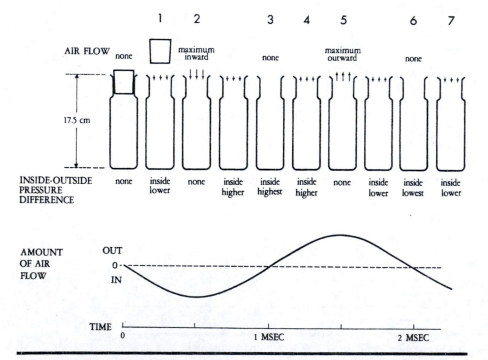

FIGURE 2-6. How a resonant oscillation begins in the air in a tube-like bottle. See text for a detailed explanation.

The form of the air oscillation depends on the way forces operate to move the air particles. In simple harmonic motion the force is proportional to the displacement (or distance) from resting position. This type of force relation also operates for the cork and bottle; the force here is a difference in air pressure at the mouth of the bottle. The sequence of forces and oscillation are illustrated in Figure 2-6. At the moment when the cork leaves the mouth of the bottle, at stage 1 in the figure, the air pressure in the bottle is lower than the outside pressure at the mouth because of the space vacated by the cork. Air flows inward in response to this difference in pressure, but the difference decreases as air flows in and causes the pressure in the bottle to rise. As air particles continue to move into the bottle, the pressure difference becomes less and less and finally becomes zero at stage 2.

The process is analogous to the pendulum; here, for the air in the mouth of the bottle, a simple harmonic oscillation of the air particles occurs in response to a force (the pressure difference) proportional to the displacement of the particles from their resting position. At the moment when the pressure difference becomes zero, the particles are still moving inward and their momentum carries them further into the bottle (in the same way as a pendulum swings past its resting position). This causes a rise in the pressure inside the bottle. The air inflow continues until the pressure is high enough, at stage 3, to stop the particle motion, and reverse it at 4; then the particles move outward and the pressure difference eventually reduces to zero at 5, but the particles now have an outward momentum and continue moving outward, reducing the pressure in the mouth sufficiently to stop the outward movement at stage 6 and produce inward movement again at 7. At that point, as the air again moves inward, the situation is like the initial movement after pulling the cork, and so we see that the cycles of airflow and pressure decrease/increase at the mouth of the bottle will continue more or less indefinitely. Actually, the cycle gradually dies out because of the damping effects of friction between the particles and of the energy dissipated in moving the air

outside the bottle mouth. The form of this oscillation is a damped sinusoid; the first cycle of oscillation is traced as a graph of the net airflow, in time along the bottom of Figure 2-6. The form must be sinusoidal because the force (pressure difference) is proportional to the net amount of displaced particles. (In the graph, the form of the sinusoidal flow changes is stretched out on a long scale to be synchronous with the bottle sequence).

Now let us account for the frequency of oscillation. This depends on the size of the bottle. A small bottle makes a high-pitched "pop"; a large bottle makes a lower-pitched "thump" or "whump." This is because the sound is produced by the propagation and repeated reflection, back and forth within the bottle, of the initial air disturbance from pulling out the cork. There are longer intervals between the reflections in a large bottle than in a small bottle, because of the longer travel time between the mouth and the bottom and, of course, longer intervals between reflections will result in a slower frequency of oscillation. This reflection model is simply an alternative way to describe the oscillatory airflow, an easier way to derive the frequency of oscillation.

We can calculate the frequency of oscillation in the bottle, using the speed of sound propagation and the distance to the bottom. We simply calculate the time between appearances of reflections of the initial pulse of pressure disturbance at the mouth. In Figure 2-6 we chose a distance giving a total round-trip travel time, from mouth to bottom and back to mouth, of 1 ms. The corresponding distance is for a bottle like a uniform tube that is 17.5 cm long.

The time sequence of the reflections of the initial pulse is as follows. The rarefaction created at stage 1 in Figure 2-6 is propagated down to the bottom, reflected by the bottom, and propagated back outward to appear at the mouth 1 ms later at stage 3. The opening at the mouth of the bottle inverts the rarefaction to a compression pulse. This pulse is propagated back down the bottle and reflected from the bottom to appear again 1 ms later at the mouth, at stage 6 in the figure. This second pulse, returned to the mouth as an outgoing pulse, is inverted there to an inflow pulse having the same airflow direction as the initial pulse at stage 1; thus the pulse disturbance is propagated and reflected, back and forth, repeatedly. There is repeated cycling of the pulse disturbance. The reflected pulses are 1 ms apart and, due to the inversion of pressure at the mouth, the airflow of every other pulse is opposite in direction to the initial pulse.

DEFINITION OF RESONANT FREQUENCY

We see in Figure 2-6 that the time for the fluctuation of the airflow at the mouth to go through a complete cycle and just begin to repeat itself in

the original inward direction requires two round-trip reflection cycles of 1 ms per round trip, giving a total time of 2 ms, or 1/500 second. This value is the period of each cycle of resonant oscillation. The cycle repeats at a rate of 500 times per second (500 Hz), and this is the *resonant frequency*. The air column in the bottle is a resonant system having a natural frequency of 500 Hz.

Outside the bottle, the air-pressure oscillation at the mouth is also radiated into the air where it continues to propagate as a sound wave that may be heard. Figure 2-7 shows how this sound is generated. The damped sinusoidal wave of the net airflow is illustrated together with the corresponding

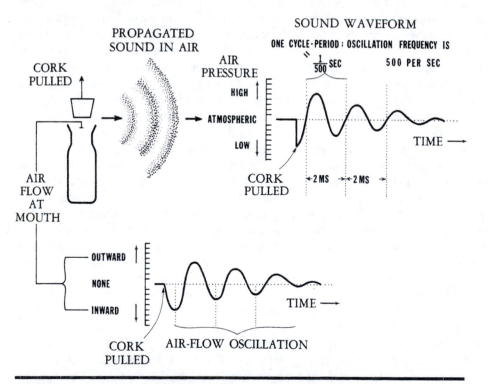

FIGURE 2-7. Diagram of oscillation of the total airflow through the mouth of a tubular bottle and the corresponding sound pressure wave produced by pulling a cork from the bottle. The main resonance of the bottle is at a frequency of 500 Hz. The horizontal scale of the wave has been compressed for the diagram (as compared with Figure 2-6, where only the first cycle could be shown on the time scale). The sound wave of air pressure and the airflow oscillation are both damped sinusoids; the pressure is at a maximum or minimum whenever the net flow is at 0 and the net flow is maximum in or out whenever the pressure is at atmospheric (see text on this relationship).

air pressure fluctuation propagated away from the bottle by the surrounding air. The dashed vertical lines on the flow and pressure lines represent identical instants in time, allowing us to observe how the flow and pressure are coordinated. It is interesting to note how the amount of the sound-generating airflow is always out of step with the fluctuations of the air pressure in the resulting sound wave: Maximum total inflow, that is, the peak at the first vertical dashed line on the inward downswing in the lower (airflow) curve, coincides with zero pressure difference from atmospheric in the upper, pressure curve; the maximum pressure above atmospheric coincides with momentary zero net flow. The direction of flow at this instant is outward and with a maximum velocity. Thus the pressure and the flow velocity are in a reciprocal relationship; it is this reciprocity that generates the sound. Although this relation is not important in purely acoustic descriptions of sounds, it is essential to the understanding of sound production per se. So, for example, the reciprocity of flow and pressure means little to persons concerned only with sound patterns, like audiologists or voice recognizers or listeners, but it is basic to understanding how the voice is generated and manipulated for communication, both in humans and animals; for more see Fletcher (1992), Chapter 14, "Pneumatically Excited Sound Generators." We will encounter this effect again in our study of phonation in the next chapters.

The resonances seen in speech sounds are caused by the same process of oscillation just described. For example, when a vowel is spoken, the vocal tract has a tube-like shape and production of a vowel is perfectly analogous to what took place in the corked bottle example. In vowel production, pulses of airflow are emitted by the glottis into the pharynx; each glottal pulse is propagated upward to the open mouth as a pressure-wave; at the mouth the pressure pulse produces an outward pulse of airflow, the escaping air particles of which now appear as a rarefaction (negative) pressure pulse for propagation back toward the vocal fold surfaces. The vocal folds act like the bottom of a bottle and reflect the rarefaction pulse; it then is propagated upward

again, and so on. Thus, the glottal pulse is repeatedly reflected back and forth between the vocal folds and the mouth. The round-trip propagation is so rapid, compared to the slow pulse-emitting rate of the glottis, that quite a few reflections can take place after each glottal pulse before the vocal folds open again to emit the next glottal pulse. Typically, ten round-trip reflections producing five cycles of oscillation can occur between successive glottal pulses of an adult male speaker.

The analogy between the corked bottle reflections and glottal pulse reflections is exact, allowing for the differences in origin and direction of pulse flow. Both have the same reflection arrangements, namely, a tube that is closed at one end, at the bottom of the bottle or at the vocal folds, and open at the other end, the mouth. The bottom-to-mouth distance of the bottle in Figure 2-6 was chosen to be the same as the average distance, from the vocal folds to the lips, in adult male speakers. Thus, the basic resonant frequency of 500 Hz for the bottle is the same as for the average adult male speaker. In speech the resonances of the vocal tract are called *formants*. The basic formant frequency of the average size adult male is 500 Hz.

The vocal tract, like any tube, has other resonances at frequencies higher than the basic one; these also affect the form of speech sounds. The resonant frequencies also depend on the shape of the vocal tract. In fact, many of the sounds of speech are distinguished by specific patterns of resonant frequencies, the *formant patterns*. In later chapters this is explained in more detail.

Our explanation above of the basis for vocal resonances begins in the time domain and converts reflection times to frequency. This approach seems highly intuitive. It is based on an analysis in Fant (1968) where it is developed further to account for the entire set of resonance frequencies as multiples of the first resonance. Other approaches employ tube wavelength-to-frequency conversion and/or a mathematical analysis of the fundamental physics. Tutorial explanations of formant frequencies according to vocal tube wavelengths will be found in Ladefoged (1996, Chapter 8) and in Lieberman and Blumstein (1988, pp. 42–49).

SPECTRUM ANALYSIS

Consider again the form of the sound wave produced by a resonant air column in a bottle, a tube, or the vocal tract. How can this wave be analyzed, that is, how can it be represented in the simple sine wave terms of frequency and amplitude as we did with the pendulum motion? We can do this by using a set of sine waves instead of a single wave.

The form of any wave can be constructed by adding together a number of sine waves of the proper amplitudes and frequencies. Sine waves that can be added to form a more complex wave are called the *components* of the complex wave. The fact that any wave, no matter how complex, can be represented by a certain set of component sine waves gives us the basis for the analysis of complex waves into their patterns of frequency and amplitude. To analyze a complex wave we find the set of component sine waves that would, when added together, produce a wave identical to the complex wave. This method, *Fourier analysis*, is how we analyze speech waves.

Speech waves often consist of resonant damped oscillations, so let us see how to represent a resonant wave by means of sine wave components. Figure 2-8 shows a damped sinusoidal wave

from a resonator whose resonant frequency is 500 Hz, together with a sinusoid of the same frequency. The resonant wave is similar to the sinusoid; however, the damped resonant wave decreases in amplitude as it dies out, whereas the sinusoid is constant in amplitude. So, obviously one component of the analysis could be a sinusoid having a frequency of the resonant frequency and the total duration of the damped oscillation. By adding to it other sinusoids having frequencies higher and lower than the resonant frequency, we can produce a wave that is sinusoidal in form and damps out in amplitude in a regular fashion. This can be partially accomplished with three sinusoids, as shown in Figure 2-9, where we approximate the 500 Hz damped sinusoid by combining sinusoids of 450, 500, and 550 Hz. The sinusoids of 450 and 550 Hz, above and below the resonant frequency, have amplitudes less than the sinusoid at the resonant frequency.

In order to represent completely the damped resonant wave it is necessary to add to the resonant frequency component a very large number of other sinusoids having frequencies both above and below the resonant frequency, and all the other sinusoids must have lower amplitudes according to their distance from the resonant frequency.

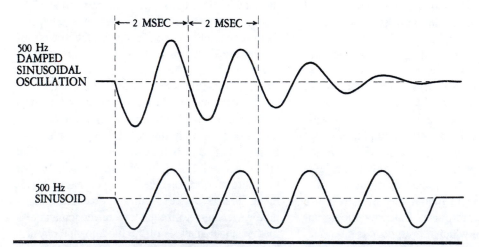

FIGURE 2-8.   The wave at the bottom, consisting of 4 1/2 cycles of a 500 Hz sine wave, is perfectly synchronous with the damped sinusoidal oscillation of 500 Hz, above. But the sine wave does not decrease in amplitude as time proceeds.

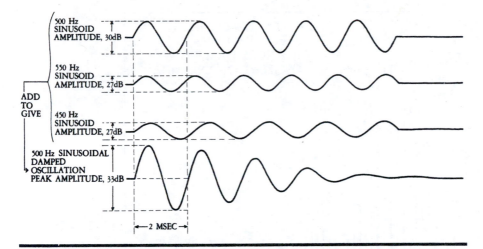

FIGURE 2-9. Three sinusoids having frequencies of 450, 500, and 550 Hz and amplitudes chosen so they add together to produce a damped sinusoidal oscillation of 500 Hz, seen in the bottom wave. During the last half of the 5th cycle of the 500 Hz wave the 450 and 550 Hz waves are positive by the same total amount that the 500 Hz wave is negative, so the result is zero amplitude. (When amplitudes are expressed in dB as I did here, two equal amplitudes combined add 6 dB to the total combined amplitude. For the first cycles the total peak amplitude in the bottom wave is, by decibel addition, 30 + 24 + 24 = 36 dB).

DEFINITIONS OF SPECTRUM TERMS

The pattern of the amplitudes of all the component frequencies of a sound is called the *amplitude-frequency spectrum* or the *power-density spectrum*. For brevity it is called simply the *spectrum*, or the *frequency spectrum*. The spectrum is the result of analyzing the sound and thus deriving its sine wave components.

The spectrum is plotted as a graph of the amplitudes at each of the frequencies, as in Figure 2-10, where I have plotted 55 components of the damped resonant oscillation of 500 Hz. Actually an infinite number of sine waves, infinitely close together in frequency, are necessary to represent a single occurrence of a resonant oscillation. The components would have amplitudes on the curved line drawn through the amplitudes of the 55 components in Figure 2-10.

The line connecting all the amplitudes is called the *spectrum envelope*. The spectrum envelope of

Figure 2-10 describes the shape of the spectrum of the 500 Hz damped resonant wave in Figures 2-7 and 2-8. The frequency spectrum represents the analysis of the wave.

In much work on speech analysis the amplitude-frequency spectrum of sound is measured and the time relations (phases) of the components are ignored. This is because the phases of the spectral components do not have large effects on the identity of the different sounds of speech. However, the phases of the components do affect voice timbre or voice quality. We use the term spectrum to mean only the amplitude-frequency spectrum.

The concept of the amplitude-frequency spectrum is used to analyze and describe sounds of all types, not just speech. Sounds whose spectra have been studied extensively range from noises, such as the roar of jet aircraft, the clatter of machinery, vehicle exhaust noise, and animal vocalizations, to musical sounds like those of bells, trumpets, violins, and opera singers.

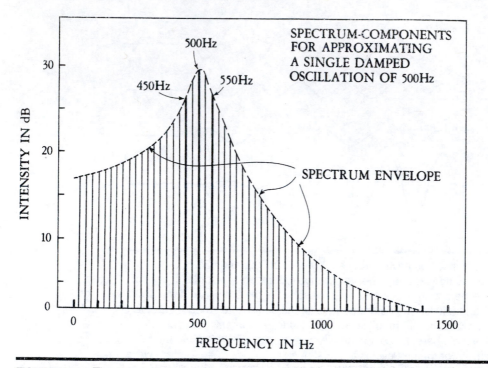

FIGURE 2-10. The top end of each spectrum line gives the amplitude (intensity) of a sine wave spectrum component of a 500 Hz damped sinusoidal oscillation. There are 55 components, one every 25 Hz. Adding all 55 of these sine waves together, even though they are of infinite duration, gives an approximation of a single damped sinusoidal oscillation of 500 Hz like the one at the bottom of Figure 2-9. The frequencies of the three sine wave segment components used in Figure 2-9 are indicated by the darker vertical lines. The spectrum envelope describes the amplitude-frequency shape for the infinite number of components that would be necessary to exactly produce the single damped oscillation.

The resonance characteristics of the vocal tract are studied by finding and plotting the shape of the spectrum envelope of the sounds emitted from the mouth. There are definite relations between the shape of the vocal tract and the sound spectrum shape, as we will see in the next chapter.

SPECTRA OF RECURRING RESONANT OSCILLATIONS

In speech, the vowel sounds are produced via the repeated "pulsing" of the vocal tract air column by a train of glottal pulses. Let us now see how a vocal tract resonance would be represented by the spectrum of repeated occurrences of damped oscillations. Go back to our pulsed-tube model of the vocal tract. Assume the tube to be pulsed repeatedly and that the pulses succeed each other very rapidly, at intervals of 10 ms. This amounts to assuming a glottal pulse rate of 100 pulses per second, a typical rate for a low-pitched male speaker. The wave produced in this way would look like the wave in Figure 2-11A, which is simply the same wave as at the bottom of Figure 2-10, but now it recurs every 10 ms. The rate or frequency of the pulses is 100 pulses per second, and it will be noted in the waveform of Figure 2-11A that the wave has two types of periodic, repeated fluctuation. First, there is a periodicity of 100 per second, that is, the wave shows a damped oscilla-

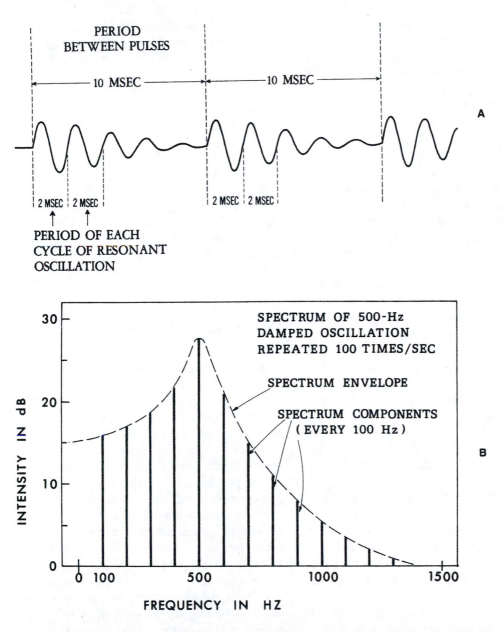

RESONANT 500-Hz OSCILLATION
PULSED 100 TIMES PER SECOND

PERIOD
BETWEEN PULSES

10 MSEC   10 MSEC

A

2 MSEC   2 MSEC   2 MSEC   2 MSEC

PERIOD OF EACH
CYCLE OF RESONANT
OSCILLATION

SPECTRUM OF 500-Hz
DAMPED OSCILLATION
REPEATED 100 TIMES/SEC

SPECTRUM ENVELOPE

SPECTRUM COMPONENTS
(EVERY 100 Hz)

INTENSITY IN dB

FREQUENCY IN HZ

B

FIGURE 2-11.   Waveform (A) and spectrum (B) of a 500 Hz damped oscillation that is pulsed at a rate of 100 times per second. In the spectrum there is a component at every multiple of 100 Hz, corresponding to the 100 per second frequency of pulsing; the most intense component, 500 Hz, corresponds to the frequency of the resonant oscillation.

tion recurring at a rate of 100 times per second. Secondly, there is the periodicity at the resonant frequency of each damped oscillation. This frequency is 500 Hz. It is the frequency of the basic formant for a 17.5 cm vocal tract.

The spectrum of this wave appears in Figure 2-11B. Compare the spectrum in Figure 2-11B with the spectrum in Figure 2-10; you will see the shape of the spectrum envelope is the same in both. This is because the spectrum envelope depends only on the physical characteristics of the air column that determine its resonant frequency and the damping. The individual components of the spectrum for the tract pulsed at 100 pulses per second are different from the components of the wave resulting from a single pulsing. Instead of a very large number of components, close together in frequency, there are components at 400 Hz, 300 Hz, 200 Hz, and 100 Hz below the resonant frequency, and components at 600 Hz, 700 Hz, 800 Hz, and so on above the resonant frequency. The frequency component of 100 Hz in this wave is called the *fundamental frequency* of the wave, or simply the *fundamental*. Because of the way the wave was produced, by pulsing at 100 times per second, the other components of the wave are all multiples of this fundamental frequency. In listening to the wave, a person will hear a fundamental pitch corresponding to the fundamental frequency of 100 Hz and will also hear a timbre corresponding to the resonant frequency of 500 Hz.

It is important that the strongest component in the spectrum is at 500 Hz, the resonant frequency, and all other components of the sound, including the fundamental component, are weaker in amplitude than the component at the resonant frequency. This is because of the resonance of the air column. It is true for the spectrum of any sound produced by a resonant system: The most intense component of the spectrum is the one at, or closest to, the resonant frequency.

Some resonant systems respond to a pulse with more prolonged vibration than an air column because their materials do not damp out the oscillations to such a great degree. A wine glass is a good example of a resonant system with rather little damping. If a wine glass is tapped very rapidly, say at 100 taps per second, then the resonant oscillations decay only a little between taps. The spectrum of this sound would show the amplitude of the fundamental frequency, the 100 Hz component, to be extremely low compared with the amplitude of the component at the resonant frequency. In listening to such a sound, the ear can still discriminate the low periodicity corresponding to the fundamental pulsing rate of the tapping and hear this as the lowest pitch of the sound wave. But the dominant tonal pitch corresponds to the resonant frequency of the glass.

Imagine a resonant system that has no damping at all. The oscillation from one pulse would continue forever and we would hear a pure tone at the resonant frequency; the spectrum of this wave would be a single component at the resonant frequency with no other components.

DEFINITIONS OF HARMONICS

At this point we need some definitions of terms used in describing spectra like the one in Figure 2-11B. When the spectrum of a wave consists of components whose frequencies are all multiples of a fundamental frequency, the spectrum is said to be a *harmonic spectrum*. This term arose because the components of the wave are synchronously (harmoniously) produced by the fundamental pulsing activity at a constant frequency. The components are called *harmonics*, and individual harmonics are always at frequencies that are simple integer multiples of the fundamental for the type of wave we are now considering. The harmonics are numbered in order from low to high frequencies, using numbers corresponding to their multiples; thus the wave component next above the fundamental is the *second harmonic*; its frequency is twice that of the fundamental. The frequency of the next component is three times the fundamental—it is the *third harmonic*, and so on, for higher-numbered harmonics. The component at the resonant frequency in Figure 2-11B is 500 Hz, which is five times the fundamental frequency, so it is the fifth harmonic of that spectrum.

The spectrum of a periodic wave is usually plotted as in Figure 2-11B, using a line for each component. Each line has a length representing the amplitude (intensity) of the wave component and a position on the frequency scale representing the frequency of the component. A spectrum plot of such component lines is called a *line spectrum*. If the spectral lines are harmonically related, that is, if they are multiples of a single frequency, the line spectrum is also a harmonic spectrum; if not, it is an inharmonic spectrum.

In speech, voiced sounds are produced with various pulsing rates of the glottis, so let us now consider what would happen to the line spectrum of the sound produced if the vocal tract were pulsed at different fundamental rates. If the glottal pulses were delivered at a rate of 200 per second, a rate often found for adult female speakers and some children, the spectrum would appear as in Figure 2-12A. Here we see the components of the spectrum are now at intervals of 200 Hz: There is a component in the spectrum at every multiple of the fundamental pulsing frequency. The spectrum envelope is still the same as before (in Figure 2-11B) because the assumed resonance characteristics have not been changed; we have only increased the rate of the pulsing that periodically excites the air column to vibrate, but the form of resonant vibration between pulses remains exactly the same and this determines the shape of the spectrum envelope.

Similarly, if the resonance is pulsed at a rate of 300 pulses per second, the spectrum envelope will again remain the same but the components, 300, 600, 900, and 1200 Hz, are located at multiples of the fundamental 300 Hz. I show this in the spectrum in Figure 2-12B.

RESONANT WAVES, SPECTRUM PLOTS, AND SPEECH WAVES

The amplitude-time wave of the pulsed 500 Hz resonator in of Figure 2-11A is somewhat like a real speech wave and the spectrum plot of the

intensities of its component frequencies in Figure 2-11B is like spectra seen when we analyze real speech. This procedure is a highly useful and standard way to show speech characteristics that are not so easy to understand by looking at the whole waveform. To solidly relate this to real speech we can go back to one of our landscape examples, the greeting "Hi Sam" by Father in Figure 1-1. We will see how the sound wave of "Hi Sam" is similar to the wave from the pulsed resonator, first in their waveforms and then in their spectrum components.

Figure 2-13 shows how we dissected out, for this explanation, part of the [æ]-sound wave from the original "Hi Sam." At the top is the region of the original soundscape; below it is the waveform of the [aⁱ s æ] part of "Hi Sam" and then, next below, a magnified projection of part of the [sæ] in "Sam." Below that we have taken out and further magnified a short section of the [æ]-vowel that covers only two of the vocal pulse cycles of the [æ]-vowel to compare with the pulses we applied to the model 500 Hz resonator to make the wave of Figure 2-11A. There is a strong similarity between the oscillations of the model's 500 Hz wave and the wave from the real [æ] in "Sam." This is because the largest oscillations in the [æ] are at a low frequency and the smaller oscillations are at higher frequencies, riding on the large low-frequency wave. The speech sounds that originate from vocal pulses are made up entirely of a combination of resonant oscillations that is radiated from the mouth as speech.

All such oscillations, large, small, fast, or slow in their fluctuations, are like the repeated ringing of a bell. In speech the ringing dies out between "strokes" (vocal pulses) much more rapidly than for a bell, but the pulses occur so frequently that we do not hear pulsing as such, only a continuous vowel sound. However, the duration of ringing is acoustically specific to nasal speech sounds as we shall see later.

At the bottom of the figure we have marked the duration, 7.3 ms, of one period of the glottal pulsing (the first cycle) and one period of the large, main resonant fluctuation, much shorter at

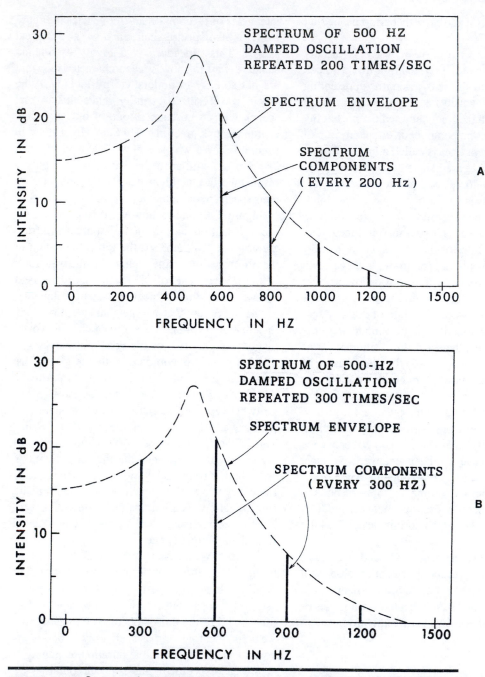

FIGURE 2-12.   Spectra of a 500 Hz damped oscillation pulsed at (A) 200 times per second and (B) 300 times per second.

FIGURE 2-13.   Illustration of the selection of segments from the [æ] wave of "Hi Sam" for analysis of wave characteristics, such as the glottal pulsing period for f0 and the oscillation period for F1.

DISSECTING
A SPEECH WAVE

Soundscape Perspective
from
Middle of "Hi Sam"

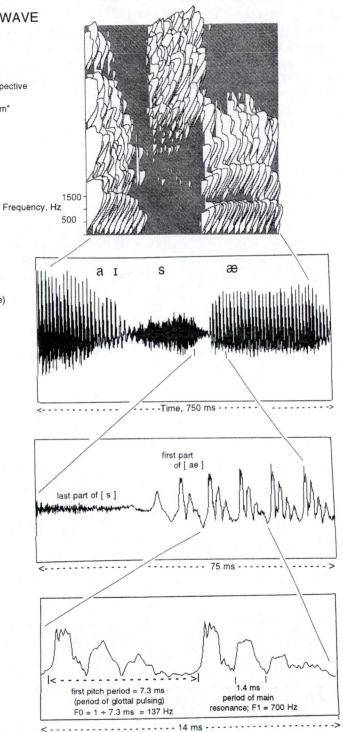

Frequency, Hz

1500

500

a ɪ   s   æ

Waveform
(amplitude over time)
from
Middle of "Hi Sam"

<----------- ------Time, 750 ms ------ ---------->

Waveform of
75 ms piece
from "Sam"

first part
of [ae]

last part of [s]

<- - - - - - - - -   - - - - - - - - - - 75 ms - - - - - - - - - - - >

Waveform of
2 pitch periods
from [ ]

|<- - - - - - - - - - - - - - - - - - >|

first pitch period = 7.3 ms
(period of glottal pulsing)
F0 = 1 ÷ 7.3 ms = 137 Hz

1.4 ms
period of main
resonance; F1 = 700 Hz

< - 14 ms - - - - - - - - - - - - - - - >

1.4 ms, in the second glottal pulse cycle. In speech analysis, the glottal pulsing period is called the *pitch period* because it corresponds to the pitch of the voice; for this speaker the pitch at this point is 137 Hz; the *voice pitch frequency is often called F0 or f0.* The shorter-period fluctuation we measured in the second glottal cycle is the period of the lowest resonance in this portion of the vowel [æ]. We notice that there are three of these in each glottal cycle, all of very similar duration, but of successively lower amplitude proceeding to the right, in time, through each cycle; the resonant frequency is the reciprocal of 1.4 ms or 700 Hz, approximately constant over these cycles, but dying out between cycles. In speech analysis the resonances are called *formants* and the lowest formant in frequency is called the *first formant,* or *F1.*

Now to compare the spectrum of this formant of this [æ] we will study only the large low-frequency oscillation and compare it with that of the 500 Hz resonator, by looking at the spectrum of the waves. The waveforms were plotted by a computer program, Edwave, which was used also to pick out the two cycles of vocal pulsing from [æ], to analyze its spectrum components, and to plot them in a graph. These [æ]-components are plotted in Figure 2-14, for the large low frequencies only, showing the vertical intensity of each component plotted at its frequency position on the horizontal scale. To plot a spectrum, the computer makes a peak at the intensity of each component and connects between these peaks with much lower points that represent the noise level in the recording of the original speech. We see that the components' peaks follow a pattern of rise and

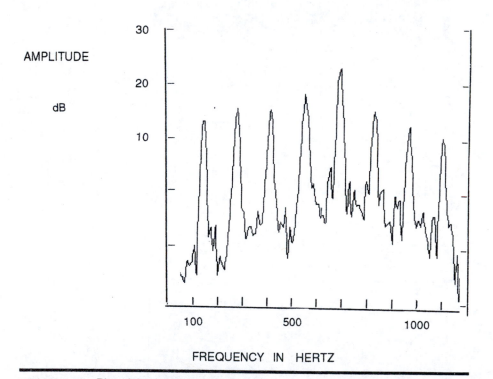

FIGURE 2-14.   Plot of the first 8 harmonics in the center of the vowel selected in Figure 2-13. Note that the strongest harmonic, harmonic 5, indicates an F1 of 700 Hz.

fall, around a maximum at 700 Hz, that is very similar to the rise-fall around 500 Hz for the resonator of Figure 2-11B. Because that spectrum can be called the "spectrum of a simple pulsed 500 Hz resonator," we can also describe this major acoustic pattern of the [æ]-vowel as "a pulsed 700 Hz resonator."

Notice how succinct and useful it is to talk about the spectrum of a resonant response rather than its waveform. First, it is simpler to specify a resonance spectrum by the two numbers, resonance frequency (at the peak amplitude or maximum amplification) and amount of amplification (also called the Q or "figure of merit"). Then, for all the other frequencies the amplitude and intensity values are predetermined, and the spectrum can be plotted and compared with that of any noise present, or with the contour of hearing at different frequencies (audiogram) of listeners with impaired hearing. If we should try to specify the resonance response waveform instead of its spectrum, we would need to measure and plot the amplitudes of the resonant wave at many instants of time. Furthermore, we could not compare that wave with the threshold of hearing at different frequencies; comparing wave amplitudes versus frequency amplitudes is trying to compare values in two totally different domains of description.

As we shall see later, the sound characteristics of different vowels and consonants can be very succinctly described just by giving their major resonance frequencies. In addition, we will see in Chapter Seventeen on speech technology that speech can be synthesized by simply feeding a track of electronic pulses into a set of resonators that are programmed to be like those in speech.

APERIODIC SPEECH SOUNDS

Up to this point I have dealt only with the periodic sounds of speech, those based on the periodic pulses of air emitted by the glottis. The aperiodic, turbulent sounds of speech are also important. The *aperiodic sounds* are, as the name indicates, sounds that do not have a periodic form of sound wave. This is because the airflow disturbances

producing aperiodic sounds are events that occur randomly in time. Aperiodic speech sounds are produced by two types of disturbance: (1) sudden transient releases of the breath pressure built up behind consonant closures, and (2) turbulence in the breath stream as it rushes through a constriction. Air turbulence is random in time, producing random, aperiodic fluctuations in sound amplitude.

Sounds produced by transients and turbulence have spectra showing components at all frequencies. The form of the spectrum depends, as with periodic sounds, on the spectrum of the source and on the resonances of the vocal tract through which the source sound passes. We will examine the production and spectra of aperiodic speech sounds later.

SUMMARY

We have seen in this chapter how sound, which originates as a disturbance of the resting positions of air particles, propagates the form of the disturbance faithfully and rapidly through the air. In speech, sound is produced by the vocal organs and propagated through the vocal tract to the outside air. The air particle motions of speech sounds are complex in form but they can be represented as combinations of the simple oscillations of simple harmonic motion, a type of motion like that of a pendulum, where the motion is caused by a restoring force that is proportional to the displacement from resting position. Simple harmonic motion produces a sine wave. The amplitude, frequency, and sinusoidal form of a sine wave sound (pure tone) define its physical and auditory character.

A natural vibrating system, such as a pendulum, a ringing wine glass, or the air in a tube like the vocal tract, responds to a disturbance from the resting state with a sinusoidal damped oscillation. This is called resonant oscillation.

The frequency of resonant oscillation of the air in a tube-like bottle, and in the vocal tract, can be explained in terms of reflections up and down the length of the air column. The form of resonant oscillation of an air column is sinusoidal because the force producing air particle motion is a pressure difference proportional to the air particle distance or total flow from the resting state.

The sound wave produced by a resonant oscillation can be analyzed by sine-wave components; the main component is a sinusoid having the same frequency as the resonant oscillation; other components having frequencies higher and lower than the main component are necessary and these have amplitudes that are less than the main component. The amplitudes of the components, when plotted on a frequency scale, represent the spectrum of the resonant oscillation.

In speech the vowel sounds are produced by a *periodic* series of pulses emitted by the glottis. Each such pulse causes damped oscillations of the vocal tract air column. The resulting wave of recurring damped oscillations is analyzed by deriving its spectrum components. The frequencies of the spectrum components depend on the pulsing rate, which determines the fundamental frequency and the frequencies of the other spectrum components. The components are harmonics, all of which are simple multiples of the fundamental frequency. The amplitudes of the spectrum components are determined by the resonant frequency of the damped oscillation and by the amount of damping. The harmonic at the resonant frequency always has the highest amplitude and the other components have lower amplitudes according to their distance from the resonant frequency.

Nonperiodic, *aperiodic* sounds also occur in speech. These are caused by random pulsing of the vocal tract by transient or turbulent disturbances in the air particle distribution.

CHAPTER THREE

VOWEL SHAPING
AND VOWEL FORMANTS

The purpose of this chapter is to explain how the vocal shapes of vowels produce the spectrum patterns of the different vowels. We need only a few concepts and rules to go from the vocal tract shape for a vowel to its spectrum envelope. The rules give relations between the formant frequencies of the vocal tract and its shape. To demonstrate these relations we use a simple tube model of the vowel tract. The tube model produces sounds with formant frequencies similar to those of vowels. The formant frequencies are related to the length of the tube and to constrictions in the tube like those formed in the vocal tract by the pharynx, lips, and tongue in speaking vowels. A set of rules is given for these relations. The rules are used to develop a set of formant frequencies for model vowels.

MODEL OF THE PHARYNGEAL-ORAL TRACT

All the different vowel sounds begin as a single common sound produced by the glottis; this sound is propagated through the pharynx and mouth to the air outside. The form of the pharyngeal and oral passages determines what the resulting vowel sound will be. We call this passageway the *pharyngeal-oral tract* or simply the *oral tract*. When the oral tract has a given shape, the vowel sound produced has a certain pattern; when some other shape is formed, a different pattern of vowel sound is formed.

Acoustic research on vowel shaping has found that a surprisingly simple model of the tract will produce artificial vowel sounds very similar to those of natural speech. The model is a shaped tube. It provides an easy way to remember the different spectrum patterns of vowels and, at the same time, it is a true physical model of how these patterns are produced.

The adequacy of the tube model was demonstrated by research comparing the sounds from models with sounds from natural speakers. First, natural vowel sounds were spoken and recorded. At the same time X-rays were made of the vocal tracts of the speakers. The shapes of the pharyngeal oral tract for each vowel were then sketched from the X-rays. Using these shapes and dimensions, tube models were made that had the same shapes seen in the X-rays. Finally, sound was passed through the tube models and the emerging sound patterns were compared with the natural vowel patterns. The agreement was good.[1]

We use the same model here to explain the main sound patterns of vowels. We start with the vowel that has the most simple shape—the neutral vowel [ə], as in the phrase, *a toy* [ətɔɪ]. For this vowel sound the shape of the oral tract is neutral. That is, the tract has no appreciable constriction at any point; it is like a tube that has the same width at all points. A simple straight tube is the model for this vowel. Figure 3-1 illustrates the relation between the tract shape and the model.

---

[1] This research began with the work of Chiba and Kajiyama (1941) and was continued in the 1950s by Dunn. Fant related vocal X-ray shapes to the acoustic theory of tube shapes and developed an acoustic theory of speech production that brought both acoustics and phonetics to bear on a unified description of speech. For details see Dunn (1950), Fant (1960, 1968), Jakobson, Fant, and Halle (1951), Lindblom and Sundberg (1971), and Stevens and House (1955, 1961), but students without technical background should first read this chapter and the next one on the spectra of vowel sounds.

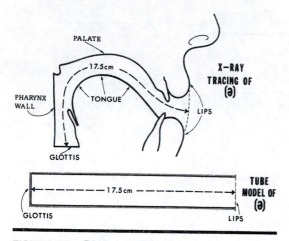

FIGURE 3-1. Diagram of an X-ray tracing of the shape of the pharyngeal-oral tract and a tube model of the tract for the neutral vowel [ə].

In Figure 3-1, an X-ray sketch of the pharyngeal-oral tract shape for [ə] shows the neutral position of the tongue and lips forming a tract that is nearly constant in width from the glottis through the lips. The length of the tract from glottis through lips is important for the vowel pattern; it is 17.5 cm long. This length is used for the model because it is the average distance through the tract from the glottis to the lips for adult males. The curvature of the tract does not affect sound propagation appreciably. Thus the tube model for this vowel is straight, of equal width throughout, and is 17.5 cm long, as shown in the lower part of Figure 3-1. The natural tract has minor deviations from equal width at the teeth and just above the glottis, but these have only minor effects on the vowel patterns.

Our object is to compare the sound pattern from the natural tract with that derived from the tube model. We do this by comparing the spectrum of sound from the model tube with the spectrum of a natural vowel sound. Each vowel sound has a characteristic shape of spectrum envelope depending on the formant frequency locations. Some simple rules relate the formant frequencies to the vowel shape, and this makes it easy to describe the sound pattern for a number of the basic vowel shapes used in producing speech.

SPECTRUM OF THE NEUTRAL VOWEL [ə]

Let us see how the spectrum envelope of the neutral vowel [ə] arises from its oral tract shape. In Figure 3-2 we can see how the spectrum of a model [ə]-vowel is formed by the tube model and compare the model spectrum with a neutral vowel spectrum spoken by the author. A speaker of English can only form a uniform, neutral vocal tract by expressing horrified disgust, as in "ughhhh," or by pretending to retch. Examine first how the sound is formed in the tube model. The sound that is inserted into the tube at the "glottis" end has a spectrum envelope that slopes downward in intensity as we go from low to high frequencies. This spectrum is an ideal one that represents the sound emitted from the glottis; it is the spectrum of the glottal sound source, the source of sound for vowels.

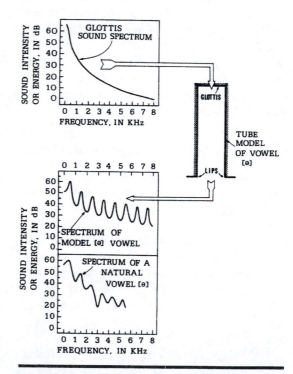

FIGURE 3-2. Illustration of the modification of the glottal sound spectrum by transmission through a tube model of the neutral vowel [ə] and comparison spectrum of a natural [ə] spoken by the author.

Now note that the spectrum of the sound coming out of the tube also slopes downward, but it is scalloped with regular peaks and valleys of sound intensity. The general downward slope of the scalloped spectrum is the same as the slope of the glottal spectrum that was inserted into the tube. However, when we compare the spectrum of the emitted sound with that of the inserted sound, we see that passage through the tube has emphasized some frequencies more than others in a very regular pattern. The first peak is at a frequency of 500 Hz; above this peak there are peaks at 1500 Hz, 2500 Hz, 3500 Hz, and 4500 Hz. In other words, *there is a peak every 1000 Hz above the first peak at 500 Hz.*

As we saw in the previous chapter, the peak at 500 Hz represents the basic resonance of a 17.5 cm tube. It is the resonance that is lowest in frequency. The other peaks represent resonances at frequencies above the basic resonance. The resonant frequencies of a tube depend on its particular shape and dimensions. For a uniform tube the resonances occur at regular frequency intervals above the lowest resonance. This pattern will be our reference for describing model patterns of all the vowels.

Going back to Figure 3-2, examine the spectrum of the natural vowel [ə] and compare it with the spectrum of the sound from the tube model. There is a considerable similarity between the two spectra. In the natural vowel, the peaks of sound intensity occur at 475, 1450, 2375, 3350, 4300, and 5200 Hz; these peaks are regularly spaced at intervals of about 950 Hz. The pattern of resonances of this natural [ə] seems to be shifted downward slightly in frequency compared with the pattern of the model [ə].

It is through acoustic modeling in this way that we know how the frequency locations of the resonant peaks in vowels depend on the length and shape of the vocal tract or, in the model, on the length and shape of a tube with the same dimensions. In the modeling process different sections of the model tube are given different diameters representing sections of the vocal tract where the lips are more or less rounded, protruded, or spread, and where the tongue is humped up

in a given location or the pharynx is constricted. Using X-ray pictures of the lip, tongue, and pharynx constrictions, the resonance patterns and spectrum envelopes of many spoken vowels have been compared with those produced by tube models constricted according to the X-ray pictures. Good agreement has been found and we conclude that the resonance patterns of natural vowels are formed by the same physical effects that determine the resonances of tubes.

DEFINITION OF SPEECH FORMANTS

Before describing how the spectrum patterns with various resonant peaks are formed for different vowels, we need some exact definitions of the acoustic terms we will use.

The resonances in sound transmission through the vocal tract are called *formants*. We define *a formant as a resonance of the vocal tract.*

The effects of the formants are seen in the spectrum pattern of a speech sound because the spectrum is strongly affected by the resonances of the vocal tract. When the effects of the vocal resonances are apparent in the spectrum of a speech sound, the spectrum peaks may be called the "formants" of the speech sound but, strictly speaking, this is not correct because it is not the sound that has formants or resonances, it is the vocal tract. The formants are not the peaks seen in the spectrum; they are acoustic properties of the vocal tract that produced the spectrum. We should always keep in mind the fact that formants are really properties of the vocal tract; this basic approach is essential when we try to explain the spectrum peaks and their possible relation to the vocal tract shape.[2]

---

[2] In practice we often want to infer the formant pattern of the vocal tract that produced a given speech sound by examining the spectrum of the sound. Then the frequencies and intensities of the formants are estimated by examining the peaks in the spectrum. However, because the formants are resonances of the vocal tract, a more principled and accurate method to measure the formants would be to read them from a plot of the transmission of sound through the actual vocal tract shape with no complication from the source spectrum.

The formants of a speech sound are numbered in order of their frequencies and are called the first formant (F1), second formant (F2), third formant (F3), fourth formant (F4), and so on, as far as needed.

The frequency locations of the formants, especially F1 and F2, are closely tied to the shape of the vocal tract as the lips, tongue, pharynx, and jaw move to articulate the consonants and vowels. The frequency of the third formant, F3, is related to only a few specific speech sounds, which are discussed later. The fourth and fifth and higher formants—F4, F5, and so on—remain rather constant in frequency location regardless of changes in articulation. First, we will concentrate on F1 and F2, especially on their frequency locations for the different vowel sounds.

The formant frequency locations for vowels are affected by three factors: the *length* of the pharyngeal-oral tract, the *location of constrictions* in the tract, and the degree of *narrowness of the constrictions*.

VOWEL FORMANT LOCATIONS AND LENGTH OF PHARYNGEAL-ORAL TRACT

The length of the pharyngeal-oral tract depends on the physical size of the speaker. The length affects the frequency locations of all of the vowel formants; this fact helps us to predict where the formant peaks in the spectrum will appear for children, women, and men. A very simple rule relates the frequencies of the formants to the overall length of the tract from glottis through lips. The rule for this relation is:

Length Rule. The average frequencies of the vowel formants are inversely proportional to the length of the pharyngeal-oral tract. In other words, the longer the tract, the lower are its average formant frequencies.

The neutral vowel formants for the average man, with an oral tract 17.5 cm in length, are at 500, 1500, 2500 Hz, and so on, with the lowest formant at 500 Hz and frequency spacing of 1000 Hz between all formants.

An easy way to remember the neutral formant frequencies is to think of the odd numbers 1, 3, 5, 7, 9, and so on, because the formant frequencies of a uniform tube that is closed at one end and open at the other, like the pharyngeal-oral tract, are always odd multiples of the frequency of the lowest formant. For example, begin with the basic formant frequency, 500 Hz, as the unit or 1; then the formant frequencies above that are $500 \times 3 = 1500$ Hz, $500 \times 5 = 2500$ Hz, and so on. This method, calculating the formants above F1 as multiples of F1, applies only as a model of a neutral tract shape.

The pharyngeal-oral tract length of an infant is approximately half the length of that of a man. Therefore, following our Length Rule about formant frequency locations, the formants of a neutral-shaped infant tract in relation to a man's would be at frequency locations that are a factor of the reciprocal of 1/2, or twice those of the man. On this basis the infant formant locations for a neutral vowel would be as follows: F1 is $500 \times 2 = 1000$ Hz, F2 is $1500 \times 2 = 3000$ Hz, F3 is $2500 \times 2 = 5000$ Hz, and so on.

Following the same procedure, a woman's vocal tract, on the average, is about 15% shorter than that of a man. The ratio corresponding to this amount of shortening is approximately 5/6. The reciprocal of 5/6 is 6/5, which is equal to a factor of 1.20, which, when multiplied by the man's neutral formant frequencies, gives the woman's values of 20% higher: F1 is $500 \times 1.2 = 600$ Hz, F2 is $1500 \times 1.2 = 1800$ Hz, F3 is $2500 \times 1.2 = 3000$ Hz, and so on.

It should also be noted that the frequency spacing between the formants can be calculated by the Length Rule, that is, simply by applying a factor that is the reciprocal of the length ratio taken relative to the 17.5 cm length.

Figure 3-3 illustrates these relations between the model tract lengths for women, men, and infants and the corresponding formant frequency positions in the spectra of model neutral vowels.

For another example of applying the Length Rule, return to Figure 3-2 and ask the following question about the natural [ə] vowel. Why were

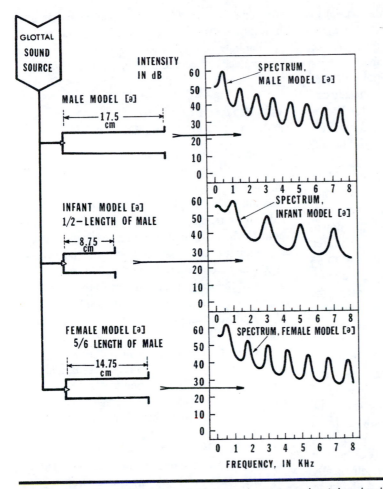

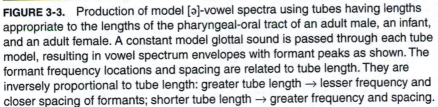

FIGURE 3-3. Production of model [ə]-vowel spectra using tubes having lengths appropriate to the lengths of the pharyngeal-oral tract of an adult male, an infant, and an adult female. A constant model glottal sound is passed through each tube model, resulting in vowel spectrum envelopes with formant peaks as shown. The formant frequency locations and spacing are related to tube length. They are inversely proportional to tube length: greater tube length → lesser frequency and closer spacing of formants; shorter tube length → greater frequency and spacing.

the formant frequencies indicated by the spectrum of the natural [ə] vowel a little lower and more closely spaced than those of the model [ə] vowel? The natural formants in this case seem to be about 5% lower than those for the 17.5 cm model; 5% lower is a ratio of 0.95, the reciprocal of which is 1.053, so it may be that the pharyngeal-oral

tract of the natural speaker was 5.3% longer than 17.5 cm.

The relation of model formant frequency locations and formant spacing to the length of the vocal tract is a useful aid in analyzing speech patterns. The Length Rule tells us approximately where we may find the formants for the very young as well as for older, larger persons. However, the neutral locations of F1 and F2 for an individual are also affected by the length proportions of the vocal tract between the oral and pharyngeal cavities (Fant, 1973, Chapter 4). In general, the location and spacing of formants F3 and above are more closely correlated with length of vocal tract than for F1 and F2. The average locations of F1 and F2 for an individual are also affected somewhat by language environment and training.

In view of the Length Rule, some very interesting questions can be asked about how children acquire speech. As children grow, their vocal tracts grow longer and their formants shift downward in frequency. In other words, as children learn to speak, over the period of about 10 to 48 months of age, the sounds they produce are gradually changing in the frequency location of the formants! How do they learn to make the correct sounds, if the results of their productions are changing in sound pattern?

This is one of the great mysteries of speech. It may be that auditory self-monitoring for speech development is unnecessary after the initial stages of learning to make a given sound. Or it may be that the child's auditory system somehow readjusts its frequency scale for listening as the vocal tract is growing. It's possible that some sort of built-in readjustment or rescaling takes place automatically in the auditory system, because, in addition to adjusting for growth changes in its own speech sounds, the child also uses adult sounds as models; adult sounds cannot correspond to the child's own proper sounds because of the large difference in size between adult and child vocal tracts. It is physically impossible for a young child to match adult speech sounds. Speculations on this question are very interesting. One theory, described below in connection with the formant/constriction rules, is that babies start to rescale their control of vowels while they imitate adults' exaggerated speech to them using the extreme "point vowels." The problem comes up again in Chapter Thirteen on theories of speech perception.

Still, not to abandon children here, we know that mothers exaggerate their vowels when speaking to their babies. We will have more insight into how mothers might do this after we see in the next section how vowel formant frequencies are linked to the place and degree of vocal constrictions.

VOCAL TRACT CONSTRICTIONS AND FORMANT FREQUENCY LOCATIONS

Having located the neutral formant positions, we now need to see how different articulatory shapes of the pharyngeal-oral tract affect the formant locations. The simplest way to do this is to consider, for modeling purposes, just the constriction points of the articulation. First, we consider just the amount of constriction, that is the narrowness at places of constriction. Figure 3-4 shows diagrams of the tract shapes for several vowels. The diagrams are based on an X-ray study by Lindblom and Sundberg (1971). The tongue positions in Figure 3-4 for the front vowels, [i, e, ɛ, æ], can be seen to form a series with progressively less constriction at the front of the palate. In addition the jaw position is more open for [ɛ, æ] than for [i, e], and the pharynx is more constricted.

The back vowels [u] and [o] differ in amount of constriction by the tongue at a place near the back of the palate, with [u] being more constricted than [o]. Also the lips are narrowly rounded for [u] but are less so for [o]. The back vowels [ɔ] and [ɑ] have progressively less lip constriction but are formed by constricting the pharynx progressively more going from [o] to [ɔ] to [ɑ]. In addition, the jaw position is more open for [ɑ].

In describing rules that relate vowel shapes to formant locations we begin with the effect of amount of constriction on the frequency of F1. A constriction also affects F2, but in different ways, which are described separately. There are two rules relating constriction and F1, one for oral constrictions and another for pharyngeal constrictions.

Oral Constriction/F1 Rule. The frequency of F1 is lowered by any constriction in the front half of the oral part of the vocal tract, and the greater the constriction the more F1 is lowered.

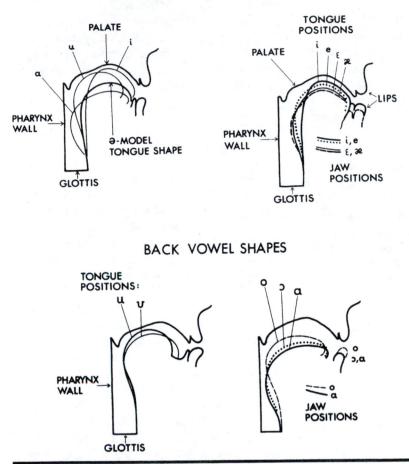

FIGURE 3-4. Diagrams of pharyngeal-oral tract shapes for front and back vowels. (Adapted from Lindblom & Sundberg, 1971)

Thus, if the tongue is somewhat humped up close to the middle of the palate or to the front of the palate instead of being in the position forming a neutral uniform area tube, then F1 is forced lower in frequency than the neutral 500 Hz. This also applies to a constriction formed at the lips or teeth.

You can hear the frequency (pitch) of F1 by snapping your finger against your throat at the top of your larynx, keeping your glottis closed (Catford, 1988, Exercise 113, p. 163). Start snapping with your tongue in an open front constriction, like for the [æ] in *add*; then keep snapping as you move your tongue toward more constriction, closer to the front of your palate, toward [e] as in *aid*, you will hear the "snap pitch" go downward with the increasing constriction. There is also a faint pitch that goes up as you move your tongue closer at the front of the palate. This weak pitch is easier to hear as a whispered pitch; it is due to F2 (see Catford, 1988, Exercise 114, cited below under the Constriction Rules/F2).

Pharyngeal Constriction/F1 Rule. The frequency of F1 is raised by constriction of the pharynx, and the greater the constriction the more F1 is raised.

As we saw in Figure 3-4, different degrees of constriction of the pharynx occur in the back vowels, going from the least pharyngeal constriction for [o] to the most pharyngeal constriction for [ɑ]. This causes F1 of these vowels to be progressively higher than 500 Hz.

The rise in F1 with increasing pharynx constriction can be heard in "snap pitch" while you move your tongue from the [æ]-position for *add* toward the [ɑ]-position for *odd* (use a General American speaker). You can also start snapping with your tongue in an [o]-position as for *ode* if you can inhibit your natural tendency to lip-rounding, which by itself lowers the F1 pitch.

Next, we give rules relating F2 frequency to vocal tract constrictions. The frequency rule of F2 depends on whether the tongue constriction is near the front of the oral tract, as for front vowels, or near the back, as for the back vowels. First we consider back constrictions.

Back Tongue Constriction/F2 Rule. The frequency of F2 tends to be lowered by a back tongue constriction, and the greater the constriction the more F2 is lowered.

If the tongue is humped up toward the back of the palate to constrict the oral tract and form one of the back vowels, [u] for example, the effect is to lower the frequency of F2. In fact, the vowel [u] is formed by humping the tongue rather close to the soft palate, and the frequency location of F2 for this vowel is very low because of the rather narrow constriction. Compared with the frequency location of F2 for the neutral vowel shape, the F2 for [u] for a man is about 800 Hz instead of a neutral F2 of 1500 Hz. The next vowel in the series of back vowels, [o], is formed with less tongue constriction and less lip-rounding than [u]; therefore, since the amount of lowering of F2 depends on the amount of constriction, F2 is at a higher frequency location for [o] than for [u]. In a typical man's [o], F2 is about 900 Hz.

When the constriction of the tongue is at the front of the palate, F2 is affected by the constriction in a way just opposite to that for back tongue constrictions. The rule relating front tongue constriction and frequency of F2 is:

Front Tongue Constriction/F2 Rule. The frequency of F2 is raised by a front tongue constriction, and the greater the constriction the more F2 is raised.

You can hear the rise in F2 very clearly if you whisper while moving your tongue between [ɛ] and [i], as in Catford's Exercise 114, p. 164. Make sure your whisper is generated deep in the throat by your glottis, not by forming a fricative-like vowel. Similarly, you can hear whispered F2 go down in pitch if you move your tongue from [æ] to [ɑ].

The front vowels can be arranged in a series where the amount of tongue constriction is least for [æ] and greatest for [i] (cf. Figure 3-4); the series is [æ], [ɛ], [e], [i]. Following our rules for the frequency location of F1 and F2 over the series of front vowels from least constricted to most constricted, the frequency of F1 decreases; however, the frequency of F2 goes from a frequency of 1700 Hz, just slightly higher than the neutral position for F2, to a high frequency for the most constricted front vowel, [i], where F2 is at a frequency of about 2200 Hz for an average man. The pharyngeal constrictions of [æ] and [ɛ] raise F1 above the neutral F1 of 500 Hz.

Our final rule describes the effects of lip-rounding on the formants as follows:

Lip-Rounding Rule. The frequencies of all formants are lowered by lip-rounding. The more the rounding, the more the constriction, and the more the formants are lowered.

To hear the formants go lower, whisper an [ɑ] and then, holding the same tongue position, round your lips inward and then out again. Actually, you can start with any whispered vowel and hear some very strange-sounding whispered vowels by rounding, unrounding, and spreading your lips in a smile.

Lip-rounding plays an important part in forming the back vowels and some of the consonants. The series of back vowels involves a series of lip positions beginning with wide-open lips for [ɑ] and progressing to more and more rounded, that is, more and more lip-constricted configurations as we proceed to [ɔ], [o], and [u]. In addition, the back tongue constrictions for the back vowels are more and more constricted going from [ɔ] to [o] to [u]. Thus, two effects cause the frequency locations of F1 and F2 to be progressively lower over the back vowel series going from the most open, unrounded vowel [a] to the [u] vowel with the most tongue constriction at the back and the most lip-rounding at the lips. The pharyngeal constriction also comes into play going from [ɑ] to [o]. The frequency of F1 begins with [a] at a high frequency and is lowered by the decrease in pharyngeal constriction for [ɔ] and [o]. The increasing back tongue constriction causes F2 to decrease between [o] and [u] while, at the same time, increasing lip-rounding causes further decrease in F2, as well as decrease in Fl.

Point Vowels and the Baby's Formant-Matching Problem

There are three extreme vowels corresponding to three extremes of oral-tract constriction: [u], most back-tongue/lips rounded; [i], most front-tongue/jaw closed/lips spread; and [ɑ], most pharyngeal/jaw open. These are called "point vowels." They occur in all languages. We might speculate that the ubiquity of the point vowels is due to fact that the articulations of these vowels are easy to see. When babies imitate father's or mother's lip and tongue positions (Kuhl, Williams, & Meltzoff, 1991), then vocalize, they may be giving themselves experience in perceptually equating their higher formant patterns, due to their smaller vocal tracts, to match the lower formant patterns of their parents.

Infants make the point vowels by about age one, possibly in response to parents' exaggerated articulation of vowels. Kuhl, Andruski, Chistovich, Chistovich, and Kozhevnikova (1997) measured the formants of mothers speaking to their babies compared with speaking to adults, in American English, Russian, and Swedish. The point vowels were selected from recorded conversations. In all three languages the mothers' vowels showed more extreme formant positions in baby-directed speech than in adult-directed speech. Apparently mothers assume more extreme articulations, making their vowels even easier to see, and thus assist their babies in solving the mismatch between vocal tract sizes.

The rules given above provide a simple framework for predicting formant patterns from vocal tract shape and for keeping in mind the relations between vowel formants and the constrictions. However, these rules have some limitations in range of operation. They operate best when a single constriction is the dominant feature of the shape of the vocal tract. Single-constriction shapes occur for the close front vowels, [i, e], and the open back vowels, [ɑ, ɔ], when they are spoken in isolation, and at points in words where the vowel shape is not greatly affected by consonant constrictions. For these single-constriction shapes different degrees of constriction cause large shifts of formant frequencies in the directions given by the rules. When there are two constrictions involved in the shape of the tract, a rule may or may not operate over the entire range of constrictions. For example, different degrees of lip-rounding have strong effects when superimposed on a front vowel shape, but have only limited effects when added to back vowel shapes. In running speech where the constriction movements of the lips, tongue, and pharynx frequently overlap each other in time, it is only during phases of single constriction dominance and during certain combined constrictions that our formant/constriction rules apply strongly. Stevens and House (1955) and Fant (1960) provide curves relating formant frequencies and degrees of constriction; these sources should be consulted for predictions of formant frequencies that are more accurate than our simple rules allow.

The purpose of the our five rules relating vocal tract constrictions and formant frequencies is to provide a simplified framework that summarizes the acoustic shaping of normal vowels. The rules may not always apply to defective speech because abnormal (compensatory) shaping of the vocal tract and abnormal vocal fold action can produce spectral patterns not explained by the rules.

FORMANTS OF MODEL VOWELS

A set of model formant frequencies for vowels is given in Figure 3-5. The set is constructed in a somewhat artificial way to serve as a mnemonic device. The end values of F1 and F2, at the ends of the front series and the back series, are set at frequencies that are fairly close to the average formant frequencies found for American men (Peterson & Barney, 1952). However, the end values were also selected to allow equal steps of either 100 or 150 Hz between formants of two

adjacent vowels. The 150 Hz steps are used for F1 and for the F2 range of the front vowels from [i] to [æ]. The 100 Hz steps are used for the F2 steps between adjacent back vowels and 150 Hz steps are used for Fl.

This results in a set of vowel formant frequencies that are easy to keep in mind, or even to reconstruct, knowing only the extreme F values and step sizes. For example, one can start by writing down just the F values for the close vowels, [i] and [u]; these are front F1 and back F1 = 250 Hz, front F2 = 2150 Hz, and back F2 = 800 Hz. Then, following the constriction rules, from close to open, go down in frequency in 150 Hz steps of F2 over the series of front vowels, next go up in frequency in 150 Hz steps of F1 over the series of front vowels, then go up in frequency in 100 Hz steps of F2 over the back vowels, and up in 150 Hz steps for the F1 values. This constructs a table of model formant frequencies for the front and back vowels.

The table in Figure 3-5 shows us that for each front vowel there is a corresponding back vowel having a similar degree of constriction and, therefore, a very similar frequency of the first formant. We might predict that when vowels are heard in a noisy situation where the noise interferes more with hearing the second formant region than the first, listeners will confuse the pairs of front and back vowels that have similar frequencies of the first formant, namely, they will confuse [i] with [u], [e] with [o], [ɛ] with [ɔ], and [æ] with [ɑ]. These confusions actually do occur very frequently in listening to speech in hissing, high-frequency noises where the second formant region cannot be heard (Pickett, 1957). We also predicted a similar result for hearing-impaired listeners who have a type of deafness where hearing is more impaired in the frequency range of F2 than in the range of Fl, a very common type of impairment. When we analyzed the errors of such listeners in identifying amplified words, we found the same types of confusions; they interconfused [i] and [u], both vowels having low F1, and [ɑ] with [æ], both vowels having high F1, but did not often confuse between

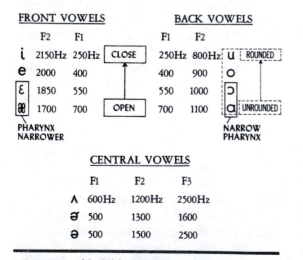

FRONT VOWELS

	F2	F1	
i	2150Hz	250Hz	CLOSE
e	2000	400	
ɛ	1850	550	
æ	1700	700	OPEN

PHARYNX NARROWER

BACK VOWELS

	F1	F2		
250Hz	800Hz	u	ROUNDED
400	900	o	
550	1000	ɔ	
700	1100	ɑ	UNROUNDED

NARROW PHARYNX

CENTRAL VOWELS

	F1	F2	F3
ʌ	600Hz	1200Hz	2500Hz
ɚ	500	1300	1600
ə	500	1500	2500

FIGURE 3-5. Model formant frequencies for front, back, and central vowels, depending on degree of constriction, open-to-close.

vowels of high and low F1 frequency. Thus, their poor hearing for F2 caused confusions, but F1 was heard well enough to prevent confusion between low F1 vowels and high F1 vowels (Pickett, Martin, Johnson, Smith, Daniel, Willis, & Otis, 1970).

CENTRAL VOWELS

Two English vowels are formed with constriction in the central part of the oral tract. These are [ʌ] and [ɝ]. The vowel [ʌ] is similar to the neutral vowel [ə], but the tongue hump is often retracted slightly back so that this vowel has a larger portion of the oral tract in front of the constriction than behind it. F1 for [ʌ] is at about 600 Hz, slightly higher than the neutral position of Fl. F2 of [ɝ] is at about 1200 Hz; as with other back tongue constrictions, F2 is lower than the 1500 Hz neutral position.

The vowel [ɝ] is formed with the tongue flexed backward at the tip forming a midpalatal constriction; this is a "retroflex" constriction. The first formant of [ɝ] is in a rather neutral position at about 500 Hz; the second formant is at about 1300 Hz. In these respects [ɝ] is similar to a neutral vowel. However, when there is a midpalatal constriction, the frequency location of the third formant is strongly affected. The third formant is lowered by this constriction. For the vowel [ɝ], the third formant, for a man, is very low, at about 1600 Hz, compared with the F3 neutral position of 2500 Hz.

SUMMARY

Acoustic research on speech production has developed a physical model of the pharyngeal-oral tract. The model represents the basics of the production of natural vowel sounds. The physical model is a tube, the length and shape of which determines the resonant frequencies (the formant frequencies) of the tube.

Five simple shape rules can be used to give model frequencies of the first and second for-

Phonology Note:
Varieties of Central Vowels

British English in the so-called Received Pronunciation (RP English) employs a rather neutral [ə:] in place of the original -er syllable or any diphthong [Vɝ], which is still preserved in the General American English spoken in the midwestern United States and Martha's Vineyard, but not generally in the northeastern states, nor in New York City where it is usually retracted to [ʌ:] (Labov, 1972). Although English does not employ a completely neutral vowel phoneme with formant frequencies at about 500, 1500, and 2500 Hz, other languages use vowel phonemes that are close to neutral. A nearly neutral vowel [œ] can easily be pronounced by a French speaker, as in the word *peur*; the F1 frequency would be about 550 Hz with F2 at about 1400 Hz; in German [œ] in *Goethe* has F1 at about 500 Hz with F2 at 1550 Hz; French words, *deux* [dø], *peu* [pø], and *pneu* [pnø], meaning "two," "little," and "tire," employ another nearly neutral vowel with F1 at about 375 Hz and F2 at 1600 Hz (Delattre, 1965). In Swedish, a French-based word for "goodbye" is *adjö* [ajø]. However, these nearly neutral formant positions are not necessarily due to articulation with a nearly uniform, neutral vocal tract configuration, because they may be lip-rounded versions of front-tongue constrictions (Ladefoged, 1993). In any language, the schwa [ə] is frequently seen acoustically with neutral formant locations when a vowel is "reduced to schwa" because it is very short in duration and the tongue reaches only a neutral position instead of the target, phonemic position that would be used for a citation of how to pronounce the vowel in phonological distinction from other vowels.

mants for the front vowels and for the back vowels. Referring again to Figure 3-5, we see that it is easy, with the rules in mind, to reconstruct a set of model formant frequencies for F1 and F2, over the back vowel series and over the front vowel series, knowing only the rules and the starting points of the formants at the extreme ends of each series.

If a listener is in noise or has hearing impairment that prevents hearing the second formant, confusions among vowels demonstrate mishearing of the second formant with retained hearing of the first formant.

CHAPTER FOUR

THE GLOTTAL SOUND SOURCE AND THE SPECTRA OF VOWELS

In . . . vowels sounded on succession of different larynx notes . . . what the ear hears is the . . . resonant characteristics of the cavities through which that larynx note has passed . . . due to the relative volume and areas of orifices produced by the different attitudes of the tongue and lips.
—R. A. S. Paget, 1924

I said earlier that consonants are more important than vowels in the phonemic word-coding of speech. In the following two chapters we are going to see how vowels work. They gain great importance when, in addition to their phonemic partnership with consonants to encode words, we examine sentences and personal voices and expression. In this chapter we mostly explain the sound spectrum patterns for the phonemic differences among vowels, the "resonant characteristics" of Paget who anticipated the importance of formants. Still, we must begin at the beginning, with the basic voice source for vowels that also conveys much personal information and conversational meaning that we take up in the next chapter.

We have looked at vowel phonemes according to vocal tract shape and its effects on the formant locations. A complete description of a vowel sound also includes characteristics due to actions of the glottis. Now we are going to combine tract shape and glottal action. First, we see how the glottis produces the glottal sound source and influences the spectrum of that sound. Then the effects of the vocal tract resonances on the glottal spectrum are presented, using the source-filter theory of vowel production. We also study the effects on the vowel spectrum of low- and high-pitched

voice, of vocal effort, and of nasalization. We describe the standard method of depicting the spectrum during speech, via spectrograms skimmed from the tops of the changing speech soundscape. Using spectrograms, we illustrate spectrum patterns for all the English vowels and diphthongs.

THE GLOTTAL SOUND SOURCE

Vowel sounds begin in the larynx, where the primary sound is formed to serve as the basis for every voiced, periodic sound. This sounding occurs by means of a rapid, repeated opening and closing of the glottis, the chink between the vocal folds, in response to the tracheal air pressure. To see how this can occur we will look into the larynx and examine the form and movements of the glottis. If we took snapshots looking down into the larynx, we would often catch the glottis presenting two widely different profiles, a narrow slot for speaking or a wide gap for breathing (see Figure 4-1).

Rapid variation of the narrow glottis aperture to produce a pulsing sound source is called *phonation*. Phonation occurs because of the vibration of a pair of shelf-like ligaments that extend out

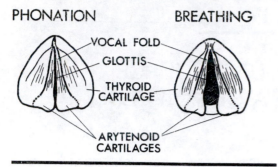

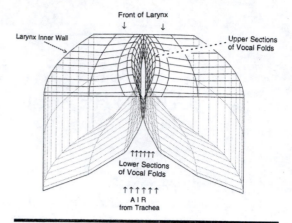

FIGURE 4-1. Diagrams of the larynx as seen from above, illustrating the positions of the arytenoid cartilages and vocal folds for breathing, on the left, and for phonation, on the right.

FIGURE 4-2. A three-dimensional diagram through the vocal folds and glottis, as used in a computer model. The view is from the arytenoids toward the front with the lower sections of the folds touching and the upper sections about to close while the lower sections will open to begin a cycle of phonation.

(Computer-generated figure from Ingo R. Titze, National Center for Voice and Speech, University of Iowa)

about 1/2 inch from the inner surfaces of the larynx into the airway. Their primitive functions are to help protect the breathing airway from intrusions, but vocalizing is so important to us that these two projections are called the *vocal folds*, not the "choking guards" or "coughing flaps."

The vocal folds are held in different postures by the arytenoid cartilages, to which the rear portions of the folds are attached. The anatomical name of the folds is thyro-arytenoid ligaments; they stretch across inside the larynx, front to back, between the thyroid cartilage ("Adam's apple") and the arytenoid cartilages. As shown in Figure 4-1, during breathing the arytenoid cartilages are held outward, keeping the glottis open at the back in a wide-open position. When phonation is about to begin, the arytenoids move inward to bring the vocal folds together; the configuration during this movement is diagrammed in three dimensions for a computer model in Figure 4-2. The top sections of the folds, open in the diagram, are then brought to touch each other and the bottom sections separate by a small space opening downward into the trachea.

THE PHONATION MECHANISM

Anatomical investigations combined with computer modeling of the aerodynamic behavior of

the vocal folds have recently elucidated many of the former mysteries of human voice production. As an introduction for students of speech production, phoneticians, and speech scientists, we will now describe some of this research. Audiologists and others who may only be concerned with the sound features related to phonation may wish to skip to the next section, "The Spectrum of the Glottal Sound Source."

The phonating behavior of the tiny organs of Figures 4-1 and 4-2 has been intensively studied to explain a wide range of voice phenomena in speaking, vocal performance, fatigue, and disorders. A very clear summary of larynx anatomy and control of the vocal folds is given by Lieberman and Blumstein (1988: 97-114). A thorough and lucid source of bioacoustic explanations of all phonation (voice) phenomena is a textbook by Titze (1994), where you will also find summaries of the vast literature on phonation. Here we are going to limit ourselves to an outline of the physical voice research on the major aspects of speech.

First, we will look at the work that led to explanations of the glottal sound source.

For phonation a cyclic interrupting action of the glottis on the air flowing through the larynx forms a train of air pulses, which is called the glottal sound source. The spectrum of this sound is the raw material of vowel sounds and so the spectrum of the glottal sound is reflected in every vowel spectrum. The particular form of the glottal sound spectrum is important in every vowel. The glottal sound spectrum depends on just how the air pulses are shaped by the vibrations of the vocal folds. For each glottal pulse, the exact form of the airflow through the glottis has an effect on the glottal sound spectrum, so we will first examine how the glottal airflow is made to pulsate and then the shapes of the pulses.

The spectrum of the glottal source has been studied by many scientists. However, only recently have we had powerful experimental techniques that promise to lead to a complete description of all the factors that affect the glottal spectrum. The purpose of the early researchers was to observe the time-course and forms of the fluctuations in glottal airflow, from which they could then calculate the glottal sound spectrum. It was (and still is) not possible to record the airflow at the glottis, but the flow variation could be calculated by observing the variation in amount of aperture of the glottis during glottal opening and closing for phonation.

The first modern observation technique, ultra-high-speed cinematography, was developed at Bell Laboratories (Farnsworth, 1940). The method was to take several thousand pictures per second through a small mirror angled to look downward toward the glottis. A series of such pictures made at the Speech Research Branch of the Air Force Cambridge Research Laboratories is shown in Figure 4-3.

The frames of these "glottal movies" show the sequence of glottal apertures between the vocal folds. To determine the waveform of glottal airflow the area is calculated for each of the apertures and the sequence of area values is converted to a sequence of amounts of glottal airflow,[1] which sequence constitutes the glottal flow wave. This method was used by W. W. Fletcher in 1950 at Northwestern University to determine glottal area waveforms in time and to study how these waveforms were related to voice intensity.

Flanagan (1958) used Fletcher's waveforms to derive the first detailed plots of the spectrum of glottal pulses. Flanagan and his colleagues at Bell Laboratories then proceeded to develop a computer model of the action of the vocal folds (Flanagan & Landgraf, 1968). Computer models produce directly their own waveforms of glottal pulses. This is because a computer model can simulate many of the anatomical and physical conditions, the interacting forces between the vocal folds and the slug of air within the glottis, and the resulting movements of the vocal folds. In the computer simulation, an input of constant subglottal pressure produces movements of simulated vocal folds and corresponding pulses of air escaping through the simulated glottis between the folds.

Many researchers have continued the tradition of creating models of airflow through the glottis. Mechanical models (Scherer & Titze, 1983) have been constructed to facilitate measurements of airflow. Various computer models have been developed to study the many factors in the vibratory activity (Ishizaka & Flanagan, 1972; Ishizaka & Matsudaira, 1968; Stevens, 1977; Titze, 1994; Titze & Talkin, 1979).

Microscopic studies of the structure of human vocal folds (Hirano & Sato, 1993) have provided

---

[1] The term airflow is called glottal volume velocity in acoustic research on speech. It is equal to the area of the glottal opening multiplied by the air particle velocity through the glottis. The air particle velocity, in a first approximation, is simply proportional to the difference in air pressure above and below the glottis. This transglottal pressure difference is approximately constant throughout a cycle of glottal action, although, of course, it is under the influence of external changes in pressure from the chest action or from any narrow constriction in the vocal tract above the glottis and may be slowly rising or falling due to these influences. Further discussions of the physics of glottal action are found in Ishizaka and Flanagan (1972) and Titze (1988, 1994).

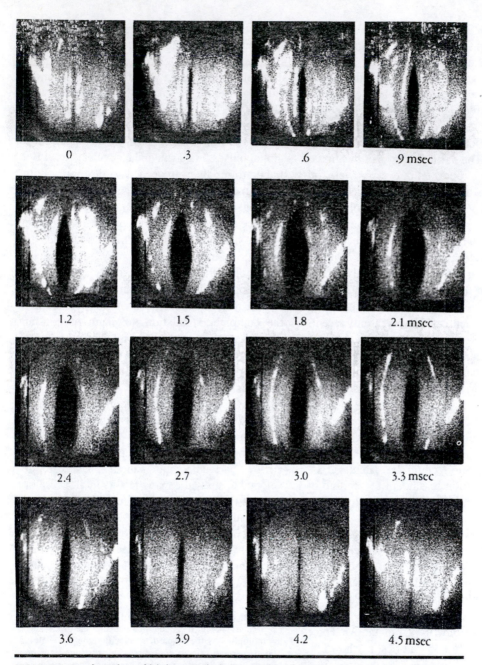

FIGURE 4-3.   A series of high speed photographs of one cycle of glottal action during phonation. The pictures were taken looking down on the glottis; the arytenoid cartilages are out of view at the bottom of each frame. The speaker was a high-pitched adult male phonating at a high fundamental frequency. The film was taken at a rate of 10,000 frames per second; only every third frame is shown.

(Photos courtesy of W. Wathen-Dunn, H. Soron, and P. Lieberman, taken at Air Force Cambridge Research Laboratories, Hanscom Air Force Base, Lexington, MA, 1962) essential information for the development of detailed theories of the dynamics of vibrating vocal folds. Each vocal fold consists symmetrically of a body of muscle and connective tissues within a cover of epithelial and mucosal tissues. One theory of the relationship between the body and cover of the vocal fold focuses on the importance of the wave of tissue deformation that travels over the surface (Hirano & Kakita, 1985). In our glottal movie frames of Figure 4-3, the wave-like movements across the cover are seen as a highlighted ridge, curving from top to bottom, which appears in the left vocal fold at frame 1.5 and moves away toward the side in subsequent frames until the ridge disappears after frame 3.3 ms. The corresponding wave in the right vocal fold is discernable but not so prominently displayed. These waves play a significant role in maintaining the movement of the two vocal folds toward and away from each other. Titze's (1994) computer model incorporated such tissue parameters, resulting in a simulation of the motions of the cover wave that is integral with the motions of the entire folds.

Other researchers have used observations of excised animal larynges to obtain more detailed information on vocal fold vibration than is practical with human larynges (Baer, 1975, 1981; Kakita, Hirano, & Ohmaru, 1981; Perlman & Durham, 1987; Titze & Durham, 1987). Baer's stroboscope observations first demonstrated the lead-lag relation of the motions of the lower and upper sections of the vocal folds. Some of these studies measured the physical properties of the laryngeal tissues, such as their elasticity and stiffness, which were then used in computer simulations of vocal fold vibration.

We will illustrate glottal pulsing using a recent research model devised by Titze, his colleagues, and their coworkers (Titze, 1994). This model and related ones in the literature are based on the previous medical and biological data about the composition of the vocal fold tissues. They have been used to explain a wide variety of voice characteristics, as well as many details of vowels and consonants. Figure 4-4 shows the model as envisioned

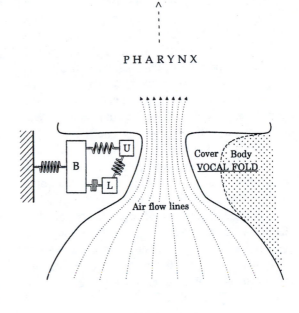

FIGURE 4-4. Model of the vocal folds seen in cross-section. This "coronal" section, like a crown, is oriented in a left-to-right crosswise plane through our downward view of the glottis in Figure 4-1. It is as if we are looking at a large X-ray through the neck, from back to front, to see the outline shape of the glottis. In the left vocal fold is a diagram of a computer model of the masses, U and L, of the upper and lower parts of the folds, connected by springs with each other and with the main mass, B, which is also mounted on a spring. The springs simulate the elasticity of all the tissues of the fold; in the actual model damping devices were connected in parallel to each spring but these are omitted for clarity of the diagram.
(Adapted from Titze, 1994)

within the vocal folds seen in a cross section through the larynx airway.

Vibration is maintained for phonation because different parts of the vocal folds move relative to each other. In a cycle of vocal fold vibration, the lower parts move apart before the upper parts, and the movement of the lower part causes the rest of the fold to move, just as one domino in a set up row moves first and the movement of that first one starts the next one moving and so on. A simple model of the vocal folds consisting of a pair of two-section pieces, one upper and the other lower, has been used by researchers to explain phonation. Each section is compliant and has mass; the upper and lower sections are modeled as held together vertically by a spring. The subglottal air pressure from the lungs pushes on the lower sections, forcing them apart. As the lower sections move farther apart they begin to pull each upper section along with the lower section it is attached to. Then the upper sections separate and the glottis becomes open. Air begins to flow through the opening, causing the pressure between the lower folds to decrease rapidly and so the lower sections begin to move inward. As they come close together, the Bernoulli effect[2] increases the speed of closure. The lower sections quickly return to their closed positions. The upper sections follow the movement of the lower ones and return to the position of touching each other. Then the cycle begins again with the lower sections being forced apart by the subglottal air pressure.

To summarize the forces in the cycle of glottal action, the subglottal pressure forces the vocal folds to open and then move outward; when the glottis is open and the pressure between the folds

drops, they reverse and then move inward; the momentum of inward movement and, finally, the increased suction of the Bernoulli effect causes the folds to close abruptly. The subglottal pressure and elastic restoring forces during closure cause the cycle to begin again.

As long as the subglottal pressure remains at a sufficiently high level and the arytenoid cartilages hold the vocal folds together, voicing phonation occurs and the glottis will continue to emit a rapid series of air pulses; one air pulse is emitted during each open-close cycle of glottal action.

A sequence of vocal-fold movements is shown via a series of coronal cross-sections in Figure 4-5, based on observations of Baer (1975, 1981); the dimensions here are expanded to emphasize the wave-like movement in the surfaces; this movement appears primarily as changing surface shapes along the top of each section, going from section 1 to section 5; the surface shape changes are due to deformation of the cover tissue of the vocal folds. For comparison, a simulated sequence of a vocal-fold cycle is given in Figure 4-6. Here we see a sequence of coronal sections plotted by computer via a biomechanical model of the vocal folds of Berry and Titze (1994). The computer vocal folds are similar to the natural vocal folds in their movements and shape changes in the upper surfaces during the opening of the glottis.

THE SPECTRUM OF THE GLOTTAL SOUND SOURCE

Now let us see how the airflow pulses resulting from the vocal-fold movements in the airstream are related to the glottal source spectrum. Figures 4-7 and 4-8 illustrate the origin of the source spectrum; Figure 4-7 shows a waveform of the glottal area for two cycles of vocal-fold vibration and the resulting waves of glottal airflow, and Figure 4-8 shows the spectrum of the glottal airflow waveform. The waves of Figure 4-7 were generated by a computer model of the vocal folds; the model incorporated typical conditions of the subglottal pressure, of the physical characteristics

---

[2] The Bernoulli pressure is a difference in pressure that must exist to maintain equal energy in a duct with varying cross-section. The total flow energy depends on the pressure and air particle velocity. The particle velocity at a constriction is higher than it is at the adjacent larger areas; therefore, because the total flow energy must remain constant, the pressure in the constricted area is lower than the pressure in the adjacent areas. A Bernoulli force exists wherever there is a difference in fluid pressure between opposite sides of an object. Two other examples of a Bernoulli force in a constricted area of flow are: (1) blowing between parallel sheets of paper held close together (they pull together instead of flying apart because the air velocity is greater and the pressure is lower between the sheets than on the outer sides) and (2) the attraction of a hose nozzle toward the bottom of a pail because of the increased velocity of the water when the nozzle is near the bottom (if the nozzle outlet is too close to the bottom, the Bernoulli suction is strong enough to completely shut off the water flow in spite of the water pressure outward through the nozzle).

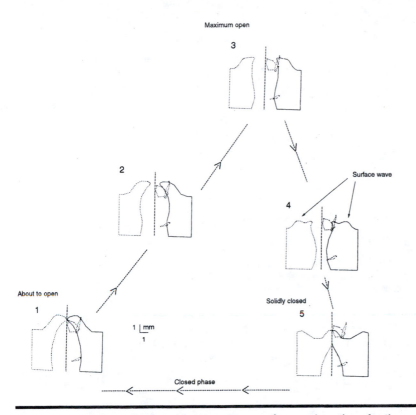

FIGURE 4-5. Schematic diagrams in sequence of coronal sections for the open phase of vocal-fold vibration, from a study of excised animal larynges by Baer (1975; 1981). The shapes were sketched by Baer to represent the changes in shape of the glottal surfaces that he observed and measured via stroboscopic illumination. The left vocal fold is drawn with a dotted line (the right fold is diagrammed symmetrically by a solid line with small dotted, angular ellipses indicating the cycle movement of three particles attached to the vocal fold). We will not discuss these local movements but focus on the shape changes in the left vocal fold. The sequence of actions affecting the width and shape of the glottis between the folds is as follows. At 1 the glottis is closed with folds just touching, having been pushed upward by the lower sections, which are spreading under the force of the subglottal pressure. The glottis above is just about to open; the upward thrust has raised the edges of the folds and these deformations from flat will now proceed outward as a wave over the upper surfaces. At 2 the upper parts have separated; at 3 they are fully opening the glottis; at 4 the lower sections are beginning to return toward the midline and the bulge of the deformation wave has moved about half the way to the side; at 5 the folds have come solidly back together, and the thrust from the lower sections has started to push up the edges of the folds, in the closed phase of the total cycle. Note that the features of the wave-like changes in shape are very small, a maximum of 2 mm for the highest point of the wave, at 1 (scale to the right of the shape). Also the maximum glottal opening at 3 is only about 2 mm. During the closure some time is required for the subglottal pressure to force the lower sections upward and begin the cycle again at 1. I have arranged the drawings to indicate a more rapid closing leg, 3–5, of the open phase.

(Drawings courtesy of Baer, 1981, adapted and interpreted by author JMP)

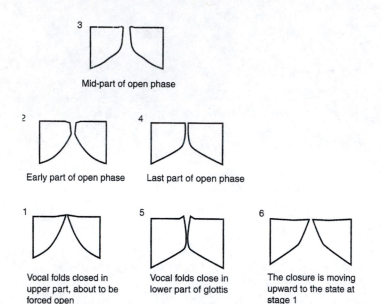

FIGURE 4-6.   Vocal-fold sequence of coronal sections for the open phase of a cycle of glottal vibration, generated via computer modeling. This sequence is similar to that in Figure 4-5 of the natural vocal folds studied by Baer, except that the computer scaling for the plot was much smaller.

(Adaptation of original diagrams from I. R. Titze, National Center for Voice and Speech, University of Iowa)

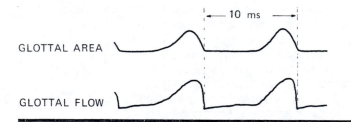

FIGURE 4-7.   The upper curve shows an example of how the area of the glottal opening varies in time in phonation and the lower curve shows the corresponding variation of the airflow through the glottis. The alignment of the sharp corners at the dotted lines shows the simultaneity of the onset of glottal closure in the area curve and the abrupt cessation of positive glottal flow. This abrupt change in flow is the change that excites oscillations in the air pressure in the upper vocal tract; this repeated cessation of flow, as the glottis opens and closes, is the basic source of voiced speech. It may also be observed that the indicated peak of glottal flow lags the peak in the glottal area. These curves were generated by a computer model of the vocal folds activated by subglottal air pressure from below. The model was adjusted with typical values of pressure and muscle tension to produce a smoothly sloping spectrum for the glottal flow wave and a fundamental frequency of 100 Hz; the period of one cycle is 10 ms.

(Model and curves developed at the Center for Auditory and Speech Sciences, Gallaudet University, by I. Titze and D. Talkin, 1978)

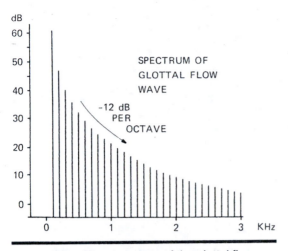

FIGURE 4-8. The spectrum of the glottal flow wave of Figure 4-7. This is an idealized spectrum, which serves well as a model of the source spectrum for the vowel sounds.

of the folds, and of the muscle tensions on the folds. This particular model of vocal-fold action was developed by Titze and Talkin (1979), who kindly furnished the curves of Figure 4-7. The pressure and tension conditions were chosen to produce an idealized glottal source spectrum having a slope with the same general pattern as found at Bell Laboratories and by other investigators in previous studies of the actual glottal spectrum.[3]

Two characteristics of the glottal spectrum are especially important: (1) the frequency spacing of the spectral components, that is, the fundamental and the harmonics, and (2) the amplitude pattern of the components over frequency. The frequency spacing depends on the repetition rate of the pulses in the glottal wave. The amplitude pattern of the spectral components depends on the exact shape of the pulses.

The spacing of the components of the glottal wave of Figure 4-8 is 100 Hz between components. This spacing corresponds to the repetition rate of the glottal pulses and to the fundamental frequency of the glottal wave. In other words, the glottal pulses repeat at a rate of 100 pulses per second, the corresponding fundamental frequency of the wave of glottal pulses is 100 Hz, and the harmonics in the spectrum of this wave are spaced 100 Hz apart. The fundamental frequency of the spectrum shown in Figure 4-8 is typical for a low-pitched adult male voice, that is, a fundamental frequency of 100 Hz.

Most of the time during phonation the vocal tract configuration does not influence the pattern of vocal-fold movement significantly. However, the vocal tract does influence vocal-fold movement whenever there are very close constrictions in the tract. Examples are points near the closures of obstruent consonants and during the most constricted portions of glide consonants. Close constrictions cause the waveform of the glottal airflow to be skewed by an increase in the duration of the glottal pulse relative to the glottal period. The amount of skew is small (see the dashed extensions of the pulses in the upper part of Figure 4-9); nevertheless, the effect on the glottal source spectrum can be considerable, shifting the spectral balance more toward the low frequencies (lower part of Figure 4-9).

This effect is seen during liquids, glides, and voiced fricatives, in very close vowels, and wherever there is very close constriction immediately adjacent to an obstruent consonant. The skewing is due to additional loading imposed by the mass of the air within the constriction, which in effect opposes the fold-closing Bernoulli force and thus delays closure. In the spectrum of skewed glottal pulses the low-frequency amplitude is increased

[3] The veracity of the glottal pulses produced by computer models has been checked by other methods. One of the best methods is to analyze actual speech waves by filtering to remove the effects of the resonances of the pharyngeal-oral tract and leave as an output from the filters the original glottal pulses. This method is called inverse filtering; the resonant frequencies and bandwidths of the main formants of a steady portion of a vowel sound are determined, then inverse filters are set at the same frequencies and bandwidths, and finally the vowel sound is passed through this inverse filter set. The output wave from the filters has the same waveshape as the pulses of glottal airflow. For examples of the resulting waves of glottal airflow see Rothenberg (1973). Inverse filtering has been used extensively to study the differences between male and female voices (Holmberg, Hillman, & Perkell, 1988, 1989; Karlsson, 1985).

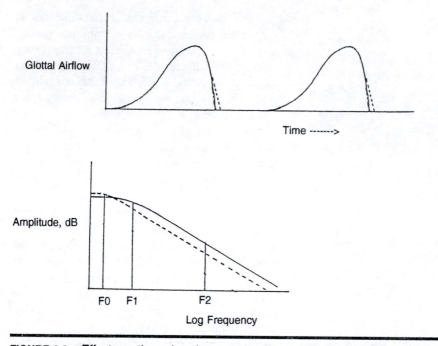

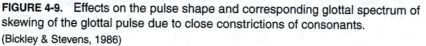

FIGURE 4-9.   Effects on the pulse shape and corresponding glottal spectrum of skewing of the glottal pulse due to close constrictions of consonants. (Bickley & Stevens, 1986)

relative to the case of the unconstricted vocal tract (Bickley & Stevens, 1986; Rothenberg, 1981).

The amplitudes of the components in the glottal spectrum have a pattern that generally decreases from low-frequency harmonics to higher ones; that is, the spectrum slopes generally downward. The intensity slopes downward at an average of 12 dB per octave change (doubling) in frequency. The spectrum of the glottal flow wave in Figures 4-8 and 4-9 therefore has a slope of −12dB/octave.

For actual glottal waves there are variations in the component amplitudes of the glottal spectrum that are related to the degree of rounding of the corners of the glottal airflow waveform, to the duration of the closure, and to other details of the glottal waveform. These relate physiologically to the style and force of speaking and to individual characteristics of vocal-fold behavior. However, an

idealized glottal spectrum with a smooth slope of −12 dB/octave is a good, standard basis for describing the spectra of voiced sounds.

Klatt and Klatt (1990) describe detailed measurements of the spectra of the voices of sixteen female speakers. They found female glottal spectra are primarily characterized in terms of the relative amplitude of the fundamental component, the amount of noise in the region of the third formant, and evidence of coupling to the trachea.

Important varieties of voice production, aside from the male and female norms resulting from clearly distinct air-pulses through the vocal folds, have been found to be related to the ways in which the arytenoid cartilages are positioned together at their tip attachments, by rotational tensions or held laterally by adducting muscles. Arytenoid positioning controls the firmness and degree of closure of a subsidiary glottis-like slit between the cartilages. Overly firm rotation and strong adduction of the cartilages results in "pressed voice"; lax adduction results in "breathy voice" where there is a steady leakage of airflow through the chink of this mini-glottis, in addition to the airflow pulses being produced by vocal-fold vibration. Voice qualities of pressed or breathy are described in terms of differences among component amplitudes in the glottal spectrum. The spectrum of a *pressed voice* has relatively high amplitude of high-frequency harmonics; a *breathy voice* has relatively low amplitude in the higher harmonics and often a relatively stronger fundamental component (Titze, 1995).

The pitch or fundamental frequency of the glottal pulsing depends primarily on the tension on the vocal folds, on the mass distribution within the vocal folds, and on the subglottal pressure. The mass overall depends on the size of the vocal folds, which in turn depends on age, sex, and the individual. For example, the vocal folds are progressively larger as we go from children to women to adult males. This corresponds to a change in voice pitch or fundamental pulse rate going from higher to lower pulsing rates as we go from the smaller vocal folds to the larger ones. High tension on the vocal folds causes high voice pitch and low tension produces low pitch. The tension control by speakers will be explained in a later chapter.

The fundamental frequency also depends on the air pressure in the oral cavity: If the difference between the subglottal and oral pressure (transglottal pressure) is less than about 3 cm H_2O then there is no vocal-fold vibration (Finkelhor, Titze & Durham, 1988, Verdolini-Marston, Titze, & Druker, 1990)

SOURCE-FILTER THEORY OF VOWEL PRODUCTION

In the formation of vowel sounds the action of the glottis produces the basic source of sound, as we have seen above; this sound is then propagated, or transmitted, to the outside air through the vocal tract. We can think of the tract as a filter or horn that amplifies some of the components of the source sound, namely those at and near the resonant frequencies of the tract. In fact, if the glottal source sound alone were propagated into open air without any resonating horn, it would sound like a rather weak hum or buzz—like the reed in a New Year's noisemaker or a tenor sax, which is not stentorian without its horn to speak through. Therefore, we explain the formation of vowels as the result of a filtering, amplifying action of the pharyngeal-oral tract on the sound source produced by the glottis. This view of vowel production is called the source-filter theory of vowel production and was first developed by Fant (1960). Fant's theory was based on the production of model vowel sounds derived from vocal tract shapes, as already described in Chapter Three. The source-filter theory helps us explain how the details of vowel spectra arise from the combination of: (1) the spectrum of the glottal sound source and (2) the filtering of this spectrum by its transmission through the vocal tract.

Recall from our discussion of vowel shaping in Chapter Three that the vowel resonant peaks depend for their frequency locations on the positions of the tongue and lips. Thus, in order to describe how the spectrum of a vowel is formed, all we need to do is describe the effect on the glottal spectrum of the resonant peaks of the vocal tract. The resonant peaks determine the filtering curve or transmission response of the tract. When we apply this filter curve to the spectrum of the glottal sound source, the resulting spectrum is the vowel sound spectrum.

In other words, it is as if the glottal sound spectrum were passed through a certain filter that determines what the vowel will be. This is illustrated in Figure 4-10, where diagrams show how the spectrum of the glottal sound source is modified according to filter curves of the oralpharyngeal tract to form the different vowel sound spectra for several vowels. The fundamental frequency is 100 Hz and thus the harmonics are at all

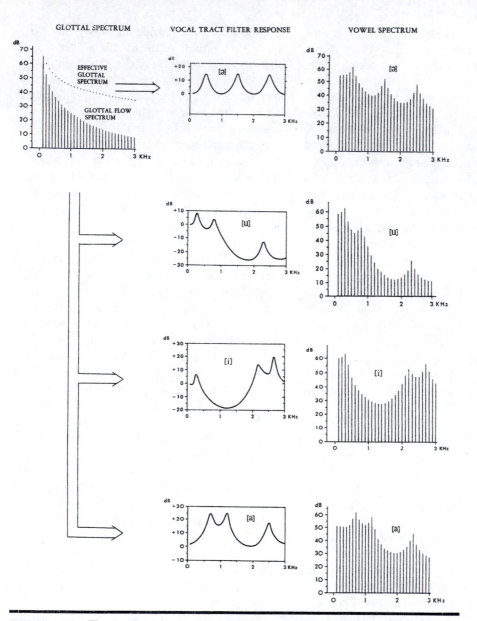

FIGURE 4-10. The production of model vowels according to the source-filter theory. An idealized spectrum that slopes −12 dB/octave is assumed as the spectrum of the basic waveform of glottal airflow. However, radiation of the vowel sound from the mouth is more efficient for high than for low frequencies, on a slope of about +6 dB/octave. This constant factor is added to the glottal flow spectrum to give an effective glottal source spectrum, the dashed curve, which slopes −6dB/octave for all the vowels. The effective source spectrum is modified by the filter responses of the vocal tract, shown for the different vowels, to produce the final vowel spectra on the right. The filter shapes were calculated from combinations of ideal resonators. (Adapted from Fant, 1960; Stevens & House, 1961)

the multiples of 100 Hz. (The effective glottal spectrum, shown as a dashed curve, has a slope of –6 dB/octave instead of the –12 dB/octave of the average glottal spectrum; the slope of the effective glottal spectrum is the sum of the –12 dB/octave glottal source spectrum and a +6 dB/octave constant factor due to the radiation characteristics of the mouth-opening in the human head; the effective source spectrum has a slope of –6 dB/octave).

The important things to note in Figure 4-10 are that the spectrum of the glottal sound source is the same for all the different vowels and this sound spectrum is then changed by the filtering of the vocal tract to produce vowel sounds that have different spectral patterns. Let us see how the different spectrum shapes are produced for different vowels.

First, examine the relations between the formant peaks in the spectrum and the overall slope of the spectrum from low to high frequencies. In the filter response for the neutral [ə] vowel (top row center graph), the slope of amplification is flat across frequencies, except for the scallops due to the amplification by the formant resonances at 500, 1500, and 2500 Hz. Each resonance has an increasing amplifying effect on frequencies going up to the resonance frequency, which then decreases above the resonance. Then an attenuation effect takes over as the frequencies go higher. However, the higher-frequency attenuation is counterbalanced by the amplification of the next higher resonance frequency because the amount of amplification at the higher resonance is a factor of the resonance frequency itself. For the neutral uniform tube shape of the model vocal tract, this higher amplification factor is exactly balanced by the amount of attenuation by distance in frequency from the lower resonance and so the net amplitude of amplification at the higher resonance is the same as at the lower one. This produces the flat-but-scalloped spectrum shape for the neutral tract filter response. When this response curve is applied to the glottal source spectrum, the result is the downward-sloping scalloped spectrum of the model neutral vowel in the top row, right-hand column.

The general slope of the spectra of the other vowels, the non-neutral ones, stems both from the spectrum of the glottal sound source and from the degree of proximity of the formant frequencies and the interactions between their amplification and attenuation responses. The slope is affected by any formants that are very close to each other. In the filter response for the vowel [u], for example (second row center), the first and second formants are close in frequency and at a low location; the two close resonances reinforce each other and thus raise the low-frequency part of the spectrum to a higher amplitude than for the neutral vowel and very high in relation to the third formant of [u].

The second important factor in the effects of the formant resonances on the spectrum of a vowel is the fact that certain frequency components are attenuated to make up for the amplification of components near the resonance frequency. This brings the total energy in the vowel in line with the energy output from the glottis. The attenuated components in a formant response are those that are higher in frequency by a certain amount, than the resonance resonance frequency. Attenuation starts above a frequency that is two times the resonance frequency and then attenuates by about 12 dB for each doubling of frequency above that. Notice in the vowel spectrum for [u] that this attenuation has greatly reduced the amplitude of the third formant (it is at a frequency of about 3 octaves above the F1 resonance frequency).

In the case of the vowel [i], the second formant is close to the third formant, and thus they reinforce each other and raise the high-frequency end of the vowel spectrum relative to the middle. However, both F2 and F3 are now very far away from F1, which is in a low position for the vowel [i]. Because of the distance between them, the reinforcing effect of the first formant on the second and third formants is much less. Actually, the second and third formants are riding low down in amplitude on the attenuation tail of the first formant. The net result on the spectrum of [i] is that the amplitude level of the spectrum in the region of F3 is still low compared with the amplitude level in the low frequencies, but it is much higher than for [u] and substantially higher than for [ə] and [a]. Thus, we see that the particular locations of formant peaks, which are determined by the shape of the vocal tract, will affect not only the location in frequency of the vowel spectrum peaks but also the amplitudes of the peaks in relation to each other and the relative strengths of F3 and higher formants. The amplitudes of components in the F1 region are greater than the amplitudes of components lower in frequency.

In addition to the effect of the tract shape on the vowel spectrum envelope, the conditions of glottal action have their effects on the resulting vowel spectrum. There are two main glottal factors: One is the fundamental pulsing rate at the voice pitch frequency, and the other is the amount of vocal effort. The factor of voice pitch affects only the frequency positions of the individual harmonic components in the spectrum and does not affect the shape of the spectrum.

The effects on the spectrum of changes in voice pitch frequency are illustrated in Figure 4-11. On the left side of Figure 4-11 is the spectrum for a voice pitch that is lower than the fundamental frequency of 100 Hz that was assumed for the vowels of Figure 4-10. The low pitch causes the spectrum components to be spaced more closely together, compared with the vowel on the right side of the figure, which has a fundamental frequency of 100 Hz. The low-pitched spectrum on the left is for a fundamental voice frequency of 50 pulses per second. Thus, the spectrum components in the vowel are at 50 Hz intervals. A voice pitch as low as 50 Hz occurs for extremely low-pitched voices as sometimes heard in male radio announcers. At the bottom of Figure 4-11 is the spectrum for a high-pitched voice where the voice fundamental frequency is 200 pulses per second. For this vowel the spectral components occur at intervals of 200 Hz and the density of components is thus more sparse.

It should be especially noted in Figure 4-11 that the general shape of the spectrum, which is determined by the positions of the formants and their relations to each other, is not changed by changes in the voice pitch. Only the spacing of

the component frequencies, that is, the spacing of the harmonics corresponding to the fundamental pulse rate, is changed by changes in voice pitch. How these components are shaped to form the general envelope of the spectrum depends only on the vocal tract shape and not at all on the frequency of the voice pulsing rate.

The fundamental frequency, in speech analysis, is often called "F zero" or F0; in this case, F does not refer to a formant. To differentiate F0 from the formants, some analysts call it f0.

The glottal wave assumed for Figures 4-8 and 4-9 had a smooth spectrum envelope with slope of −12 dB/octave. The spectra of real glottal pulses do not have such a smooth spectrum slope, but the 12 dB slope is a good representation for average speech spoken for specimen or citation purposes. In more relaxed phonation the glottal pulses are more rounded on the corners, causing the glottal spectrum to slope downward more steeply. A typical spectrum slope for this type of phonation is −15 dB/octave; this value would correspond to a relaxed conversational level of vocal effort. If the style of speaking is very forceful, the glottal pulses can have very steep sides and sharper corners, because of higher subglottal pressure on the opening of the vocal folds and higher Bernoulli suction before the closing. With such high effort, the glottal spectrum slope will be more shallow than −12dB/octave, say about −9dB/ octave (see Fant, 1959; Flanagan, 1958; Martony, 1965; Rothenberg, 1973).

Figure 4-12 shows the effect of a change in vocal effort on the vowel spectrum of a model [a] vowel. For the purposes of the figure we assume that there is no change in the voice pitch and no change in the shape of the vocal tract. The left-hand spectrum is for the vowel spoken softly on a pitch of 100 Hz, that is, the glottal pulsing rate is 100 per second and vocal effort is low; the right-hand spectrum is for the same [a] vowel at the same pulse rate but with a high amount of effort and producing a higher amplitude of sound. For low vocal effort the spectrum is steeper in slope and the level is low in amplitude. On the right side of Figure 4-12 we see an effect of high vocal

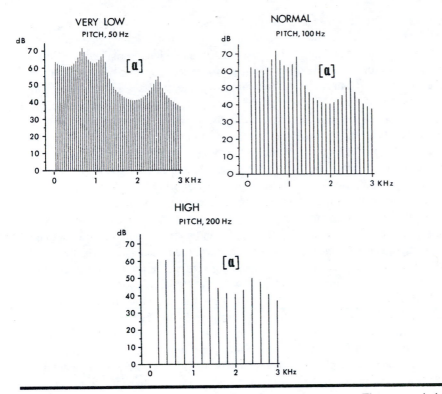

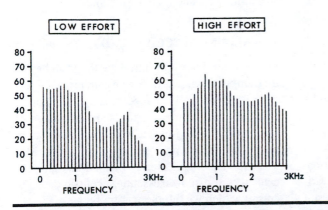

FIGURE 4-11. Effects of voice pitch on a model vowel spectrum. The general shape of the spectrum (spectrum envelope) is constant, but the harmonic spacing changes with fundamental frequency (pitch).

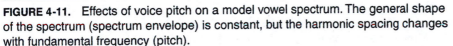

FIGURE 4-12. Effects of vocal effort on the vowel spectrum. Note that the overall slope of the vowel spectrum is steep for low effort and more gradual for high effort. The second and higher formants are relatively more intense under high vocal effort. See text for further explanation.

effort on the vowel spectrum. In constructing these model [a] spectra, the oral tract response was the same as that for [a] in Figure 4-10; the slope of the source spectrum was –15 dB/octave for low effort and –9 dB/octave for high effort. The fundamental voice pitch frequency was kept the same at 100 Hz. The vocal tract shape has remained the same, as for an [a] vowel, and so the spectrum peaks occur at the same locations. However, for higher effort the voice is louder and the spectrum slope has changed considerably; the spectrum slope is more shallow with higher amplitudes at the high frequencies, and the amplitudes of the formant peaks of the spectrum are higher than for normal effort, but the fundamental component is lower in amplitude. In other words, the increased voice loudness with high effort is due to increases in the amplitudes of the resonant oscillations.

In addition to the effects of glottal pulse shape on the overall slope of the glottal spectrum, the individual spectrum components are affected in amplitude by the general time features of the glottal wave. Each cycle has a pulse corresponding to the open portion of the glottal cycle and a flat portion corresponding to the closed portion of the glottal cycle. The ratio of the open portion to the closed portion and the degree of symmetry of the opening and closing legs of the pulses cause variations in component amplitudes above and below the average slope of the spectrum. These variations give a scalloped effect to the source spectrum envelope by lowering the amplitude of about every fourth or fifth harmonic. In addition, there is often a narrow depression in the source spectrum, somewhere in the region between 600 and 1000 Hz, which is due to absorption of sound by the subglottal spaces.

Research on glottal function is currently concerned with relating these aspects of the glottal waveform to various conditions of phonation. Systematic rules about the glottal spectra for various styles and types of phonation should result from this research, but at present we do not have these rules.

Individual anatomic structure of the vocal folds and voice training can also affect the spectrum of the glottal pulses. However, at present we do not have enough systematic knowledge to explain how these individual characteristics arise. In general, a highly efficient, "strong" speaking voice is attributable to a steep offset of the glottal pulse just before the closed portion of the pulse cycle and not to the vocal tract resonances per se; the resonances are more strongly excited by a more efficient shape of glottal pulse, that is, pulses with steeper offsets (Fant & Lin, 1991). Professional singers probably employ both steep glottal pulses and formant resonance adjustments. Tenor singers were found to adjust the frequencies of the upper formants, F2 and above, in singing vowels, to produce more amplitude than is seen in their ordinary speaking versions of the same vowels (Titze, Mapes, & Story, 1994). Singers may adjust their pharynx to raise the amplitude of the vowel spectrum in the region F3 to F5 (Sundberg, 1973). This type of increase in voice loudness and penetrating quality (the clarion tenor, for example) is probably accomplished mainly via mutual resonant reinforcements among the higher formants, in a manner similar to the mutual amplification between F1 and F2 ordinarily seen in the spoken vowel [ɑ]. So the strong voices of singers may result from the combined effects of a steep glottal pulse that increases amplitude and a manipulation of formant frequencies to further increase the mutual spectrum of F2 and higher formants.

VISUALIZING SPEECH SOUNDS

In this section we will introduce the sound spectrogram, our major tool for visualizing and measuring the spectrum of speech. A spectrogram of a spoken word, for example, shows a pattern of spectrum changes for that word that can be compared with the changes seen in other words. This is the fundamental, primary method that phoneticians use to discover essential acoustic constituents by which we tell the words apart.

The movements of speech cause shifts in the shape of the oral tract and in the source of sound, so we would expect the spectral patterns of speech to change over time. In fact, the rapid articulation of speech causes rapid changes in the shape of the vocal tract, so we would expect the spectrum patterns of speech also to fluctuate. Consider, for example, that the lips and tongue move rapidly between the consonant constrictions and the more open vocal tract shapes for the vowels. This causes the formants of the vowels to move rapidly from one frequency location to another. We need to look at the formant changes caused by these articulations; we also want to measure the formant frequencies at the more steady points, for example, to characterize the vowels. In addition, when the vocal tract becomes very constricted, forming turbulent aperiodic sounds, there are, of course, corresponding changes in the sound pattern. In fact, it happens fairly often that the sound suddenly shifts from vowel-like pulsing periodicity to aperiodic turbulence to form a fricative consonant. An example is at the end of the word "yes" where there is a sudden shift from the pulsing or buzzing sound of the vowel [ɛ] to the hissing of the [s]. Rapid changes occur also in the amplitude of sound during different phases in the formation of the vowels and consonants, depending on the amount and type of constriction in the vocal tract. We shall also see later how the expressive and rhythmical aspects of speech are embodied in changing patterns of the frequencies and amplitudes of speech.

Thus, many of the most important characteristics of speech can be seen in the spectrum patterns as they change in time. The process of sound spectrography operates on speech waves, or any other waves for that matter, to analyze their spectra and make a picture of the spectral changes showing the patterns in time, frequency, and intensity. We often need a permanent record so we can measure and study these patterns. Also we need to examine all the components of speech at once. We do this via sound spectrograms.

Spectrography analyzes the spectrum by measuring successive segments or portions of sound waves to find the amplitude of sound for each frequency component of every segment. This array of amplitudes and frequencies, plotted in the time-sequence of the segments, is a spectrogram.

The spectrum analysis to obtain the data is done by filters. A filter is a system that can be tuned as an analyzer to isolate one or more frequency components of a complex wave. The wave segment to be analyzed is fed through the filter and the amplitude of the electrical output of the filter represents the amplitude of the component of the wave that is isolated by the filter. Both analog and digital methods of filtering were used in making the spectrograms in this book; the spectral data and spectrograms reproduced here from the original edition were made using the analog Kay Elemetrics Sona-Graph™. The new 3-D "perspectrograms" and horizontal spectrum plots were made on a personal computer with programs provided by the Sensimetrics Corporation in their SpeechStation. For a listing of other programs available see Appendix A.

Figure 4-13 illustrates how a spectrogram is derived from the total landscape of a syllable "bub" taken from the phrase "buh, buh, buh" of Figure 1-3 (it is the middle syllable there). Here the complete landscape of "bub" is on the left; then in the middle, by raising the plane of the landscape, the formants, F1, F2, and F3 are made easier to identify and track across the syllable because some of the features irrelevant to the formants are too weak to appear above the raised plane. On the right, the plot has been reduced to two dimensions by darkening in proportion to sound amplitude and not plotting anything below the high plane. The frequency axis is calibrated so that one can measure the formant frequencies against a scale. This is the standard spectrogram.

Examine the spectrogram derived in Figure 4-13. The vertical frequency scale is in kilohertz (kHz) or thousands of Hertz. The dark bars in the vowel, below a frequency of about 3 kHz, are due to the peaks in the spectrum caused by the three lowest formants (resonances of the vocal tract). These formants change in frequency as the speech is articulated. Above these formants we can see another dark bar at about 3.5 kHz; this is due to the fourth formant. Its frequency does not change greatly with articulation, as do the frequencies of the three lower formants.

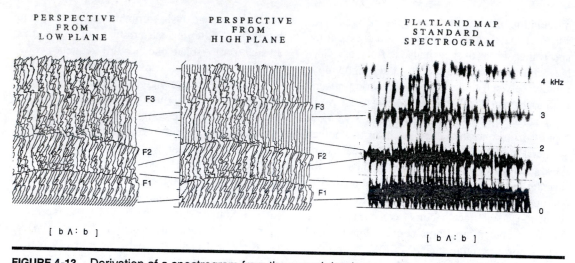

FIGURE 4-13.   Derivation of a spectrogram from the speech landscape of the word "bub."
(Spectrograms plotted via SpeechStation2 from Sensimetrics Corporation)

The formant locations stand out boldly in the spectrogram because the computer analysis process is especially designed for this. The filter for this type of display in the spectrogram is intentionally made sufficiently wide in its frequency coverage so that the individual spectrum components of these sounds do not appear individually in the spectrogram. Only when the total sum of the energy of several components within the filter reaches a rather high level is the paper marked to indicate the presence of a high amount of energy. This allows the instrument to skim effectively over the top of the spectrum and pick off the areas of high amplitude, namely, those places where the formant peaks occur in the spectrum. The result is a very effective display of some of the most important spectrum changes. Especially prominent are the formant frequency changes, as they occur in time. The occurrence of aperiodic sounds, such as fricative consonants, also stand out. All these patterns are explained more in later chapters.

ANATOMY OF A SPECTROGRAM

Spectrograms are the most popular with speech researchers of any of the various ways to portray speech events. Most of the computer programs for looking at speech can plot the amplitude of the speech wave, in time synchrony with the spectrogram. An example of this type of plot is given in Figure 4-14. Here the amplitude wave is given equal space with the spectrogram because the designer of the display (Edwav shareware by Timothy Bunnell at Gallaudet University and now at the A. I. Dupont Institute) wanted to have a method by which to manipulate segments of the speech wave based on joint changes in the wave and in the spectrum pattern. For example, by looking for the time-points in the spectrogram where the pattern changes from vowel formants to a stretch of high-frequency friction and then back again to vowel formants, one could mark out a fricative sound precisely on the wave itself. This friction wave segment could then be removed, saved, and used alone as a test sound in a speech listening experiment. Or such a marked-out segment could be replaced in the speech wave with some other sound segment for a perception test of the importance of the interchanged segments. As we shall see in Part Two of our study, many experiments like this have told us a great deal about how acoustic speech communication works.

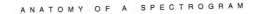

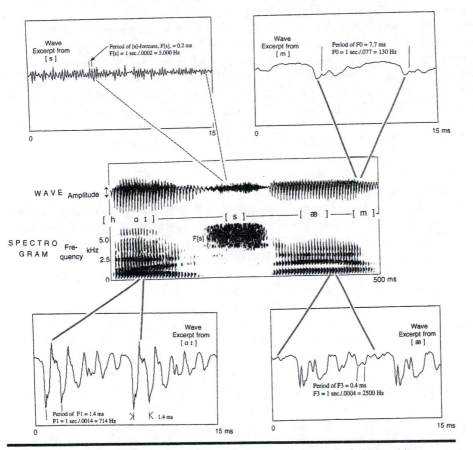

FIGURE 4-14. The wave anatomy that underlies a spectrogram. Relationships between wave segments of the [ɑɪ], [s], and [m] of "Hi Sam" and the corresponding spectrogram. Note that the F1 period (from which to calculate F1 frequency) is measurable from the waveform and even the higher formant oscillations can be seen and estimated in frequency by measuring their periods of oscillation.

Some Wave Features That Underlie Spectrogram Features

Let us take a closer look at relations between wave and spectrogram so we can know the acoustic basis of a spectrogram. I have designed Figure 4-14 to examine some features of speech waves that correspond to formants and friction sounds in the spectrogram. We have plotted together, using Edwav, the wave of sound amplitude and the spectrogram of "Hi Sam" spoken by the Father for the speech landscapes of Figure 1-1. Then, from Father's amplitude wave I selected and expanded four short sections, each about 15 ms in duration: one from the [ɑɪ] in "Hi," then another from the [s]-friction, a third one from the [æ] of "Sam," and a fourth at the end of the utterance, a bit of the [m]-wave. These wave sections are plotted in four panels and labeled so you can identify the wave oscillation patterns for the vowel formants and one of the formant frequencies in the friction of the [s].

I selected some of the wave features that are related to important spectral features, measured their wave characteristics, and then calculated the corresponding spectrum features and values. The selected wave segments and where they occur in the wave or spectrogram are indicated by the slanted lines of expansion leading into each panel. The total extent of each panel is 15 ms. Each expansion of the voiced sounds covers one pitch period of about 8 ms indicated by the slanted lines. Within the unvoiced [s]-segment (upper left panel) I marked a period of one predominant wave-oscillation, that is apparently due to the main formant resonance of the [s]-sound; excitation of this resonance appears to be random in time and amplitude. The marked period was 0.2 ms, which calculates to a frequency F[s] of 5000 Hz, as you will see recorded in the panel.

Going clockwise around the panels, similar marks and calculations were made for the [m]-, the [æ]-, and the [ɑɪ]-sounds. In the [m] I marked and measured one period of the fundamental frequency, F0, which is the predominant wave (greatest amplitude of fluctuation).

It is very important for the remainder of our course of study to have a thorough understanding of spectrograms. At this point the student can accomplish this easily by interactive experience, doing the wave excerpting and expansion procedures of our Figure 4-14 on various utterances, using one of the PC speech-processing programs, such as SpeechStation, Edwav, CSRE, WavEd, CSpeech, or the like (see Appendix A).

Spectrum Plots Related to Spectrograms

In addition to being able to see the frequency positions and course of the formants in time, as in the spectrogram, we also want to be able to examine the individual components of the spectrum at points of interest. For this purpose sound analyzing programs allow us to pick out selected time points on the spectrogram and make a plot of the detailed spectrum at each of these points. Each of these plots is called a spectral section or simply a spectrum.

In Figure 4-15 we see the sounds of "Hi Sam" in another utterance and spectrogram like the soundscape of Figure 1-1, and we have supplemented the two-dimensional picture with four spectrum plots by SpeechStation to show the exact amplitudes of the frequency components of the sounds [ɑ] and [ɪ] of the [ɑɪ]-vowel of "Hi," and the [s] and [m] of "Sam." The section for [ɑ] has its frequency axis oriented in the same upward direction as in the spectrogram and the formant effects are labeled and keyed between the two plots. In the other spectrum sections the plots are rotated clockwise toward the orientation used on computer screens, where frequency is usually plotted horizontally and amplitude vertically.

You will note that the two vowel spectrum sections show a general downward slope of amplitudes with increasing frequency of components, as expected on the basis of the downward spectrum slopes we have seen in the glottal sound source and the resulting vowels of Figure 4-10. In order to make the middle and higher sound components appear in spectrograms, a "pre-emphasis" or so-called "spectral flattening" is applied by the computer before the analysis. Usually speech researchers retain the pre-emphasis when plotting spectrum sections. However, persons concerned with the actual amplitude levels within the sound spectrum, such as audiologists and communication engineers dealing with noise interference, will plot unflattened spectra via the pre-emphasis switch in the computer program, as we have done here using SpeechStation.

In Figure 4-15 there are several spectral sections taken at time points in the utterance "Hi Sam" shown in the soundscape and the spectrogram. The spectral sections clearly show the individual components of sound and their amplitude relations to each other. Also, the spectrum components are pictured on a linear scale of frequency so their frequency locations can be measured and formant frequencies can be estimated; the fundamental frequency of periodic sounds can be measured by counting the frequency intervals

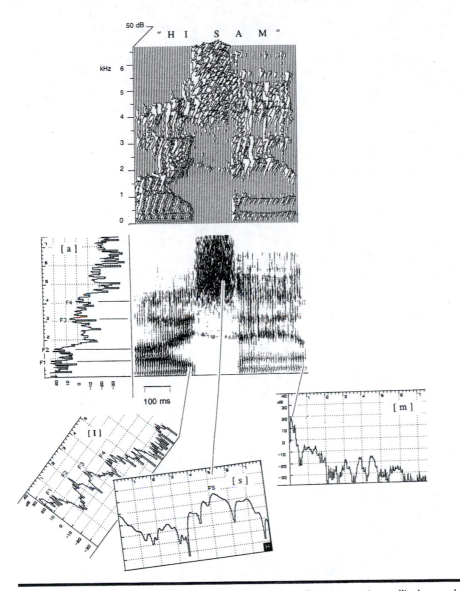

FIGURE 4-15. Derivation of spectrum sections, plots of component amplitudes and frequencies, related to a spectrogram of "Hi Sam."

between components. This may be done by measuring the span in frequency of several successive components and then dividing by the number of intervals spanned. This gives the frequency spacing between components, which is the same as the fundamental frequency, as we saw earlier. Some PC analysis programs will calculate the

fundamental automatically and even plot it as a "pitch track" on each spectrogram. Using Speech-Station to analyze pitch a table of pitch values in the utterance is presented with the pitch track.

The process of constructing a spectrogram in Figure 4-15 is another very instructive path to understanding. This is actually better done with an animated graphics example that is available as an interactive computer exercise in the Course Unit on spectrograms in Sensimetrics' Speech Production and Perception I. This course, for CD-ROM PCs, is described in Appendix A.

SPECTROGRAMS OF VOWELS

Spectrograms of spoken examples of the vowels [i], [ɑ], and [u] are shown in Figure 4-16 to illustrate the variables in vowel formation. The vowels were spoken by an adult male in words beginning with [h] and ending with [d]. Next to the spectrogram of each vowel is a spectral section taken at one time point during the vowel. The spectrograms and sections were made on a Kay Sonagraph adjusted to apply as pre-emphasis an upward tilt to the spectrum above 500 Hz of 3 1/2 dB/octave. The sections show the effects on the spectrum envelope of the

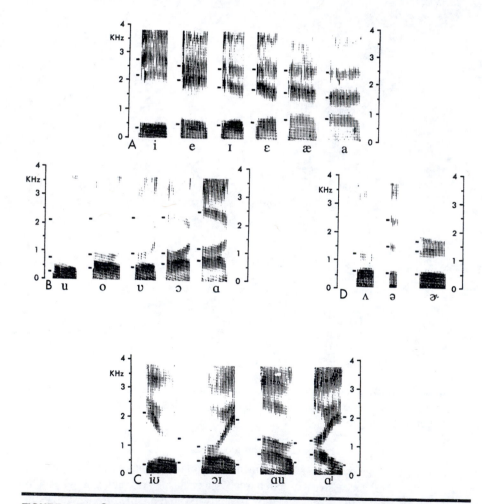

FIGURE 4-16. Spectrograms of examples of the vowels and diphthongs of American English (Vs), spoken in [hVd]. The formants of the vowels are indicated by the bars at the left side of each spectrogram. Each formant was measured at the vowel's mid-point in time. For the diphthongs in the bottom row of spectrograms the formants were measured at the beginning (left) and the end (right).

vocal tract shape differences between [i], [ɑ], and [u]. The sections also show the effects on the glottal source spectrum for low and high-pitched voices: The voice pitch is reflected in the frequency spacing of the harmonic components, with wider spacing for high pitch than for low pitch. The effects of high vocal effort appear in the amplitudes of F2 and F3 between 1 and 3 kHz, which are seen to be much more intense relative to the F1 region for high effort versus low effort.

The pitch of the voice can be seen in a spectrogram as well as in the spectrum sections. In the spectrogram there is a pulse of sound energy for each pulse of the glottis, which forms the source of the vowel sound. On the spectrogram each glottal pulse appears as a striation running vertically from low to high frequencies. The striations are darker at frequencies where the intensity is stronger, namely at and near the formant frequencies. The striations succeed each other in time exactly in synchrony with the glottal pulses. Since the glottal pulses are more widely spaced in time for a low-pitched voice, the spectrogram pulses are farther apart for vowels spoken on a low voice pitch. For the high-pitched voice the glottal pulses and the striations in the spectrogram are more closely packed together, because for a high-pitched voice the glottal pulses succeed each other more rapidly in time.

Spectrograms of all of the vowels and diphthongs are shown in Figure 4-16, as spoken by an adult male in syllables beginning with [h] and ending with [d], except for [ə], which was spoken in the phrase *a toy* [ətoi]. The speaker used his native General American dialect except for the vowel [a], where he imitated a native of Massachusetts saying the word *hard*. Going across the top row A of spectrograms, we go through the series of front vowels starting with [i] and going through [ɪ], [e], [ɛ], [æ], and [ɑ]; you will note that the second formant comes down from high to low frequencies through this series of front vowels, and the first formant rises from a low to a high frequency position through the series. You will also note that two of the front vowels, namely, [ɪ]

and [ɛ], are shorter in duration than the other vowels. Of course, any vowel can be deliberately shortened or prolonged in pronunciation, but, as they occur in naturally spoken English, certain vowels have shorter durations than the other vowels. The average durations of vowels in stressed one-syllable words, spoken by American talkers, was found to be about 230 ms for the long vowels and 180 ms for the short vowels (Peterson & Lehiste, 1960). The vowel durations in Figure 4-16 are similar to these values.

The second row of spectrograms (Figure 4-16B) shows the sound patterns of the back vowel series starting with [u] and going through [ʊ], [o], [ɔ], and [ɑ]. You will note in this series that both the first and second formant resonances go from low frequency positions to higher frequency positions. In the series of back vowels there is one short vowel, [ʊ].

Figure 4-16D shows the spectrograms of the three central vowels [ʌ], [ə], and [ɚ]. The short central vowel is [ə]. The diphthongs [ɪʊ], [ɔɪ], and [ɑu] and [ɑɪ] are shown in row C; they are longer in duration. Diphthongs are similar to double vowels, and they include a glide in articulation from one vowel position to another. In the spectrograms of the diphthongs you can see both the first and second formant frequency positions changing in time as the vocal tract shape changes from one vowel configuration to the other.

Distinct types of formant movement patterns for vowels produced in consonant-vowel consonant (CVC) syllables were classified by Lehiste and Peterson (1961) according to the relative durations of three components: onglides (formant movements from the release of the initial consonant to the vowel target), targets (in which formants were steady-state or movement was relatively slow), and offglides (formant movements from the target to consonant closure). The short monophthongs contrasted with the long monophthongs primarily in the relative durations of targets and offglides. Short vowels contained relatively short targets and longer offglides, while long vowels had relatively long targets and shorter offglides. That is, long vowels remained near their target positions for a greater proportion of the syllable than did short vowels.

The diphthongized vowels [eɪ] and [oʊ] and the retroflex vowel [ɚ] all had a single target and extensive offglides, while the true diphthongs could be divided into five distinct components: onglide, target 1, glide, target 2, and offglide. The first target was typically longer than the second; however, the glide between targets was longer than either target.

NASALIZATION OF VOWELS

The vowel sounds of English are spoken with the velum raised against the walls and back of the pharynx to shut off the nasal passages from the pharynx and oral tract. However, speakers of American English often seem to nasalize their vowels slightly by allowing the velum to remain slightly open. Nasalization also occurs in vowels that are adjacent to nasal consonants, especially in the portions of the vowel immediately next to the consonant. Vowel nasalization is used phonemically in many languages, but not in English. Later in the chapter we describe some nasal vowels as phonemes of French and, in Chapter Ten, nasal vowels of Gujarati, a language of India.

In pathological speech, such as that of a person who has a cleft palate, which opens the oral tract into the nasal passages, or a person with an undeveloped velum or abnormally sluggish velum action, there may be extreme nasalization of all sounds. Persons who were born deaf sometimes speak with nasalized sounds.

The important acoustic effects of nasalization have been determined through research on vocal tract models (House & Stevens, 1956). Electrical models were built of the cavities of the nasal tract and the oral tract, and the two tracts were connected together through circuits representing greater or lesser amounts of opening between them. It was found that the main effect on a vowel of an opening at the velum is to produce changes in the filter curve of the oral tract. One effect was that the first formant became broader and less peaked than before, because of the damping of the formant resonance by the loss of energy through the opening into the nasal tract.

Another change due to opening the velum is to apply negative resonant peaks to the oral tract response. In the mathematical representation of these nasal+oral tract filters the *negative resonances are called zeroes and the positive resonances are called poles*. Zeroes are antiresonances; they are exactly the opposite of resonances in their effect on the spectrum. Instead of reinforcing and amplifying the spectrum at and near the resonant frequency, an antiresonance selectively absorbs sound so that it greatly reduces the amplitudes of components at and near the antiresonant frequency. Further, acting just opposite the *attenuation* of components above a formant resonant frequency, a zero *amplifies* components that are sufficiently above the antiresonance frequency and in proportion to component frequency. In addition, for each zero there is an extra pole introduced. The amount of these effects depends on the amount of opening between the pharyngeal-oral tract and the nasal tract. In other words, the nasalization effects on the spectrum depend on the amount of coupling between the two tracts. The amount of coupling also affects the frequency positions of the zero and extra pole. Thus the effects of nasalization on a vowel depends on its non-nasal formant frequencies, determined by the oral tract shape, and on the frequencies of the zeroes and poles introduced by nasal tract coupling, determined by the amount of coupling.

The effects on the vowel spectrum have been summarized by nasalization researchers as follows: (1) The presence of a low-frequency zero below F1 tends to make the spectral peak in the region of F1 appear to be higher in frequency than it would normally be. Thus the effects of nasalization on F1 are to reduce and broaden its amplitude peak, and this moves the apparent F1 in this region to a higher frequency position. The amount of frequency shift in the apparent F1 is 50 to 100 Hz; (2) the nasal coupling can also cause zeroes in the region of F2 and F3, and often this reduces the peakedness of these formants or completely flattens the peaks.

Some effects of nasalization are diagrammed in Figure 4-17, showing spectrum envelopes for a natural [ɑ] and for the same vowel heavily nasalized. The talker spoke the [ɑ] continuously, maintaining fairly constant positions of tongue and jaw while opening and closing the velum to nasalize and denasalize the vowel. The peaks due to the formants are numbered 1, 2, and 3 for the normal [ɑ]. For the spectrum of the nasalized [ɑ], z's are drawn to indicate spectral regions that appear to be influenced by zeroes in the vocal tract response. In this case it appears that a low-frequency zero at about 600 Hz has produced a spectral dip at that frequency and that two higher zeroes have radically altered the normal spectrum at points near the third resonance. The positions of these zeroes may be typical for heavily nasalized [ɑ] but should not be considered to hold for milder degrees of nasalization, nor for other vowels, since the pharyngeal-oral shape and amount of velar opening interact to determine the frequency positions of the formants and zeroes.

PHONEMIC NASAL VOWELS

Many languages exploit for phonemic purposes our ability to control the opening of the velar port. Or, to put it another way, some languages expand their vowel "vocabulary," their phonologic vowel inventory, by opening the velar port during some of their vowels. Such a language uses nasalized vowels to distinguish within pairs of words that are otherwise the same. It uses nasal vowels that are produced with shapes of oral configuration similar to the oral shapes of some of its non-nasal vowels.

Gujarati, an Indo-Aryan language widely spoken in Northwest India, uses a set of five non-nasal vowels, all of which are employed phonemically in opposition to the same vowels nasalized, to make the complete set of ten vowels. Hawkins and Stevens (1985) chose these vowels for an intensive study of the acoustic cues to the nasal-nonnasal distinction. To identify the possible acoustic cues, Hawkins and Stevens analyzed examples of all

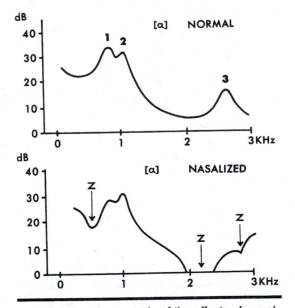

FIGURE 4-17. An example of the effects of vowel nasalization on the vowel spectrum. The spectrum envelopes of a normal [ɑ] and a heavily nasalized [ɑ] were plotted from spectral sections. The first three formants are labeled in the normal vowel. In the nasalized vowel, there are three local reductions in spectrum level, indicated by "z's"; these are the result of the addition of anti-resonant zeroes to the vocal tract response, due to a wide-open velar port.

ten vowels, uttered in Gujarati words by a native speaker.

We will compare the Gujarati nasalization of [a] to [ã] with our heavy nasalization of American [a] to [ã] in the previous figure, to see if the nasalization has similar effects for the two speakers. Figure 4-18 plots Hawkins and Stevens' spectrum analysis of Gujarati [a] and [ã]. You can see that the F1 region (1000 Hz and below) is strongly suppressed and it contains no predominate peak, like the F1 peak at 700 Hz in the non-nasal [a]. The non-nasal F2 peak at 1200 Hz is weaker by about 11 dB in the nasal and at a slightly lower frequency. These effects are very similar to those seen in our heavy nasalization in Figure 4-17.

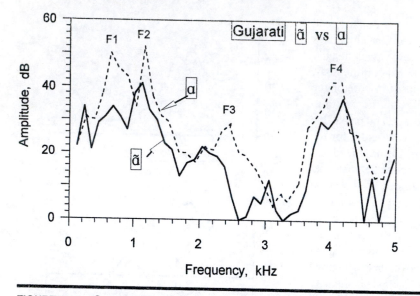

FIGURE 4-18.   Comparison of the Gujarati nasalized [ã]-vowel, plotted with solid lines, and the oral vowel, plotted with dashed lines. Note that the nasal vowel spectrum is generally lower in amplitude and has different peaks and valleys compared with the oral [a]. Data replotted from Hawkins and Stevens (1985). See text for further comparisons.

The third formant F3 in Gujarati [a] at about 2500 Hz (an adult male speaker) is very heavily suppressed and lowered in frequency to about 2100 Hz in the nasal [ã]. In the American nasalized [ã] in the previous figure the F3 region lacks any prominent peak due apparently to the addition of two zeroes by the nasalization.

French Nasal Vowels

French is the most widely known example of a language that uses vowel nasalization phonemically. To look at some examples of nasal vowels, French-speaking phonetician Noel Nguyen provided spectral data for some of the non-nasal/ nasal vowels that differentiate pairs of words in his own speech. Then I made spectrum plots and assembled one pair in Figure 4-19 to illustrate the differences between nasal and non-nasal. The figure shows spectra of the nasal from the pair [ɛ, ɛ̃] in Nguyen's spoken French words *paix, pain.*

First, it should be noticed in Figure 4-19, scanning over the two spectra, plotted with dashed lines for the [ɛ] and solid lines for the [ɛ̃], that the formants, F1, F2, and F3, indicated above the dashed-line plots, are well-defined by prominent peaks in amplitude. This is true for both vowels.

Going over the solid-curve spectrum of nasal [ɛ], however, the corresponding formant peaks near those of the non-nasal F1, F2 peaks don't seem to stand out so clearly. Their formant peaks are not as sharply peaked; they have flatter tops.

Comparing [ɛ̃] relative to [ɛ]: The F1 peak is broadened; F2 appears as a broad hump extending from about 1100–1750 Hz instead of the narrower peak at 1625 Hz for [ɛ]; both F1 and F2 are weaker by 5 to 8 dB; F3 has been weakened 11 dB; the F4-F5 region is greatly lowered, 20 dB, possibly due to a zero near the 3125 Hz point. Similar results were seen for other pairs of French nasal–non-nasal vowels.

We conclude that nasalization effects on vowel spectra are similar between speakers and languages. This is due to the similarities of the vocal

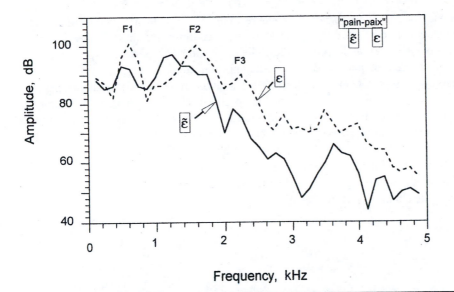

FIGURE 4-19. Comparison of the nasal French vowel in the word *pain* (bread) with its counterpart non-nasal, oral vowel, [ɛ] in the word *paix* (peace). The nasal vowel is plotted with solid lines and the oral vowel with dashed lines. Note that the nasal vowel spectrum is generally lower in amplitude and has different peaks and valleys compared with the oral [ɛ] in *paix*. Further details of comparison are described in the text. (The spectra were obtained from a 25.6 ms sample taken in the center of the vowel and analyzed by computer; the plots connect the amplitude values for each 125 Hz step across the frequency scale. The words were spoken and analyzed by Noel Nguyen of the Psycholinguistics Department in the University of Geneva, Switzerland).

tracts of all human speakers. Hawkins and Stevens (1985) designed a vocal-tract model to synthesize nasal vowels; it simulated variations in the velar port opening between tubes that were sized like the oral and nasal tracts. The model produced synthetic nasal and non-nasal vowels that were identified correctly by Gujarati-speaking listeners as their non-nasal vowels when the velar port was closed and as their nasal vowels when the velar port was open. The flattening of the F1 region appeared to be the major nasal characteristic controlling perception.

SUMMARY

The spectral characteristics of vowels are caused by the combination of the spectrum of the glottal source sound and the resonances of the pharyngeal-oral tract. The source-filter theory of vowel production considers the glottal source spectrum to be shaped, or filtered, by the response of the vocal tract, independent of glottal actions affecting the source spectrum. Factors that affect the source spectrum operate through changes in the pulse form of the airflow through the glottis in forming each glottal pulse. Vocal-fold tension affects primarily the fundamental pulsing rate. The airflow velocity within the glottis causes a suction force (Bernoulli force) between the folds, which affects the pulse shape. The pulse shape is also subject to secondary effects whenever there is a very close constriction in the pharygeal-oral tract.

The spacing in frequency of the components of glottal spectrum depends on the voice pitch, the fundamental glottal pulsing frequency; the slope of the glottal spectrum depends on the pulse shape, which is sensitive to the amount of vocal effort.

The formant resonances of the vowels and diphthongs, and the effects of changes in pitch and vocal effort, are exemplified in spectrograms of natural speech.

The articulation of speech causes the sound spectrum to change rapidly over time. To observe these changes we use computers to analyze and display the spectrum. Two modes of analysis are used: In a spectrographic mode, computers display spectrograms showing the changes over time of the resonances, or formants, of the vocal tract; in a spectral section mode they display and plot the individual components of the spectrum at a specified point in time.

Vowel sounds may be nasalized by opening the velar port; this causes a reduction in F1 amplitude and the insertion of antiresonances (zeroes) and extra formants in the transmission of the pharyngeal-oral tract, thus altering the vowel spectrum. Some languages use vowel nasalization to distinguish words phonemically.

CHAPTER FIVE

PROSODIC AND TONAL FEATURES

"I remember the melody, if not the words.
—Anonymous

INTRODUCTION: TELLING WHAT AND HOW

Speech has special voice features that are inherent to communication. When we talk with someone we usually want to convey two things: some objective information or the WHAT and some sort of attitude or HOW we feel about it. Both of these aims are accomplished by speaking with special variations of voice pitch and rhythm, called *prosodic features*. We tell WHAT by choosing words and putting them in phrases that are spoken melodically according to certain rules. These rules for the WHAT content of our message are code rules of our language that distinguish among words and signal the grammar of a sentence. These melodies are patterns of rhythms, tones, and timing of the syllables. These patterns are a linguistic code; they are specific to one's native language and usually different from those of other languages.

Another type of melodic coding is for expressive, affective purposes. It tells HOW we feel about the WHAT, our temper or humor about it, and often our intentions in saying it. Consider, for example, how we can agree, *Yes*, in a wide variety of attitudes using different tonal glides of voice pitch. A long, upward-gliding *yes* can mean, *OK, is that really true? Tell me more.* A shorter up-gliding *yes* means, *OK, I'm listening.* A downward-gliding *yes* means, *Yes, I agree.* A long, drawn-out *ye . . . s* with a steady voice tone can indicate boredom or impatience. These are only a few of the things we can convey just by tonal variations of *yes*

in certain situations. This type of tonal expression with speech is a form of communication that uses a social code. This code is not a formal linguistic property of our language; it is an expressive code. A song is another example of expressive speech. The melody of a song conveys a mood or emotion that is not a formal part of the language, as are the words and phrases.

Phoneticians look for the expressive and linguistic codes of speech in the tonal patterns of the voice pitch and in variations in the syllable stresses and timing to form rhythmic patterns. Both in everyday conversation and in formal discourse these prosodic variations are used linguistically for what we say and expressively for emphasis, attitudes, and intentions about what we are saying. Our study here of the phonetics of rhythm and tone concentrates primarily on their linguistic functions, but we also present some extra-linguistic facts and some tonal forms that are used expressively. In talking to each other we like to color what we think and feel; we affirm, claim, disagree, condemn, emphasize, distinguish, convince, approve, and disapprove. These affective meanings, the HOW signals, are accomplished by well-established patterns of the pitches and rhythms, the melodies, of speaking.

In this chapter we look at the prosodic sound patterns and their mechanisms of production by the larynx and other articulators. Then subsequent chapters describe production of the vowels and consonants that are fitted into the prosodic patterns.

PARENTING SPEECH

A fascinating thing about prosodic features is they are probably the very first speech patterns we hear, in the womb before we are born. Fetuses in the womb begin to respond to sound stimuli in the third trimester. The lower speech frequencies, 100 to 500 Hz, are available to be heard above the noises of blood circulation. The mother's voice in this range is well above the noise.

After birth our parents express their affection or disaffection by talking to us with exaggerated prosodics. Linguists call this style of speech *parenting*, *caretaker*, or *infant-directed* speech. People call it *baby-talk*. As we learn our language, parents, caretakers, friends, and teachers all use special prosodics to encourage and correct us.

To look at some parenting speech I analyzed the pitch variations in the recordings of my neighbors with which we began Chapter One. While reading a story book, some phrases of Mother and Son showed wide changes in pitch, as we see in Figure 5-1.

How did we get that way? Why do parents and caretakers almost universally use baby-talk to infants and very young children? There is a lot of acoustic evidence on the evolutionary, survival significance of infant-directed speech (Fernald, 1992). For a description of how motherese can aid the baby to acquire its native language, see Chapter Fourteen.

PROSODIC FEATURES OF LANGUAGE FORMS

Of primary importance to us will be the linguistic melodic patterns of speaking that code differences in word meanings and grammar. But the

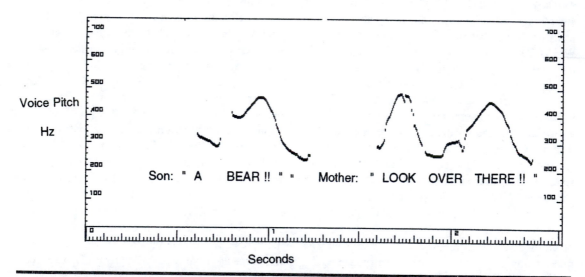

FIGURE 5-1. Pitch contours of Son (7 yrs) and Mother while reading a story and looking at a cartoon of a bear among people in a train station. The son's *a bear!!* is in his usual pitch range of 250–480 Hz. Mother's normal conversational pitch ranges from about 125 to 250 Hz but here with *Look over there!!* she points out another part of the cartoon with a pitch range raised to her son's level. Both Son and Mother use extreme rises and falls in pitch, expressing their delight in finding new characters in the cartoon.

(Voice pitch tracks derived and plotted via SpeechStation2 from Sensimetrics Corporation)

tunes come before the words in early child speech. Prosodic patterns of the ambient language of the family appear in the infants' speech before phonemic sounds are mastered and well before the first word is spoken. For example, French babies use more upward intonation than English babies. And parents often hear their toddlers talking nonsense to themselves, propounding statements, asking questions, and making arguments that are amusingly devoid of specifics. For a general review of infant prosodics research see Vihman (1996).

Infants also use prosodic patterns they hear as an early way to latch onto the spoken word as an essential unit in language structure. Word boundaries are not clearly marked in speaking. The listening infant must learn to discern, to "segment out," the word patterns from the continuous stream of speech sounds. One source of information is the prosodic patterns of the utterance, because prosodic variations are used by adult speakers both to differentiate and to emphasize words and phrases. There is strong evidence that infants 3 to 9 months old depend on prosodic integrity of the utterance to detect phonemic changes that would signal word differences. This evidence was developed by Jusczyk and his co-workers (reviewed in Jusczyk, 1997, pp. 137–158). Investigators of language development in children have called this "prosodic boot-strapping" because, given that word-boundaries are not clearly marked out in the fluent flow of consonants and vowels, it would seem impossible for the child to learn words in the absence of prosodic patterns correlated with the grouping of the sounds into words.

Prosodic features play a strong role in the linguistic code for communication. Further proof of their vital function for the adult is seen in cases of abnormal or defective prosodics. For example, foreign speakers of English who articulate well all of the vowels and consonants are not easily understood unless they speak with correct English rhythms and intonation. The reason for our difficulty is that utterances are formed under definite rules of rhythm and intonation. These prosodic rules are unique for every language. Different languages share many phonemes in common, but the articulations of these common vowels and consonants are tailored for each language to fit its prosodic rules. Understanding speech depends partly on listeners' correct rhythmic entrainment, their expectations of prosodic patterns, as an aid to deciphering the fitted-in articulations for the phonemes.

Another example of the importance of rhythm and intonation sometimes appears in the speech of deaf persons: They can be taught to produce good individual speech sounds, but their speech can still be nearly unintelligible if the sounds are not expressed within the overall rhythmic and tonal rules of the language. In the field of artificial speech, as in reading machines for the blind and in computer talk-back applications, the correct programming of the prosodics has been found to be necessary for good intelligibility (see speech synthesis in Chapter Seventeen on speech technology).

Prosodic patterns usually extend over several successive phoneme episodes or segments, and thus are said to be *suprasegmental*. They are produced by certain special manipulations of the sound sources and the shaping of the vocal tract. The source factors operate through actions of the speech breathing muscles and the vocal folds; the shaping factors operate through the movements of the upper articulators, the excursions of the jaw, tongue, and lips. The acoustic patterns of the prosodic features are found in systematic variations of the duration, intensity, and fundamental frequency (pitch), and in the spectrum patterns of the individual sounds. Our aim in this chapter is to give a basic explanation of how some of these prosodic patterns are produced. We begin with the glottal source and then proceed to describe other factors.

We are mainly interested in the prosodic features that convey linguistic information. Stress and intonation are the most important of these. By means of stress we differentiate similar forms that have different meanings; for example, compare the two phrases *That's just insight* and *That's just in sight*. In the first phrase there is a stress on *sight* but *in* is unstressed; in the second phrase this relation is reversed, giving an entirely different meaning. By means of intonation patterns we differentiate grammatical functions; an example is the rising intonation of a question as contrasted with the falling intonation of a statement. One can state *That's just insight*, using a downward glide in pitch, or one can query *That's just insight?*, using an upward glide.

In addition to syllable stresses used in the language to differentiate meanings, stress is used by speakers to emphasize words or phrases considered to be especially significant. This is called emphatic stress. For example, the statement *That's just insight* can be spoken with emphasis on any of the three words, *that*, *just*, or *insight*, depending on which word the speaker wants the listener to give special attention to.

Speakers' manipulations of their glottal source for prosodic features has been intensively studied to define the physiological and acoustic conditions of stress patterns and intonation patterns (Ladefoged, 1963, 1967; Lieberman, 1967). This work has established some basic mechanisms of prosodics. These experiments are now described. We include some details about the research techniques.

GLOTTAL SOURCE FACTORS IN STRESS AND INTONATION

There are two main factors responsible for production of the glottal source variations for prosodic features: (1) the tension on the vocal folds and (2) the subglottal air pressure. These affect the characteristics of the glottal sound source, especially the pulsing rate (fundamental frequency) but also the source amplitude and the source spectrum.

Subglottal Air Pressure

Increasing expiratory force on the lungs causes a corresponding increase in the subglottal air pressure. The increase in subglottal pressure causes an increase in the rate of repetition of the airflow pulses emitted by the glottis; that is, the fundamental frequency increases. Pitch increase via subglottal pressure may be caused in two ways. First, the increased elastic stretch on the folds as they are forced farther apart by the increased subglottal pressure can cause a faster closure movement. Second, the lateral displacement of the folds may be kept constant by increased muscle tension and this may increase the stiffness of the folds and reduce their local mass, causing them to move at a higher rate (see Chapter Four and Titze, 1995). Increased subglottal pressure can also cause a faster rate of inward movement of the folds just before glottal closure, because of an increased Bernoulli effect; this causes a more sudden closure and results in a greater efficiency of pulse excitation of the air in the upper tract. Thus, subjectively, the pitch[1] and loudness of the voice are both increased by increases in subglottal pressure.

Also, a sharper voice timbre will result if the increase of pressure causes the glottal closures to be more sudden. Everyone experiences these effects when shouting louder and louder to attract someone's attention. The loudness goes higher but so do the pitch and timbre of the voice.

There are some familiar examples of the relations between the air pressure on a flexible slit-like opening, such as the glottis, and the characteristics of the wave pulses produced. One example is the noise-making horns used to celebrate New Year's Eve. The harder you blow, the higher is the pitch (frequency) and loudness (amplitude). A similar situation exists in speech when a steady note is sung and then outside pressure is suddenly put on the chest of the singer to increase the subglottal pressure. This causes an immediate rise in pitch and loudness. Children sometimes use this effect in play, pushing and pounding on chests to make each other sing unpredictable songs.

---

[1]In acoustic writings on speech the term *voice pitch*, or simply *pitch*, means the fundamental frequency of the vocal fold vibration in producing a glottal sound source. In the field of hearing, the sensation of pitch is found to depend largely on the fundamental frequency of the sound stimulus. Thus, the pitch sensation and the frequency of a sound signal, although closely related, are not the same thing. In the speech literature, however, pitch and fundamental frequency are used synonymously, and we will use these terms in the same way.

As a first step in the study of intonation and stress Ladefoged measured the relation between the subglottal pressure and voice pitch (Ladefoged, 1963). The chest-push effect was used to measure this relation. The procedure was as follows. The subject intoned a vowel sound in a relaxed manner, keeping vocal force relatively constant; the experimenter pushed on the subject's chest, using different amounts of force, causing the subject's voice to rise and fall; the voice sound wave and the subglottal pressure were both recorded during these maneuvers. The subglottal pressure was picked up by means of a small balloon located in the esophagus just behind the trachea of the subject. The mouth of the balloon was connected to a flexible plastic tube that was swallowed down a short way into the esophagus. The other end of the tube was attached to a pressure-sensing device that measured the pressure in the tube. This pressure was recorded graphically by a continuous tracing of the increases and decreases in pressure. It was found to be nearly the same as the pressure recorded directly through a large hypodermic needle inserted into the larynx just below the vocal folds.

The voice pitch was measured by deriving the fundamental frequency from the sound wave of the vowel intoned by the subject. The fundamental frequency was measured electronically and recorded simultaneously with the subglottal pressure. The results of these measurements are shown in Figure 5-2. Each point in the figure shows the fundamental frequency corresponding to a given amount of subglottal pressure. The fundamental frequency is plotted on the vertical scale in Hertz. The subglottal pressure is plotted on the horizontal scale in centimeters of water (cm H_2O; multiply by 9.806×102 to obtain the pressure in metric units, dynes per square centimeter). The 16 points clustered in the lower left part of the graph are results without any external pressure on the speaker's chest; they represent the normal, rather forceful low frequency range of this speaker. His normal fundamental frequency ranges from 89 Hz to 100 Hz and his subglottal pressure ranges from about 13 to 16.5

cm H_2O, a somewhat higher than average range of pressure. The remaining points on the graph show the voice fundamental and subglottal pressure for instances of the peak pressures resulting from the pushes on the chest of the speaker while he was phonating. It will be seen that the higher the subglottal pressure, the higher the fundamental frequency of the speaker's voice. This relation approximates a straight line when the fundamental frequency is scaled logarithmically as it is on this graph; a line is drawn through the points for comparison. The scatter of points around the straight line is probably due to variations in the speaker's vocal fold tension just before his chest was pushed. The change in voice fundamental frequency in Figure 5-2 averages about 4.5 Hz per cm H_2O; this is based on a total change of about 45 Hz over the 10 cm range from 14 to 24 cm H_2O.

The next step in Ladefoged's study of intonation and stress was to find out how different stress patterns are produced by different patterns of subglottal pressure, depending on whether the stress is located on the first syllable or the second syllable of a word and also depending on whether the word is spoken in a statement or in a question. The words chosen were pairs of two-syllable words in which the word was a noun when the stress was on the first syllable, but the same word was a verb when the stress was on the second syllable. These were spoken in short sentences, for example, *That's a digest* and *He didn't digest*; or *That's a survey* and *He didn't survey*. Each of these sentences could be spoken either as a statement, that is, with a downward contour of intonation on the final word, or as a question, with a rise in intonation.

It was found that the pattern of subglottal pressure was related to the location of the stressed syllable in the phrase. These effects are diagrammed in Figure 5-3, where we see the patterns of subglottal pressure and fundamental frequency for the four sentences with the word *digest*. Examine the subglottal pressure pattern under the word *digest* [daidzest] spoken as a noun with stress on the first syllable (upper curves of subglottal

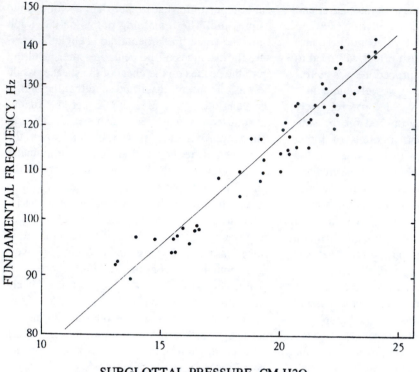

FIGURE 5-2.   Relation between voice fundamental frequency, plotted on a log scale, and subglottal pressure. Subglottal pressure was varied by unexpected pushes, with various force, on the speaker's chest, while he was phonating a vowel intended to be steady. The group of points between about 89 and 100 Hz are from the speaker's normal phonations, before he was pushed.
(Adapted from Ladefoged, 1963)

pressure). Then do the same for *digest* spoken as a verb with stress on the second syllable (lower curves). You will note that the stressed syllable is always spoken with a higher subglottal pressure. The pressure increase on the stressed syllable seems to be greater for the statements on the left than for the questions on the right.

Now examine the intonation patterns above the pressure patterns. These show the voice pitch during the vowels and the duration of each vowel. For the statements, on the left, we see that the general trend of pitch is downward-going from the beginning of the statement to the end. Also, we see that the stressed syllable has the longest

vowel duration of any in the sentence and that the noun in the statement has a very high pitch on the stressed syllable. On the other hand the verb in the statement has a more level pitch on the second, stressed syllable. because it appears that the expression of the statement depends on an overall decline in pitch or, in the case of a stressed final syllable, the implication of a decline that is counteracted by the stress effect on pitch.

When the same sentences are spoken as questions, the pitch of the voice rises continuously from the beginning to the end of the question. For the noun in the question neither the duration nor the pitch of the stressed syllable is higher than

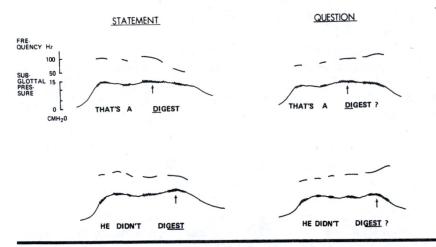

FIGURE 5-3.   Relations between contours of voice fundamental frequency and subglottal pressure for statements and questions with two different patterns of word stress. The stressed syllable is underlined and indicated by an arrow under the contour of subglottal pressure. Each intonation contour is plotted above its contour of subglottal pressure. It can be seen that the stressed syllables correspond to peaks in the pressure contours and that the intonation contours rise for the questions and tend to fall for the statements.

(Adapted from Ladefoged, 1963)

that of the following unstressed syllable because of the rising intonation contour on the final unstressed syllable. The rising contour is required to express the question. In the verb form of the word in the question, the second syllable, that is, the stressed syllable, has a longer duration and higher pitch.

We see from these comparisons that the patterns of voice pitch and duration, corresponding to stressed versus unstressed syllables, are dependent on whether the general pattern of intonation expresses a statement or a question.

Now examine the subglottal pressure patterns in relation to the intonation curves of the four sentences. The striking thing to note is that the subglottal pressure is relatively constant and does not show a trend corresponding to the intonation contour; that is to say, the subglottal pressure is not generally falling during the statements and it is not generally rising during the questions. This is especially evident in the noun, *DI*gest, where the

subglottal pressure falls somewhat, but the pitch rises between the two syllables.

What is it then, that controls the voice pitch to produce the rising intonation of a question in contrast to the falling intonation of a statement? It must be the tension on the vocal folds and not primarily the subglottal pressure.

Vocal Fold Tension for Intonation

The major factor controlling voice pitch is the tension on the vocal folds; muscular control of this tension is applied through small muscles in the larynx. At the time of Ladefoged's study, there were no methods for measuring the vocal fold tension to determine its exact role in control of voice pitch. On the assumption that any changes in pitch not accounted for by changes in subglottal pressure would be due to changes in vocal fold tension, Ladefoged concluded that the overall pattern change in vocal fold tension is somewhat more simple than would be indicated by following all the fundamental frequency changes seen in the acoustic signal. It also appeared that the strongest stress of a syllable in a phrase is produced by a combination of an increase in vocal fold tension and a peak in subglottal pressure.

We can now summarize our main points about stress and intonation as follows:

1. Phonetic patterns for different stress patterns and different intonational expressions are based on an interplay between manipulations of the vocal fold tension, the peaks of subglottal pressure, and the durations of the vowel and consonant articulations.
2. The voice pitch reflects both the vocal fold tension and the subglottal pressure. When there is an increase in either the vocal fold tension or the subglottal pressure or both, there is a corresponding increase in the voice fundamental frequency.
3. During the utterance of a phrase, if the changes in voice fundamental frequency caused by changes in the subglottal pressure are taken into account, the resulting "basic" curve, reflecting the effect of vocal fold tension, is a relatively simple curve compared to the curve of changes in fundamental frequency.

We see then that there is a complex interaction between the stress patterns of speech and the intonation or inflectional patterns of speech. The resulting acoustic patterns of vowel duration, pitch, and intensity are also rather complex but there is evidence that the basic factors of subglottal pressure and vocal fold tension operate in relatively simple ways.

Breath Group Theory of Intonation

Experimental work by Lieberman (1967) led him to propose a simple theory of how the basic patterns of subglottal pressure and vocal fold tension produce the effects of stress and intonation. The theory states that speech is based on two simple actions, the grouping of words into breath groups and the marking of these groups by stress and intonational changes.

Words, phrases, or sentences are grouped into *breath groups*. A breath group is a section of utterance that is produced between two respiratory inspirations. The typical breath group is produced on a pattern of change in subglottal air pressure that rises just before the beginning of the breath group and then remains fairly constant except during the last part of the group, when the subglottal air pressure falls gradually during the final part of the breath group and then falls abruptly to end the group. In breath groups where the speaker has no reason to emphasize the final word or syllables, fundamental frequency usually falls during the final part of the breath group because of the fall-off in subglottal pressure.

Lieberman proposed that this relatively simple manipulation of the breath stream, and a state of rather constant vocal fold tension throughout the breath group, is the basic maneuver for speaking called the *unmarked breath group*. Short statements, such as *That's a digest* or *That's just insight*, are produced by one unmarked breath group. Longer statements would consist of a series of such breath groups.

The unmarked breath group is considered to be the simplest way to produce an utterance with the least amount of muscular effort expended to maintain phonation. In this sense the breath group is universal for all languages, although some languages, dialects, and individual habits may involve simple variations on this "archetypal" breath group. For explanations of the "primitive" biological status and linguistic significance of the breath group concept, see the textbook of Lieberman and Blumstein (1988, p. 199 ff.).

An example of an utterance spoken as an unmarked breath group is shown in Figure 5-4. The utterance was the statement *Joe ate his soup*, with the main stress on *Joe*. It will be seen that the fundamental frequency and the subglottal pressure tend to parallel each other. The final syllable *soup* has a fundamental frequency contour, which

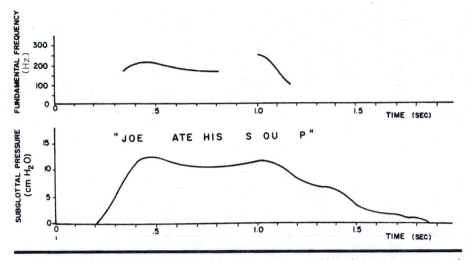

FIGURE 5-4. Contour of fundamental frequency (top graph) and concurrent curve of subglottal pressure (bottom graph) for an unmarked breath group. (From Lieberman, 1967)

starts at a high pitch level but falls very rapidly under the influence of the falling subglottal pressure, probably supplemented by a decrease in vocal fold tension. Relatively simple variations on the basic breath group produce the stress patterns specified by the language and modified by the speaker in expressive or emphatic patterns. For example, to express a question, the speaker may raise vocal fold tension during the last portion of the breath group and thus maintain fundamental frequency at a constant level instead of allowing it to fall under the influence of the declining subglottal pressure.

The pattern of syllable stress within the breath group is generally dominated by a momentary increase in the subglottal pressure during the stressed syllable. The rise in pressure produces an increase in the fundamental frequency, in the loudness, and in the level of the high frequency part of the vowel spectrum. The stressed syllable also shows increased duration in relation to the other syllables of the breath group.

The main stress of the breath group corresponds to the peak subglottal pressure of the group. The syllable that follows the peak may have a slightly subnormal pressure because of the lower level of elastic recoil of the lung tissues. There is a rapid reduction in lung volume during the peak stress that causes the lung tissues to become less distended and therefore to exert less recoil pressure. This lowering of subglottal pressure following peak stress is usually not compensated by an increase in vocal fold tension and so the voice fundamental frequency is lower on post-stress syllables.

An example of an utterance spoken as a *marked breath group*, marked for a question, is shown in Figure 5-5. The utterance was *Did Joe eat his soup?* The breath group is *marked* by the rising fundamental frequency on the final syllable, which occurs despite the falling subglottal pressure. The rise during *soup* must have been caused by an increase in vocal fold tension.

Within a given language there may be variations in the manipulation of vocal fold tension and in the subglottal pressure pattern of the breath group. For example, Lieberman believes that, in contrast to the relatively constant vocal fold tension maintained in breath groups by American speakers, speakers of British English tend to begin

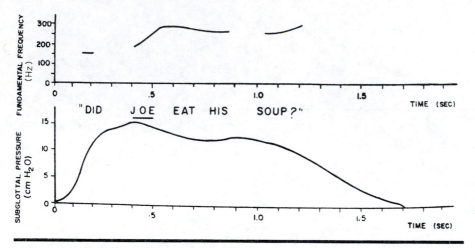

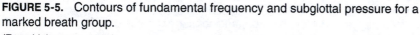

FIGURE 5-5. Contours of fundamental frequency and subglottal pressure for a marked breath group.
(From Lieberman, 1967)

a breath group with rather high vocal fold tension, which tends to decrease throughout the breath group. Ladefoged's data in Figure 5-3 were obtained from a speaker of British English; this speaker's contours of subglottal pressure do not appear to fall greatly and thus his falling intonation on statements may have been realized primarily by a decrease in vocal fold tension.

Controversy over the Breath Group Theory

The breath group theory of intonation is attractive because of its simplicity, but other research, partly by Ladefoged and his co-workers, has indicated that the production of intonation and stress may be considerably more complex. Vanderslice (1967) asked, "Is it the larynx or lungs that controls pitch?" and Ohala (1977) has reviewed the counterevidence. A primary difficulty is the fact that the subglottal pressure and vocal fold tension are not completely independent of each other. The vocal fold tension has some influence on the subglottal pressure. This is because the vocal fold action controls the flow of air from the lungs, which in turn can affect the subglottal pressure (Ohala, 1974, 1977). For example, a temporary vocal fold adjustment, for a higher pitch and inten-

sity of a stressed syllable, can reduce the airflow and raise the subglottal pressure; thus, the higher pitch may have been caused by the increased vocal fold tension and not by the accompanying increase in subglottal pressure. The conclusion reached by Ohala is that changes in vocal fold adjustments are the primary factor in producing the pitch change in stressed syllables. He has carried out further studies, measuring the effective degree of resistance of the vocal folds to airflow by monitoring the volume of air in the lungs (Ohala, 1977).

The breath group theory pointed to a basic, primitive mechanism for the general phenomenon of declining intonation. In conversation and discourse, intonation patterns, superimposed on declination by the laryngeal tensions on the vocal folds, are used to signal our attitudes and intentions, as we will discuss later in the chapter. First, let us examine how these intonational patterns may be controlled by the laryngeal and breathing mechanisms.

Larynx Muscle Actions for Stress and Intonation

The actions of the muscles of the larynx that control the tension and thickness of the vocal folds have been studied in relation to stress and intonation patterns. The action of muscles is studied by means of an electrical technique called *electromyography* or EMG. In EMG studies of the larynx the muscle activity is picked up through small electrode wires, inserted into the muscle(s) to monitor the electrical activity of each muscle. The amount of electrical activity in a muscle is correlated with the amount of tensioning force that the muscle is producing; thus, a muscle's EMG activity may be taken as an indicator of the amount of contracting force it is exerting.

The stretching forces exerted on the vocal folds are from two sets of muscles: (1) a set of muscles within the larynx, called *intrinsic laryngeal muscles*, which act directly on the front-to-back tension of the vocal folds, and (2) a set of muscles in the neck called the *strap muscles*. The strap muscles control the vertical position of the larynx as a whole. The vertical position affects the vocal folds by varying the stretching tension from below. If the larynx is held high, there is more stretching tension on the folds from the tissues of the trachea, which attach to the folds from below. If the larynx is held low, this stretching force is less.

In EMG studies of the control of intonation, simultaneous recordings are made of the pitch, the subglottal pressure, and the electrical activity of the intrinsic and strap muscles of the larynx. There have been quite a few such studies, but, because of the somewhat invasive nature of the EMG technique, only a limited number of speakers have been used, and sometimes not all of the muscles were monitored. This research is still in progress and there has been some controversy about how the results should be interpreted. A simplified version of this work follows. The student who wants to go into detail should first read Hirano and Ohala (1969), where the muscles and techniques are described, then Lieberman, Sawashima, Harris, and Gay, (1970) and Atkinson (1978). Atkinson's interpretation of the findings, which is a modified version of the breath group theory, is presented here.

Recall that the contour of change in pitch (the intonation contour) varies in downward or upward trend, depending on whether the talker is making a statement or asking a question. The intonation contour also varies in shape, depending on the stress pattern of the words spoken. The stress pattern is determined jointly by the stress patterns of the words and by the intent of the talker, who may selectively emphasize or deemphasize one or more of the words. These same linguistic maneuvers have been used to produce different contours in the studies of the relations between intonation contours, laryngeal muscle action as seen in EMG, and subglottal pressure.

The first general finding is that, in statements, the subglottal pressure seems to be the main controlling factor; in other words, the falling pitch contour of a statement is related to a falling contour in the subglottal pressure; this relation is extremely close in the low range of pitch, which tends to occur at the end of the unmarked breath group that is used for a statement having no strong emphasis on the final portion. This relation of subglottal pressure to pitch is significant for other types of statements as well. In contrast, the relation between laryngeal muscle activity and pitch is weak for statements. For questions, on the other hand, the situation is reversed. The rising intonation contours of questions were found to be accompanied by increasing amounts of activity in the intrinsic laryngeal muscles that tension the vocal folds. Also, in the part of a question where pitch is high, this relation is more close, and here the subglottal pressure seems to be a weak or ineffective factor in changing the pitch.

The strap muscles of the larynx appear to coordinate with the other two factors to adjust the pitch range in the following way: The strap muscle, which lowers the larynx, is active when the pitch is low, producing a slackness in the vocal folds, which is thought to increase the sensitivity of pitch to the subglottal pressure. When the pitch is high, the larynx-lowering strap muscle is inactive. (High and low pitch here refer to the high and low regions of normally spoken statements and questions). Thus, the strap muscles might be thought of as adjusters or facilitators for the use of the high and low ranges of the conversational voice, whereas the intrinsic muscles are primarily responsible for pitch variations within the high range and the subglottal pressure is responsible for variations within the low range.

Both laryngeal and subglottal factors can act together, however. For example, at the end of a breath group the fall of pitch with falling subglottal pressure may be prevented by increased tension from the intrinsic muscles, thus producing a marked breath group where questioning intonation is needed at the end of the breath group. Furthermore, when a syllable in a marked breath group is emphasized by the talker, a syllabic increase in subglottal pressure may be superimposed on a high tension, high-pitched portion of the breath group, or on a low-tension, low-pitched portion; the increased pressure will have more effect, raising the pitch of the syllable, if it is in a low-pitched portion of the breath group.

Intensity and Spectrum in Stressed Syllables

Thus far we have dealt primarily with the voice pitch factor in the stress patterning of speech. Other sound features from the glottal source factors in stress are the sound intensity and the spectral balance between low- and high-frequency regions. Intensity and spectrum balance are discussed just briefly.

The spectrum balance of a vowel sound can be affected by the amount of vocal effort, as noted in Chapter 4. An increase in vocal effort increases subglottal pressure and results in a steeper glottal flow wave with sharper corners. The spectrum of this wave has a shape that slopes downward more gradually than the spectrum of the more rounded glottal flow wave produced with lower subglottal pressure. Stressed syllables are spoken with greater vocal effort. Thus, on stressed syllables the source spectrum slopes downward less steeply than it does for unstressed syllables. Increased vocal fold tension might also affect the spectrum balance by boosting the high frequency end of the glottal spectrum. Stressed vowels consequently have relatively more intense amplitude in the region of F2, F3, and higher formants. This effect

was demonstrated by Lieberman (1967). These effects on the formant amplitudes are shown in speech landscapes of the word "subject" said with the two different stress patterns in the sentence "Do they refuse to subject to subjects like math?"

We may *summarize the major sound-source factors* in prosodic features as follows:

1. The fundamental voice frequency (or pitch) of vowels, responding to the amount of subglottal pressure and vocal fold tension, is higher in stressed syllables than in unstressed syllables. In addition, voice pitch shows a contour of variation (intonation contour) over the syllables of a phrase that corresponds to the grammatical function of the phrase.
2. The intensity of the vowels in stressed syllables is higher than in unstressed syllables.
3. The relative intensity of F2, F3, and higher formants is greater in vowels of stressed syllables.

DURATIONAL PROSODIC FEATURES

In addition to the glottal source factors of pitch, intensity, and spectrum, there are important durational variations that arise from prosodic conditions. We have already noted in Figures 5-2 and 5-5 that syllable stress causes a lengthening of the vowel. Durational features involve the control of the tongue and lip articulations in coordination with the presence or absence of phonation. This coordination is subject to a wide variety of prosodic influences, such as the number of syllables in a word; the location of stress; emphasis; boundaries between words, between phrases, between clauses, and between sentences; and the influence of word importance and meaning/content. These factors in articulation cause certain systematic changes in the durations of vowels and consonants, changes that have been well studied for two important reasons. First, physiologically minded phoneticians needed data that indicate how the temporal patterning of speech is organized by the brain and motor system. Second, the need for good artificial speech in computer talk-back systems, and also in text-to-speech for the blind, led to intensive searches for specific prosodic rules governing the durations of consonants and vowels. Basic data and initial rules have been published by Klatt (1975, 1976) and by Umeda (1975, 1977); Lindblom and his colleagues (Lindblom, Lyberg, & Holmgren, 1977) have studied duration patterns to arrive at principles of motor organization. The following account is based on all of this work.

Syllable Duration and Position in Breath Group

In an early study of durational prosodics, Stetson (1928; 1951, p. 113) measured the durations of syllables occurring in either initial position or final position in a breath group. Final position in the breath group was found to be associated with longer duration. Initial single syllables had a mean duration of 280 ms compared with final syllables of 310 ms. Two-syllable rhythmic units had a mean unit duration of 480 ms in initial position and 600 ms in final position in the breath group.

Vowel Duration Effects

Vowels are greatly affected in duration by a number of factors, such as the identity of the following consonant, the rate of speaking, the syllable stress, the number of syllables in the word, the position of the vowel in the phrase or sentence, the type of word, and the importance or emphasis assigned to the word by the speaker. Umeda (1975) was the first to study a large range of these effects, using extended reading from text. She found that the longest vowels were those in stressed syllables occurring at the end of phrases, clauses, or sentences. These are called prepausal stressed vowels; on the average they ranged from 150 ms for [ɪ] to 212 ms for [ɑ]. In contrast the same vowels in "function" words (that are not usually stressed), such as *in* and *on*, were much shorter, averaging 52 ms for [ɪ] and 97 ms for [ɑ]. The position and word type thus cause vowel duration changes by large factors, as great as two or three to one.

Another major factor in vowel duration is the characteristics of the consonant following the vowel. Vowels are shortened when followed by voiceless stop consonants; a typical amount of shortening was about 20 ms but the prepausal stressed vowels were shortened by an average of 40 ms. A following nasal consonant lengthens the preceding vowel if it is not prepausal and not one of the lax vowels, [ɪ, ɛ, ʌ]. Diphthongs follow rules similar to the vowels.

The importance of a word also affects its duration, especially the duration of the stressed vowel. Umeda found that a given stressed vowel is longer in words having a high meaning content, such as nouns and main verbs, than it is in words that carry little content and are more predictable from the context, such as articles and prepositions. Furthermore, when an initially unpredictable word, *father*, occurred repeatedly in the read text, the stressed vowel [ɑ] was much longer the first few times the word occurred than later.

Consonant Duration Effects

The durations of consonants are also affected by syllable stress, emphasis, the position of the consonant in the word, and grammatical conditions, as shown by Umeda (1977). The duration of the consonant was taken as the constricted or closed time as seen on spectrograms. This was measured for stops, nasals, fricatives, and [l] and [r]; the burst durations after stops were not included as part of the stop durations but were measured separately.

First consider the stop and nasal consonants that occurred between two vowels, that is, single intervocalic consonants. The average duration for types of these intervocalic consonants ranged from 25 ms to about 90 ms, depending on the location of adjacent syllable stress, of a word boundary, and on the specific consonant. The shortest average durations occurred for [t, d, n] (25, 26, 34 ms), within a word and following a stressed vowel. The longest average durations occurred for intervocalic [p, b, m] (89, 90, 86 ms), initiating a word that was a stressed syllable or a word that began with a stressed syllable. The condition of stop voicing, that is, voiced [b, d, g] versus unvoiced [p, t, k], had no effect on the consonant occlusion duration when the consonant was word initial and stressed; for poststressed stops within a word, the average occlusions for [b] and [g] were 10 and 8 ms shorter, respectively, than for [p] and [k]; the [t] and [d] in this position were very brief flaps with no difference in average duration, as is typical for American speakers.

The occurrence of a pause after the consonant had a large lengthening effect on fricative consonants. This is similar to the prepausal lengthening effect seen for vowels, but it did not occur consistently among nonfricative consonants. Consonants following a pause were predominantly [s, sh, f, m, n, l]; these were all shortened in this postpausal position.

As with vowels the duration of consonants is longer in words having a higher content of meaning, about 20 ms longer for [m] and for the stops [t, b, d], and 40 ms for [f].

It might be expected that the degree of change in duration of a consonant would be proportional to its inherent duration, that is, that long consonants, such as fricatives, would show more variation than short consonants, such as stops. However, an analysis of the amount of variation in duration of single intervocalic consonants showed no relation to the average duration of the consonant class. Rather, the widest variation occurred under conditions where there could be a wide variety of prosodic influences, such as more or less word emphasis and more or less blending (coarticulation) across word boundaries.

The unvoiced stop consonants are accompanied by a release burst of noise during the transition between the opening point of the occlusion and the point at which the voicing of the vowel begins. As seen for the occlusions, the duration of these bursts depended on prosodic conditions of word boundary, stress, pause, and meaning/content. One major series of conditions causes an increase in both burst duration and occlusion duration, generated by factors of intersyllabic pause, word boundary, and stress locations relative

to the stop. However, if the stop is at the end of a word, there is little burst duration regardless of different occlusion durations; if it follows a nasal consonant, the burst duration may be normally long or short, but with proportionately much shorter occlusion duration.

Fant, Kruckenberg, and Nord (1991) and Fant and Kruckenberg (1995) studied stress durational effects in Swedish, English, and French. They measured the durations of all the syllables and phonemes in the oral readings of a brief (1-minute) passage from a Swedish novel by a native speaker of each language. The French and English readings were translations of the Swedish passage. These data were examined to describe how syllables are lengthened by stress and shortened by unstress, of various degrees, and in various utterance locations. Other prosodic phenomena, such as inter-stress intervals, isochrony and auditory prominence, are considerably elucidated. Within syllables, French CV units, consonants and their following vowels, accounted for the syllable-lengthening of stress. In Swedish, VCs, vowels and their following consonants, accounted for most stress-lengthening of syllables. In English, CVs and VCs are lengthened about equally. English and Swedish stress-induced lengthening is greater than in French. French unstressed vowels show much less shortening and vowel-reduction toward neutral in their formant patterns, than do Swedish and English (Delattre, 1969).

Rules Describing Durational Effects

Klatt (1973) noted that there was a limit to the temporal compressibility of vowels when they are affected by a combination of two shortening factors, namely, when followed by an unvoiced consonant and/or by an additional syllable, compared with the long vowel seen in a monosyllable that ends in a voiced consonant. He later expressed this incompressibility in a formula (Klatt, 1975), which was also applied as a rule to adjust consonant durations for various shortening effects (Klatt, 1976).

Lindblom and colleagues (1977) and Umeda (1977) have also proposed rules expressing lengthening and shortening effects for vowels and consonants. The Lindblom rules are the most general; they are mathematical statements of the operation of three principles: (1) The greater the number of subunits in a unit of speech, the shorter is each subunit, (2) each subunit is shorter up to a limit of compressibility, and (3) the number of subunits following a given subunit has a greater shortening effect than the number of preceding subunits. These principles are seen to operate for both small and large subunits, that is, for vowels and consonants as subunits of syllables, for syllables as subunits of words, and for words or phrases as subunits of sentences. Word-final and phrase-final (prepausal) lengthening are thus accounted for as being less shortened, by principle (3).

Going even further, Lindblom and colleagues (1977) proposed a tentative theory of motor organization of any sequence of syllables. The theory invokes only two principles to account for the various durational phenomena seen. One principle puts a limitation on the number of units that can be held in motor memory waiting to be performed. The other principle involves economy of effort for performing the transitions between adjacent units. For more on this theory, see Chapter 10.

Rules like these are used to improve the intelligibility and naturalness of artificial speech produced by computer from printed text or typed sentences. They also have important implications for further research on how the brain organizes the production of speech and controls the speech movements. Furthermore, these rules may have considerable potential for application in speech training and therapy.

ORAL TRACT SHAPING FACTOR

Thus far in our study of prosodic features we have described two factors in prosodic variations. First, the voice source is the origin of changes in pitch, intensity, and spectrum, depending on the prosodic stress patterns of words and phrases; second,

the articulatory movements of the vowels and consonants produce differences in the durations of vowels and consonants depending on stress patterns and position in sentence or phrase. These two factors, that is, the voice source variations and the timing of articulatory movement, are the most important factors for the prosody of English.

In addition, there are some systematic differences in oral tract shape depending on stress and emphasis; the shape differences result in vowel formant differences, as we see in Figure 5-6. In English these are highly correlated with differences in pitch, intensity, and duration, and the formant differences do not seem to be as noticeable as the intensity differences. Thus, the oral tract shape differences do not seem to be of primary importance in the communication of English stress patterns. Nevertheless, these articulatory shaping differences are an interesting feature of some languages, and they have been well-studied because they are important for understanding the motor organization of speech and historical sound-changes in languages. Let us look at these effects briefly.

The effect of stress on oral tract shape is audible if one listens carefully to words like *ob*ject versus ob*ject* spoken in sentences like *That's an object* and *He didn't object*. In *ob*ject the [ɑ] of the first syllable sounds [ɑ]-like in quality and has formant frequencies similar to those of a specimen [ɑ] vowel; however, in ob*ject*, the "[ɑ]" is very different in quality; it sounds more like the neutral vowel; in fact, the formant frequencies are shifted toward the positions for the neutral [ə] vowel. Another such pair of words is *re*ject versus re*ject* in *A reject is bad* and *To reject is bad*. A similar effect occurs in Swedish between certain pairs of words where the stress patterns are the only word-differentiating factor. In general, the effect is for an unstressed vowel to have a partially neutralized, reduced vowel quality.

This effect, where the unstressed version of a vowel has more neutral formant positions than the stressed vowel, is called *vowel reduction*. There are languages that do not show vowel reduction in unstressed vowels. A review of acoustic studies of

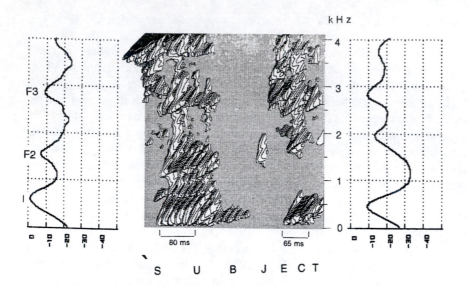

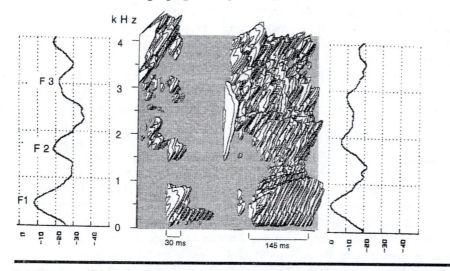

FIGURE 5-6. Speech landscapes and vowel spectra showing the effects of syllable stress on the formants, particularly F2 and F3. The vowel spectra of the two "sub" syllables (on the left) show a large stress difference, with F2 and F3 amplitudes much higher relative to F1 in the lower left spectrum plot (stressed) than in the upper left plot (unstressed). Comparing the vowels of the two "ject" syllables on the right, the unstressed vowel (upper right spectrum) is not simply a neutralized version of the stressed vowel below; it appears to have been fronted, bringing F2 and F3 closer together and raising their amplitude relative to F1. You will also see that the stressed versions of the vowels are longer in duration; measured durations appear below each vowel.

(Perspectrograms and average pre-emphasized spectra plotted via SpeechStation2 from Sensimetrics Corporation) vowel reduction in different languages is given by Lehiste (1970, pp. 139–142).

There are several acoustic studies of vowel reduction in English and Swedish. Tiffany (1959) used 20 American talkers speaking short test sentences; Lindblom (1963) used a Swedish talker speaking selected syllables in a "carrier" phrase that had different stress patterns. These studies measured the formant frequencies and durations of the stressed and unstressed versions of nearly all the vowels of English and Swedish, keeping the adjacent consonants constant. The results of the Swedish study showed very consistent reduction of the duration of the unstressed vowel relative to its stressed version and displacement of the frequency of F2 toward a more neutral position. For example, the F2 of long stressed [ih] in the syllable *did* was about 2200 Hz, but in the short unstressed [ih] F2 was shifted downward (toward the neutral position of 1500 Hz) to about 2000 Hz; in the syllable [dɔd] the long stressed [ɔ] had a low F2 of about 850 and the F2 of short unstressed [aw] was shifted upward to 1150 Hz. The displacement of F2 toward neutral was fairly regular in that it was correlated to a significant degree with the amount of decrease in duration relative to the long stressed version of the vowel. On the other hand, in the American study some of the vowels showed the expected neutralization of F2 but others did not; the duration and pitch changes were quite consistent: There was longer duration and higher pitch on the stressed versions of all the vowels.

There are several differences between these two experiments that might have produced the discrepancy in F2 neutralization, but perhaps the most important difference is that meaningful sentences were employed in the American study in contrast to the somewhat artificial carrier phrases of the Swedish study. Furthermore, the stress variations in the American study were produced by the talkers by means of emphasizing or not emphasizing the words containing the test vowels, that is, by attempting to signal the importance attached to key words. In the Swedish experiment the talker may have been operating more as a strictly rhythmic producer of stress and thus the extent of his articulatory movements toward a given vowel position might have been more consistently subject to foreshortening on the shorter vowels. In a later Swedish experiment (Stalhammar, Karlsson, & Fant, 1974), the long Swedish vowels, spoken in connected speech, showed small neutralization effects, but the short vowels showed larger, more consistent neutralization.

Gay (1978) carried out a study of vowel reduction where both the rate of utterance and the stress were systematically varied. The talkers were American phoneticians and they were instructed to try to maintain vowel identity in the unstressed versions of the vowels and not to reduce them all the way to neutral. The unstressed vowels were found to be shorter and lower in pitch than their stressed versions, for both rapid and slow speech. There was some neutralization in formant frequencies in the slowly spoken unstressed vowels compared with the formants of rapidly spoken stressed vowels of about the same duration as the unstressed vowels. However, the rapid rate of speaking per se did not produce formant neutralization; the rapidly spoken stressed vowels, although shorter than the slowly spoken stressed vowels, were not neutralized in formant frequencies; the same was true of the unstressed vowels. This result implies that the mechanisms controlling the articulators operate differently in producing rate changes and stress, even though both affect vowel duration. Slis (1975) found that stress produces an earlier movement toward the initial consonant of a stressed syllable compared with an unstressed syllable.

On the whole it appears that the oral tract shape of a vowel may be affected not only by the stress pattern but also by the vowel system of the particular language, and even by the momentary need of the speaker to communicate a word as clearly as possible. The intention of the speaker as a factor in vowel shaping is implied by one of the duration findings of Umeda, mentioned earlier, and by the low degree of vowel reduction by Gay's speakers, who were instructed to maintain vowel identity in their unstressed syllables.

INTONATION IN DISCOURSE

Our conversations and speeches are intended to communicate not only information about events, persons' actions and objects, but also our attitudes about them. The information governs our linguistic choices and grammatical formulations, the formal, linguistic phonology, but the empathetic, expressive, attentive, and intentional aspects of speaking, interpretations and attitudes about the information, are of equal if not primary importance to us. In linguistics both the information and these more personal aspects of social intercourse are conveyed by speech melodies or tunes called intonation patterns. Perhaps the very first tunes we hear as infants are those special changes in pitch of "motherese" that we described earlier.

Language communities in general evolve systems of intonational signaling, usually distinctive to each language, that speakers use to express their attitudes and feelings about what they are saying. In other words, intonations are conventionalized and made part of the social language system; in discourse they are used with reference to speakers' and listeners' shared beliefs about topics and statements. For any given discourse, the pragmatic, affective, or even emotional outcomes are the result of the participants' attitudes conveyed by the use of the formal, linguistic intonation conventions.

Considering the wide variety of languages, communities, and what they might be about, there are of course many systems of linguistic analysis of meanings in discourse, making up the rich and fascinating field of pragmatics under study by linguists. The phonetic system of tunes used in native English has been analyzed by M. Y. Liberman and his colleagues. As an example we will describe part of an English discourse model of Pierrehumbert and Hirschberg (1990), which we will call the PHH model of intonation.

The PHH model aims to codify the intonation patterns commonly used in interpersonal discourse. Intonation is used by speakers to focus the hearer's attention to particular words or meanings and to express attitudes and intentions about the spoken information. The model's units are the simplest possible code levels of relative pitch: high-pitched peaks, H; low-pitched regions, L; and combinations of these events with stress (*) and end of utterance (%). At the same time the pitch patterns used must conform to the stress patterns of the words and the grammar. Speakers compose tunes of voice pitches that are special intonational phrases that have boundary marks. The boundaries of a tune phrase may be determined by its sequence of pitches as well as by non-tonal stress factors, such as duration and articulatory reach of the vowels. The tunes themselves are composed of three types of intonation change or accents: (1) *pitch accents*, on the stressed syllable of the focal or emphasized word of the phrase; (2) *phrase accents*, which signal the end of a phrase and the beginning of the next; and (3) *boundary tone*, which signals the end of the utterance.

To look at how we can use the PHH model to describe the intonational signaling in a discourse, I recorded a brief interchange, with myself as Talker A and also as Talker B in the following dialogue:

TALKER A, THE AUTHORITY: "Only a millionaire can have a house with round-windowed sun-lighted rooms."

TALKER B, QUESTIONING AUTHORITY: "Only a millionaire?"

TALKER A, FLATLY FINAL: "Only a millionaire."

The tracks of voice pitch for the interchange are plotted in Figure 5-7, where we may examine the crucial changes in voice pitch. Keep in mind that the PHH model is designed to codify the changes used by speakers to emphasize particular words and to express attitudes over particular phrases. In the top half of the figure we can first see that the Authority statement starts with a rather high pitch and a large swing down and up while the subsequent parts are spoken with a generally lower pitch level and perhaps with less variation.

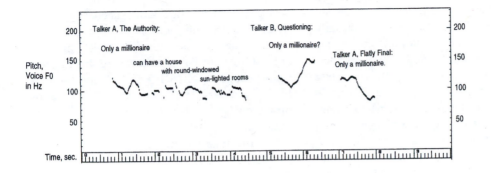

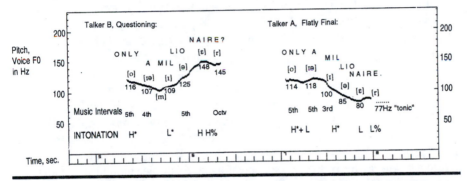

FIGURE 5-7. Analysis of a dialogue to illustrate the Pierrehumbert/Hirschberg (PHH) model for characterizing intonational patterns of voice pitch. The top panel gives the texts spoken in relation to the pitch track of each part of the dialogue. There are three utterances, Talker A making a statement, Talker B questioning A, and Talker A answering in a part re-statement with finality. The texts are adapted material from Pierrehumbert and Hirschberg (1990) acted out and analyzed by the author. The bottom panel expands the tracks of the question and the answer, for the analysis. Vowels and their pitch values are indicated on each track. See text for details of the PHH intonation analysis to arrive at the accent codes indicated by the different H and L symbols contrasting the question and answer. Talker A's initial, authoritative propositional statement, analyzed to illustrate application of PHH intonation analysis to an extended utterance. The utterance is presented as a spectrogram where some of the vowels are indicated for orientation and with a pitch track plotted below. Under the pitch track we give average pitch values of vowels at peak and valley features identified for the PHH analysis of the tunes the talker used within each of the four phrases of the utterance. A discussion of each of the four tunes is given in the text.

(Utterance text material adapted from Pierrehumbert & Hirschberg, 1990; acoustic plots, data analysis, and values via SpeechStation2 from Sensimetrics Corporation)

Then when Talker B questions A's statement, "Only a millionaire?", his voice pitch is generally very high and swings down and up to an extreme on the emphasized word "millionaire." Furthermore, there is a striking contrast between Talker B's Questioning swings of pitch and Talker A's final drop in pitch to confirm his original meaning; here Talker A emphasizes "Only" and signals finality with a very steep drop to an extreme of low pitch at the end of "millionaire."

In the bottom panel of Figure 5-7 I have stretched the two contrasting pitch plots and shown the location of each vowel and its pitch so we can see exactly how I codified with the PHH model. At the bottom of the plots are the accent codes for the intonation contours, or phrase tunes of Talker B's Questioning phrase and Talker A's single-phrase restatement.

The Question begins with a high tone H on the stressed (*) vowel [o], a combination indicated by H*. This vowel is pitched at 116 Hz, compared with the speaker's overall mean of about 100 Hz. The high tone is set off for stress and from the following questioning rise in intonation by falling to a nadir low tone, L, reached during the [m] of "millionaire." The steep questioning rise during *millionaire* places the correct lexical stress on the last syllable with a high tone, H, at 148 Hz and virtually simultaneous with a boundary tone, H%.

Talker A's restatement emphasizes *only a* with a high-pitched stressed level, H*, 114–118 Hz, and then confirms *millionaire* with a very steep drop to the finality of an LL% tone of only 80 Hz, with only a slight rise and lengthening of [r] to breathiness, perhaps as the vestige of the proper lexical stress on the final syllable of the word.

Another interesting way to describe these melodies is to treat them as musical tunes. To try this I converted pitches of the phrases to relative musical intervals by assuming an octave scale to span the difference between the lowest pitch, 77 Hz, reached in the breathy phonation of [r] indicated by the dotted lines at the end, and the highest pitch, 148 Hz, reached at the height of the questioning. The pitches of the phrase tunes in these terms of music interval positions within this

octave are noted in the bottom panel of Figure 5-7 under corresponding vowels of the phrases. You can hear these phrase melodies by playing in the key of C on your guitar or keyboard: for Talker B, Questioning ----- G ↘F ↗G ↗C; for Talker A, Flatly Final ----- G G ↘E ↘C. (The up-arrow means go up for that note and the down-arrow means go down). You will hear one of our most used basic tune contrasts, the Question and the Answer. In music these eight notes might be called a question-answer motif ending with a resolution on the tonic note of the scale.

However, in their study of Japanese tone patterns Pierrehumbert and Beckman (1988) found that, although the tonal relations of accentual types were proportionately scalable and consistent arbitrary ratios were used, these were not integral ratios like those in music.

The PHH model is intended to codify many more extended speech melodies than the single-phrase utterances we have just analyzed. To do this, the same coding system is simply applied to each successive phrase of an extended utterance. We take Talker A's original authoritative-style statement as an example, plotted in Figure 5-8. Here we have plotted the pitch track underneath a broadband spectrogram in the course of which we have identified some of the vowels for orientation between the spectrogram and the pitch track. The scale of the pitch track is the same, 10 Hz per division, as previously. A normally rather laconic speaker, A's entire statement ranges within only 36 Hz, from 116 Hz at its peak to a low of 80 Hz near the end. Nevertheless, his pitch variations are expressive of the relationships he intends to impart to Talker B for a possible rejoinder.

Adopting PHH analysis for Figure 5-8 we may break the continuous, total statement into four phrases, each with a different intonation melody. We will characterize these as the Initial Phrase (1), *Only a millionaire*; an Intermediate Phrase (2) *can have a house*; another Intermediate Phrase (3), *with round-windowed*; and Terminal Phrase (4), *sun-lighted rooms*. I have coded the phrases in PHH-terms below the pitch track. In

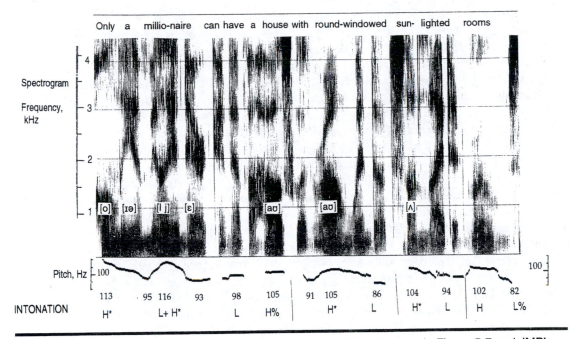

FIGURE 5-8.   Relations between the spectrographic analysis of the utterance in Figure 5-7 and JMP's use of PHH model of intonation and the corresponding pitch track.

addition, the F0 values of corresponding vowels are given at each crucial peak or valley.

Phrase 1 has its primary or focal stress, also that of the entire utterance, on the middle of *millionaire*, signaled by the H peak together with the stress mark (*); notice though that *only*, since it expresses Talker A's upcoming exclusionary proposition, also receives some emphasis by starting with a high pitch. The phrase pitch level averages 104.5 Hz.

Intermediate Phrase 2 emphasizes *house* by means of a low-to-high contour skipping up to the [aʊ] from the low start of the phrase. This intonation resets to begin lower than the previous average phrase level of pitch, at an intermediate level lower than the long, strongly stressed word to come, but higher that the ending pitch level of the previous phrase, signaling that more is being said about the *millionaire*. The L H* contour of Phrase 2 breaks from Phrase 1 but also still continues a high relationship at a mean level of 105 Hz.

Phrase 3 intermediates downward, starting a pitch declination toward finality, but preserving a *house*-qualifying stress on *round* as to the *windows*, with a H*+L contour. The mean pitch has dropped to 96 Hz.

Phrase 4 stresses the *sun* in the *rooms* with the tune H*+L plus H+L% to emphasize the final referent, *rooms*, the parts of the *house* that A is talking about. The final low pitch, signified by L%, finishes the multi-phrase statement at 82 Hz.

Discourse intentions and interactions of speakers of English are conveyed by voice melodies of the above types. New items or topics may be indicated by resetting talkers' ranges. Still, the same simple classification of peak and low regions of pitch, in conjunction with the stress patterns of the lexical word and the desired word-emphasis, seems to cover many of the contingencies of informational discourse (Pierrehumbert & Hirschberg, 1990). For some further uses of prosodic models to analyze informational speech, see the special issue of *Phonetica*, edited by Barry, Diehl, and Kohler (1993).

An interesting study to generate emotional expression in synthetic speech was carried out by Janet Cahn, for her MS thesis at MIT. She used adjustments of intonation (pitch patterns), speaking manner, and voice qualities, as indicated by the research literature of previous acoustical analyses of emotions in speech. These adjustments were programmed automatically by an "Affect Editor" to simulate six different emotions: Angry, Disgusted, Glad, Sad, Scared, or Surprised. Listeners were able to correctly identify the intended emotions in 54% of the thirty sentences they heard, far above the chance level of 17% correct (for the six possible emotions). The best emotion score was obtained on the five Sad sentences at 91% correct, the worst was for Disgusted (42%). Disgusted and Angry were frequently confused with each other, possibly because of their common low amount of hesitation. Some of the Sad speech features were: a breaking voice with pitch discontinuities and hesitations, breathiness, and a restricted pitch range with smaller than normal lowering of pitch at the end of the sentences (Cahn, 1990).

PACING, RHYTHMS, AND LANGUAGES

People rarely speak in unexpected fast bursts, nor do they suddenly slow down to a crawl. The overall pace of speaking usually remains rather steady over appreciable periods of time. Probably this makes it easier to communicate, because the listener can "lock on" and keep in step with the speaker, or even anticipate the pacing of what will be said.

Pacing and rhythmic patterning are important features of every language. Pacing provides a steady progression for organizing articulations. Rhythmic patterning provides the framework for the speaker's detailed timing of articulatory movements and a corresponding framework for the listener's perception.

Individual languages exhibit distinctly different temporal pacing in their spoken phrases and sentences. For example, French sounds as if it is paced with equal time between syllables; Swedish and English, on the other hand, sound as if they are paced with equal time between stresses. So, French is said to be *syllable-paced*, or syllable-timed; Swedish and English are said to be *stress-paced*, or stress-timed.

Why should languages exhibit such differences? How can they be accounted for? A likely possibility would be that they are due to interaction between steady pacing and the rhythmic, stress-pattern differences among the languages. Pacing differences might be "forced" by the typical lexical stress patterns of each language. In French words, syllable stress is not specified by the dictionary; any syllable of a word may be spoken with primary stress; the only word-stress rule is that pre-pausal syllables receive a minor stress, usually expressed with a pitch rise. In contrast, English and Swedish words have stress patterns specified in the lexicon and, to be understood, must be spoken as specified.

Fant and colleagues (1991), described above, also developed data from which to try to pinpoint the sources of the syllable-paced impression of French versus stress-paced Swedish and English. They concluded that there is less acoustical contrast between stressed and unstressed syllables in French, compared with English and Swedish where the stress-patterns of words are specified and highly important. French shows less vowel reduction, both in duration and formant pattern, and therefore sounds like a rapid succession of rather evenly emphasized syllables. Swedish and English, on the other hand, especially Swedish, have highly prominent stressed syllables and weak unstressed syllables, and therefore sound like a slower succession of rhythmic phrases.

TONE LANGUAGES

Many persons speak languages that employ patterns of pitch variation to distinguish between different meanings of words that have the same pattern of consonants and vowels. Tone features in tone languages are segmental and phonemic in function. That is to say, the tones for a word are specified in the lexicon, the dictionary of a tone language. Thus, the tones are segmental features and strictly speaking not prosodic or suprasegmental. But tones are produced by the same glottal mechanisms for voice-pitch variations and so can be expected to interact with suprasegmental prosodic variations. One of the tone languages, Mandarin Chinese, is the most popular world language; it is spoken by more than 800 million, compared with about 400 million speakers of English and 300 million each of Spanish and Russian (Burling, 1992, pp. 89, 91). An example of a tonal difference in Chinese (from Ladefoged, 1993, pp. 252–256) is [ma], which means *mother* if spoken with a level, high pitch but, if spoken with a falling high pitch, it means *scold*.

Japanese is one of the tone languages that has been studied very intensively to discover its tonal codings. We will illustrate with one example from the work of Pierrehumbert (Pierrehumbert & Beckman, 1988). Figure 5-9 compares the pitch tracks of two utterances, pitch-accented and unaccented, with identical phoneme sequences of [mai] and [me]. When [mai] is pitch-accented, the solid pitch track in the figure with a high peak on [mai] and a following low pitch on [me], it means "good-tasting beans." But when [mai] and [me] are unaccented, spoken with the same pitch level, the dashed track in the figure, the meaning of [mai] switches to "sweet" and the meaning of [me] is "candies." Thus the makeup of a meaning unit in Japanese may be unchanged in its phonemes, here the sequences /mai/ and /me/, but signify different meanings depending on relative pitch levels.

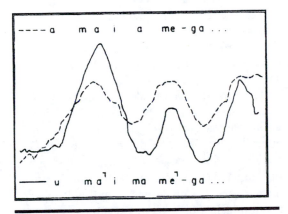

FIGURE 5-9. An example of contrasting pitch tracks in Japanese that differentiate utterance meanings solely on the basis of tonal differences on the same phoneme sequence. The sequences [mai] and [me] receive an accented High-Low relation (solid pitch track) to mean "good-tasting beans" to contrast with the meaning "sweet candies" when the two sequences are unaccented and equal in pitch.

(From Pierrehumbert & Beckman, *Japanese Tone Structure*, MIT Press, Cambridge, MA, 1988.)

SUMMARY

The rhythms and intonations of a language are formed under definite rules and these prosodic rules have fundamental functions in the code of every language. The prosodic features are produced by special manipulations of the glottal sound source, by the timing of articulatory movements and by the shape-configuration of the vocal tract. The source factors operate through actions of the speech breathing muscles and the vocal folds; the timing factors operate through the movements of the upper articulators. The two main factors in the glottal source variations for prosodic features are: (1) the tension on the vocal folds and (2) the subglottal air pressure. These affect the fundamental frequency, the amplitude, and the source spectrum. Increasing the subglottal air pressure increases the fundamental frequency or pitch of the voice and also the intensity. The pressure increase is produced by increasing the expiratory forces on the lungs.

The relations between the subglottal expiratory mechanism for controlling intonation and the mechanism of the muscle tension on the vocal folds have been studied experimentally to explain the acoustic effects seen as features of stress and intonation. The intonation contour for a statement generally shows a down-going pitch, which may be correlated with a decrease in subglottal pressure toward the end of the statement. However, superimposed on this may be variations in the pitch due to the syllable stress of the utterance and the speaker's emphasis. For expressing a question, the pitch contour rises during the utterance because of increased vocal fold tension and, again, the stressed syllable will have a higher pitch than the other syllables. The stressed syllable generally corresponds to a peak in the subglottal pressure that, other factors equal, will raise the syllable pitch.

A breath group theory of intonation has been proposed, which states simply that the intonation contour will naturally always fall toward the end of a breath group because of the lower subglottal pressure just before taking a new breath of air. Then this basic breath group contour can be marked as a question through an increase in vocal fold tension to raise the pitch or maintain it at a higher level than dictated by the subglottal pressure. The theory assumes, in its simple form, a high degree of independence of the two factors, vocal fold tension and subglottal pressure, in determining pitch. Some investigators believe that the vocal fold tension factor is the dominant factor, not the breath group cycle. A recent study of the vocal fold tension through electromyography indicated that the breath group theory had to be modified such that the intonation contours are controlled primarily by vocal fold tension in the high-pitched parts of a contour and by subglottal pressure in the lower-pitched parts of a contour. The vertical position of the larynx is thought to be an adjusting factor determining which control factor dominates, the vocal fold tension or the subglottal pressure.

Another glottal source factor related to stress and intonation is the sound intensity and the spectral balance between the low and high regions of the glottal source spectrum. Increased subglottal pressure will increase the intensity of the glottal source sound and raise the high frequency part of the source spectrum relative to the low frequency part. Thus, stressed vowels may have a higher amplitude in F2 and the higher formants than unstressed vowels.

In addition to the glottal source, there are important durational variations that arise from prosodic conditions. In general, a syllable is longer in final position in a breath group. Within breath groups, at places where pauses may occur at the end of phrases and clauses, the vowels are longer. If a word is an unstressed function word, the vowels are shorter. The characteristics of consonants that follow a vowel have a strong effect on the preceding vowel duration. In particular vowels are shortened when followed by voiceless consonants. The importance of a word also affects its duration, especially in the duration of the main vowel of the word. Consonant durations are also affected by factors of the syllable stress and the position of the syllable in the utterance, in similar ways to the effects on vowel duration.

Rules describing the prosodic effects on the durations of vowels and consonants have been formulated by phoneticians who are interested in these rules for synthesizing correct speech expression and for explaining the motor organization of speech production. In general, these rules express the fact that the greater the number of subunits in a larger unit the shorter is each subunit up to a limit of compressibility. Another general rule is that the number of subunits that follow a given consonant or vowel has a greater shortening effect than the number of preceding subunits. One theory explains these rules on the basis that only a limited number of units can be held in the motor memory waiting to be performed and, second, that a principle of economy of effort applies for performing the sequence of units.

Tonal changes in the pitch of the voice are employed by languages and speakers to fulfill discriminative and contrastive functions at all levels of speech communication: phonemic, lexical, grammatic, attentional, and attitudinal.

CHAPTER SIX

CONSONANT FEATURES, GLIDES, AND STOPS

There . . is something gross and brash and materialist about consonants:
They are made by banging things together, rubbing, hissing, buzzing.
Vowels . . are pure music—woodwind to the consonantal percussion.
—Anthony Burgess, *A Mouthful of Air*, 1992, p. 68

Here we begin our study of the acoustic patterns of consonants. The main acoustic features of consonants and how each feature is produced are described, beginning with the classification of consonants according to their articulatory features. Next, consonant production and vowel production are compared, and the acoustic patterns corresponding to each of the different articulatory features are described. The "woodwind" glissandi of glide consonants are explained and compared with diphthongs and stop consonants. Further chapters describe the buzzing of nasals, the banging stops, the hissing fricatives, voicing murmurs, and the places in the mouth where all these sounds are made.

ARTICULATORY FEATURES OF CONSONANTS

A group of consonants that are articulated with the same pattern or feature forms a description class for the group. Thus, sets of consonants can be thought of very succinctly in classes according to how the vocal organs are adjusted and moved in making them; these classes are often called *articulatory features*. Examples are the class *glide*, containing consonants like [j, w, r], which in English are all produced with a relatively continuous movement of the tongue to a partial constriction; or *stop*,

containing examples like [b, d, g], which are produced with a rather sudden movement to a complete obstruction.

The articulatory features of consonants are of three types: (1) features of manner of articulation, (2) the voicing feature, and (3) features of place of articulation. The manner and voicing features are types or states of articulation that can occur with any place of articulation; the voicing feature is either voiced or unvoiced; the manner features are glide, stop (plosive), nasal, and fricative. There are three subsidiary types of glide articulation: semi-vowel [w, j], lateral [1], and retroflex [r]. There are three general places of articulation—front, middle, and back—and at each general place there are two or three subsidiary places. The English consonants are shown in Table 6-1 arranged in rows corresponding to place of articulation and in columns corresponding to manner of articulation. You may already be familiar with articulatory classification of consonants from a study of general phonetics. If not, you should memorize the classification because it is so commonly used in discussing consonants and it forms the basis for our study here.

Consonants differ from vowels in two main ways: (1) in vocal tract shaping and (2) in sound sources. The sound source for vowels is always periodic, but a consonant may be produced with a

TABLE 6-1. The English consonants, grouped by types of articulatory production and some corresponding distinctive features (italics). In the distinctive features system, the voicing feature is the default state, and the voiceless consonants are produced with Glottis Spread.

ARTICULATORY FEATURES	NAME OF FEATURE						DISTINCTIVE FEATURES
	Nonobstruent		*Obstruent*				
	Sonorant		*Interrupted*		*Continuant*		
Manner	Glide	Nasal	Stop		Fricative		*Articulator*
		Ported					*Velar Port*
			Voiced	Voiceless Glottis Spread	Voiced	Voiceless Glottis Spread	
			?			h	*Glottis*
Place of Articulation							
Front							
Bilabial	w	m	b	p		ʌ	*Lips*
Labiodental					v	f	
Middle							
Dental					ð	θ	*Tongue Blade (Coronal)*
Alveolar	l	n	d	t	z	s	
Palatal	r (retroflex)				ʒ	ʃ	
Back							
Velar	j	ŋ	g	k			*Tongue Body (Dorsal)*

periodic sound source, an aperiodic sound source, or a combination of periodic and aperiodic sources. Aperiodic sources of consonant sound are caused by constrictions in the vocal tract. Consonants often include aperiodic sound because the tract constrictions for many consonants are so narrow that the airflow of the breath stream becomes turbulent. Turbulent airflow generates an aperiodic sound. The periodic sound source for consonants is the airflow fluctuations resulting from the periodic movements of the vocal folds, just as for vowels.

The vocal tract shaping of consonants constricts the tract to a larger degree than for vowels.

The stop consonants, such as [p, b, t], obstruct the breath stream completely during a portion of the articulatory gesture. The fricative consonants, such as [ʃ, s, z], are formed with a very narrow constriction. Even the glide consonants, [w] and [j], constrict the oral tract more than do the corresponding close vowels, [u] and [i].

The constriction differences cause important general differences in sound pattern between consonants and vowels. The openness of the oral tract during vowels gives them the general characteristic of strong, voice-pulsed sound. In contrast, the constrictedness of consonants causes them to have weaker voiced sound, aperiodic sound, or absence of sound. These differences are discussed briefly now, and again later in more detail for the various types of consonants.

The stop or plosive consonants [p, t, k, b, d, g] are produced by a movement that completely occludes the vocal tract. During the occlusion there is either complete silence or only weak, low frequency sound. There is a complete silence for an unvoiced stop; during the occlusion of a voiced stop there is only the sound of the very lowest harmonics as long as voicing is maintained during the occlusion. As we shall see later, certain conditions often suppress the voicing of voiced stops.

When the occlusion of a stop consonant is released to form a following vowel, a transient and, for unvoiced stops, a burst of noise-like sound occur during the release. Thus, in contrast to the continuous, strong, voiced sound of vowels, the stop consonants have an interval that is silent, or nearly so, followed by a release burst of sound.

The nonplosive consonants are the glides [w, j, r, l], the nasals [m, n, ŋ], and the fricatives [s, ʃ, f, θ, z, ʒ, v, ð]. These are produced by movements that form partial constrictions of the vocal tract. Partial constriction causes either a reduced voiced sound during the constriction or, for fricatives, a noise-like aperiodic sound caused by a turbulent sound source. The voiced sound produced during the constrictions of the glides and nasals is weaker than for vowels, especially in the region of F2 and above. Usually, the noise-like

sounds of the unvoiced fricatives [s, ʃ, f, θ] have more energy at middle and high frequencies, above 2 kHz, than at lower frequencies; in contrast, voiced sounds always have more energy in the low frequencies, below 1 kHz, than at higher frequencies.

DISTINCTIVE FEATURES

Certain acoustic features correspond to the articulatory features, and, in turn, the acoustic features are heard by the listener to distinguish each consonant from all the others. The relations among articulatory, acoustic, and perceptual features form a theory of distinctive features. A theory of distinctive features constructs category systems for phonemes; the categories are designed to cover all languages. Each feature category is derived by joint consideration of three levels of linguistic analysis: the perceptual distinctions that work in the language, the corresponding acoustic differences, and their articulatory origins. Thus, the purpose of distinctive feature theory is to provide a single consistent framework across languages for specifying the phonology, that is, the vowels and consonants and how they work to communicate (Chomsky & Halle, 1968; Halle, 1992; Jakobson et al., 1951; Stevens, 1994). In Table 6-1 we displayed the English consonants according to their articulatory features and, in italics around the periphery, according to distinctive features of English phonology. Not all the distinctive features of the theory are used here because we are dealing only with consonants and with no other languages. The names of distinctive features used by linguists are printed in slanted italics while the names of consonant articulatory features are in straight-up fonts.

Distinctive feature theory has been highly useful in the study of the sound patterns (phonology) of the world's languages. However, our purpose is more limited. We will deal mostly with English and primarily with physiological and acoustic phonetics. Thus, our description in the following

Phonology Note:
The Variegated Universe
of Consonants

The languages of the world employ a fantastic variety of consonant maneuvers, a phenomenon that may be appreciated by looking at the articulatory features found necessary for the Stanford Phonology Archiving Project (pp. 10–25 in Crothers, Lorentz, Sherman, & Vihman, 1979) or in Ladefoged's *Preliminaries to Linguistic Phonetics* (1971). There are at least 20 different places of articulation, all combinable with some or all of the degrees and types of constriction and sound sources. However, it is also remarkable that certain types of features are favored, used much more frequently when all languages are surveyed. Obstruent consonants, that is, articulations that more or less block the vocal tract temporarily, seem to be employed for distinctions most frequently. For example, I counted 409 different obstruents, compared with only 139 non-obstruents, in the phoneme index of the UPSID (see our Chapter One). Obstruent examples occurred in descending numbers in the classes stops, fricatives, affricates, clicks and glottals, and non-obstruents classed as approximants (glides), nasals, and flaps. Is it that obstruents, especially stops, can somehow be performed more easily and are more distinctive phonetically?

chapters of the acoustic patterns of consonants follows a classification according to articulatory features rather than distinctive features.

GLIDE CONSONANTS AND DIPHTHONGS

We concentrate first on the manner features, then on the voicing feature, and finally on the place features. This order is the order of importance of the features in their phonemic function in English (Carterette & Jones, 1974; Denes, 1963). We can begin our study with glide consonants, taking advantage of the fact that glides are similar to the vowels we have already studied.

Let us look first at the articulatory actions for the glide features and their corresponding acoustic features: the contrast between glide consonants and diphthongs and voiced stops, and then the differences among the voiced glides [w, j, r, l]. The unvoiced continuant [ʍ] is discussed in the next chapter.

The semivowel glide consonants, [w] and [j], when combined with vowels, are similar to diphthongs; the differences are that the glide consonants are produced with a constriction that is greater than the closest vowels and the articulatory movements to and from the glide constriction are faster than the movement between the two vowels of a diphthong.

Let us examine how the glide consonants are produced. The production of a consonant involves four important physiological factors: (1) the constricting effect of the consonant articulation on the oral tract, (2) the subglottal air pressure, (3) the air pressure in the mouth, and (4) the state of the vocal folds. Figure 6-1A shows the action of each of these factors in the production of the phrase *a Y* [əwaɪ]. This phrase contains the glide [w] and the diphthong [aɪ] for comparison.

Each of the first four numbered rows in Figure 6-1 represents the movement, state, or pattern of one of the four factors. The last row (5) shows a spectrogram of the sound patterns of the phrase marked with lines to show how the sound patterns are related to the four production factors. The articulatory factors are schematic; the spectrogram was made from the utterance of an adult male speaker.

In row 1 the basic phases of the oral tract movement are traced. These are as follows: open during vowels, transitional closing from vowel to consonant, constricted phase of the consonant, and transitional opening from consonant to vowel. The movements shown are schematic; the forms of movement shown are based partly on inferences from acoustic patterns and partly on high-speed motion pictures of lip and tongue movement (Fujimura, 1961; Houde, 1968; Kent & Moll, 1969; Perkell, 1969; Truby, 1959).

In row 1 of Figure 6-1A, the oral tract is initially in an open position for the neutral vowel

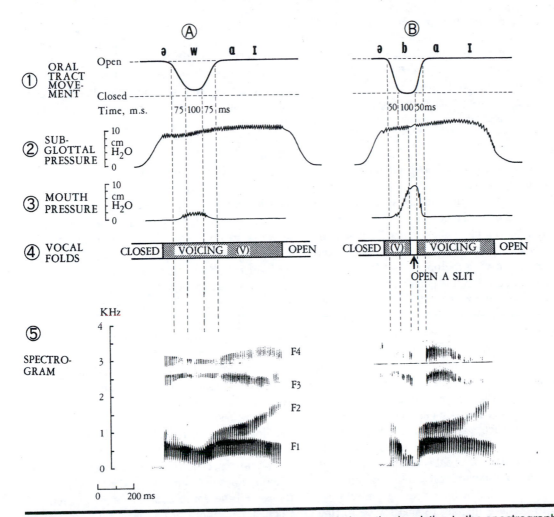

FIGURE 6-1. The patterns of articulation, air pressure, and phonation in relation to the spectrographic acoustic patterns for the phrases *a Y* [əwaɪ] and *a buy* [əbaɪ]. A full explanation of each numbered line, 1 through 5, is given in the text. The acoustic patterns are of actual utterances and the other patterns are drawn schematically (pressure curves after Netsell, 1969). They illustrate typical conditions for such utterances. The pressure unit cm H_2O is equal to 9.806×10^2 dyne/cm^2.

[ə]. About 60 ms after the start of the vowel, the lips and tongue begin to move toward constriction for [w]. The transition time from open to narrow constriction is about 75 ms; the constriction lasts about 100 ms; the opening transition is about 75 ms. The total duration of the consonant movement is about 250 ms. During the period of narrowest constriction, the amount of constriction changes only slowly, compared with the rapid

transitions to and from the constriction. After the opening transition of [w], the diphthong [aɪ] lasts about 350 ms. The oral tract is more constricted during the [ɪ] portion than during the [a] portion. These durations are typical for utterance in a citation style of a short vowel, glide consonant, and a stressed diphthong.

The open phases of vowels can vary considerably in duration, depending on regional accent, the identity of the vowel, the consonants with which it is coarticulated, and whether it is stressed or unstressed or receiving special emphasis. For the various consonants, the closed time, or the constricted time, is generally in the range of 75 to 150 ms; longer times can occur on fricative consonants. On the average the duration of the period of constriction per consonant in rapid, fluent speech is about 100 ms.

Keeping in mind the basic open-constricted movement cycle, as sketched in row 1, we can explain how these movements will affect the sound patterns. First, there must be speech sound generated by sound sources. Rows 2 and 4 indicate how these sound sources are produced and how they fit in with the open-constricted movement cycle to produce the phrase *a Y*.

The subglottal air pressure and the vocal fold action produce sound that is modified by the open-to-constricted cycle of the oral tract movement. In Figure 6-1 the articulations are coordinated in time, as shown schematically in rows 1 through 4; the schematic curves of air pressure are modeled after natural pressure curves first published by Netsell (1969). The corresponding sound patterns are shown in the spectrogram below. Before phonation of the [ə] begins, the vocal folds are brought close together (row 4) and the subglottal pressure begins to rise (row 2). When this pressure is high enough, the vocal folds begin their opening and closing action to produce the basic sound source for the vowel [ə]. This voicing action continues until, at the end of the phrase, the subglottal pressure becomes too low to produce any vocal fold action. The pressure variations generated by the pulses of glottal airflow are seen as the small oscillations in the subglottal pressure. The average subglottal pressure is rather constant through the vowel [ə] and through part of the consonant constriction. It then rises to a maximum and falls off again during the [aɪ]. This rise is a major factor in producing the stress on the second syllable of the phrase; another feature in the stress is a higher voice pitch in the [ɪ]-phase of the diphthong, which may is seen in the more dense striations toward the end of the spectrogram.

Row 3 indicates the amount of air pressure in the mouth relative to atmospheric pressure as zero. When the articulation is fairly open, as it is for all vowels, the pressure in the mouth is zero; however, whenever the articulation becomes constricted, there is a rise in the air pressure behind the constriction. The state of pressure during consonant constrictions depends on specific patterns of articulation, and this pressure is extremely important in generating certain sound patterns for the consonants. For the consonant [w] there is a considerable amount of lip constriction, and thus there is a small rise in pressure. The rise is small because the lips do not close completely.

The spectrogram shows how the sound patterns of the phrase are related to the articulation events above. When the voicing excitation of the oral tract begins, F1 is located at about 500 Hz, F2 at 1000 Hz, and F3 at 2500 Hz. The low F2 position may be due to a slight back constriction by the tongue. The formants drift downward from these positions for about 60 ms until the lips and tongue begin to move rapidly toward the [w] constriction. Then both F1 and F2 turn down in frequency because of the increasing constriction at the lips and the more back-constricted tongue; these changes in F1 and F2 frequencies are what we would expect according to the F1 and F2 constriction rules of Chapter 3. As the transition continues and the constriction becomes greater, the frequency positions of F1 and F2 become lower and lower. These changes in the formant locations are the formant transitions for [w]. As indicated by the dashed vertical lines, the formant transitions are correlated in time with the changes in constriction in row 1, which cause the formants to move to lower and lower frequencies with more and more constriction during the onset of the [w] consonant and to rise again as the lips open and the tongue moves toward the [a] position. The lip constriction also causes F3 and F4 to go down in frequency and to be greatly reduced in intensity; F1 and F2 are also lower in intensity during the narrowest part of the constriction. During and after the opening transition from the constriction, the tongue articulation moves to [a] then to [ɪ], causing F2 to rise farther and F1 to fall again for the [ɪ].

Soundscapes of the phrases *a wire* and *a buyer* are shown in Figure 6-2. The intensity and frequency changes that differentiate [w] from [b] are made more vivid by splitting the perspective in the middle of the consonants, effectively using opposite perspectives on the onset versus offset sides of the consonants.

The timing of the formant transitions is an important aspect of the glide consonant sound. The basic transition, caused by the movement into and away from the constriction, takes about 75 ms. This is seen most directly in the F1 transition, because the frequency of F1 is more closely related to the amount of constriction. If the vowel formants are located far from the glide consonant formants, then the F2 transitions may require more than 75 ms while the F1 transition lasts only about 75 ms.

The glide [w] differs in three ways from the vowel [u]. First, the lips constrict more for [w] than for [u]. This causes lowered intensity of F1 and F2, and great reduction of the intensity of F3 and the higher formants. Second, [w] may be formed in front of any tongue position; the tongue position is affected by the adjacent vowels. A slight back constriction of the tongue may accompany the [w] constriction at the lips. The vowel [u], on the other hand, requires a narrow back tongue constriction in addition to lip constriction. Third, the speed of oral tract movement is faster in producing [w] than in movements between two vowels; this is seen by comparing the speeds of F1 transition in Figure 6-1. The F1 transition on the opening of [w] into [a] is much faster than the F1 transition from [a] to [ɪ]. These differences are typical of the differences between glide consonants and diphthongs.

GLIDE AND VOICED STOP

Now that we have seen how the glide consonant [w] is produced, and how it is different from vowels and diphthongs, we need to compare it with other consonants. First, we compare [w] with [b].

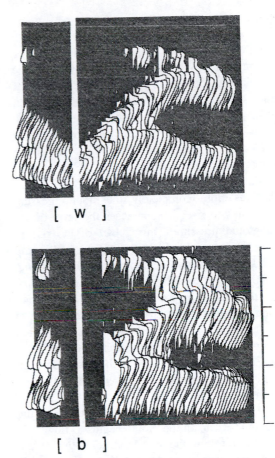

[w]

[b]

FIGURE 6-2. Soundscapes on a high plane of the phrases *a wire* (top) and *a buyer* (bottom). Each soundscape has been split in perspective in the middle of the consonant at the vertical gap. This procedure reveals the slopes of intensity changes, looking backward and forward in time from the consonant. These slopes are an important aspect of the glide/stop distinction. The slopes are gradual for glides and steep for stops. (Plots via SpeechStation2 from Sensimetrics Corporation)

The consonant [b] is a voiced stop produced at the same place of articulation as [w], that is, by a constriction of the lips. Figure 6-1B is a schema of the production of [b], in the phrase *a buy*, for comparison with the production of [w].

We see that the vocal folds are again closed at first and that the subglottal pressure rises in time.

When the subglottal pressure is high enough, vocal fold voicing action begins, thus producing the source sound for the vowel [a]. This pulsing continues throughout the vowel and through the transitional phase from open to constricted. So far all is similar to [w]. The similarity ends, however, at the point where the constriction of the lips to form the [b] reaches an amount of constriction sufficient to impede and then block the breath stream. Then the air pressure in the mouth immediately begins to rise, as shown in row 3. After the lips close completely, the mouth pressure continues to rise; it approaches the level of the subglottal pressure. During part of the rise in mouth pressure there is still enough pressure drop across the glottis to maintain vocal fold voicing, although at a decreasing pulse rate (because of the decreasing pressure drop across the glottis). Finally, the pressure drop is not large enough to cause vocal fold movement and there is a period of complete silence. The silence lasts about 25 ms until the lips begin to open in the transition from the completely closed state toward the following vowel.

As soon as the lips are even slightly open, the dammed-up air in the mouth begins to flow very rapidly through the lips, and soon the mouth pressure goes back down to zero, the atmospheric base line. The release of this pressure takes only 10 to 20 ms. This release of the pressured air in the mouth produces two sounds: an abrupt transient of increased sound pressure followed by a very brief burst of turbulent sound. The turbulent sound occurs when there is sufficient air velocity, through the barely parted lips, from the brief airflow outward in response to the higher than atmospheric air pressure inside the mouth.

During all this time the vocal folds are still held together in a position ready for voicing, probably forming a slit; as soon as the air pressure in the mouth has dropped far enough, there is a sufficient difference between the lower mouth pressure and the higher subglottal pressure for voicing action to resume. In other words, as the mouth pressure

goes down because of airflow through the opening lips, and the pressure drop across the glottis becomes large enough, the vocal fold voicing begins again for the following vowel. Voicing then continues throughout the rest of the transition to the vowel and during the vowel phase.

As the vowel continues, the subglottal pressure curve reaches a maximum, for stress on the [aɪ], and then begins to decline especially toward the end of the vowel.

Now examine the sound patterns of the phrase *a buy* in row 5 of Figure 6-1B. Note that the formant transitions are very similar to the transitions for [w], except that they seem to be cut short by the closure of the lips. Theoretically, F1 reaches zero frequency at the moment of complete lip closure, and thus the F1 transition just before the occlusion of [b] can reach a lower frequency than that of [w]. This is sometimes seen when a voicing pulse happens to occur during the final 10 ms or so of the closing movement of the lips.

While the lips are completely closed, there is no sound present except weak sound in the very low frequencies, at the fundamental frequency, and perhaps at the second harmonic; these frequencies are low enough to be transmitted at low intensity through the closed lips and the cheeks. The sound in the region of F2 and above is completely suppressed by the closure of the oral tract; indeed F2 and the higher formants are partially suppressed and lowered in frequency during the last phase of the transitional part of the consonant movement because of the progressively smaller lip opening.

At the end of the closed phase when the lips part and the mouth pressure releases through the lips, the release transient and a very brief, 10 ms burst of turbulent sound are seen in the spectrogram. Just before this pressure release, during the latter part of the closed phase, the vocal fold voicing has stopped and there is complete silence. After the release burst has dissipated enough of the mouth pressure, voicing begins again and there are corresponding vertical striations in the spectrogram, one for each airflow pulse emitted by the glottis. The lips continue to open and the tongue has already moved toward the [a] position. As the lips continue to open F1 rises, producing a transition to a level of about 650 Hz for the [a], and the F2 frequency also rises to about 1150 Hz. The reappearance and upward transitions of F3 and F4 are also seen. After the transition interval is over, the formant frequencies remain at rather steady locations until the formants begin moving toward the [ɪ] part of the diphthong.

Now compare the two consonants [w] and [b]. We see that their sound patterns differ mainly in that sound is very weak or absent during the complete closure of the [b] and there is a release-burst of sound upon opening, whereas for [w] there is strong low frequency sound present throughout and no transient burst with the opening movement. These differences arise in the oral tract movement: The [b] movement closes the tract rapidly and completely but the [w] movement goes only as far as a narrow constriction and then begins to open again. Because the [b] closes completely and rapidly, three acoustic features of a voiced stop are produced: (1) weak or absent low frequency sound, (2) a brief burst of air pressure release just before voicing begins again for a following vowel, (3) a rapid F1 transition and (4) very steep decrease toward closure and increase upon opening, in the vowel intensity, compared with the more gradual changes of [w]. The transition is typically 50 ms for a stop versus 75 ms for a glide.

The formant transitions associated with [w] and [b] are very similar in direction. This is because the transitions are produced by constricting the oral tract at the lips.

In the speech soundscapes of Figure 6-2, the differences between glide and stop in steepness of the intensity changes at onset and offset of the constrictions are easy to see. The glide [w] has much more gradual changes going from the vowel into the onset of constriction than does the stop [b]. The same difference in steepness is seen in the offsets of the consonants going into the following vowel.

GLIDE AND STOP AT MIDDLE PLACE

We now examine the production of the glide [j]. This glide is produced by a movement of the tongue to form a constriction with the palate, behind the place on the alveolar ridge where the occlusion for [d] is formed.

In Figure 6-3 we have schematized the factors in production of the glide [j] in contrast to the voiced stop [d], using two phrases, *a yacht* in Figure 6-3A and *a dot* in Figure 6-3B. The constrictive movements for [j] and [d] are similar to those of [w] and [b] in Figure 6-1; in other words, the tongue makes a glide-consonant movement toward and away from the palate for [j] that is very similar to the movement of the lips in forming [w]; for [d] the tongue makes a stop-consonant movement to and away from the alveolar ridge that is very similar to the movement of the lips for [b].

The same patterns of manipulation of the subglottal pressure, mouth pressure, and vocal fold action also occur for [j] and [d] as for [w] and [b].

Therefore, the sound patterns seen in the spectrograms of [j] and [d] are similar to those seen in the spectrograms of [w] and [b] except for a difference caused by the difference in the place of constriction. This difference is seen largely in the transitions of F2. According to the formant constriction rules for F2, constriction at an alveolar or front palatal position causes F2 to rise in frequency, but constriction of the lips causes F2 to decrease in frequency. For F1 the constriction has the same effect at both locations: a lowering of the F1 frequency during the transition from vowel to consonant and a rise in F1 frequency during the transition from consonant to vowel. The F2 transitions in *a yacht* and *a dot* show a rapid rise in frequency during the onset of the consonant constrictions and a rapid fall in frequency at the offset into the stressed vowel [a].

The words *yacht* and *dot* end with the consonant [t], which is an alveolar unvoiced stop. The production of this consonant is explained later.

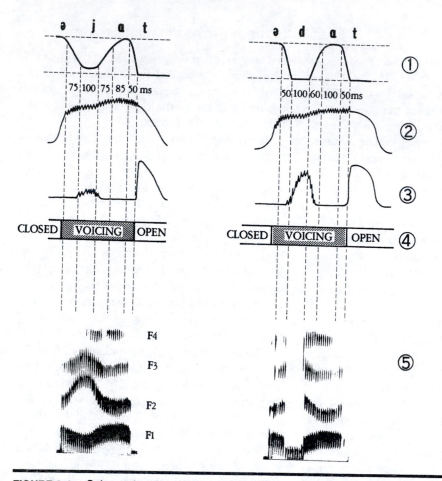

FIGURE 6-3. Schematic relations of factors in the production of alveolar glide and stop consonants, exemplified in the spoken phrases *a yacht* [əjɑt] and *a dot* [ədɑt]. A full explanation of each line, 1 through 5, is given in the text for Figure 6-1 and this figure. The pressure unit cm H_2O is equal to 9.806×10^2 dyne/CM^2.

Here, however, we can see that [t] has formant transitions in the same direction as those of the other alveolar stop [d], as we might expect. Also notice that the mouth pressure rises suddenly during the [t] occlusion and voicing stops completely; the reasons for this are discussed later.

LATERAL AND RETROFLEX GLIDES

The lateral alveolar consonant [l] and the retroflex palatal consonant [r] are very similar to glide consonants in the speed of movement, the degree of oral tract constriction, and the action of the vocal folds. Phoneticians sometimes classify [l, r] as liquids rather than glides. However, liquid is an auditory term not necessarily related to articulation. Thus, we have classified [l, r] as glides, based on their transition speed. These two consonants differ from each other, and from the other glides, in the manner in which the tongue is shaped to form the constriction. For [l] the tongue tip makes contact with the alveolar ridge but is shaped to leave lateral openings, one on each side of the contact area. For [r], the tongue is flexed back and curved upward (retroflexed) so that the tip forms a moderate constriction at the palate.

The acoustic effects of [l] and [r] articulation can be seen in the spectrograms of Figure 6-4, where they can be compared with [w] and [j]. The transitions between the vowels and the consonant constrictions have a similar duration for all four consonants, as seen especially in the F1 transitions. The amplitude is low during the constrictions, especially for F2 and higher formants, because of the greater constriction compared with the more open vowels.

The frequency courses of the formant transitions differ among the four consonants, especially in F2, F3, and F4. First compare the formant transitions of [r] and [l]. For the movement to the [r] constriction, there is a large F3 transition downward to about 1300 Hz, because of the increasing constriction of the oral tract at the middle of the palate by the retroflexed tongue tip; there is also a slight downward transition in F2 and F4. For the movement to the [l] constriction, there is a slight downward transition in F2 but little or no transition in F3 or F4. These aspects of [r] and [l] contrast with [j]. For [j]

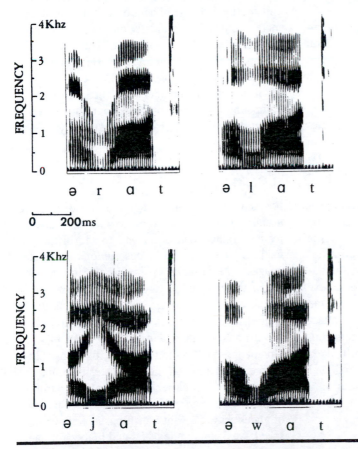

FIGURE 6-4. Spectrographic acoustic patterns of the glide consonants exemplified in the phrases *a rot* [ərɑt], *a lot* [əlɑt], *a yacht* [əjɑt], and *a watt* [əwɑt]. See text for description of the important acoustic differences and similarities among these consonants.

there are upward transitions of F2, F3, and F4 going from [ə] to the constriction and downward again for the [a]. For [w] F2 makes a large downward transition to the constriction, but F3 is not affected in frequency; F4 makes a smaller downward transition than F2.

The F1 transitions are similar for all the glides, and the transition duration is about 75 to 100 ms. The [l] has two discontinuities in the spectrum and amplitude, which are seen especially in the F1 and F2 regions. This is because the tongue tip makes, holds, and then releases its contact with the alveolar ridge. The other glides [r, w, j] are not articulated with a tongue-tip contact and therefore their formant transitions change smoothly in time, without discontinuities.

The F2 transitions of [w] and [j] are in opposite directions because of the opposite effects on F2 frequency of the labial constriction for [w] compared with the alveolar constriction for [j]. The F3 transitions for [j] are opposite the direction of those for [r].

The formant pattern of [l] during the constriction is prominent in the region of F3 and F4, in contrast to the other glides. The formants of [l] vary in location depending on the adjacent phonemes, as is described later.

Palatal glides can easily be trilled. Trills are not phonemic in English but they are often part of the vocal repertoire of children. A trilled [r] or [l] is produced by a vibration of the tongue tip toward and away from the palate, causing a rapid alternation in the spectrum between a pattern for a very narrow constriction and the pattern seen for the untrilled glide. Probably a Bernoulli suction effect between palate and tongue is a factor in producing trilled consonants. The alternation rate of trills is usually in the range of 20 to 30 per second, and thus two to three trill cycles may occur during a glide constriction of 100 ms (1/10 second).

EFFECTS OF UTTERANCE POSITION

The examples of [w, j, l, r] thus far have been in an intervocalic position, that is, between two vowels. A consonant may also occur initially at the beginning of an utterance or finally, at the end. Spectrograms of initial and final glide-like consonants are shown in Figure 6-5. The patterns of the initial glides are very similar to the constricted and releasing phases of the intervocalic glides in Figure 6-4; also the patterns of the final glides are like the onset-constriction patterns of the intervocalic glides. The constricted phase of the initial glide consonant may be more brief than for the intervocalic glide because sound-source production by the glottis may not start at the very beginning of the oral tract constriction. In the examples of final position, [r] and [l] are more diphthong-like and drawn out in duration of the constriction because phonation is not shut off but merely allowed to gradually die out; the formant transitions are slower and the discontinuity seen for initial [j] is not seen for final [l] for one of the speakers. The position of a glide consonant is often adjacent to another consonant, forming a compound consonant or consonant cluster. Then the glide consonant articulation strongly affects the adjacent vowel.

SUMMARY

For acoustic phonetic study the consonants are usually classified according to their articulatory features rather than according to the distinctive features used for linguistic descriptions across languages. The articulatory features of consonants are of three types: features of manner of articulation, voicing, and place of articulation. Features of the articulation of glide consonants are: (1) a speed of articulation that is faster than that for diphthongs but lower than that for stops, (2) a degree of constriction that is greater than that for vowels, and (3) occurrence of lateral and retroflex forms of tongue articulation. The acoustic patterns of glides show formant transitions of intermediate speed, weak amplitude of F2 and higher formants during the constriction phase, and characteristic F patterns depending on lateral (F2), retroflex (low F3), labial (low F2), or alveolar (high F2)

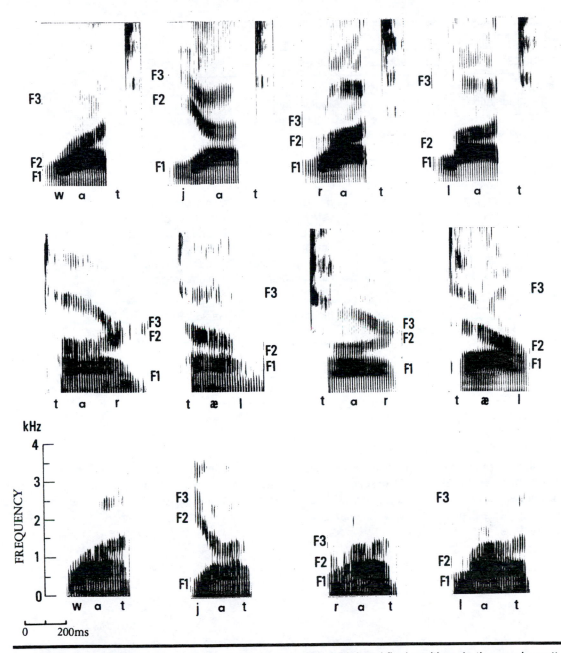

FIGURE 6-5. Acoustic patterns of the glide consonants in initial and final positions in the words *watt* [wɑt], *yacht* [jɑt], *tar* [tɑr], and *tal* [tæl]. The important points to note are described in the text. Two different male speakers spoke each word; the speaker for the top row of spectrograms has very even, regular glottal pulses and highly resonant formants, compared with the speaker in the bottom row, who was the author.

TABLE 6.2. Main features of glide consonants compared with voiced stops and diphthongs

FEATURES	DIPHTHONGS	GLIDES	VOICED STOPS
Timing			
Oral articulation	Slow	Medium-fast	Fast
Type of constriction	(No narrow constriction)	Brief constriction	Brief closure
Spectral			
Intensity during constriction	(No narrow constriction)	Strong	Weak
Spectrum during constriction	(No narrow constriction)	Low frequencies strong up to about 600 Hz; midfrequency energy weaker than in diphthongs	Very low frequencies; fundamental alone, lowered in pitch; no energy in F2, F3 and higher regions
Formant transitions	Slow formant transitions between the two component vowels	Medium-fast transitions appropriate to place, lateral opening, or retroflexion	Rapid formant transitions

constriction characteristics. The faster closing and opening between vowel and stop consonant occlusion causes steeper changes in adjacent vowel offsets and onsets than for the more gradual glide constrictions.

A summary of the main articulatory and acoustic features of diphthongs, glides, and voiced stops is given in Table 6-2.

CHAPTER SEVEN

CONSONANTS: NASAL, STOP, AND FRICATIVE MANNERS OF ARTICULATION

This chapter presents descriptions of the articulation and acoustic features for three more manners of articulation that produce phonemic distinctions among the consonants: the features nasal, stop (or plosive), and fricative. These three manner-features are extremely important in most languages. In English, for example, they have been calculated to account together for about 80% of all the consonantal distinctions among words (Denes, 1963).

The nasal consonants have some acoustic similarities to glides, so we will describe the nasal manner of articulation before discussing how nasals differ from glides. The nasals are also compared with voiced stops. Fricative consonants are then described, especially as compared with stops.

NASAL CONSONANTS

The nasal consonants [m, n, ŋ] are articulated by a combination of two movements: (1) movement of the tongue or lips to completely occlude the oral tract and (2) lowering of the velum. Velar lowering introduces an opening from the pharynx into the nasal passages; this opening is called the velopharyngeal port or simply the *velar port*. The oral occluding movements for the nasals are similar to those for the corresponding voiced stops [b, d, g] in that the constricting movement of the tongue or lips is rapid and a complete oral occlusion is formed. Because of this similarity some linguists classify the nasals as stops having the feature of nasalization.

During the interval when the oral tract is completely occluded by the articulation of a nasal con-

sonant, the sound produced by the glottal action of phonation is propagated through the velar port and the nasal passages and out through the nose. This sound from the nose is called a nasal murmur; its spectrum is dominated by low frequency sound determined mostly by the main resonance of the large volume of the nasal passages constricted by the small nose openings. The nasal passages of a speaker remain constant in shape and size for the different nasal consonants. For this reason the murmur spectrum does not differ greatly among [m, n, ŋ]; however, there are some differences due to the different lengths of the connected but closed oral tract, longest for [m] and shortest for [ŋ] (see Chapter Nine).

NASAL-GLIDE-STOP DIFFERENCES

Figure 7-1 compares the nasal and glide consonants showing spectrograms of the phrases *a wire*

Phonology Note: Voiceless Nasals

All the nasal phonemes of English are voiced. English speakers, however, usually know how to utter a voiceless version of "m" [m̥]; they frequently use a voiceless nasal [m̥] to begin exclamations like "hmmm" [m̥mm], expressing thoughtfulness or dubiousness, and an intervocalic version in "uhumm" [m̥m̥m], signaling agreement or "yes" without opening one's mouth (Catford, 1988 Ex. 25). Among languages using voiceless nasals as distinctive phonemes are Burmese, Yao, Hopi, and Aleut (Maddieson, 1984:239).

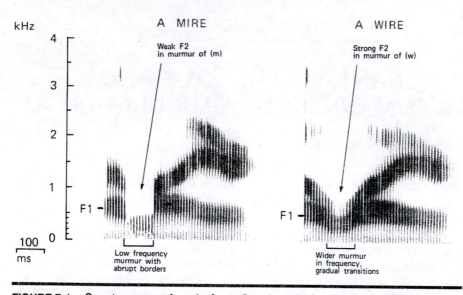

FIGURE 7-1. Spectrograms of *a wire* [əwaɪr] and *a mire* [əmaɪr] to compare the formant patterns and constriction murmurs between glide and nasal consonants. The changes in sound between vowel and constriction are more abrupt for the nasal. The strongest part of the murmur ranges up to about 800 Hz for the glide but only to about 300 Hz for the nasal.

[əwaɪr] and *a mire* [əmaɪr]. The spectrograms show differences between nasal and glide consonants in the transitions to and from the consonant constrictions and also during the murmurs of the constriction intervals. The strong low-frequency portion of the nasal murmur is similar to that in the glide constriction intervals except that in the nasal murmur it is limited to the region below about 300 Hz, whereas the strong low-frequency energy in the constriction of glides ranges up to about 800 Hz. The nasal murmur has abrupt borders compared to the more gradual transitions of the glide constriction from vowel to constriction and back to vowel. The abruptness of onset and offset of the nasal murmur results from two circumstances: (1) the suddenness of onset and offset of the oral occlusion and (2) the nasal port is already wide open at the onset of the occlusion and remains so throughout.

There are important differences between nasals and glides in the spectrum of the murmur sound above the low frequency part. The nasal murmurs are much less intense above 800 Hz than are the murmurs of the glides, and the pattern of formant frequencies in this upper region is not so highly distinctive among the nasals [m, n, ŋ] as it is among glides.

We next compare the nasal and voiced stop consonants. The nasal versus stop acoustic differences are somewhat complicated, but they can be easily understood if the production factors are kept in mind. There are three main acoustic differences between voiced stops and nasals: (1) the stops have release bursts but the nasals do not; (2) the nasals have stronger intensity of the constriction murmur; and (3) the vowels adjacent to nasals are nasalized, but not for stops. The movement of the oral tract for nasals is similar to that of stops, with rapid transitions, abrupt onset and offset of occlusion, and an occlusion interval of about 100 ms. However, during the occlusion interval of nasals there is present the relatively strong, low frequency sound of the murmur compared with weak or absent sound during stop occlusions. The murmur and nasalization patterns can be compared in Figure 7-2. Let us now see how all these acoustic differences are produced.

Release Bursts and Murmur Intensity

During the closed period of voiced stops, the vocal folds continue to open and close, emitting pulses of subglottal air into the closed oral cavity. As this continues, the air pressure in the mouth increases until it is high enough to stop phonation or until the release of the oral closure. At the moment of release the oral pressure is higher than the atmospheric pressure. Thus, upon release, there is a burst consisting of a transient (momentary), step-like increase in the pressure of the air in front of the lips and following formant resonances; then phonation starts for the following vowel sound. In contrast, the release of a nasal consonant is not accompanied by a burst because, due to the open state of the velar port, there has been no build-up of air pressure in the oral-pharyngeal cavity during the oral occlusion.

The first event in the burst is the *release transient*, step-like, instantaneous increase in sound pressure. This is followed by damped oscillations at resonant frequencies (formants) determined by the location in the vocal tract of the sound source (the step change) and the vocal tract shape at that moment. The voiced stop release bursts are brief, lasting only 10 to 20 ms. The release burst of the [b] in Figure 7-2 was visible on the original spectrogram but cannot be seen in the reproduced figure.

The nasal murmur during the oral occlusion of the nasals is more intense than the constriction murmurs that are seen during voiced stops. The reason is that much more sound can radiate through the nostrils during the nasal consonant than can radiate through the walls of the closed vocal tract during the voiced stops.

Thus, there are two main differences distinguishing nasals and voiced stops that stem from the articulatory conditions during the oral occlusion: (1) the absence or presence of a release burst and (2) the intensity of the murmur.

On the release (or opening) of the oral occlusion of nasals the oral opening movement is a little slower compared with releases of stops. This difference is due to the air pressure in the mouth during stop closures compared with the lack of this pressure on nasals because of the open velar port and nose. The pressure of air behind the stop closure causes a slightly faster opening movement just after the release than is seen for the nasals (Fujimura, 1961).

Nasalization of Vowels Adjacent to Nasal Consonants

The movement downward of the velum for a nasal consonant begins well before the beginning of oral tract movement toward occlusion, and thus the opening of the velar port is already accomplished by the time the oral tract becomes closed. The velar port also remains open during the release and opening of the oral occlusion. The lead and lag of velar opening and closing, preceding and following the oral tract occlusion, are typically about 100 ms. This causes nasalization of portions of vowels for about 100 ms preceding and following the oral occlusions of nasal consonants.

The effects of the leading and lagging nasalization are seen in Figure 7-2 by comparing the vowels adjacent to the stop in *a buyer* with the vowels adjacent to the nasal in *a mire*. Nasalization of vowels introduces extra resonances and antiresonances into the response of the oral tract to the frequencies of the glottal sound source; this is because in addition to the open vowel configuration the velar port is partially open, adding the nasal cavity as a shunt to the overall system. This shunt has frequency-tuning effects on transmission of the glottal sound through the oral cavity. These vowel nasalization effects are mainly caused by changes in the response of the oral tract, not by the added sound coming out of the nose, a sound that is negligible because of its low

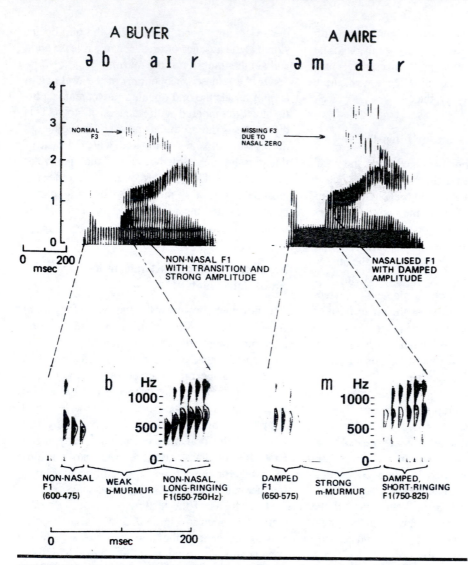

FIGURE 7-2. Spectrograms of *a buyer* [əbaɪr] and *a mire* [əmaɪr] to compare the acoustic patterns of nasal versus voiced stop consonants. In the upper spectrogram, the stop has a very weak murmur during the occlusion interval and a release transient and the nasal has a strong murmur but no release transient. Nasalization adjacent to the nasal causes differences in the vowel spectrum compared with that adjacent to the stop. In the bottom spectrograms, the constriction murmurs and the adjacent transitions of the vowels are presented on an expanded time scale. The expansion makes visible the individual formant-ringing intervals of the vowel. These ringing intervals have been outlined by hand on the spectrogram and look like "lozenges" that are straight on the left leading edge and round on the right trailing edge. Because nasalization damps the ringing of F1, the lozenges are thinner (shorter ringing time) near the nasal than the stop.

amplitude in the frequencies above about 500 Hz, relative to the vowel sound.

In acoustic descriptions of the response of the vocal tract, the resonances (or formants) are called *poles* and the antiresonances are called *zeroes*; these terms are used in describing the effects of nasalization on the vowel spectrum. The frequency response of a zero is the exact opposite to that of a pole or resonance. A zero attenuates glottal source components that are close to the antiresonance frequency, just as a resonance amplifies frequency components of the source that are close in frequency to the resonant frequency as we saw in Chapter Four. Just as a resonance attentuates frequencies that are sufficiently above the resonance frequency (at a rate of 12 dB per octave), so a zero amplifies frequencies that are sufficiently above the antiresonance frequency at the same rate, amplification of 12 dB per octave. The overall response of the vocal tract is made up of the sum of both the amplifying and attenuating effects of the poles (resonances) and the zeroes (antiresonances). If a vocal tract pole and zero have the same frequency, there is no net effect on the source spectrum.

Nasalization of a vowel introduces a pole at a very low frequency, below the fundamental F0, which amplifies the fundamental, and a zero at a frequency just above the pole, which reduces the energy in the spectrum above the fundamental, in the F1 region. If the normal oral tract F1 is low in frequency, for example, as in close vowels, such as [u] and [i], the zero can cancel the F1 resonance, leaving a flattened spectrum instead of an F1 peak. If F1 is normally high, as in open vowels [ɑ] and [æ], the zero reduces the spectral energy in an area between the fundamental and F1. The zeroes often show in the spectrogram as light patches or light areas in the F1 region, and these can be seen in Figures 7-2 and 7-3. Nasalization also introduces zeroes in the regions of F2 and F3.

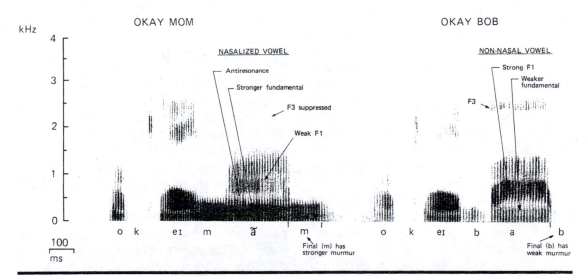

FIGURE 7-3. Spectrograms of *Okay Bob* and *Okay Mom* to compare initial and final voiced stop and nasal consonants. The lag and lead of the velar opening for the nasal consonant causes complete nasalization of the [ã] in *Mom* in contrast to the "normal" [ɑ] in *Bob*. The important effects of the nasalization are noted in the spectrograms and discussed in the text.

In areas of the spectrum where zeroes are present the spectrogram has missing or depressed harmonics, and there is an overall broadening in frequency bandwidth of any formant resonances. There is also a reduction in intensity of the oral formants. This effect can often be seen by comparing the vowel formant intensities near the nasal murmur with those near non-nasal stop consonant closures, where there is no nasalization. These effects are clearly visible, especially in the expanded sections of the spectrograms in the lower half of Figure 7-2. The F1 intensity is weaker adjacent to the [m] than the [b] and the apparent F1 transitions are less extensive (starting and ending frequencies of the F1 transitions are given in parentheses on the spectrogram). Also the resonant ringing of F1 is damped out more rapidly: In the expanded spectrograms the ringing period of the formant forms a lozenge-shaped pattern, which has been hand-outlined on the spectrogram for each formant pulse. It will be seen that the formant-ringing lozenges are thinner, that is, shorter in time, near the [m] than near the [b].

The frequency locations of the poles and zeroes due to nasalization depend greatly on the amount of opening of the velar port. The velar port changes in size, from small to larger before the oral occlusion and from large to smaller during the opening of the occlusion. These changes in amount of velar opening cause changes in the frequency locations of the poles and zeroes; this makes the spectral effects of nasalization extremely variable, depending on the time course of velar movement and the particular combination of vowel and consonant.

The F1 formant transitions of nasal consonant articulation are often somewhat overridden by the changing pole-zero pattern from nasalization. This is seen in Figure 7-2, comparing the F1 transitions adjacent to the closures of [b] versus [m]. The F2 transitions in Figure 7-2 are not so much affected by nasalization as are the F1 transitions.

Figure 7-2 also shows a case of suppression of F3 by a zero where, after the [b], the F3 of the following vowel starts immediately upon release of the [b] occlusion. On release of the [m] occlusion, however, F3 is apparently suppressed because it is seen only after a delay of about 50 ms.

The effects of nasalization on F2 and F3 vary considerably depending on the combinations of particular vowels and consonants, but the suppressions seen above are typical for [ɑ] combined with [b] and with [m].

Initial and Final Nasals and Stops

Initial and final nasal consonants are similar to the intervocalic nasals in timing and spectral pattern. Examples are shown in the spectrograms of Figure 7-3. When a syllable begins and ends with a nasal consonant, the lag and lead of nasalization often cause the entire vowel to be nasalized. Compare *mom* and *bob* in vowel pattern; note that the formants are weaker throughout the nasalized [ã] of *mom* compared with the [ɑ] of *bob*. A weak or blank area below F1 indicates the presence of a zero in the oral tract response caused by nasal coupling. This zero reduces the amplitude of F1. A pole of lower frequency than this zero increases the amplitude of the fundamental compared with its amplitude in the unnasalized vowel.

FRICATIVE CONSONANTS

The fricative consonants are similar to the stop and nasal consonants in the general timing of the open-constricted cycle of articulation. The difference is that, instead of being produced with a complete occlusion of the oral tract during the consonant gesture, fricatives are produced with a narrow constriction. The breath stream, passing through the constriction, becomes turbulent because of friction of the airstream within the constriction and/or by passing over an obstruction to smooth flow, such as the teeth. This generates a hissing sound, which is the hallmark of the fricatives.

The main differences between the sound patterns of the alveolar voiced fricative, stop, and glide are compared in Figure 7-4. In the spectrograms we see that the vowel formant frequencies and their transition are similar for the [d] and [z]. This is because of the similarity of the tongue

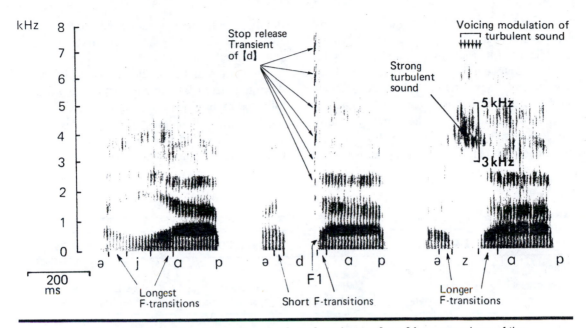

FIGURE 7-4. Spectrograms of *a yap* [əjɑp], *a dap* [ədɑp], and *a zap* [əzɑp] for comparison of the acoustic patterns of glide, stop, and fricative. Acoustic features are noted on the spectrogram and further discussed in the text.

articulations. However, during the fricative constrictions for [z] there is a strong, continuous, turbulent sound between 4 and 5 kz but a complete silence in this high frequency region during the occlusion of the [d].

The high frequency turbulent sound during the constriction of the [z] is caused by turbulence of the airstream as it passes through the narrow constriction between the tongue and the alveolar ridge. Air turbulence produced in this way, by various kinds of narrow constrictions in the vocal tract, is the typical source sound for all fricative consonants. At the source it is a random noise having a spectrum with approximately equal amplitude, on the average, at all frequencies. The amplitude at each frequency varies randomly, from moment to moment in time. This randomness can be seen in the spectrum of the [z] sound in Figure 7-4; the spectrogram of a sound with randomly varying amplitudes at each frequency of the sound has a mottled appearance as compared with the striated appearance of periodically

pulsed sounds, such as vowels. However, a closer examination of the [z] sound reveals that there is also a partial periodicity of amplitude. This is often seen in voiced fricatives because the vocal folds are held fairly close together throughout the consonant constriction and the airflow through the folds causes them to vibrate toward and away from each other, more or less as in vowel phonation, and this modulates the airflow supplied to the fricative constriction above, thereby modulating the turbulence amplitude produced.

The overall spectrum shape of the fricative sound received outside the mouth is determined by the size and shape of the oral cavity in front of the constriction. The spectrum of fricatives is usually much more intense in the frequencies above about 2.5 kHz than at lower frequencies. The spectra of fricatives are discussed in more detail under the topic of the shape and place features of consonants (Chapter Nine).

The formant transitions in F1 and F2 during the closing and opening movements should be compared between [z] and [d]. It will be seen that the transitions are slightly longer and slower for [z] than for [d]. Perhaps this difference is because the tongue must form a certain shaped narrow passage against the palate in order to produce the fricative turbulence of [z], and this adjustment requires a controlled slowing down of the constricting movement compared with the movement for [d], which can attain occlusion simply by collision with the palate; there is some evidence from an x-ray study that this may be the case (Perkell, 1969).

Note in the figure that the release of [d] has a sharp transient containing energy up to 7.5 kHz followed by brief formant ringing at F1, F2, F3, and F4, and a silent gap of about 15 ms before the first vocal fold pulse of the vowel and its very strong F1. This delay in voicing may have

TABLE 7-1. Summary of main features of nasals, glides, voiced stops, and voiced fricatives.

FEATURES	NASALS	GLIDES	VOICED STOPS	VOICED FRICATIVES
Timing				
Oral articulation	Rapid Brief closure duration	Medium Brief closure duration	Rapid Brief closure duration	Rapid Brief closure duration
Velar articulation	Velar port opening leads oral closing Velar port closing lags oral opening	Velar port remains closed	Velar port remains closed	Velar port remains closed
Spectral				
Murmur intensity	Strong	Strong	Weak	High frequency turbulence
Murmur spectrum	Low frequency resonance of nasal passages up to about 300 Hz; very weak above this	Low frequencies strong up to about 800 Hz; midfrequency pattern stronger than nasals; different F patterns among glides but not among nasals	Very low frequencies (fundamental alone); no energy in F2, F3 or higher regions	Strong in high frequencies (above 2.5 kHz)
Formant transitions in adjacent vowel	Nasalization during the transitions, may obscure expected transitions; F1 of adjacent vowels is weakened	Long formant transitions appropriate to speed, place, and retroflexion (r articulation only)	Short formant transitions	Somewhat longer formant transitions than for stops
Overall spectral changes	Abrupt onset and offset, without a release transient	Gradual, smooth changes	Abrupt and with a release transient	Change from periodic to random turbulence that is amplitude modulated; no release transient

occurred because the last half of the occlusion period was de-voiced, indicating a high mouth pressure that had to be dissipated before vowel voicing could begin. A similar release gap in voicing does not appear after the [z].

Figure 7-4 also includes a spectrogram of the phrase *a yap* so that the alveolar glide [j] can be compared in rate and extent of formant transitions with [d] and [z]. The transitions have been marked on the spectrograms. It will be seen that the transitions of [j] are more extended than those for [d] and [z].

There is an additional manner of fricative articulation, called affricate, which includes the consonant sounds [tʃ], as in *church*, and [dʒ], as in *judge*; sometimes affricates are considered to be unitary phonemes, the sounds of which are symbolized by [č] and [ǰ]. The affricates are produced like fricatives that are preceded by an occlusion instead of a more open articulation. The occlusion is formed at the same place as the ensuing constriction for the friction part, which is usually of shorter duration than in a fricative.

SUMMARY

Table 7-1 summarizes the articulatory and acoustic features of all four manner distinctions among consonants: nasality, glide, stop (plosive), and fricative.

CHAPTER EIGHT

CONSONANTS: THE
VOICED-UNVOICED CONTRAST

The phonemes /b, d, g, z, ʒ, v, ð/ are said to be voiced in contrast to the phonemes /p, t, k, s, ʃ, f, θ/, which are unvoiced. In phonology the corresponding distinctive feature is called voicing. The term *voicing* refers to the vibratory action of the vocal folds, which produces voicing periodicity in the speech wave, as explained in Chapter Four. Voicing is usually present during the constriction of voiced consonants and absent during the constriction of unvoiced consonants. This difference is controlled by muscles in the larynx that hold the vocal folds in either a closed position for voicing or in an open position for unvoiced. The position of the folds also produces other acoustic differences (other than presence or absence of voicing) that distinguish voiced versus unvoiced consonants.

PRODUCTION OF THE VOICED-VOICELESS DISTINCTION

To illustrate how the essential sound differences arise between voiced and unvoiced consonants, a schematic picture of the action of the oral tract articulators together with the subglottal pressure pattern, the mouth pressure, and the position of the vocal folds was constructed. Figure 8-1 shows this picture for [b] and [p] using the phrases *a buy* and *a pie*. Note that the first line, showing the oral tract movement, is similar for the two phrases, but the closure movement is a little faster for [p] than for [b]. The transitional movements for [b] and [p] are complete in about 50 ms. The subglottal pressure curve too is the same in general. However, in the mouth pressure there is an important difference during the occlusion: The pressure rises slowly for [b] but rapidly for [p]. This is

---

Phonology Note:
Laryngeal Varieties of Consonants

Most languages make use of consonant voicing differences. English is heavily dependent on this feature (Denes, 1963), and it is the only laryngeal feature we employ distinctively. Other types of laryngeal/glottal distinctions for consonants in the world's languages are aspiration, breathy voice, slack voice, creaky voice, and stiff voice. These types of laryngeal action and the languages using them in stop consonants are surveyed by Henton et al. (1992). Stevens (1977) provided a physical analysis of how laryngeal actions may accomplish the various glottal features found in phonological studies.

---

because of the difference in vocal fold position during the occlusion.

The voiced-voiceless distinction originates in a difference in the posture of the vocal folds. This difference produces the main acoustic differences between the voiced and unvoiced stops. In row 4 it can be seen that during the closed phase of the consonant [p], the vocal folds are in a wide-open position in contrast to [b], where they remain closed in a position to produce voicing. The wide-open position on [p] affords little or no resistance to the flow of air into the mouth and so the mouth pressure rises rapidly to become equal to the subglottal pressure. Also, because the vocal folds have been opened wide at about the same time as the lips close, there is no vocal fold pulsing at all

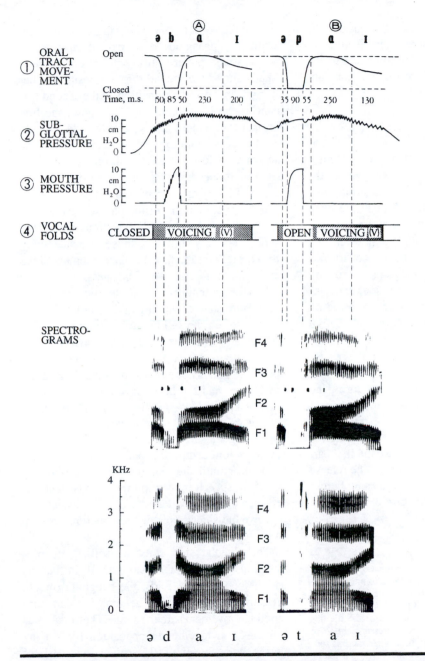

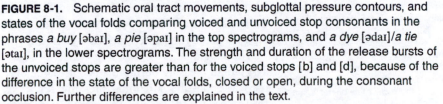

FIGURE 8-1. Schematic oral tract movements, subglottal pressure contours, and states of the vocal folds comparing voiced and unvoiced stop consonants in the phrases *a buy* [əbaɪ], *a pie* [əpaɪ] in the top spectrograms, and *a dye* [ədaɪ]/*a tie* [ətaɪ], in the lower spectrograms. The strength and duration of the release bursts of the unvoiced stops are greater than for the voiced stops [b] and [d], because of the difference in the state of the vocal folds, closed or open, during the consonant occlusion. Further differences are explained in the text.

during the closed phase because the vocal folds are too far apart; furthermore, there is little or no pressure drop across the glottis because the mouth pressure is virtually the same as the sub-glottal pressure (Netsell, 1969).

ACOUSTICS OF CONSONANT VOICING

At the end of the closed phase of [p], when the lips just begin to open to form the following vowel, the high mouth pressure is released and a strong flow of air travels from the trachea through the open vocal folds and out through the small lip opening. The release of the high mouth pressure and the subsequent rush of airflow from the trachea through the mouth and out through the narrow lip opening causes an intense transient sound, essentially a step-like change in pressure, followed by turbulent sounds (friction and aspiration) before the vowel begins. We call the transient and following friction and aspiration, all together, the release burst of the consonant.[1]

The lip-opening transition continues during the friction and aspiration phase before voicing begins for the following vowel. The part of this transitional phase that is voiced is thus shorter than it is for the voiced consonant [b], because the first part is occupied by friction and aspiration. The release interval for [b] shows a weak transient before the first voice pulse but no friction or aspiration,

because the vocal folds are held together, thus preventing any strong now of air from the trachea.

The sound pattern during the unvoiced burst usually shows the second formant position rather strongly and also the transition of the second formant as the lips open more and more; the first formant energy does not appear strongly until the vocal tract is again excited by voice pulses. The lack of first formant energy during the burst is believed to be due to sound absorption in the region of F1 by the trachea and lungs.

In the spectrogram for the phrase *a pie* in Figure 8-1, note that the F2 transitions associated with [p] are very similar to those associated with [b]. This reflects the fact that the movement of the lips is similar for the two consonants.

It is the switching of the sound source between the pulsing state of voicing and complete silence and the strong, noise-like airflow on release that distinguish the voiced from the unvoiced stop consonant. In the case of the voiced consonant, vocal fold pulsing continues for some time during the closure and the burst on the release is short and weak, whereas for the unvoiced consonant there is complete silence (no vocal fold pulsing) during the closure and the burst on release is strong, of longer duration, and the F1 energy does not appear until the beginning of the following vowel. In speech perception these consistent differences in sound pattern are used by listeners to perceive the voiced-voiceless distinction between stop consonants.

The alveolar stop consonants [d, t] are produced just like the labial stops [b, p] in that the actions of the vocal folds, the subglottal/mouth pressure effects, and the general form of constricting movements are the same. The vocal folds remain close together in a position for voicing during the occlusion of [d], as they do for [b]; for [t] the vocal folds are pulled open at the start of the occlusion and then brought back together during the opening transition, just as we saw for [p].

The subglottal pressure curve is also the same. The mouth pressure during the occlusion quickly rises to equal the subglottal pressure for [t] as for [p], but for [d] the mouth pressure rises more

---

[1]During the [p] release the subglottal pressure shows a dip of about 1 cm H_2O, which is not seen on the release of [b]. This dip is probably due to the fact that the vocal folds are still wide apart, allowing a high airflow to occur. At this point in time the mouth and trachea are connected through a rather wide-open glottis. Just before this, at the moment before the lips open, the mouth pressure and subglottal pressure are equal and there is no airflow out of the trachea. When the lips suddenly move apart, a high flow occurs from the trachea but the relatively massive chest and lung tissues cannot move inward quickly enough to maintain the subglottal pressure. This would cause the pressure to fall momentarily until the chest catches up and the glottis closes for voicing the vowel. During the burst interval of [p], the vocal folds start to move back toward the voicing position and, when the mouth pressure reaches a low enough level through the dissipation of the burst-flow, the voicing action of the vocal folds begins again for the following vowel.

slowly, just as for [b], and does not reach equality with the subglottal pressure before the release of the occlusion occurs.

The form of the constricting movement is about the same for all of the stop consonants. Transition from open to occluded and from occluded to open takes place in about 50 ms, and the duration of the occlusion is about 100 ms. The contact of the tongue with the palate covers a greater area and has a slightly longer duration for [t] than for [d]; the tongue contact of [t] extends backward somewhat from the alveolar ridge, whereas [d] has a narrower region of contact along the ridge.

Now examine the sound patterns of [d] and [t] in the phrases *a dye* and *a tie* in the bottom row of Figure 8-1. In their source characteristics, the sound patterns of [d] and [t] are the same as the corresponding patterns of [b] and [p]. That is, for the voiced stops the periodic sound source operates throughout the consonant, as long as the transglottal pressure conditions permit, that is, as long as there is enough pressure drop across the glottis to cause vocal fold vibration. Sometimes the pressure drop is low and voicing stops (called de-voicing). On release of the voiced occlusion a weak and brief transient burst occurs, which sometimes produces a very brief, turbulent noise source. The transient excites the resonances of the oral tract and the brief noise burst may also exhibit these resonances.

For the unvoiced stops, the wide open state of the vocal folds does not permit periodic voicing. There is no sound source operating during the occlusion (complete silence), and then at the release there is a transient followed by strong noise from the turbulence at the narrowest part of the constriction as it is just opening. Because the vocal folds only begin to close after the release of the occlusion, there is a strong turbulent now of air during most of the opening transition of the oral tract; the turbulent sources on releases of [t] operate for 40 ms or more and excite the resonances of the oral tract shape. Finally, when the vocal folds are sufficiently close together, voicing action can resume for the

following vowel and voicing striations are seen in the spectrogram.[2]

In studies of the perception of stop voicing, the delay between stop release and the onset of voicing is called voice onset time (VOT) (Lisker & Abramson, 1967). VOT is defined for stops as the time elapsing from the release of the occlusion to the beginning of voicing. VOT is short for voiced stops, about 0 to 20 ms, and long for voiceless stops, 30 ms or more.

The difference in vocal fold adjustment for voiced versus unvoiced stops is the main cause of the acoustic differences. However, there are other articulatory differences that also contribute to the voicing distinction. We have noted that the tongue contact extends farther back for [t] than for [d]. The duration of the closed interval is usually slightly longer for unvoiced stops than for voiced stops. In addition, the larynx position is higher for unvoiced consonants than voiced consonants, which would tend to make the mouth pressure higher and to stretch the vocal folds to produce a slightly higher pitch in adjacent vowels. Furthermore, a higher tension may consistently exist in one or more of the articulating factors of unvoiced stops and an enlargement of the mouth cavity may occur during the occlusions of voiced stops.[3]

---

[2]A detailed discussion of the acoustic factors in stop production is given by Fant (1973, Chapter 7). To summarize: The unvoiced bursts have three sound sources: transient, frication, and aspiration. Frication is produced by turbulence at the consonant constriction; aspiration is produced by turbulence at the glottis. We may speculate that the aspirant turbulence is produced as the glottis becomes narrower during its closure toward the voicing position. All of these effects of the source conditions and the corresponding features in the sound patterns that differentiate voiced from unvoiced consonants are the same for all the stop consonants.

[3]Some linguists prefer the terms *lax* or *lenis* for voiced and *tense* or *fortis* for unvoiced, referring to evidence that the constrictions of unvoiced consonants are articulated with more force or tension than for the voiced consonants. This is true, but the present author believes this may be only a secondary, synergistic effect, necessary to contain the higher air pressure in the mouth that occurs on unvoiced consonants because of the wide-open posture of the vocal folds. The primary factor is believed to be the open or closed posture of the vocal folds as described in the text. However, the issue should not be considered closed: Malécot (1970) provides an

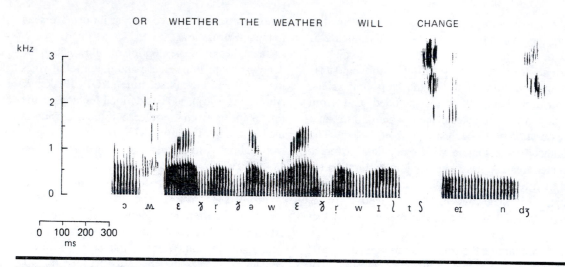

FIGURE 8-2. Spectrogram of the phrase *"or whether the weather will change"* to illustrate differences between unvoiced [ʍ] and voiced [w].

The voicing contrast of stops is produced as just described in English and some other similar languages, such as German, Swedish, and Dutch. In some other languages, however, there are phonemic stop contrasts not used in English, such as pre-voiced and unaspirated unvoiced. These are produced by mechanisms of vocal fold adjustment, articulator tension, and timing coordination, which are different from those we have given. For an advanced discussion of some of the possible mechanisms, see Fujimura (1972) and Stevens (1977).

The oral shape conditions and the corresponding formant patterns differ between stop consonants that are articulated at different locations in the oral tract, as we would expect. A main difference appears in the frequency transitions of F2. For the labial stops we saw that, other conditions being equal, F2 is lowered in frequency by the labial constriction. For the alveolar stops F2 is raised by the constriction. Further description of pattern differences related to place of articulation are given in Chapter Nine.

In formal citation we can distinguish pairs of words like *weather* and *whether*, *witch* and *which*, although these contrasts are usually not well marked in informal speech. The second of each of these word pairs begins with a voiceless version of [w] that is symbolized as an upside-down w [ʍ]. The voiceless source of sound is produced by a wide-open glottis and a back constriction sufficient to generate a turbulent sound that is shaped in spectrum by a glide-like movement of the lips from constricted to open. During the glide transition to the following vowel the vocal folds move from the open position to a close position for voicing. In Figure 8-2 we can compare [w] and [ʍ] in the phrase *or whether the weather will change*. The sound spectrum at the first part of the noise phase of [ʍ] in *whether* is concentrated in the low frequencies, but as the lips begin to move toward a more open position the noise sound contains higher frequencies; this transition is similar to the opening transition of the [w] in *weather*.

interesting review and Slis (1975) proposes a neuromuscular theory of stop-voicing phenomena, which states that the acoustic features of unvoiced stops and tense (long) vowels are due to stronger neural commands to the articulators than for the voiced stops and lax (short) vowels.

VOICED VERSUS UNVOICED FINAL CONSONANTS

When final consonants occur in a pre-boundary position, that is, immediately before the end of a word, phrase, or sentence where a pause may occur, the vowel preceding the consonant is considerably longer if the consonant is voiced than if it is unvoiced. The pre-boundary vowel lengthening effect of voicing the final consonant is large,

being on the order of 50 to 100 ms. The effect is largest if the vowel is the last one in the utterance.

An illustration of these effects is given in Figure 8-3 showing spectrograms of the sentences *Take a cap in the cab* and *Take a cab on the Cap* (a peninsula on the French Riviera). Each sentence was spoken fluently without any pauses. The durations of the consonant constrictions and the preceding vowels are given in ms on the spectrograms. The vowel before the phrase boundary

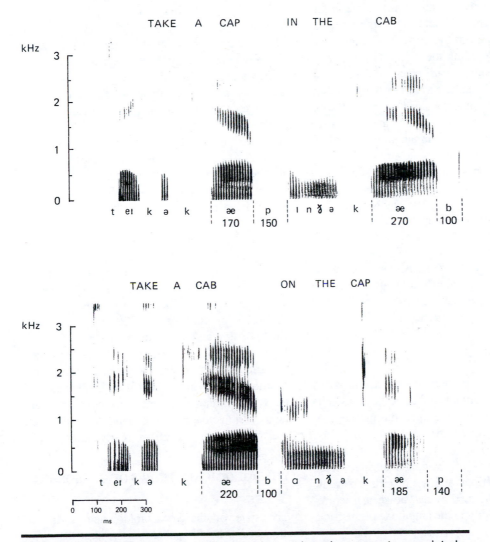
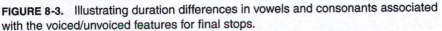

FIGURE 8-3.   Illustrating duration differences in vowels and consonants associated with the voiced/unvoiced features for final stops.

[b] in the second sentence is 220 ms in duration, but the vowel before the phrase boundary [p] in the first sentence is only 170 ms, giving a lengthening effect of 50 ms due to the voiced consonant. For the utterance final vowels, the [æ] of *cab* in the first sentence and the [æ] of *Cap* in the second sentence, the lengthening is 85 ms, a very large durational difference.

The durations in the first and second sentences of Figure 8-3, including release bursts of the intervocalic [p] and [b], respectively, show a 50 ms shortening effect of voicing, a fairly large difference due to the phrase-final position of these consonants; it is equal to the amount of lengthening of the vowel preceding the voiced [b]. It is as if there is a tendency toward equal syllable length between *cap* and *cab*, and thus the vowel duration of *cap* loses the amount gained by the following consonant. However, this is not the case when the two syllables are final in the utterance, where the shortening of consonant closure is 40 ms but the vowel lengthening is much greater, 85 ms.

Vowels before syllable-final consonants that are not pre-boundary also show a lengthening effect depending on voiced versus unvoiced consonant, but it is a much smaller difference, being on the order of the difference in duration of closure.

The timing coordinations between the vocal folds and the upper articulators that produce the voicing effects have been described by Slis and Cohen (1969) and Slis (1975).

VOICED AND UNVOICED FRICATIVES

The production of the voiced/unvoiced contrast in fricatives is very similar to that of the stops: The vocal folds are held wide apart during the constriction interval for unvoiced fricatives and close for voiced fricatives.

The vocal folds often vibrate during voiced fricative constrictions and the resulting periodic modulation of the airflow can be seen in corresponding periodicity in the amplitude of the frication sound.

The characteristics of voiced and unvoiced fricatives are illustrated in Figure 8-4, showing spectrograms of the clauses *the base of the bays* and *the bays at the base*. Each clause contains two phrases, one of which is at the end of the utterance with voiced [z] and unvoiced [s] in phrase-final boundary positions. This allows us to compare the durations of the preboundary sounds at both utterance positions as we just did for the stops [b] and [p]. The durations of the fricative constriction intervals and preceding vowels are given on the spectrograms.

First, it should be noted in Figure 8-4 that the vocal folds do not always vibrate during the voiced fricative: The utterance-final [z] in the first clause shows no little or no low-frequency sound and no correlated periodicity in the higher frequencies, whereas the intervocalic [z] in the second clause shows pronounced periodic low-frequency sound and a considerable amount of periodicity in the middle and high frequencies of the turbulent frication. The mid- and high-frequency periodicity is difficult to discern because it is superimposed on the random amplitude fluctuations of the turbulence; therefore, the pulses of the low-frequency sound have been marked on the spectrogram at middle and high positions to make it easier to look for the pulse correlations.

The durations of the constrictions and the preceding vowels show strong effects of the consonant voicing, similar to those seen for the stops. The lengthening of the vowel by the voicing of the following consonant is 120 ms in utterance-final position and 30 ms in the non-final but pre-boundary position. The shortening of the consonant constriction by voicing is 80 ms in utterance-final position and 35 ms in non-final. Lengthening of the syllables due to utterance-final position is very large: 330 ms longer than in non-final position for the syllable *base* and 360 ms longer for *bays*.

PHYSIOLOGICAL STUDIES OF CONSONANT VOICING

The state of the vocal folds, held apart for unvoiced or held together for voiced, is the major factor in the voicing feature of consonants. How is this accomplished in speech production? Because

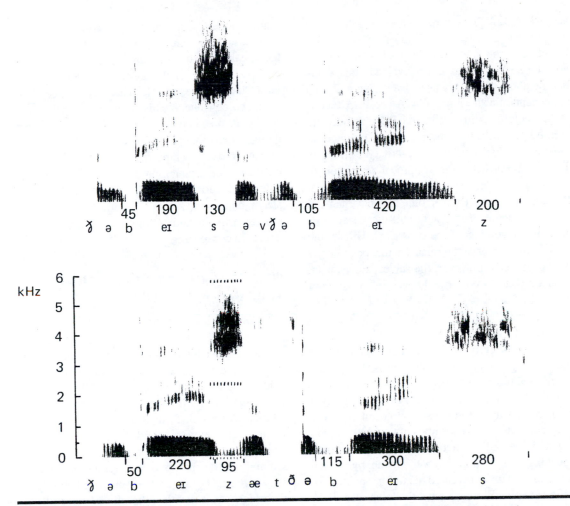

FIGURE 8-4. Illustrating characteristics of voiced and unvoiced fricatives in different positions in utterance. Durations and frication-periodicity are indicated on the spectrograms.

of its high importance, linguistically in the voicing distinction and prosodically in the control of intonation and stress, the physiology of vocal-fold positioning and tensioning has been extensively studied by many researchers. In presenting some of their findings it is convenient to think of voiced as the default state of consonants and unvoiced as the state that marks the "voicing" distinction (for production/perception evidence on this view, see Pickett, Bunnell, & Revoile, 1995).

In one of the earliest studies of actual muscle actions using modern electronic techniques, Hirose

and Gay (1972) recorded the control activity of positioners of the vocal folds during speech. The positioning activity was recorded from electrodes inserted in two muscles: (1) an abductor muscle that is anatomically arranged to pull the vocal folds apart, the posterior cricoarytenoid muscle (PCA), and (2) an adductor muscle that pulls the folds together, the interarytenoid muscle (IA). The subject spoke phrases that contrasted in the voicing of consonants, such as /əpʌp/, /əbʌp/, /əpɪb/. Each phrase was spoken a number of times and a computer was used to add up the muscle activity signals received from small electrodes in each muscle (averaged EMG activity). It was found that the adductor IA was active during vowel phonation and during voiced consonants but the abductor PCA was active during unvoiced consonants. Furthermore, the IA and PCA tended to be reciprocal in action: As PCA activity increased to open the vocal folds to produce an unvoiced consonant, the IA activity decreased. That is, because of the reciprocal relaxation of the adductor interarytenoid muscles, the abductor PCAs do not have to overcome the active tension of the adductors in order to pull the vocal folds apart for unvoicing of the consonant. Hirose and Gay did not observe the related actual positions of the vocal folds; however, the subject's consonant acoustic patterns confirmed the correlated state of the folds.

Flanagan and his co-workers (Flanagan, Rabiner, Christopher, Boch, & Shipp, 1976) studied the activity of PCA and IA together with the opening and closing of the glottis. The glottal opening was observed and recorded by the trans-illumination method, that is, by passing light from above the glottis to a photocell beneath. Very accurate time recordings of the glottal opening and the muscle actions that occurred upon speaking single phrases were made by digital recording. These revealed that, for an intervocalic unvoiced consonant, the abductor PCA muscle began activity 20 to 30 ms in advance of the glottal opening and continued to act while the glottis was open, until (at about 40 or 50 ms before the following vowel) the IA muscle activity began, starting to move the folds back together, and the PCA muscle ceased acting. This brief study indicated that the muscles controlling the vocal fold positions are very precisely activated in time to produce the voicing differences between consonants.

A recent review and discussion by Löfqvist (1995) deals specifically with the timing of muscle activities in unvoicing movements, that is, open-then-close glottal gestures, of the vocal folds for unvoiced consonants. The reciprocal actions of PCA (open) and IA (close) were confirmed for many phonetic contexts. The crico-thyroid (CT) muscle also participates via active tensioning of the vocal folds to assist unvoicing. There appears to be a separate glottal gesture to "open," or at least toward more open, for each occurrence of an unvoiced consonant. This was seen even in clusters of unvoiced consonants. In other words, even though there may be no need for the glottis to retreat from an open posture, over a succession of unvoiced consonants, there is an active, muscle-controlled narrowing of the glottis between adjacent consonants. It is as if the glottis moves momentarily toward a voicing position between unvoiced consonants.

PHYSIOLOGICAL STUDIES OF FRICATIVE VOICING

In order for a long frication sound to be produced, as seen in fricatives, a continuing supply of high airflow is necessary. This tends to be incompatible with voicing phonation because the vocal folds are held together throughout the constriction, restricting the flow. Experimenters have studied this problem, measuring the air pressure behind the constriction and the degree of adduction of the vocal folds for stops and fricatives. Comparing the amount of air pressure behind the constriction, it is highest for unvoiced stops and next highest for unvoiced fricatives, voiced fricatives, and voiced stops, in that order (Collier, Lisker, Hirose, & Ushijima, 1979). Thus, the air pressure in the mouth is higher for voiced fricatives than for voiced stops; the higher pressure is probably necessary for the airflow for the friction sound. There is some evidence that the vocal folds are held more open during voiced fricatives than during voiced stops (Sawashima, 1968; Sawashima & Miyazaki, 1973). This would seem necessary to allow enough airflow to produce a frication sound. Sometimes there is no voicing during voiced fricatives; then the only contrast with unvoiced fricatives is durational shortening and weaker frication for the voiced fricative.

Collier and colleagues also studied the action of the muscles controlling the position of the

TABLE 8-1.   Summary of the main features of the voiced/unvoiced contrast in stops and fricatives.

FEATURE	VOICED STOPS	VOICED FRICATIVES	UNVOICED STOPS	UNVOICED FRICATIVES
Timing				
Preceding vowel	Long preceding vowel when in pre-boundary position	Long preceding vowel when in pre-boundary position	Shortened preceding vowel when in pre-boundary position	Shortened preceding vowel when in pre-boundary position
Constriction	Brief oral closure	Brief oral constriction	Longer oral closure	Longer oral constriction
Release	Brief release transient, 10–20 ms	No transient on release	Strong release transient and aspiration, 30–70 ms	No transient on release
Spectral				
Constriction	Very low-frequency sound during closure, but this may be absent (de-voiced)	Very low frequency sound during constriction and correlated fluctuations in mid- and high-frequency regions; these two features may be absent	Silence	Strong mid- and high-frequency sound
Release	Weak transient on release of closure but no aspiration	No transient on release	Strong release transient; following oral resonances during aspiration showing formant transitions in F2 and F3	No transient on release

vocal folds in voiced and unvoiced fricatives and stops in Dutch. They concluded that voicing was accompanied by less activity in the abductor muscles than the activity seen on unvoiced consonants, confirming the results for stops in English found by Hirose and Gay (1972). However, there was less activity in the adductor muscles (they pull and hold the folds together) on the fricatives than on the stops, indicating that the folds are positioned farther apart for fricatives than for stops, apparently to allow more airflow and thus produce frication sound. This was later confirmed with actual observations of glottal opening (see Löfqvist, 1995).

SUMMARY

The features of consonant voicing are summarized in Table 8-1.

CHAPTER NINE.

CONSONANTS: FEATURES OF PLACE OF ARTICULATION

Up to this point in our study of the consonants we have described the acoustic features that arise from the manner of articulation and from the source of sound. In manner of articulation we looked at the formants of glides, stops, and nasals, and the turbulent sounds of fricatives; for the source of sound we studied the low-frequency features of the voiced source and the characteristics of unvoiced sources. A final factor in shaping the sound patterns of a consonant is its *place of articulation* in the vocal tract. A consonant may be articulated at any place at which a constriction can be formed. Almost any manner or source can be employed in combination with any place of constriction. Thus, the linguistically distinctive sounds that result from using these many different combinations are remarkably diverse.

Here, for our acoustic study we will look only at the major place patterns seen in English consonants. These places we have called front or labial, middle (alveolar and palatal), and back (velar).

Phonology Note: Places of Articulation

Linguists have found, thus far, 16 different places of consonant articulation in the world's languages (Ladefoged & Maddieson, 1988). For stops, the alveolar and dental places are used somewhat more frequently than the velar place, followed by bilabial, palatal, uvular, and, least of all, complex simultaneous places of labial+velar (Henton et al., 1992).

The place of articulation affects the shape of the vocal tract, so we would expect that many of the acoustic differences between places of articulation will be seen in differences in the formant patterns. Furthermore, in forming consonant constrictions the vocal tract must move between open and constricted at different places, causing varied types of transitions in the formant frequencies. Thus, the place features of the consonants are associated with transitional changes in spectral patterns, whereas the manner and source features tend to be more constant in spectral pattern and characterized by sudden on-off changes in the gross features of the spectrum. However, the complete pattern of a speech sound depends on the source as well as its relation to the vocal tract shape. Some of these relations are discussed in this chapter. First, we look at the transitions in the formants that are related to the distinction between labial place of articulation and alveolar place; then we see how different adjacent vowels affect the formant transitions for different places of consonants, and how the spectrum of fricatives depends on their place of articulation.

FORMANT TRANSITIONS OF ALVEOLAR VERSUS LABIAL CONSONANTS

Recall from Chapter Three that alveolar constrictions cause F2 frequency to rise and labial constrictions cause F2 frequency to fall, and the frequency change of F2 is dependent on the amount of constriction. When an alveolar consonant is articulated, the closing movement goes from open to more constricted and the opening movement goes from constricted to more open.

Therefore, with an alveolar consonant we expect F2 frequency to rise in frequency during the closing movement and fall in frequency during the opening movement. And for a labial consonant F2 frequency would fall during the closing movement and rise during the opening movement. These effects are illustrated in Figure 9-1, showing spectrograms of the alveolar and labial stops and a glide: *a tot, a dot, a yacht,* in the top row and *a pate, abate, await* in the lower row.

These examples were selected so that a neutral vowel precedes each consonant. Note that the F2 frequency of this vowel rises during the closing movement to the alveolar consonants in the top row of the figure, but F2 falls before the labial consonants in the bottom half of the figure. Upon the opening to the vowel following the consonants, F2 falls in frequency after the alveolar consonants in the top row and in the bottom row F2 rises toward its frequency in the following vowel, upon the opening movement from the labial consonants. It will also be noticed that the F3 frequency tends to parallel the transitions in F2 frequency. Comparing the unvoiced stops in the top row with the voiced stops below, it can also be seen that the transition in F2 frequency is visible during the aspiration period of the release burst of the unvoiced stops.

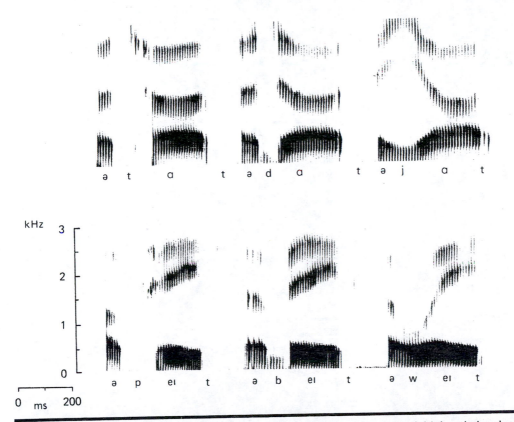

FIGURE 9-1. Spectrograms to compare intervocalic stops and glides at the labial and alveolar places of articulation. Note that alveolar versus labial place is differentiated by the direction of transition in F2: During the closure from the neutral vowel [ə] preceding each consonant, for alveolar place (top row), the vowel F2 transitions to a higher frequency, but for labial place (bottom row) F2 transitions to a lower frequency. During the opening of each consonant into the following vowel, F2 transitions go opposite to their closing direction, falling in frequency for the alveolars and rising for the labials, for both [ɑ] and [eɪ].

CONSONANT PLACE: TRANSITIONS WITH DIFFERENT VOWELS

As we have seen in Figure 9-1, the distinction between labial and alveolar place of articulation can be signaled simply by the direction of transition of the second formant. However, when we consider vowels other than the [a] and [eɪ]

combined with all three places of stop articulation—labial, alveolar, and velar—the distinctions become more complex. We can best appreciate these differences by examining some further visualizations of the spectral patterns and formant changes in Figures 9-2 and 9-3.

In the perspective spectrograms of Figure 9-2 we focus closely on the consonant release and the

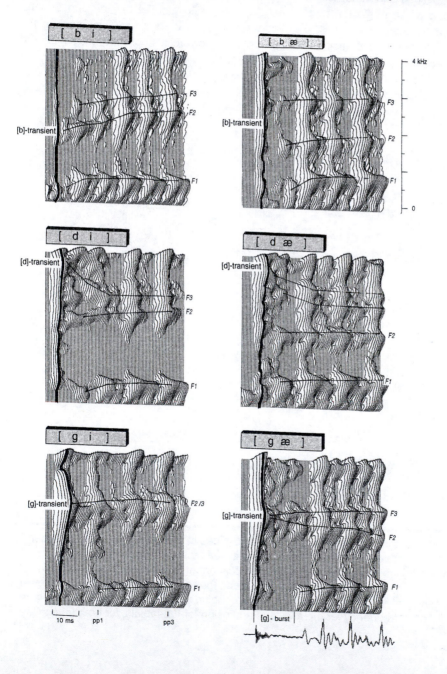

early part of the vowel following, because, as we shall see in later chapters, perception research has shown the release burst and early vowel transition to contain the crucial cues to the distinction of stop place. The consonants [b], [d], and [g] were spoken in single utterances of the form [əCV]. The stressed CV was spoken in a citation style at an average rate of 450 ms per syllable. V was either of two front vowels, the close vowel [i], or the open vowel [æ]. The sample taken contained the release burst and three to five pitch periods of the following vowel.

Examine the frequency transitions of the peaks of F1, F2, and F3, which have been traced over the crests of each pitch period of the vowels. For the labial and alveolar stops, the F2 transitions differ in direction with the vowels [i] and [æ], in the same way that they did with the [a] of the previous figure, namely, that the direction of transition of F2 on opening is upward for the labials and downward for the alveolars. On the other hand, with the velar stop [g] the transition of F2 is also downward on the opening of the consonant as it was for the alveolar stop. Here we must examine F3 to see a definite difference. The F3 opening transition from [g] tends to be divergent from the F2 transition instead of parallel to it, as it was for the alveolar stop. This is especially noticeable in the lower row of Figure 9-2 on the vowel [æ]. Initially, the F3 transition is flat and then rising to give a divergent pattern.

Another important feature of the stops that is distinctive for place of constriction and release, is the burst of sound upon the release of the constriction. The sound of the release is due to a step-like increase in sound pressure as the oral air

FIGURE 9-2. Perspectrograms for comparing labial, alveolar, and velar voiced stops spoken in [əCV] with front vowels [i] and [æ]. Examine the spectra of the transients, marked by the heavy vertical curves, and the following transitions of the formants marked with light straight lines that trace the peaks of the formants in each pitch period of the vowel. The labial place [b] is distinguished by upward transitions following the transients in both F2 and F3 and by a diffuse, weak transient spectrum. The velar place of [g] is distinguished from the alveolar [d] by an F3 transition that is divergent from the F2 transition and by a release transient that is "compact" in the peak part of the spectrum. At the lower left the time scale is indicated and the instants of pitch-pulse onsets are marked, for the [gi] above. At the lower right, underneath the perspectrogram of [gæ], the waveform of the [g]-burst is plotted in synchrony with the spectra above. Note that the resonant frequency that dominates the [gæ] transient spectrum at about 2500 Hz corresponds to a relatively long, rapid oscillation in the waveform; there are about 15 cycles of transient strong oscillation or ringing in the first 6 ms, followed by 14 ms of aspiration that also shows weak oscillations at about the same frequency. See text for more complete discussion.[1]

---

[1] Technical details on the construction of the perspective spectrograms: The spectral patterns are "waterfall" plots made with SpeechStation 3.1 of Sensimetrics Corporation. Each panel plots 100 spectra taken at successive 0.5 ms intervals. The spectra are plotted with a perspective-generating slant instead of the normal spectrum scale of vertical frequency versus horizontal amplitude. Thus vertical distances of frequency depend on the concurrent amplitude. The frequency scale at the upper right has been displaced upward so you can estimate formant frequencies at the highest peak amplitudes of the spectra; it should not be used for intermediate or low-amplitude peaks. The smoothing or averaging over the individual components of each spectrum was obtained by using a very short segment of the waveform for each spectrum. The segments were selected by a 6.4 ms Hamming window and spectrum-analyzed by Fourier analysis (FFT). The effective window was 3.2 ms, resulting in amplitude values averaged over approximately 3 successive harmonics (an effective analysis bandwidth of 313 Hz). Waveform features: Below the [gæ] spectrogram I have plotted the waveform of the syllable onset to show the release burst followed by the first four pitch periods of the vowel that are included in the perspectrogram.

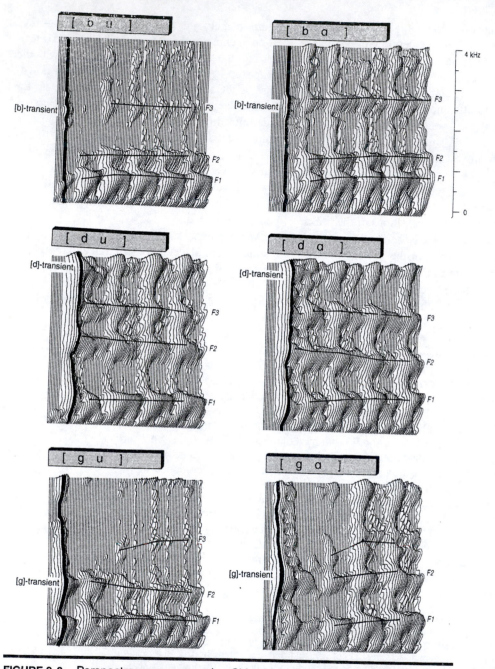

FIGURE 9-3. Perspectrograms comparing CVs of labial, alveolar, and velar voiced stops followed by back vowels. Here velar place is distinguished by flat or upward F3 transitions and very strongly resonant transients (conditions same as Figure 9-2).

pressure contained by stop obstruction is suddenly freed by the opening of the stop; this step excites the air pressure in the vocal tract to oscillate, producing a wave called the *release transient*. In Figure 9-2, at the lower right, a transient wave is seen as the very first fine oscillations, lasting about 6 ms in that case, in the waveform plotted below the [gæ] spectrogram.

The spectrum of the transient depends on the shape of the vocal tract at that moment, which in turn depends on the place of the constriction together with the anticipatory shape of the following vowel.

For acoustic comparison of these release transients among places/vowels, the spectral contours of the time-samples with the highest amplitude values are heavily outlined in Figure 9-2. All spectra of the figure are plotted with an upward-tilted bias relative to the flat base, by applying a high-pass pre-emphasis of +6 dB/ octave. This is a common standard bias that "flattens" the overall spectrum representation for easy comparisons between spectra. It is also used in the time-frequency-amplitude plots of spectrograms (as in Figure 9-1).

Notice in Figure 9-2 that the total stop burst spectrum, transient spectrum and following aspirate frication vary among [b], [d], and [g]. This serves as another differentiating factor among the three places of articulation. Examine carefully the bursts for their frequency extents and frequency locations. It will be seen that the labial bursts cover a fairly wide frequency band from about 1500 Hz upward, but that they are very weak, consisting only of a transient without any aspiration at all. The release bursts of [d] on the other hand are much stronger and, following the release transient, they have strong energy, which becomes stronger, going up from 2000 Hz. Finally, for [g] the release bursts are rather strong, but the strongest energy in them is located at about 2500 Hz and is not spread out in frequency as much as it is for the alveolar [d]. Thus, comparing the spectra, the labial burst is diffuse and weak, the alveolar burst is diffuse and stronger in the high frequencies, and the velar burst is compact and strong in the mid-frequencies.

The same stop consonants are combined with back vowels in Figure 9-3. The F2 transitions exhibit the same difference between [b] and [d] as they did with the front vowels, namely, that for the labial [b] the F2 opening transition is upward in frequency, whereas for the alveolar [d] the situation is just the opposite, the opening F2 transition is downward. The frequency of F3 can be seen to move more or less in parallel with F2 for the alveolar consonant [d]. For the velar consonant [g] the F2 transitions are similar to those for [d], with the opening transition downward in frequency. The frequency of F3 upon the opening transition is either level or diverging upward from the F2 transition. The consonant release bursts before the back vowels show a similar difference between [b] and [d] to that seen with front vowels, that is, the [b] bursts are weak and the [d] bursts are strong in energy at F2 and above. However, the [g] bursts are not compact in frequency as with the front vowels; they show downward F2 opening transitions from low F2 starting positions because of the back constriction. The F2 starting position is strongly resonant in the release burst; in contrast, the [b] bursts do not show the low F2 starting frequency at all. Comparing the F2 bursts and the starting F2s between [d] and [g], it is seen that, for the same vowel, the F2 starting position is much lower in frequency for [g] than it is for [d].

These features of place of voiced stops are also seen in unvoiced stops, but the opening F2 transitions take place largely during the relatively longer aspiration intervals of the voiceless release bursts.

Fant (1973) described the production factors leading to the spectral differences at the release of stop consonants depending on different places of consonant constriction. Immediately after the opening transient, the airflow relieving the mouth pressure passes through the still narrow constriction, generating a frication turbulence noise. The size and shape of the cavity in front of this noise source determine the spectrum pattern of this frication. The alveolar [t] and [d] have a small front cavity, which acts as a high pass filter that transmits more turbulence energy in the higher frequencies than for the velar constrictions for [k] and [g], which have a larger cavity in front of the constriction and thus have a main concentration of energy in the burst at a lower frequency. The [p] and [b] consonants have no front cavity in front of the release point and this causes a diffuse spectrum in the release frication, that is, a spectrum pattern where there are no very prominent peaks.

After the opening movement has proceeded far enough, the constriction no longer produces a sound source and then the source shifts to the glottis. For unvoiced consonants an aspirant source is generated by the airflow through the glottis, still open but beginning to close down for the following vowel; the resultant aspiration phase shows formants determined by the shape of the oral-pharyngeal tract, at first without F1 because of the open glottis. For voiced consonants the release frication, which is generally weaker because of the lower air pressure in the mouth, is followed by voicing phonation.

PLACE FEATURES OF NASAL CONSONANTS

In the nasal murmur that occurs during the oral occlusion intervals of [m, n, ŋ], the spectrum pattern is determined mainly by the sound transmission of the pharyngeal-nasal tract, secondarily affected by the closed oral cavity. The oral cavity may then be viewed as a side branch of different lengths depending on the place of occlusion. The length of the oral side branch is greatest for [m], shorter for [n], the shortest for [ŋ]; this length affects the frequency of an antiresonance (zero) in the transmission of the pharyngeal-nasal tract, which consequently affects the spectrum of the murmur. The frequency of the zero tends to be inversely related to the length of the oral side branch and is at about 800 Hz for [m], 1500–2000 Hz for [n], and about 5000 Hz or above for [ŋ]. The murmur spectrum is strong in amplitude in the region below 500 Hz and relatively weak above 500 Hz. Thus, the differences in murmur features, mainly the location of the zero corresponding to

nasal place of articulation, are not very prominent. The formant transitions in adjacent vowels appear acoustically to be more distinctive than the differences in murmur spectrum (Fant, 1960; Fujimura, 1962; House, 1957; Malécot, 1956).

The formant transitions of the nasal consonants would be similar to those of the stops articulated at the same place, except for the fact that nasalization occurs in the intervals preceding and following nasal consonants. As explained in Chapter 7, this nasalization inserts variable zeroes, in the transmission of the oral tract, in the region of F1 and F2. This makes it difficult to analyze out the different spectrum features that might be related to the tongue and lip articulations. However, early research indicated that consistent place differences must exist among the spectral patterns in vowel-to-nasal transitions because listeners can correctly identify these transitions as for [m, n] or [ŋ] (Malécot, 1956, Table 5). More recent perception tests on the integration of the murmur and transition cues for the [m,n]-distinction, initially before [ɑ,u] or [i], indicated that the transitions may be slightly more distinctive than the murmurs, for [ɑ] and [u] but not for [i]; interactions between place of vowel articulation and place of consonant may be responsible for these differences (Repp, 1986). An excellent condensation of perception research on [m,n] is given in Kent and Read (1992).

PLACE FEATURES OF FRICATIVE CONSONANTS

It will be recalled that the fricative sounds are produced by forming a constriction through which the strong airflow becomes turbulent and produces a random, noise-like sound. This frication sound has random fluctuations in amplitude and covers a broad range of frequencies (like a white noise). This is the source sound for fricatives. The place at which the constriction is formed and the shape and size of the front cavity between the constriction and the air outside the lips have a frequency-filtering effect on the source sound in much the same way that vowel shape acts as a filter to form the vowel spectra from the source sound produced by the glottis. The back cavity, behind the constriction, does not strongly affect the fricative spectrum.

One general filtering rule that determines the spectra of the different fricative sounds is that the low-frequency resonances of the shaping cavity are at frequencies inversely related to the size of the cavity (Heinz & Stevens, 1961). These lower resonances are the strongest fricative resonances. Figure 9-4 illustrates this principle with a spectrogram of a specially chosen phrase (spoken by an adult male) that includes each of the unvoiced fricative consonants followed by a back vowel; the phrase is *How Shaw saw it thaw for him.* For the first fricative in the phrase, [h], the sound source is at the glottis and thus the front cavity is the largest of the five fricatives. In the spectrogram the frequency location of the strongest part of the fricative sound has been marked with brackets. Notice that, as the front cavity becomes smaller, that is, as we go from the largest [h] to [ʃ] to [s] to [θ] to [f], the position of the strongest resonances moves upward in frequency. The strongest resonances are in a region around 1 kHz for [h], 3 kHz for [ʃ], 4 kHz for [s], 5 kHz

for [θ], and a range from about 4 1/2 to 7 kHz for [f]. The [f] sound also has weak low frequency turbulences that extend all the way down to about 1 kHz as indicated by the first left-hand bracket in the spectrogram next to [f]. For female and child speakers all the resonances would be shifted upward because of the smaller size of the oral tract.

The spectrum pattern of the [h] sound varies because of two factors. First, the vowel shape to follow the [h] is beginning to be formed before the production of the frication; this shape will change for different vowels and thus affect the spectrum of the [h]. Second, for the close front vowels the source of the [h] turbulence may be at a velar or upper pharyngeal location rather than low in the pharynx or at the glottis. Then the cavity in front will be rather small and the intense part of the frequency spectrum will be located in the region of F2 and F3 of the following vowel, which will be at a much higher location than for the [h] before [a] seen in Figure 9-4.

In the last syllable of the phrase in the spectrogram (Figure 9-4), a "voiced [h]" is seen at the beginning of the *him*. This sound appears to be completely voiced at a very low frequency and

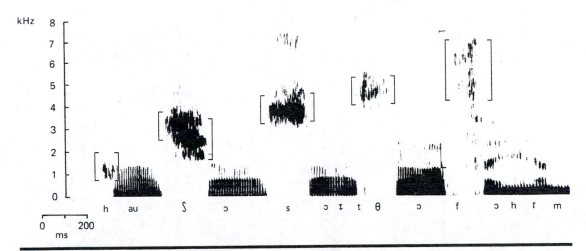

FIGURE 9-4. Spectrogram of a special phrase having a series of fricative consonants going from large to small front cavity. The main resonant frequencies of the fricatives are bracketed and are seen to rise in frequency as the front cavity becomes smaller and smaller.

TABLE 9-1. Summary of spectral features corresponding to place of consonant articulation[a].

CONSONANT CLASS	PLACE OF ARTICULATION						
	LABIAL	DENTAL	ALVEOLAR	PALATAL	VELAR	PHARYNGEAL	GLOTTAL
Glide — Constriction/vowel transition	[w] Low F2/upward F2		[j] High F2/down-ward F2	[j]			
Voiced stop — Transient/vowel transition	[b] Diffuse, weak/upward F2		[d] Diffuse, high-frequency/downward F2		[g] Compact mid-frequency/diverging F2 and F3		[ʔ] Transient form-ants same as following vowel
Unvoiced stop — Transient/aspiration	[p] Diffuse/upward F2		[t] Strong, high-frequency/downward F2		[k] Strong, compact, mid-frequency/diverging F2 and F3		
Nasals — Murmur/vowel transition	[m] Zero c. 800 Hz/nasalized upward F2		[n] Mid-frequency zero/nasalized downward F2		[ŋ] High-frequency zero/nasalized diverging F2 and F3		
Fricatives — Frication (strong for unvoiced, weaker for voiced)/vowel transitions	[v, f] Diffuse spectrum, strongest around 5–7 kHz/upward F2	[ð, θ] Diffuse spectrum strongest in frequencies around 5 kHz and above/downward F2	[z, s] Strong spectrum at 4 kHz and above/often no vowel transitions	[ʒ, ʃ] Strong spectrum at 3 kHz and above/often no vowel transitions		[h] Weak spectrum, 1 kHz and above having formants of following vowel/no transitions	

[a] All transitional features are considered only as seen on consonant release. Two phases of each consonant type are described, separated by a slash. For example, for the glide type the two phases are the constriction and the following transition into the vowel, characterized for [w] by low F2 frequency and upward transition of F2, respectively.

the F1 and F2 resonances are like those of the following [ɪ]. However, the formants appear to be excited irregularly compared with the vowel. This is probably because the glottis is held only partially closed for the voiced [h] instead of completely closed as for a vowel.

The different voiced fricative consonants, [ʒ, z, v, ð] and voiced [h], are produced at similar locations to the unvoiced ones that we have just discussed and, therefore, their frequency spectra are also governed by the size of cavity in front of the constriction. The friction sounds of voiced fricatives are usually somewhat weaker in intensity than in the unvoiced fricatives because the vocal folds are held closer to a voicing position and the total airflow available for producing turbulence at the constriction is therefore lower than for the unvoiced fricatives, where the vocal folds are held wide apart.

SUMMARY

A summary of the main acoustic features of the places of consonant articulation is given in Table 9-1.

CHAPTER TEN

THE FLOW OF SPEECH

I do not believe that a division of the flow of speech . . . has the slightest justification . . .
—E. W. Scripture, 1902

This chapter is about the flow of speech. We have already seen how consonants and vowels flow into each other, in the transitions between the consonant constrictions and the vowel openings. Now we look briefly at further types of interaction in the flow of articulations and we also examine some properties of fluent speech.

The smooth flow and coordination of the articulatory movements of speech are so basic to its production that I regret having to relegate this topic to the end of our study of speech production. Nine chapters have taken speech apart and now this one tries to put it back together again. This can be done only to a small extent. At some future time it will be possible to organize acoustic phonetics from the movement flow as the fundamental starting point. This approach would be more natural and it could simplify explanations of how spoken messages are perceived and understood. In the meantime, rather than wait for a complete motor theory of speech production, great progress can be made, as in the past 50 years, using the analytic concepts of acoustics and linguistics. These concepts presently work best when articulation is held still in order to study the spectral patterns, which are then seen to change with the flow of changing articulations. If we could begin with the flow of articulations, then transitions and so-called coarticulatory effects would be the primary patterns, not the fixed vocal tract shapes with which we began our study of vowels in Chapter Three. For new theoretical approaches based on the movement flow of speech see Chapters Fourteen and Fifteen.

Speech patterns are typically in transition much of the time. In casual speech, the vowel formant frequencies are usually in transition on the way to or from positions that are more neutral than the vowels of carefully enunciated speech. The bursts of noise of consonants show changes in spectrum under the influence of adjacent articulations. As an example, examine the spectrograms of the sentence in Figure 10-1: *The branch droops and strikes the steel track*. First note in the top spectrogram that the second formants of the vowels are almost always in transition; F2 rarely stands still. The first formant also moves up and down because of the consonant constrictions, and to different positions for the vowels.

The third formant goes through extensive changes during the [r] sounds, where the formants are traced with lines in the top spectrogram. All of the [r] sounds begin with F3 at a very low position, about 1.6 to 1.8 kHz, with the following [u] and [a] causing lower starting frequencies for F3 than the [æ]. The F3 transitions are all upward toward the normal F3 position of about 2.5 kHz. The starting position of F2 in [r] varies greatly with the following F2 position for the vowel. These are coarticulatory effects on the spectrum patterns of [r].

The [s] sounds in Figure 10-1 are more fully displayed in the lower spectrogram where the frequency range is extended to 8 kHz. The main

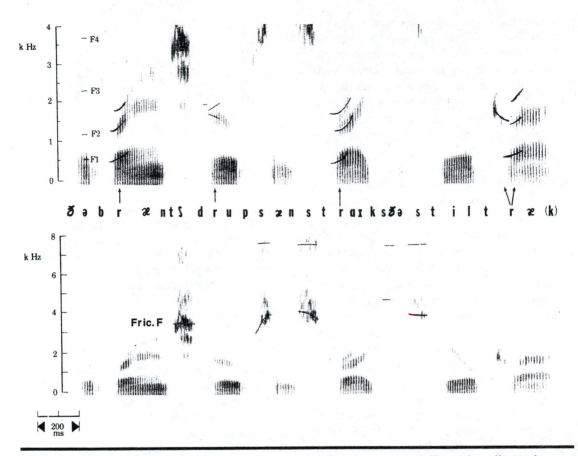

FIGURE 10-1. Spectrogram of *The branch droops and strikes the steel track*, illustrating effects of coarticulation on the spectra of [r] sounds (top spectrogram) and [s] sounds (bottom spectrogram). The [r] sounds are strongly influenced by the nature of the vowels that follow them, as can be seen from the lines tracing the formants. In the bottom spectrogram the main resonances of the [s] sounds have been traced; here we see that the sound following [s] had a large effect on this resonance. See the text for a detailed description of these coarticulatory effects.

resonances of the [s]'s are traced with lines. The upper resonances, above about 5 kHz, are relatively steady in frequency, but there are frequency transitions in the lower resonances. The [s] in *droops* has a large upward transition in its lower resonance. The transition is rapid in the first 50 ms and goes from 2.9 to 3.8 kHz; this transition occurs because the [s] begins while the lips are still only partly open in transition from the preceding closed position for [p], and thus the [s] cavity is strongly rounded but becoming less rounded as the lips open rapidly over a period of about 50 ms. The first [s] in *strikes* is influenced by the following [t] and [r] articulations and has a downward transition from 3.9 to 3.6 kHz; the second [s] in *strikes* has a steady resonance at 4.5 kHz. The [s] in *steel* has a steady low resonance at 3.75 kHz.

COARTICULATION

Coarticulation is the term used to refer to the influences of the articulation of one sound on the articulation of other sounds in the same utterance.

For example compare the spoken words *seep* and *sweep* in Figure 10-2. In *seep* the [s] has very little sound energy below 3.5 kHz but in *sweep* the [s] energy extends down to about 2 kHz. This is because of the coarticulation of [s] with the following [w]; the [w] needs to be formed by close rounding of the lips and, in order to achieve that at the proper time, the rounding movement must begin during the [s], in anticipation of the [w]. Lip-rounding lowers the resonance of the mouth cavity in front of the [s] constriction and causes more low frequencies in the source sound to be transmitted out of the mouth than in *seep*, where the lip open area during the [s] is larger and the mouth cavity in front of the [s] constriction is more open. In fact, a careful look at the [s] in *sweep* shows that for the first 50 ms it was nearly the same as in *seep*, with a main resonance at about 3.7 kHz versus 4.0 kHz for *seep*; however, during the last 60 ms the low frequency resonance of the [s] in *sweep* moves downward about 500 Hz under the influence of the coarticulation with [w].

A similar effect is seen when [s] is coarticulated with other labial consonants. Compare the [s] sounds in the words *sane*, *stain*, and *Spain* in Figure 10-3. In *sane* and *stain* the spectra of the [s] sounds are limited to frequencies above about

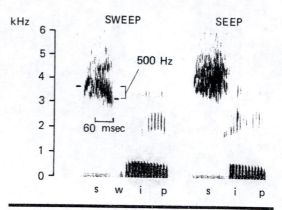

FIGURE 10-2. Spectrogram of the coarticulatory effect on the [s] spectrum of anticipatory lip-rounding for the following [w] in *sweep* for comparison with the [s] in *seep*. The lip-rounding causes a lowering of about 500 Hz in the frequency of the lower [s] resonances over a period of about 60 ms.

3.5 kHz, but in *Spain* the low-frequency edge of the [s]-spectrum sweeps downward just before the [p]-closure, as the lips move rapidly together. The effect is similar to the effect of [w] on [s] in the previous figure.

Coarticulation also affects final consonants, as can be seen in Figure 10-4, where we compare

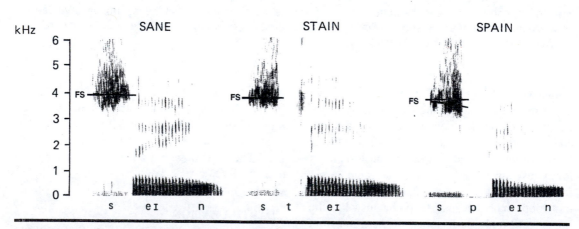

FIGURE 10-3. Spectrograms of *sane*, *stain*, and *Spain* for comparing the coarticulatory effects of following sounds on the spectrum of [s]. The frequency center of the low resonance of [s], FS, has been traced; this frequency is about the same in *sane* and *stain*, but has a downward transition before the [p] in *Spain* because of the anticipatory rounding of the lips during the [s].

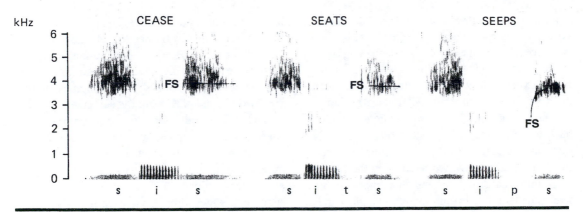

FIGURE 10-4. Spectrograms of *cease, seats,* and *seeps* for comparing the effects of preceding articulations on the spectrum of [s] in final position. The frequency center of the low resonance, FS, has been marked with a tracing through the final [s]'s; this frequency is constant at about 3.9 kHz for both *cease* and *seats,* but has a very large upward transition, from about 2.8 to 3.8 kHz, in *seeps.* See text for explanation.

the words *cease, seats,* and *seeps.* In the final [s] of *seeps* there is a coarticulation effect on the [s]-spectrum because of the preceding articulation of [p]. The [s]-constriction of the tongue is prepared during the interval when the lips are closed; when they start to open, the [s] sound begins, but because of the initial presence of lip constriction, the [s]-sound begins with a spectrum pattern extending much lower in frequency than in *cease* or *seats.* As the lips open farther, the low-frequency edge of the [s]-spectrum moves upward in frequency for about 40 ms until, during the final 120 ms, the spectrum is about the same as for the other final [s]'s.

These are examples of the coarticulation of two adjacent consonants. In the preceding chapter we saw how the place of articulation of a consonant affects the formant transitions of the adjacent vowels. There are also some coarticulation effects between a consonant and the preceding vowel. In other words, coarticulation is the rule in speech production; sounds unaffected by adjacent ones are exceptions.

How does coarticulation take place? Are there principles and rules of coarticulation? Obviously, these would be very important in explaining speech production. It seems in general that the movements of the tongue and lips are free to over-

lap in time but they must also be under sequential timing control in order to produce sufficiently intelligible utterances. Indeed, the tongue articulation for a vowel-consonant-vowel sequence can vary depending on the positions that the tongue must attain, the "target" positions, for the particular vowels and consonant. Let us examine some explanations of how articulations might interact.

There are two main factors behind coarticulatory effects: (1) the specific vocal tract shapes to be attained and (2) the motor program for performing the sequence of speech units: consonants, vowels, syllables, and phrases.

One major aspect of speech motor programs seems to be that they are anticipatory. That is, the movements for a sequence of sounds, syllables, and words seem to be organized so that later articulatory patterns are prepared for. Thus, current parts of an utterance are affected by what is soon to come. A similar anticipatory principle was seen in Chapter Five on prosodic features, where the evidence on consonant and vowel duration shows that these durations are shortened depending on the number of elements to follow within each hierarchical subunit of the utterance: consonant cluster, syllable, word, or phrase.

This anticipatory procedure might be expected to be a good way to program a sequence for communicative effectiveness, given the breath group structure of speech (Chapter Five). If there were no tailoring of early sounds depending on the number of sounds to follow, given the limited breath expenditure available before another breath must be taken, then it would frequently happen that proper phrasing and flow of utterance would have to be interrupted to take a breath. An arbitrary interruption would disturb intonation contours and lead to misinterpretation by the listener of grammatical structures and phonemes. Alternatively, the later-occurring sounds would have to be crowded in and spoken too rapidly for clarity.

MODEL OF SPEECH MOTOR PROGRAMMING

A general theory of motor programming was suggested by Lindblom and co-workers (1977), based on a previous principle derived by Klatt (1973, 1976). The theory is called the short-term memory (STM) model. The model proposes that there is a short-term storage of the neural instructions for speech movements; the contents of this storage are continually updated as instructions leave the store to discharge the actual movements, and new instructions enter for later discharge in proper sequence. The size of the store is limited; because of this, storage space must be economized; thus, every segment in store may be compressed in duration whenever a new segment is entered. However, there is a limit on this compressibility because of the time required for effective target reaching of articulations and the transition times between targets. For example, the gestures for stop consonants must reach full occlusion to produce audible stop-gaps and release bursts; the gestures for fricatives must reach a close constriction for an audible turbulence to be generated.

Consequences of the limits on compressibility are that the vowels and consonants of early monosyllabic words are shortened more in anticipation of increased numbers of later segments than are the segments of early bisyllabic words; similarly, early trisyllabic words suffer less shortening than bisyllabic words. This is because storage is in terms of numbers of syllables and not so much of the limited capacity is needed to store a word with fewer syllables. There is continual readjustment for economizing the allotted storage space depending on the number of phonemes, syllables, words, and phrases in the sentence.

The STM model for motor programming of speech accounts quantitatively for the general amounts of shortening seen and the limits. However, the final segments of an utterance are generally less subject to shortening than earlier segments, suggesting that the earlier segments, which are not so close to being played out of storage, can sacrifice more space to those on their way in. This seems to be another example of the operation of the anticipation principle. Further studies are needed to measure this effect and incorporate it into a general model of speech production for connected utterances.

THE SYLLABLE AS COARTICULATION UNIT

As mentioned in Chapter One, the most fundamental unit of speech seems to be the syllable. On the articulatory side, the syllable is produced by the alternation between open and constricted phases of the upper vocal tract. If the syllable is basic to articulation, then the effects of coarticulation would be secondary ones, explainable in terms of the organization of the syllable (Stetson, 1928, 1951). In other words, all the coarticulatory influences of a consonant on nearby consonants and vowels would depend on the particular way in which that consonant gesture and constriction must be carried out as dictated by the motor control program of the syllable cycle in which it functions as a constriction.

Kozhevnikov and Chistovich (1965) adopted the syllable as a unit for speech production studies of coarticulatory effects within and between syllables (1965, pp. 123–142) and as a basis for a motor theory of speech perception (see Pickett, 1985, for a detailed review, and Chistovich, Pickett, & Porter, 1998).

One study of coarticulation of the consonant and vowel movements of the tongue indicated that the syllable unit of motor organization is a consonant-vowel unit (Gay, 1977). The movements of the tongue were studied by making x-ray motion pictures. It was found that the anticipatory tongue movements for the second vowel of a VCV sequence never began until the consonant closure had been attained. Also, substantial movement toward the second vowel target occurred during the consonant occlusion, and this had a large effect on the position and shape of the tongue upon release of the occlusion. On the other hand, the vowel preceding the consonant had little effect on the position of the tongue at the moment of closure. In other words, there seems to be a great deal of coarticulation between consonant and following vowel as a unit and little or no carryover coarticulation of a vowel on a following consonant. Or to put it another way: What the vowel following a consonant is going to be has a large effect on the consonant release shape and what the consonant is going to be has an effect on a preceding vowel; but what the last vowel was has little effect on the coming consonant. It appears that the timing of anticipatory adjustments is geared to start the adjustments mainly during consonant constrictions. Thus, the programming for syllables seems to go in simple CV units. Further confirmation of this finding would establish a very important principle.

EFFECTS OF RATE OF UTTERANCE

The speed of speaking is another important aspect of the flow of speech. Speed of articulation can vary greatly depending on the different styles and dialects of different speakers. Furthermore, we may articulate very rapidly if we are in a hurry and the message is more or less redundant to the situation.

These variations in rate of articulation cause appropriate compression or expansion in time of the sound patterns. Examples are shown in the spectrograms of Figure 10-5. To look at compressions I spoke the phrase *anticipation of downstream articulations* at increasing rates of fluent utterance. The slowest rate is in the top of the

figure and the fastest rate is at the bottom, with the intermediate rates ranged in order in between. For the slowest rate, my style of speaking was exceedingly deliberate, with each word spoken almost as if isolated from the adjacent words, but without pauses and with words joined in a fluent manner; 13 syllables were spoken in 4.5 seconds, yielding a syllable rate of 2.9 syllables per second (s/s). The next faster rate was a little faster but still rather deliberately slow (3.1 s/s). The next rate was in my "formal" style, as if lecturing in class (4.5 s/s). The fourth rate was normal conversational (5.0 s/s); this rate is based on only 12 syllables because of the omission of the [ə] vowel in the "-tion" syllable of *anticipation*. The fifth rate was fast conversational (5.6 s/s). The fastest rate seemed to me to be the fastest I could speak with clear articulation (6.7 s/s).

First note that overall the change in rate from the most deliberate to the "fastest clear" articulation is rather large, a factor of 2.3:1. What segments have shortened to achieve this compression? It might be expected that, since consonant movements must often attain a specific occlusion or narrow constriction, increases in rate of utterance would tend to be absorbed more by the vowels than the consonants.

To test this for my utterances of Figure 10-5, I measured the durations of all of the consonant constrictions and vowels and calculated the percentages of compression between two pairs of rates. First, going from my slowest rate (2.9 s/s) to "lecture" style (4.5 s/s), both consonants and vowels were compressed 33%. Then, from "lecture" to my fastest rate, the vowels were compressed 50% but the consonants only 26%.

ASSIMILATION BETWEEN ADJACENT CONSONANTS

An important type of time compression occurs between consonants that are adjacent across a boundary between two syllables within the same breath group; these consonants are especially interesting because their timing reflects the motor programming of syllables and phrases. Examples

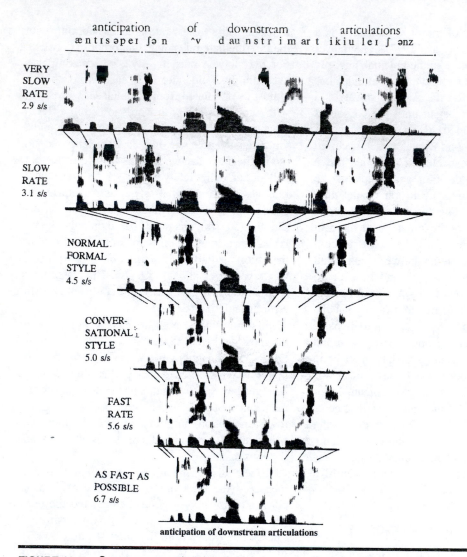

anticipation of downstream articulations
æ n t ɪ s ə p e ɪ ʃ ə n ˄v d aʊ n s t r i m a r t ɪ k i u l e ɪ ʃ ə n z

VERY SLOW RATE 2.9 s/s

SLOW RATE 3.1 s/s

NORMAL FORMAL STYLE 4.5 s/s

CONVER-SATIONAL STYLE 5.0 s/s

FAST RATE 5.6 s/s

AS FAST AS POSSIBLE 6.7 s/s

anticipation of downstream articulations

FIGURE 10-5. Spectrograms showing the compression in time of the phrase *anticipation of downstream articulations* spoken fluently at increasingly faster rates of utterance. The rates are given in syllables per second (s/s). The lines between spectrograms connect equivalent time-points in the stream of each utterance to help illustrate the amount of compression.

are double consonants, like the [pp] in *top pole*, and abutting different consonants, such as [pk] in *dropkick*, [dp] in *tadpole*, and [dk] in *sidekick*. At slow and moderate rates of utterance, the two consonants can be articulated separately (although the first consonant may not be released before the following one reaches occlusion). At faster rates of

utterance the articulation of the first consonant advances more into the following one, and at a very fast rate there remains only the single consonant at the beginning of the second syllable.

Stetson (1928, 1951; reprint by Kelso & Munhall, 1988) demonstrated these changes in an extensive series of articulatory recordings. He measured the durations of double (e.g., *pp*) and abutting (e.g., *pk*) consonants, and the durations of their syllables, under different rates of utterance. The rate was varied by two methods: (1) by speaking slowly and then gradually faster in successive repetitions of the test words and (2) by speaking normally but with some of the syllables stressed and others unstressed. A typical slow rate was 2.5 syllables per second (s/s) with a corresponding syllable length of 400 ms: At this rate both consonants were articulated as two separate consonants but with no release of occlusion between. When the rate was increased, at a mean rate of 4 s/s (250 ms syllables) the majority of these consonants had become single, the first member of the pair having been absorbed into the second (Stetson, 1951/1988:93).

The same type of "singling" of double consonants across the syllable boundary also occurred for unstressed syllables in which a final consonant was prescribed and a following heavily stressed syllable absorbed the preceding final consonant into its own initial consonant; the majority of these unstressed syllables were 250 ms in duration; that is, they occurred at a momentary rate of 4 s/s (Stetson, 1951/1988:142). This was the same rate at which singling occurred when caused by gradually increasing the rate of utterance of a series of syllables with equal stresses. The normal rate of prescribed single-consonant syllables had a mean of about 5 s/s, compared with the slowest "singles from doubles" of 3.5 s/s (1951/1988:143).

The occlusion durations of single consonants were typically 100 to 140 ms (Stetson, 1951/1988:86). The occlusion durations of the double consonants had a mean of 200 ms for same-member articulation, e.g., [pp], [dt], but only 150 ms for two-member articulations, such as [dp, bd], where the consonant movements can overlap (1951/1988:102). Thus, the two consonants were similar in timing to two overlapped single consonants with the degree of overlap being greater when it was possible anatomically.

The phonological implications of shifts of consonant function with stress and tempo are extremely interesting. Stetson (1945, 1951, cited

Phonology Note: Motor Coordination

There has been a renaissance of interest in relationships of speech gestural coordinations to phonological phenomena. Stetson (1928) had early demonstrated a bimodal distribution of utterance rates between performance of complete final consonants and their sudden skipping ahead into initial position, as rate of utterance is increased. This was interpreted by Kelso, Saltzman, and Tuller (1986) as due to optimum movement coordinations (phasing) between components of consonant gestures. Preferred phase values are believed to correspond to peak energy efficiencies. Similar relationships are found in other types of coordinated motion cycles, such as tapping of rhythms and stride cycles in walking or running (Kelso et al., 1986; Saltzman & Munhall, 1989). For speech, Tuller and Kelso (1984) measured the phasing of upper lip and lower jaw, as speakers repeated CVs, while varying rate and placement of syllable stress. Constant phasing of the CV gestures was maintained across the durational changes. Nittrouer, Munhall, Kelso, Tuller and Harris (1988) repeated these measurements with an added variable of intervocalic syllable-initial or syllable-final position and found that, although there were timing regularities dependent on rate, stress, and position, the phasing of lip movement to the jaw cycle was not consistent across these conditions. Tuller and Kelso (1990) studied the perception of consonant position in syllable as a function of rate-forced changes in phasing between the gestures of glottal opening-closing and lip closing-opening. They concluded that the coordination of a final consonant in a syllable is unstable in the mid-to-high ranges of utterance rates that occur in fluent speech. This is because final consonant gestures are not energy efficient at higher syllable rates. They also speculate that inefficiency of final consonant gestures may be the basis of linguistic phenomena of "CV dominance" (our phrase) as indicated, for example, by the preponderance of CV syllable-forms in most languages and in infant babbling (also see Kelso et al., 1986).

in Kelso and Munhall, 1988, p. 148) pointed out that only languages with strongly marked syllable stresses, and the resulting long, stressed syllables, seem to make extensive use of syllable-final consonants. He cited as examples English and German, which are heavily stressed and employ many syllables of CVC form as compared with French where there is less variation in syllable duration and fewer CVC syllables. Browman and Goldstein (1992) investigated the advantages of an articulatory-based approach to phonological representations of consonants and developed an articulatory model of phonological phenomena that can be used to synthesize speech that is produced by a computer program (see Chapter Seventeen, Articulatory Synthesis). For a discussion of relationships between phonetics and phonology, see Keating (1991) and Ohala (1990, 1992). See also Port (1986), Kelso and co-workers (1986), and reviews of stress by Harris and Bell-Berti (1984) and Beckman, Edwards, and Fletcher (1992).

The occlusion durations of intervocalic coronal consonants were found by Dart (1991) to be independent of speaker variation of the place of occlusion and of apical versus laminal tongue contact. There was no dependence of occlusion duration on place or on laminality of occlusion, although there were, of course, large effects on spectral properties. In languages where coronal place is distinctive, the corresponding spectral properties appeared to be enhanced, compared, for example, with French and English where they are not distinctive. We should also note that the relative constancy of occlusion duration for the variety of coronal articulations employed for [t, d, n] by French and English speakers (Dart, 1991: 88, 95) implies that the shape and movement of the tongue to achieve occlusion is dynamically programmed as a unit with the palatal architecture.

SUMMARY

The articulations of speech overlap each other and this causes the formant patterns to be in transition much of the time. The spectrum patterns of consonants are affected by anticipatory adjustments for the following consonant or vowel. These phenomena are called coarticulation. The motor program for performing a sequence of sounds, syllables, and words appears to anticipate the number of remaining units to be performed and shortens current and soon-to-be performed units in proportion to that number, but retains the reachability of the consonant constrictions and the identifiability of the stressed syllables.

Studies of the movements of the tongue between coarticulated consonant and vowel suggest that the syllable unit of coarticulation is consonant-vowel (rather than vowel-consonant), because the anticipatory movement for a vowel does not begin until the consonant occlusion has been attained.

Rapid rates of utterance cause more overlap of articulations and a consequent shortening (compression) of the durations of consonants and vowels. Very fast utterance appears to shorten the vowels more than the consonants, perhaps because the consonants must attain constriction positions that are sufficient to produce noticeable bursts and transitions. Adjacent consonants at a boundary between two syllables respond to increases in the rate of utterance via consistent patterns of overlapping articulations. The timing of syllable production exhibits certain resonant rate preferences.

SPEECH DECODING BY HUMAN AND MACHINE: FROM SOUND STREAM TO WORDS

When we hear someone speak we listen for a message and we usually understand. How is this done? How do we unravel the speech sound-stream to understand a message? Answering this question is the task of acoustic research on speech perception. A general answer, arrived at after several decades of experimental studies, is that humans employ special decoding processes to convert the patterns of the sound-stream back into a string of phonemes that define the words of the message (Liberman, 1996).

Part Two of our study of the speech sound code explains how the sound patterns are decoded by the listener. We begin with perception studies of the vowels, proceed with research on consonant perception, and then we study the theories that have been proposed to explain decoding of speech sounds. Finally, as a sort of capstone to our acoustic knowledge of the speech code, we show how it is applied to study impaired hearing for speech and in computer technology for communication.

Up to this point we have studied how phonation and articulatory movements produce a flow of speech sound, patterned in intensity, frequency, and time. These patterns communicate with listeners who perceive the speaker's message. The final communication link in the speech chain is a perceptual process leading to the listener's understanding. How does the listener decode the stream of speech sound to reconstruct the speaker's message? What aspects of the sound flow are the important ones?

CUES FOR PERCEIVING SPEECH

In research on speech perception the basic problem is to discover which aspects of the sound pattern are the essential ones, the ones used by listeners to identify a given unit of speech. The essential stimulus patterns in a perceived event are called cues. Speech cues are the necessary acoustic patterns of speech that are sufficient to cause a person to correctly perceive a given sentence, phrase, word, syllable, or phoneme.

Summary of potential acoustic cues from articulatory features.

ARTICULATORY FEATURES	ACOUSTIC CUES
Prosodic functions	
Syllable stress pattern	Vowel pitch, duration, spectrum and intensity (in order of importance)
End of phrase or sentence	Longer duration of vowel and continuant consonants
End of statement	Falling pitch
End of question	Level or rising pitch
Word importance	Longer duration in more important words
Vocal effort	Increased intensity of F3, and higher formants, relative to F1
Vowel features	
High (constricted) versus low (more open)	First-formant frequency, F1, low versus high in frequency
Front tongue constriction	High second-formant frequency, F2; stronger in F2, F3, F4 amplitude
Back tongue constriction	Low second-formant frequency, F2; weaker in F3 and above
Retroflex tongue (r)	Low third-formant frequency, F3
Tense versus lax	Long versus shorter duration
Nasalization	Raised F1 frequency and wider F1 bandwidth
Consonant features	
Glide versus oral-occlusive, [w, j] versus [b, d, m, n]	Long versus brief formant transitions; onset and offset envelopes more gradual for glides than occlusives
Retroflex tongue [r] versus other glides and nasals	Large F3 transition to or from low frequency
Lateral	Low frequencies strong and broadband, broad deep valley between F2 & F3
Nasal	Low-frequency murmur is narrowband, very weak midformants. Adjacent vowel affected by nasal coupling (F1 weakened and raised in frequency)
Stop	Silent interval, rapid brief formant transitions
Fricative	Longer constriction interval showing weak or absent low-frequency sound, relatively strong high-frequency, random amplitude sound
Voiced versus unvoiced	Stops: release-burst weak and brief versus strong and longer; following vowel F1 onset early versus delayed; intervocalic interval short versus long; preceding vowel long versus short for final stop at a boundary
	Fricatives: short versus longer high-frequency sound; weak versus strong high-frequency sound; duration cues same as for stops
Place of articulation	Direction of F2 transition; location and transitions of release-burst spectrum; compact-diffuse, spreading, or parallel transitions of F2 and F3; spectrum of fricative sound

CHAPTER ELEVEN

PERCEPTION OF VOWELS: DYNAMIC CONSTANCY

WINIFRED STRANGE

In this chapter and the next we present certain key research studies aimed at finding what types of perceptual processes enable phonetic perception. Here, for vowel perception the questions considered are how the spectral formant patterns may be integrated; how the different vowel patterns of men, women, and children may be perceived as the same vowel; and why a constant vowel is perceived despite changes in its formant pattern, due to coarticulation, in different phonetic contexts. It is concluded that the changing formants themselves, over their trajectories between consonants, are the key information that is processed into a constant vowel perception. Thus, the above theme: "dynamic constancy."

Articulatorily, vowels are relatively slow gestures of the tongue, lips, and jaw by which a speaker assumes a particular vocal tract posture. Thus, vowels are long in duration, relative to consonants, and vowels form the nuclei of spoken syllables. Prosodic information (the intonation and stress pattern) of an utterance is specified by changes in fundamental frequency, intensity, and duration of the vowels. All vowels are produced with a relatively open (unconstricted) vocal tract; thus, the only source of sound is a periodic "buzz" generated at the larynx by the vibration of the vocal folds.

As described in earlier chapters, the distinctive vocal tract postures associated with particular vowels determine the resonance characteristics of the open vocal tract and thus shape the spectral envelope of the vowel sound. Resonance peaks or formants occur at different frequencies for different vowels, depending on the size and shape of the pharyngeal and oral cavities, and the overall length

of the vocal tract from the larynx to the lips. The vocal tract posture that characterizes a particular vowel is often referred to as its *articulatory target*, while the associated formant pattern is called its *acoustic target*. Vowels can be further divided into monophthongs (simple vowels) and diphthongs (complex vowels). Monophthongs are vowels with single articulatory targets, whereas diphthongs are usually described as a sequence of a primary or dominant target plus a following secondary target, with a smooth transition between the two targets.

Vowels can be sustained by maintaining the articulatory target in a "steady-state" for a period of time. The acoustic signal associated with such a sustained vowel also has a steady-state formant pattern, that is, formant frequencies remain constant over time. In ongoing speech, however, the vocal tract is typically in constant motion; tongue, lips, and jaw are moving continuously throughout the "vocalic nucleus" of each syllable. Thus, the formant patterns also change throughout the course of the syllable.

In English, vowels produced in consonant-vowel-consonant (CVC) syllables can be distinguished articulatorily by their relative durations and by differences in the pattern of movement within the syllable nucleus, as well as by their articulatory targets. Acoustically, then, in addition to each vowel having a distinctive target formant pattern, vowels also differ in their "intrinsic" duration (Peterson & Lehiste, 1960) and in the temporal pattern of formant movements (Lehiste & Peterson, 1961). Four American English monophthongs are classified as short: /ɪ, ɛ, ʌ, ʊ/. The remaining monophthongs, /i, æ, ɑ, ɔ, u/ and the retroflex vowel /ɚ/, are classified as long vowels (although /i/ and /u/ tend to be somewhat shorter than the other long monophthongs). The diphthongized vowels /eɪ/ and /oʊ/ and the "true" diphthongs, /aʊ, aɪ/ and /ɔɪ/, are also classified as long vowels.

Distinct types of formant movement patterns for vowels produced in CVC syllables were classified by Lehiste and Peterson (1961) according to the relative durations of three components: *onglides* (formant transitions from the release of the initial consonant to the vowel target), *targets* (in which formants were steady-state or movement was relatively slow), and *offglides* (formant transitions from the target to consonant closure). The short monophthongs contrasted with the long monophthongs primarily in the relative durations of targets and offglides. Short vowels contained relatively short targets and longer offglides, while long vowels had relatively long targets and shorter offglides. That is, long vowels remained near their target positions for a greater proportion of the syllable than did short vowels.

The diphthongized vowels /eɪ/ and /oʊ/ and the retroflex vowel /ɚ/ all had a single target and extensive offglides, while the true diphthongs could be divided into five distinct components: onglide, target 1, glide, target 2, and offglide. The first target was typically longer than the second; however, the glide between targets was longer than either target.

In exploring the "acoustic cues" associated with the perception of vowels, early studies concentrated primarily on how perceivers distinguished steady-state formant patterns associated with sustained monophthongal vowels. As described earlier, studies with synthetic speech stimuli determined that listeners could differentiate steady-state patterns that differed only in the center frequencies of the first and second formants (F1 and F2, respectively). In fact, back vowels such as /u, ʊ, o/ could often be distinguished on the basis of the frequency of a single-formant synthetic pattern (Delattre, Liberman, Cooper, & Gerstman, 1952). Further research on how the formant patterns of

steady-state vowels are perceived is discussed in the next section.

PERCEPTION OF STEADY-STATE VOWELS

Acoustical analysis of natural vowels indicates that the center frequencies of the first three formants vary systematically for vowels produced with different tongue, lip, and jaw positions. However, perceptual studies using synthetic stimuli have shown that most vowels can be simulated perceptually by two-formant patterns, in which one or the other formant constitutes a weighted average of two or more formants in natural vowels. For instance, in one such study, listeners were asked to match two-formant patterns to "standard" synthetic vowels that included four formants with frequencies matching those of natural (Swedish) vowels (Carlson, Granstrom, & Fant, 1970). The frequency of F1 of the two-formant pattern was fixed at the frequency of the standard F1 and subjects adjusted the second formant (F2′) until they heard a vowel that was perceptually equivalent to the four-formant standard pattern. For back and central vowels, subjects adjusted the frequency of F2′ to a frequency near the F2 of the standard. For front vowels except /i/, F2′ was adjusted to a frequency intermediate between F2 and F3 of the standard. For /i/, the F2′ of the pattern that most closely matched the standard perceptually had a frequency at or above the F3 of the standard.

These findings and the earlier study by Delattre and co-workers (1952) suggest that when formants are close in frequency, as F1 and F2 are for back vowels, and F2 and F3 are for front vowels, they are integrated perceptually such that the "effective" formant is equivalent to an average of the two close spectral peaks. Ludmilla Chistovich and her colleagues (cf., Chistovich, 1985) have conducted extensive research on spectral integration effects in the perception of steady-state vowels. Their work has shown that when two or more spectral peaks occur within a *critical distance* on a psychophysical frequency scale known as the

Bark scale,[1] the perceived quality of the vowel is equivalent to a pattern with a single spectral peak at the *"center of gravity"* of the cluster of formants. That is, the *effective* formant frequency is a weighted average in frequency and amplitude of the spectral peaks within a range of 3.0–3.5 Barks. Within this critical range, the relative amplitudes of spectral peaks affect the center of gravity; the effective formant frequency is shifted toward the frequency of the higher amplitude peak. When the frequency distance between spectral peaks exceeds 3.5 Barks, the formants are perceptually distinct and changes in their relative amplitudes do not affect perceived vowel quality.

In summary then, steady-state vowels are perceived primarily on the basis of the location of the peaks in the spectral envelope. Most vowels can be differentiated perceptually by the frequency of the first two formants, F1 and F2. However, when two or more formants occur within a range of about 3.5 Barks, they are perceptually integrated into a single spectral prominence with an effective formant frequency that corresponds to the center of gravity, in terms of amplitude and frequency, of the cluster of formants. Thus, front vowels /i, ɪ, ɛ, æ/ are perceived on the basis of the frequency of F1 and F2′ (a weighted average of F2 and F3, and for /i/ F4). Back vowels /u, ʊ, o, ɑ/ are perceived on the basis of the center of gravity of F1 and F2.

The research described above indicates that the amplitude and frequency pattern of the first two or three formants provides the primary "acoustic cues" for the perception of steady-state vowels. Recall that formant frequencies are determined by the size and shape of the vocal tract cavities. Thus, the *absolute* frequencies of formants differ considerably for the same vowel spoken by different speakers with different sized vocal tracts. That is, the *same* articulatory target produced by different speakers results in *different* acoustic targets. The differences are especially apparent for vowels produced by men, women, and children. On average, men's formant frequencies for a particular vowel are lower than those of women because men's vocal cavities are larger. Children's vocal tracts are smaller than adults' so their formants are higher than those of adult women (Peterson & Barney, 1952).

Figure 11-1 illustrates the variation in formant frequencies of vowels spoken by different speakers. In this figure, vowels are represented as points in an F1/F2 space. Thus, each symbol represents one vowel produced by either a man, a woman, or a child. The ovals surround most of the instances of each vowel category spoken by 33 men, 28 women, and 15 children (Peterson & Barney, 1952). Notice that there is a great deal of variation in the frequency of F1 and F2 within a vowel category. Also, you can see that there is overlap in vowel categories such that *different* vowels (spoken by different speakers) sometimes have the same F1 and F2 frequencies. Despite this overlap in acoustic targets for different vowels and variability in acoustic targets for the same vowel, listeners are nevertheless able to identify speakers' intended vowels correctly. The fact that the acoustic target for the same perceived vowel differs across speakers of different age, size, and gender is often referred to as the "speaker normalization problem." How is it that listeners identify vowels spoken by men, women, and children correctly, despite the variability in the absolute frequencies of the formants?

One answer to this question was first proposed in the late 1800s and continues to be explored in empirical studies of vowel perception (cf., Miller, 1989, for a review of this approach). The Formant-Ratio theory of vowel perception proposes that vowel identity depends upon the *intervals between formants* (i.e., formant ratios) rather than on absolute formant values. For instance, high front vowels such as /i/ have very low first formants and very high second formants; thus, the ratio of F2 to F1 is quite large. In contrast, the interval

---

[1]The critical band scale. A Bark is a frequency distance or bandwidth of about 100 Hz in the region up to about 2 kHz, then increasing to about a bandwidth of 500 Hz at approximately 10 kHz.

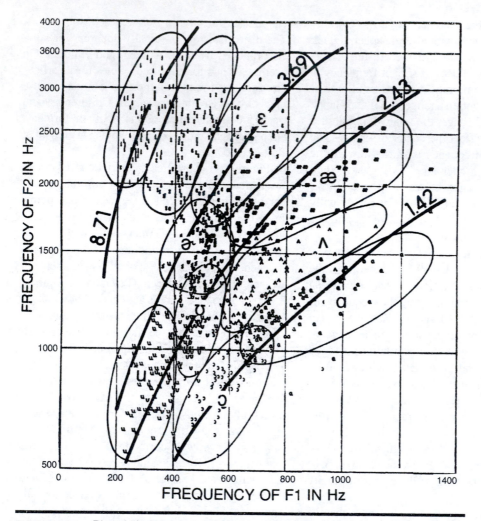

FIGURE 11-1. Plot of the F1 versus F2 positions of the vowels of the varied speakers in the classic 1952 study of Peterson and Barney. One of each of the vowels of 76 American speakers was measured and plotted. Miller (1989) constructed the heavy curved lines at constant ratios of F2/F1: 8.71 for /i/; 3.69 for /ɛ/, /ɚ/, /u/; 2.43 for /æ/, /ʊ/; and 1.42 for /ɑ/, /ɔ/. These ratios appear to be part of the basis of listeners' rescaling to perceive constant vowels and would correspond to partial compensation for the vocal tract length ratios between men, women, and children. Further explanation in text.

(Adapted via axis label changes from Miller, 1989, with permission)

between F2 and F1 is very small for low vowels such as /ɑ/. Figure 11-1 includes four constant F2/F1 ratio lines through the F1/F2 space: 8.71, 3.69, 2.43, and 1.42. Notice that the instances of the vowel /i/ cluster around the 8.71 line, whereas

the instances of /ɑ/ cluster around the 1.42 line. Thus, regardless of the absolute value of formant frequencies for /i/ spoken by men, women, and children, the *relationship between F2 and F1* is similar for a particular vowel and differs across vowels. However, this figure also demonstrates that more than one vowel can have the same F2/F1 ratio. For example, /æ/, /ʊ/, and /u/ clusters all fall near the 2.43 line. Thus, F2/F1 ratios are also ambiguous with respect to perceived vowel identity. Therefore, while vowels may be perceived on the basis of the relative values of F1 and F2 frequencies, there must be additional information that listeners use to "solve the speaker normalization problem." Research that explores the nature of this "additional information" is discussed in the next section.

SPEAKER NORMALIZATION IN VOWEL PERCEPTION

Theories about how listeners identify vowels spoken by different speakers can be divided into those that emphasize the role of "intrinsic specification" of vowels and those that focus on "extrinsic specification" of vowels (Nearey, 1989). *Intrinsic normalization models* hypothesize that there is sufficient information within the acoustic pattern of the vowel itself to allow the listener to identify it unambiguously, if all the important aspects of the spectral pattern are represented in an appropriate way (Peterson, 1961). Alternatively, *extrinsic normalization models* claim that listeners judge the identity of vowels on the basis of a "frame of reference" that is established from preceding (and perhaps even following) speech patterns (Joos, 1948). According to this approach, information about the size, age, and gender of the speaker available in the ongoing speech pattern is used as a basis for interpreting acoustically ambiguous vowels. Empirical evidence that supports both models has been obtained in studies of vowel perception, using both synthetic and natural speech.

Working within the intrinsic normalization theory, several researchers have explored the contribution of upper formants (primarily F3) and of the fundamental frequency (F0) to the specification of vowel identity. Extending the notion that vowels are perceived on the basis of formant ratios, Miller (1989) proposed that vowels spoken by

men, women, and children can be represented unambiguously in a three-dimensional "auditory-perceptual space" defined by three intervals (measured in logarithmic units of frequency:[2] F3 – F2, F2 – F1, and F1 – SR, where SR is a "sensory reference" estimated from the F0 for the speaker). Syrdal and Gopal (1986) proposed a similar representation of vowels in a two-dimensional space in which the coordinates are F1 – F0 (in Bark) and F3 – F2 (in Bark). Both Miller and Syrdal and Gopal reported that the overlap between vowel categories in the Peterson and Barney vowel corpus (shown in Figure 11-1) was reduced or eliminated when such transformations were performed. These results indirectly support the hypothesis that perceivers utilize both F3 and F0 information in differentiating vowels spoken by men, women, and children.

Studies of the perception of synthetic vowel stimuli in which F0 was systematically manipulated have provided direct evidence that the identification of vowels is influenced by F0. Lehiste and Meltzer (1973) synthesized vowels simulating productions of men, women, and children, based on average formant values for the three groups reported by Peterson and Barney (1952). Each vowel set was synthesized at three F0 values, corresponding to average male, female, and child values. If listeners "normalize" vowels produced by men, women, and children on the basis of their F1–F0 ratios (as well as ratios between upper formants), then we would expect vowel perception to be most accurate when both F0 and the formant frequencies were those of a speaker of the same age and gender, that is, when the F1–F0 ratio was appropriate. Table 11-1 presents the results of listening tests reported by Lehiste and Meltzer (1973).

As expected, the synthetic vowels with female formant frequencies were identified most accurately when the F0 was appropriate for a female (see the second row). However, vowels containing male formants were identified equally well when synthesized with a male F0 or a female F0

_____
[2]Intervals of log units = ratios of linear units.

TABLE 11-1. Identification of synthetic vowels with formants appropriate for men, women, and children synthesized at three fundamental frequencies (from Lehiste and Meltzer, 1973). (Underlined values are for stimuli with F0 and formant values appropriate for a speaker of the same gender and age.)

FORMANT FREQUENCIES	FUNDMENTALFREQUENCY		
	MALE (132 HZ)	FEMALE (223 HZ)	CHILD (264 HZ)
Male	<u>76%</u>	77%	43%
Female	54	<u>82</u>	43
Child	44	77	<u>68</u>

(first row). Finally, vowels with formants appropriate for a child were actually identified better when synthesized with an adult female's F0 than when synthesized with a F0 appropriate for a child (third row).

These results indicate that fundamental frequency does affect the identification of steady-state vowels. However, the best perception was not always obtained for synthetic vowels that contained F1–F0 ratios most appropriate to a speaker of a particular age and gender.

Ryalls and Lieberman (1982) reported similar results in a study in which synthetic vowels with men's and women's formant values were synthesized at three F0s: typical for the gender (135 Hz for men, 185 Hz for women), lower than typical (100 Hz), and higher than typical (250 Hz). For both sets of vowels, identification of stimuli synthesized with typical and lower fundamental frequencies was better than identification of vowels synthesized with the 250 Hz F0.

These results argue against the hypothesis that listeners normalize vowels on the basis of a ratio of F0 and F1. Vowels produced with high F0s (250 Hz or greater) tend to be less well perceived, regardless of whether formant frequencies are those of a child's, a woman's or a man's vowels.[3]

In summary, these studies demonstrate that variations in F0 of synthetic steady-state vowels influence the way listeners perceive the formant frequency patterns. But in exactly what way does F0 affect vowel perception? Keith Johnson (1990) has suggested that F0 influences vowel identification *indirectly*, rather than directly, in that listeners use F0 as a cue to the identity of the speaker. Johnson investigated shifts in vowel perception using synthetic stimuli in which target syllables were embedded in carrier sentences with different F0 contours (i.e., different intonation patterns). When listeners identified two utterances as being produced by the *same speaker* with two different intonation patterns, syllables with different F0s (but the same formants) were identified as the same vowel. Alternatively, when syllables with the same formants *and the same F0* were perceived as being spoken by different speakers, listeners heard a difference in the vowel. These results suggest that F0 influences vowel perception, not because F1–F0 ratios are used in the intrinsic specification of vowels, but rather because F0 determines speaker identity. In turn, the perceived age and gender of the speaker is part of the "frame of reference" within which vowels are identified. We will discuss these "extrinsic normalization" theories of vowel perception below, but first, let us consider some research on how upper formants may be utilized in the intrinsic specification of vowels spoken by different speakers.

In an early study, Fujisaki and Kawashima (1968) reported that changes in F3 affected the

---

[3]This is probably due to the fact that spectral peaks are less well defined when harmonics are widely spaced (see Chapter Four and Figure 4-11). That is, when the voice pitch is very high, harmonics may or may not occur at or near the resonance frequencies of the vocal tract; therefore, the spectral envelope is less well specified and formant frequencies can appear to be shifted.

perception of synthetic Japanese vowels, especially when F3 shifts were accompanied by shifts in F0. More recently, Nearey (1989) investigated the influence of upper formants (F3, F4, and sometimes F5) on the perception of synthetic English vowels in two conditions, when F0 remained constant, and when F0 also changed in accordance with changes in upper formants. He reported that categorization of synthetic vowels with different F1/F2 patterns changed when upper formants were shifted up in frequency, when F0 was shifted upward, and when both F0 and upper formants were shifted upward in frequency. For F1/F2 patterns appropriate for a small vocal tract, the combined shifts of upper formants and F0 yielded a greater difference in vowel perception than when either was shifted alone. For the F1/F2 patterns appropriate for a large vocal tract, changes in upper formants alone had little effect on vowel categorization, while changes in F0 alone and F0 and upper formants together shifted the perception of F1/F2 patterns in the expected direction. However, none of the effects of upper formants and F0 were as great as would be expected on the basis of a Formant-Ratio model of speaker normalization.

We turn now to research supporting extrinsic specification models of speaker normalization. According to this approach, listeners interpret the formant patterns of vowels in reference to the larger speech context in which they occur. That is, individual vowels are perceived relative to the patterns of formant frequencies at a speaker's entire vowel inventory (Joos, 1948). While the formants of the same intended vowel produced by different speakers may vary in absolute frequency, the relationship among formant patterns of different vowels spoken by the same speaker remains relatively constant. So, for instance, for any speaker, whether man, woman, or child, the vowel /i/ has a higher frequency F2 and a lower frequency F1 than the vowel /ɪ/ spoken by that same speaker. Furthermore, for any speaker, the vowel /i/ has the highest frequency F2 of all his or her vowels, the vowel /ɑ/ has the highest frequency F1, and so forth. Thus, as a listener hears the speech of a par-

ticular speaker, the *overall ranges of formant frequencies* are established by vowels that mark the articulatory extremes (/i/, /ɑ/ and /u/), often referred to as the "point vowels."

To demonstrate that the frame of reference established by the acoustic characteristics of (preceding) speech affects vowel perception, Ladefoged and Broadbent (1957) examined the identification of vowels in synthetic /b-Vowel-t/ syllables as /ɪ, ɛ, æ/ or /ʌ/ when the ranges of F1 and F2 frequencies contained in a precursor sentence were varied. They found significant shifts in identification of the test syllables with changes in the formant frequencies of vowels in the sentence. For instance, when F1 was shifted downward in the precursor sentence, the syllable heard as /bɪt/ (when presented in the original sentence) was perceived as /bɛt/ more often. Alternatively, when the F1 range was shifted upward in the sentence, the /bæt/ syllable was heard more often as /bɛt/. These shifts in vowel identification are those predicted if listeners were interpreting the F1 values of the test syllables *in relation to the range of F1 values contained in the preceding sentence.*

Nearey's (1989) study demonstrated that the overall range in F1/F2 frequencies of a set of synthetic steady-state vowels presented in citation form (as lists of isolated vowels) can also affect vowel identification responses. He synthesized two sets of F1/F2 patterns, a Low set (with frequencies within a range associated with adult male vowels) and a High set, in which F1 and F2 frequency ranges were shifted upward by 32%. He reported the results in terms of the "center of gravity" and range of F1/F2 patterns categorized as /ʊ/ (which has formant frequencies in the midrange of each speaker's vowel space in natural speech).

In the context of the High set, F1/F2 patterns with higher frequencies were identified as the vowel /ʊ/. That is, there was a shift in the /ʊ/ category in the direction expected if listeners identified ambiguous vowels in relation to the overall range of formants present in the stimulus set. However, the shift in the perceived /ʊ/ category was only about half as great as would be predicted if subjects were categorizing vowels on the basis of this extrinsic factor alone.

Other studies have shown the influence of sentence context on vowel perception using natural speech. For instance, Dechovitz (1977) reported that the perception of vowels in /b-Vowel-t/ syllables produced by an adult male was altered when the syllables were embedded in a sentence produced by a 9-year-old child. The man produced the syllables with the same stress, speaking rate, and F0 as the child; only the formant frequencies differed. Errors were consistent with the hypothesis that the vowels in the man's syllables were categorized in relation to the formant frequencies of the child's vowels in the sentence.

Researchers have also shown that when the speaker producing isolated vowels or vowels in CVC syllables varies from trial to trial in a listening test (Mixed Speaker test), errors in vowel identification are somewhat greater than when the same speaker produces all the syllables within a block of trials (Blocked Speaker test) (Assmann, Nearey, & Hogan, 1982; Macchi, 1980; Strange, Verbrugge, Shankweiler, & Edman, 1976). This suggests that vowels are misidentified in the Mixed Speaker condition because there is no opportunity to normalize for speaker differences, whereas in the Blocked condition, speaker normalization across trials is possible. However, this explanation of the results may not be accurate. Verbrugge and his colleagues reported that identification of vowels on Mixed Speaker tests did *not* improve when each trial was preceded by the same speaker's productions of the point vowels, /i/, /ɑ/, /u/, as would be predicted from an extrinsic normalization model. In addition, identification of vowels in Mixed Speaker tests was remarkably accurate in some studies (Assmann et al., 1982: Macchi, 1980), suggesting that extrinsic normalization is not *necessary* for identification of naturally spoken vowels.

Summarizing the research on speaker normalization, studies have shown that perceivers can and do utilize both intrinsically specified information (F0 and upper formants) and extrinsically specified information (formant ranges given by

sentence context or the stimulus set) in categorizing synthetic F1/F2 patterns that simulate vowels produced by men, women, and children. Research with naturally produced vowels has also demonstrated the influence of sentence context and stimulus set effects on vowel identification. However, the fact that naturally produced vowels are often highly identifiable even when there is no opportunity for extrinsic speaker normalization suggests that there may be sufficient information within the target syllable itself to specify the intended vowels of different speakers unambiguously, despite the ambiguity in F1/F2 values.

In the next section, we discuss the perception of vowels spoken in continuous speech. We mentioned earlier that vowels rarely occur as sustained, steady-state postures when produced at normal to rapid rates in ongoing speech. Rather, they are continuously moving gestures that overlap temporally with the gestures associated with preceding and following consonants. As discussed in Chapter Ten, this is called that *coarticulation*, and refers to the fact that in continuous speech, the posture of the vocal tract and movements of the articulators at any point in time are determined by more than a single phonetic segment. This results in large variations in the formant patterns in syllable nuclei identified as the same vowel in different consonantal contexts. How do listeners perceive the intended vowels of a speaker in the face of this acoustic variability? This question is basic to our understanding of vowel perception.

PERCEPTION OF COARTICULATED VOWELS

First, let us consider the nature of the variability in the F1/F2 formant patterns of vowels produced in CVC syllables. In an early acoustic study of vowels spoken in nonsense bisyllables of the form /h CVC/, Stevens and House (1963) demonstrated that steady-state acoustic targets are not often reached at syllable centers. For example, the /ɛ/-vowels in the words bet and get have very different F2 targets or trajectories but both vowels sound like /ɛ/. Figure 11-2 presents the F1/F2 plots of

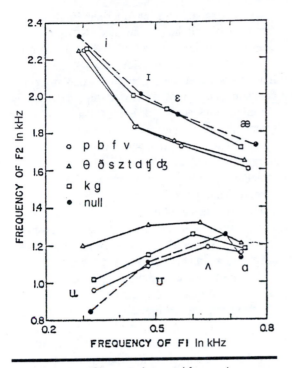

FIGURE 11-2. Changes in vowel formant positions with changes in adjacent consonants. (From the study by Stevens & House, 1963)

vowels spoken in 14 consonantal contexts and in two "null" contexts (as isolated vowels, #V#, and in /hVd/ syllables) by three speakers. The figure shows average F1/F2 values for each of 8 vowels in labial contexts (/p, b, f, v/), alveolar/palato-alveolar contexts (/θ, ð, s, z, ʧ, ʤ/), and velar contexts (/k, g/) separately.

As this figure shows, formant frequencies (especially F2 values) are shifted from target values produced in null contexts. These shifts result in a "shrinking" of the F1/F2 vowel space, such that formant patterns of different vowels are more similar to each other. That is, there is a reduction in the acoustic contrast among vowels when they are produced in consonantal context that reflects a failure of the articulators to reach the "canonical" target positions when coarticulated with consonants. Notice also, that differences in the place of articulation of preceding and following consonants result in different amounts of reduction. F2

values for front vowels are lower in the context of labial and alveolar contexts, than in velar contexts. In contrast, F2 values for back vowels are shifted upwards more when preceded and followed by alveolar and velar consonants, than in labial contexts. These changes reflect the fact that F2 frequencies of vowels in CVC syllables tend to shift toward consonantal F2 loci, that is, the frequency of the formant at, or projected to, the center of the consonant constriction period.

Bjorn Lindblom (1963) referred to these acoustic effects of coarticulation as *target undershoot*. He hypothesized that speakers' articulatory "intentions" underlying the production of vowels is the same for all contexts, speaking rates, and levels of linguistic stress (i.e., the neural commands to the articulators are invariant for each vowel/phoneme). However, as these articulatory intentions are carried out at increasingly rapid rates (as in continuous speech at normal to rapid rates), "the speech organs fail, as a result of the physiological limitations, to reach the positions that they assume when the vowel is pronounced under ideal steady-state conditions. In the acoustic domain, this is paralleled by undershoot in the formant frequencies relative to the bull's-eye formant pattern" (Lindblom, 1963, p. 1779).

According to Lindblom's Target Undershoot theory, the amount of formant undershoot depends only on the duration of the syllable, that is, on the timing of the sequential articulatory gestures associated with consonants and vowels within the syllable: the shorter the syllable duration, the greater the target undershoot. Thus, target undershoot should increase as speaking rate increases or as lexical stress decreases (both of which result in shorter duration syllables). Lindblom reported acoustical measurements of 8 Swedish lax (short) vowels in 3 consonantal contexts—/bVb/, /dVd/, and /gVg/—that supported this prediction.

With respect to the *perception* of coarticulated vowels, Lindblom hypothesized that listeners compensate for target undershoot in order to recover the canonical vowel targets. That is, identification of vowels in CVC syllables with moving formant patterns (formant trajectories) showed "perceptual overshoot." Lindblom and Studdert-Kennedy (1967) demonstrated this compensatory perceptual overshoot in a study with synthetic CVC syllables in which F2 and F3 formant trajectories were varied in four sets of syllables: fast and slow /w-w/ syllables (100 ms and 200 ms), and fast and slow /j-j/ syllables. (Recall that F2 and F3 loci are low for /w/ and high for /j/.) In each set, the frequency of F2 and F3 at the center of each syllable (formant maxima or minima) varied in 20 steps from high values appropriate for /ɪ/ to low values appropriate to /ʊ/ (F1 patterns remained constant). The stimuli were presented in random order and subjects were asked to identify the vowel in each stimulus as /ɪ/ or /ʊ/.

Results of these identification tests demonstrated compensatory perceptual overshoot in that the boundary between /ɪ/ and /ʊ/ responses differed for vowels in /w-w/ and /j-j/contexts. As predicted, the /ɪ/-/ʊ/ boundary shifted toward higher F2/F3 values in /j-j/ contexts (i.e., subjects heard mid-range values as /ʊ/) and toward lower F2/F3 values in /w-w/ contexts (subjects heard midrange values as /ɪ/). Furthermore, the shift in the /ɪ/-/ʊ/ identification boundary was greater for the "fast" /w-w/ syllables than for the "slow" /w-w/ syllables, as would be predicted if perceivers used syllable duration to "estimate" the amount of target undershoot.

These results suggest that the perception of coarticulated vowels is not based exclusively on the frequencies of F1, F2, and F3 in the center of syllables (formant maxima or minima) where they approach their canonical values most closely. Rather, the direction and slope of formant transitions into and out of the syllable nucleus affect the perceived identity of the vowel. Lindblom's Perceptual Compensation model proposes a relatively straightforward formula by which target undershoot can be computed on the basis of preceding and following consonant formant loci, canonical vowel targets, and syllable duration. However, this formula is based on the assumption that articulatory and acoustic target undershoot increases systematically as syllable duration decreases.

Acoustical analyses of American English coarticulated vowels has called this assumption into question. Studies by Gay (1978), Kuehn and Moll (1976), Moon and Lindblom (1994), and others have shown that the amount of articulatory and acoustic undershoot of vowel targets differs in complex ways across different speakers and different speaking styles. Some speakers appear to reach articulatory and acoustic vowel targets even in rapid speech, while other speakers show more target undershoot in rapid speech than in slow speech. That is, some speakers speed up their articulatory gestures or begin the vowel gesture earlier (relative to the initial consonant gesture) and thus produce the same F1/F2/F3 values at syllable centers in normal and rapid speech.

Other studies have shown that changes in syllable duration due to speaking rate and lexical stress do not lead to the same amounts of target undershoot. For instance, Gay (1978) reported that vowels produced in unstressed syllable position showed more target undershoot than those produced in stressed position, in both slow and rapid speech. Thus, rapidly produced stressed vowels contained less undershoot than slowly produced unstressed vowels, even when syllable durations were equal. Finally, the amount of target undershoot appears to vary even within a single speaker depending on speaking style (Moon & Lindblom 1994). Speakers show less acoustic undershoot of coarticulated vowels in their carefully produced speech (as when speaking under noisy conditions or to a foreigner) than in their casual speech even when syllable durations are equivalent.

Listeners are thus faced with an apparently formidable problem in interpreting the formant patterns in syllable nuclei. A model in which perceptual compensation for undershoot is based on syllable duration alone is not adequate to explain how perceivers identify coarticulated vowels. And yet perception of coarticulated vowels appears to be quite easy for listeners. In fact, vowels in CVC syllables are sometimes identified more accurately than vowels produced in isolation. For instance, Winifred Strange and her colleagues (Gottfried & Strange, 1980; Strange, Edman, & Jenkins, 1979;

Strange et al., 1976) found that vowels produced in several CVC contexts were identified more accurately than vowels produced in isolation (#V#) by the same panel of talkers, which included men, women, and (in some studies) children. This finding was unexpected, because F1/F2 formant patterns of different vowels coarticulated vowels were *more* similar to each other than were different isolated vowels.

Other studies in which isolated vowels and vowels in CVC syllables spoken by the same panel of talkers were compared reported no such advantage of coarticulated vowels (Assmann et al., 1982; Macchi, 1980). Both isolated vowels and coarticulated vowels were identified with almost no errors. However, isolated vowels were never identified *more* accurately than coarticulated vowels, even though formant patterns at syllable centers were more distinct in F1/F2 space.

Finally, Verbrugge and Shankweiler (1977) reported accurate identification of vowels in /p-p/ syllables produced in both rapid and slow sentences in stressed or destressed sentence position when the syllables were presented in their original sentence contexts. Acoustical analysis of the stimuli showed that F1/F2 patterns at syllable centers were more reduced for destressed syllables than stressed syllables. That is, F1/F2 values for different vowels were more similar to each other for destressed vowels. However, listeners did not have difficulty identifying the intended vowels.

This evidence that coarticulated vowels are perceived accurately even when F1/F2 frequencies fail to reach acoustic target values and vowel categories overlap in F1/F2 pattern suggests that listeners use other acoustic cues to differentiate vowels when they are produced in ongoing speech. As described in the beginning of this section, naturally produced English vowels are differentiated by their intrinsic durations and by the temporal pattern of the formant trajectories into and out of the syllable nucleus. Perceptual studies of coarticulated vowels have shown that these acoustic differences provide important information to the perceiver.

One kind of evidence for the perceptual importance of intrinsic duration has been provided by experiments in which duration information is either removed or is misleading. For instance, when equal duration segments of vowels are excised from CVC syllables and presented alone, the vowels are often misidentified (Jenkins, Strange, & Edman, 1983; Strange, Jenkins, & Johnson, 1983). Furthermore, when (short) CVC syllables are excised from rapidly produced sentences and played alone (as if they were produced slowly in lists), identification errors also increased (Johnson & Strange, 1982; Verbrugge & Shankweiler, 1977). Significantly, syllables containing intrinsically long vowels were misperceived as short vowels; for example, /æ/ was misheard as /ɛ/, /e/ was misheard as /ɑ/, and /ɑ/ was misheard as /ʌ/. This pattern of errors demonstrates that listeners are judging the vowels on the basis of their "normal" durations. The earlier finding that excised syllable nuclei are misperceived suggests that formant trajectory information is important for accurate perception of coarticulated vowels.

To examine the contribution of all these acoustic cues to vowel identity, Winifred Strange and her colleagues developed a technique in which target information (available in syllable nuclei), duration information, and dynamic spectral information (formant trajectories) were manipulated independently in modified versions of naturally produced syllables. CVC syllables were stored in a computer as digital waveforms. Then several different stimulus conditions were generated by deleting portions of the syllable and changing the temporal relationship of remaining portions. *Silent-Center* syllables were constructed by silencing the entire central portion of each syllable, leaving only the initial and final transitional portions (the onglides and offglides) in their original temporal relationship but separated by the silent gap. These syllables were heard as CVC syllables with a "hiccup" or glottal stop in the middle. Notice that these syllables retained the dynamic spectral information and relative duration information for the original vowel, but target information provided by the syllable nucleus was missing.

In another condition, the duration between initial and final transitional portions was modified so that syllables containing intrinsically long vowels and those containing intrinsically short vowels were the same length. Thus, in these *Neutral Duration Silent-Center* syllables, only dynamic spectral information remained; duration and target information was no longer available. Figure

11-3 illustrates these modified syllable conditions for one long vowel (left) and one short vowel (right). In addition, two *Centers Alone* conditions were made by deleting both initial and final transitional portions. In one, relative duration differences were retained; in another, all nuclei were made the same (short) duration.

Subjects were asked to identify the vowel in each of the modified syllable conditions and identification responses were compared with those for the original unmodified CVC syllables. In several studies, using stimuli with different consonantal contexts and different speakers, identification of vowels in Silent-Center syllables was found to be remarkably accurate (Jenkins et al., 1983; Parker & Diehl, 1984; Strange, 1989; Strange et al., 1983). Indeed, in some cases, listeners identified the vowels in Silent-Center syllables *as well as they did the vowels in the original unmodified syllables*. Thus, when dynamic spectral information and relative duration information was present, vowel perception remained highly accurate despite the fact that the "vowel" nucleus of the syllable was absent. When duration information was also removed (Neutral Duration Silent-Center syllables), listeners misidentified vowels in Silent-Center syllables more often. However, perception was still better than in the Centers Alone condition in which (equal duration) syllable nuclei were retained and initial and final transitions were removed. In other words, when duration information was absent, dynamic spectral information was better than nucleus target information for identifying the vowels.

These results demonstrate that formant onglides and offglides of CVC syllables *together* provide critical information about the identity of coarticulated vowels. Furthermore, this information appears to be independent of information about formant targets and relative vowel duration. In fact, these studies demonstrate that vowel targets in syllable centers are neither sufficient nor necessary for the accurate perception of coarticulated vowels.

Studies with synthetic speech have also demonstrated the importance of formant trajectories in

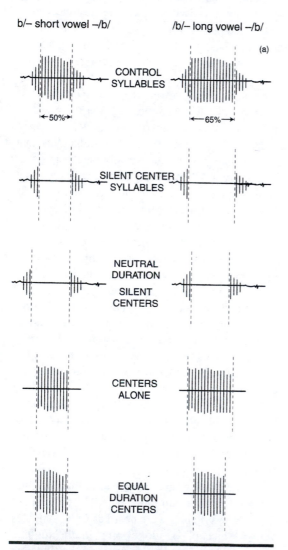

FIGURE 11-3. Stimuli types for studies of the relative importance of cues in the centers of vowels versus the cues in the onglides and offglides.

vowel perception. For instance, Huang (1985) showed that synthetic CVC syllables with short steady-states and long offglides were heard more often as short vowels than syllables with long steady-states and short offglides, as would be predicted from trajectory patterns found in naturally produced syllables (Lehiste & Peterson, 1961). DiBenedetto (1989a, 1989b) demonstrated that the *temporal* trajectory pattern of F1 influenced the perception of front vowels /i, ɪ, e, ɛ, æ/. Synthetic syllables in which F1 maxima were reached early relative to the total duration of the syllable were heard as lower in tongue height than syllables in which F1 maxima were attained later in the syllable. Again, this perceptual result matched DiBenedetto's findings about temporal trajectories in naturally produced syllables.

In summary, the perception of coarticulated vowels appears to be based on dynamic spectro-temporal patterns within the syllable. The formant pattern at any one point in the syllable does not adequately specify the intended vowel. Rather, the acoustic information for the identity of coarticulated vowels is carried in the changing formant pattern.

SUMMARY

In this chapter we explored some problems associated with understanding how vowels are perceived when they are spoken by different speakers, in different consonantal contexts, at different rates of speaking, and at different levels of lexical stress. Studies of the perception of synthetic steady-state vowels demonstrated that vowel quality was determined by the pattern of spectral peaks. The relative frequencies of the first two or three formants differentiate steady-state vowels produced by a single talker (or by a computer). However, when two or more spectral peaks are within a critical distance (3.0 to 3.5 Barks), they appear to be integrated perceptually so that the effective formant frequency is at the center of gravity of the cluster of spectral peaks.

Because formant frequencies are a function of the size and shape of the vocal cavities, spectral patterns of the same vowel spoken by men, women, and children differ markedly in absolute frequency of spectral peaks. While the *relative* frequencies of F1 and F2 (formant ratios) are more similar across speakers of different age and gender, there is still no simple one-to-one correspondence between (static) spectral patterns and perceived vowel category. Research on the "speaker normalization problem" has provided evidence for both intrinsic and extrinsic normalization models of vowel perception. Fundamental frequency affects the perception of formant patterns, perhaps by providing information about the age and gender of the speaker. The range of formant frequencies in preceding speech also determines how listeners categorize vowels in acoustically ambiguous stimuli. However, the identification of naturally produced vowels is often highly accurate even when listeners have no opportunity for extrinsic speaker normalization.

Experiments on the perception of coarticulated vowels have attempted to explain how perceivers solve the "target undershoot problem" in production. A simple perceptual compensation model cannot account for how listeners perceive vowels accurately despite complex variations in their nuclear formant patterns across different speaking rates, different speaking styles, and different levels of lexical stress. Studies with both modified natural speech and synthetic speech demonstrate that intrinsic duration differences and dynamic spectral parameters (i.e., spectral and temporal relationships defined over the formant trajectories) provide important information for the identification of vowels in continuous speech.

CHAPTER TWELVE.

PERCEPTION OF CONSONANTS: FROM VARIANCE TO INVARIANCE

WINIFRED STRANGE

Consonants are produced by rapid articulatory gestures that are superimposed on the slower, more global movements for the vowels. The co-ordination of consonant gestures with vowel gestures is organized in syllable units where the vowels are the syllable nuclei and the consonants occur at the onsets and offsets of syllables. Consonant gestures, marking the syllable borders so to speak, make temporary constrictions in the vocal tract, sometimes narrowing it enough to cause turbulent, noise-like sound, or even blocking it completely. Thus the sound patterns of consonants often involve changes in the formants, due to the reconfigurations of the tract shape between consonants and vowels, as well as abrupt silences and/or bursts of noise.

Earlier, in the summary tables for Chapters Six through Nine, we noted differences that would enable listeners to identify the consonants according to the familiar phonetic contrasts of manner of articulation, voicing, and place of articulation. For instance, very rapid formant transitions distinguish stop consonants from glides, which have more gradual transitions. Voiced stops in initial position contrast with initial voiceless stops in Voice Onset Time (i.e., F1 cutback and duration of aspiration noise). Labial, alveolar, and velar stops can be distinguished by differences in onset and direction of F2 transitions and/or differences in the frequency of the noise burst. For a given phoneme the absolute values (the frequencies, amplitudes, and durations) of such acoustic fea-tures differ depending on preceding and following vowel contexts, on the rate of speaking, and even on the gender and age of the speaker.

Now we will describe some of the remarkably direct, efficient ways in which listeners use these consonant cues, as revealed in speech perception research. First, it was found that consonant per-ception seems to employ an immediate catego-rization of the cues in terms of consonant identity, rather than a comparative weighting or careful discrimination of the cue-qualities themselves. Then we explore how such disparate cues are combined in perceiving C-identity, considering transitional formant patterns in cooperation with noise-burst and durational cues. Finally, the oper-ations of the cues are found to be instrinsically affected by the context of adjacent phonemes and the rate of speaking.

PERCEPTUAL BOUNDARIES OF CONSONANT CATEGORIES

Synthetic speech stimuli were exploited further to explore the *perceptual boundaries* of consonant categories. To do this, series of synthetic CVs were generated in which acoustic features were varied in equal steps along a continuum from val-ues associated with one phonetic category to val-ues associated with another phonetic category. For instance, in one early study, a continuum of stop-vowel syllables was constructed where the syllables differed only in the direction and extent of the second formant transition, as shown in Figure 12-1 (Liberman, Harris, Hoffman & Griffith, (1957). The F2 transitions ranged over a [b]-[d]-[g] continuum. As the figure shows, the second formant transition (F2) changed in small, evenly spaced steps from a low onset frequency (and rising transition) typical of a labial stop (#1), through intermediate onset frequencies (with slightly rising or straight second formants) typical of an alveolar stop preceding /e/, to a relatively high onset frequency (and falling formant transition) typical of a velar stop in this context (#14). Throughout the series, adjacent stimuli differed in *equal* physical steps (120 Hz) of onset frequency of F2.

When presented this series of synthetic speech patterns, most listeners reported hearing all 14 stimuli as clear cases of either "bay," "day," or "gay." As expected, the consonant was identified as /b/ when the F2 onset was low; as /d/ when F2

onset was intermediate, and /g/ when F2 onset was high. This demonstrated that differences in the F2 onset frequency and transition were *sufficient* to differentiate labial, alveolar, and velar stop consonants in CV syllables when no other cues were available.

Another synthetic continuum of stimuli was developed at Haskins Labs to study perceptual cues to consonant voicing. This series systematically varied Voice Onset Time cues for voicing in initial stops (Abramson & Lisker, 1967). The stimuli were three-formant C + [ɑ] patterns that differed in the onset of the first formant (F1), relative to the onset of the upper formants (F2 and F3), over a range from 150 ms of "prevoicing" (−150 VOT) through simultaneous onset of F1, F2, and F3, (0 VOT) to 150 ms of F1 cutback and aspiration (+150 VOT). Successive stimuli differed in equal steps of 10 ms of VOT. On the prevoicing side, adjacent stimuli differed in the duration of

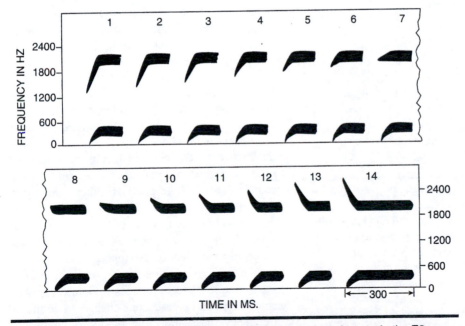

FIGURE 12-1.   Formant patterns of a series of stimuli designed to study the F2 formant transition as a cue to identification among the consonants /b,d,g/. The series forms a continuum based on changing only the onset frequency of F2. F1 has the same onset frequency for each stimulus, producing a transition that was chosen to be heard as a voiced stop-vowel syllable with V=[e].

(From Liberman, Harris, Hoffman, & Griffith, 1957, with permission)

VOT STIMULI SPECTROGRAMS

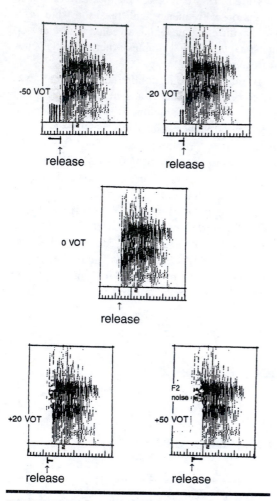

FIGURE 12-2. Spectrograms of [bɑ] and [pɑ] syllables illustrating the variations of VOT in a series of synthetic syllables used by Lisker and Abramson to study the cues for stop voicing. All times are in ms. The time scale marks are 10 ms intervals. For the 0 VOT stimulus in the center of the figure, the vowel begins immediately after the release transient marked with an arrow below the time scale. Two of the stimuli where voicing leads the release, –50 and –20 VOT, are shown in the top row, and two stimuli with cutback and aspiration noise in F2, +20 and +50 VOT, are shown in the bottom row. (The syllables shown are not the ones used by Lisker and Abramson but were made for graphic illustration from a natural syllable).

the F1 "voice murmur" preceding the onset of F2 and F3. On the "postvoicing" side, F2 and F3 were excited by aperiodic noise (F2 noise) prior to the onset of F1. Figure 12-2 presents spectrograms of five of the stimuli of the labial VOT series, –50 VOT, –20 VOT, 0 VOT, +20 VOT, and +50 VOT.

As with the place continuum, subjects consistently divided this VOT continuum into voiced and voiceless consonant categories. Stimuli with little or no aspiration noise and with F1 transitions beginning simultaneously or shortly after F2/F3 onset (–150 to +20 VOT) were heard as voiced, while stimuli with more aspiration and F1 cutback (+30 to +150 VOT) were identified as voiceless.

CATEGORICAL PERCEPTION OF SPEECH CONTINUA

While generating these acoustic continua, the Haskins researchers noticed an unusual phenomenon. When listening to each series, a change from one syllable-stimulus to the next sometimes caused no change in the consonant heard, while at other points on the continuum, the same change was heard as an abrupt change in consonant to the next consonant of the series. Equal physical differences were not *perceived* as equal across the entire range. Rather, perception of the physical continuum appeared to be *discontinuous*. Some differences along the acoustic continuum yielded no change in the perceived consonant; over a range or consonant field, several adjacent stimuli sounded identical. In contrast, other changes of the very same amount of VOT or F2 onset produced an abrupt change in voicing or place of the stop. The use of acoustic cues in stop consonant perception seemed to be uniquely categorical: Unlike the mixing of light waves or a tone sweeping in frequency that produces smooth changes in color or pitch, a graduated change in formant-frequency onset+transition produced jumps between constant impressions of consonants.

Why, in listening over the entire series of [b]-[d]-[g] stimuli, does the perception not go in continuous steps, beginning with a very clear [b], and then intermediate sounds between [b] and [d], then to a clear [d], and then some intermediate perceptions between [d] and [g], and finally to very clear [g]?

To test these curious discontinuities further, the investigators studied the degree of perceived differences across continua. They asked whether indeed it was very difficult to hear differences between syllables within the consonant fields of the continuum, differences that varied by the same amounts as the differences that were heard clearly as different consonants when placed across the boundaries between the fields. They designed an experiment that compared the identification and discrimination of stimuli along several synthetic continua. In the first study, Liberman and coworkers (1957) used the 14-step [be-de-ge] continuum of Figure 12-1. In an *Identification test*, the 14 stimuli were presented several times each in random order. The subjects' task was to *label* the consonant of each stimulus as "b," "d," or "g." In a separate *Discrimination test*, the subjects' task was to detect any difference at all between pairs of stimuli that differed in F2 onset and transition by the same amount. That is, *regardless* of whether the consonants they heard were of the same or different, was there any difference between the sounds of a pair? To make it clearer to subjects what they were supposed to do, an *ABX Discrimination* task was utilized, where after a pair, AB, is presented, either A or B is repeated as "X" and the listener decides whether X is the same as A or as B.[1]

Performance on both these tasks confirmed their informal observations that perception of the F2 continuum was discontinuous. First, identification tests showed that subjects divided the continuum into three phonetic categories, with steep slopes in the function at the boundaries between categories. (Category boundaries are defined as the 50% crossover point in identification functions.) That is, almost all of the stimuli with F2 transitions intermediate between patterns typical of natural "b" or "d" or "g" were nevertheless consistently identified as one of these consonants. (Stimuli #1 to #3 were heard as "b"; #5 through #8 as "d," and #11 through #14 as "g." Boundaries between /b-d/ and /d-g/ categories were located between stimuli #3 and #4 and stimuli #9 and #10, respectively).

More interesting were the results of the discrimination test, which also revealed discontinuous perception of the acoustic continuum. Discrimination functions contained *peaks* of accurate discrimination for cross-category comparison pairs, (i.e., pairs identified as different consonants, such as #3 and #5) and *troughs* of relatively poor discrimination for most within-category pairs (i.e., pairs identified as the same consonant such as #5 and #7 or #1 and #3). *Relative* discriminability was thus predictable from identification performance; discrimination of F2 transition differences was highly accurate only when those differences cued a change in phonetic category. Within-category acoustic differences of the same magnitude were discriminated poorly, in some cases no better than chance. The Haskins researchers dubbed this pattern of correlated performance on identification and discrimination tests *Categorical Perception*.

This pattern of perception was also found for the voicing distinction between stops cued by VOT (Abramson & Lisker, 1967; Lisker & Abramson, 1967b). In this study, the Identification test was the same as before. However, to test relative discrimination, an *Oddity Discrimination* test was used.[2] Discrimination of three levels of VOT difference was tested: 20 ms VOT, 30 ms VOT, and 40 ms VOT.

---

[1] In this task, triads of stimuli are presented. The first stimulus (A) and the second stimulus (B) of each triad differ by a fixed number of steps on the physical continuum (e.g., 2-step pairs compare #1–#3, #2–#4 . . . #12–#14). The third stimulus (X) is a repetition of either A or B. Subjects respond by saying whether X is the same as A or as B. All possible AB pairs are presented several times in random order in all four possible orders of ABX stimuli (ABA, ABB, BAA, BAB). Performance is scored in terms of the percentage of correct responses on each AB comparison; chance level of performance is 50% in this task. Thus, the *relative* discriminability is assessed across the stimulus continuum, all of which differ by the same amount acoustically for AB comparison pairs.

[2] As in the ABX test, triads of stimuli are presented in which two stimuli are identical and one differs. However, in the Oddity task, the different stimulus can occur first, second, or third and the subjects' task is to decide in which position the "odd" stimulus occurs. All six possible orderings of stimuli are included (AAB, ABA, BAA, BBA, BAB, BBA) for each comparison pair. Chance level performance is 33% correct.

Figure 12-3 presents the results of these tests. As the upper portion of the figure illustrates, the identification function is flat within categories, but becomes very steep at the boundary between voiced and voiceless categories. In fact, only two stimuli adjacent to the phonetic boundary (+20 VOT and +30 VOT) were labeled with less than 90% accuracy. Discrimination is highly accurate only on cross-category comparisons. Discrimination of within-category pairs is much poorer; it is close to chance on the voiced end of the continuum and only slightly better on the voiceless end of the continuum. Again, this illustrates that VOT was perceived *categorically*, in that discrimination performance was discontinuous. Furthermore, relative discriminability was predictable from perceivers' performance on the identification task. Peaks of highly accurate discrimination occurred only across voicing category boundaries.

This pattern of perception differs markedly from identification and discrimination of stimuli from vowel continua. In an early study, Fry, Abramson, Eimas, and Liberman (1962) synthesized a 13-step two-formant continuum of steady-state vowels in which both F1 and F2 frequencies varied from [ɪ] to [ɛ] to [æ]. Over the continuum F1 moved from lower to higher frequencies, while F2 simultaneously varied from higher to lower frequencies in equal steps. On Identification tests, subjects divided the continuum into the three vowel categories. However, the stimuli between the "good" cases of [ɪ] and [ɛ] and between good [ɛ] and [æ] were not labeled consistently from trial to trial, resulting in gradually sloping identification functions. More importantly, discrimination functions showed no large peaks or troughs. Rather, both cross-category and within-category comparisons were discriminated

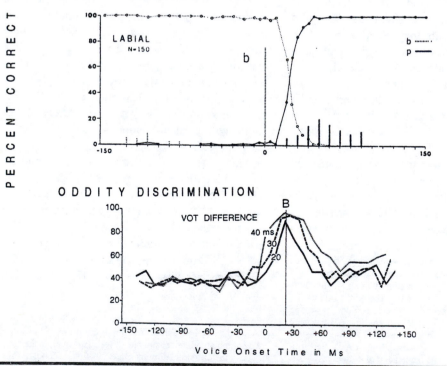

FIGURE 12-3. Categorial perception of stop voicing on a continuum of voice onset time (VOT).

(Adapted from Abramson & Lisker, 1967, with permission from Haskins Laboratories)

very well (e.g., performance on all 2-step pairs was greater than 90% correct). This pattern of identification and discrimination performance is referred to as *continuous perception*, because discrimination accuracy is not predictable on the basis of the vowel category boundaries, and discrimination throughout the continuum is uniformly high.[3]

The Haskins investigators pointed out that the difference in categorical versus noncategorical perception between consonants and vowels might be related to a difference in the motor conditions of articulation. The consonants are produced by discrete motions that must attain certain targets, for example, closures at certain places for the stop consonants and a state of closed or open glottis for producing the voiced/unvoiced distinction. The alveolar stop consonants must attain a closure at the alveolar position. There are no stop consonants that are produced in between the labial and alveolar closure positions.

For the vowels, on the other hand, the tongue position can assume a large number of different positions in the front vowels, for example, from very close [i] to less close [ɪ], and so on over different degrees of closeness between [ɪ] and [e] and [ɛ] and on to the most open front vowel [æ]. Thus, it would seem that the degree to which categorization of perception occurs along the acoustic dimensions of the cues depends on whether the sounds are produced categorically (consonants) or noncategorically (vowels). Perception seems to correspond to the nature of articulation rather than to the continuum of acoustic cues. The Haskins group suggested that speech perception might involve a process in which the articulations that would be necessary to produce a heard acoustic pattern are the basis for the perception. This "motor" theory of speech perception is discussed further in the next chapter.

Subsequent studies showed that the acoustic cues for vowel categories were perceived less continuously when the vowels were shorter in duration or when the vowels were placed in CVC contexts and included moving formant patterns. For instance, Pisoni (1973) compared the perception of two steady-state vowel continua—long vowels (300 ms) and short vowels (50 ms)—with two consonant continua—a VOT series [b-p] and a place series [b-d]. For the place series, transition onset and direction varied simultaneously for both F2 and F3 from lower to higher values.

Figure 12-4 shows results for the four 7-step continua. Superimposed on the curves of identification performance (shown by the solid and dashed lines) are the results of an AX Discrimination test (shown by the dotted lines).[4] To shorten these tests, only three 2-step comparison pairs from each continuum were examined: one cross-category pair, #3–#5, and two within-category pairs, #1–#3, and #5–#7.

Notice that the major difference in discrimination performance across the four continua was the accuracy of discrimination of within-category pairs. For the two consonant continua, within-category discrimination was near chance (50%), as would be predicted from identification. In contrast, the within-category pairs of the long vowel continuum were discriminated nearly as well as the cross-category pair (> 80% accuracy), demonstrating nearly continuous perception. Discrimination of the short vowel continuum was less continuous. While within-category discrimination was less accurate than cross-category discrimination (75% versus 90% correct), it was nevertheless well above chance. Thus, this study again demonstrated that the acoustic cues for voice and place contrasts in stop consonants were perceived categorically, while acoustic cues for vowels were

---

[3] This pattern is more typical of the perception of simple acoustic dimensions such as the frequency of sine wave stimuli (pure tones). In tests of frequency perception, the ability to detect differences between two frequencies is much more accurate than one's ability to absolutely identify the frequency of individual pure tones.

[4] In an AX discrimination task, pairs of stimuli are presented and subjects respond "same" or "different." Chance level of performance is 50%. Subjects are instructed to respond "different" if they detect any difference in the stimuli, regardless of whether the speech sounds they hear are of the same or different phonetic categories.

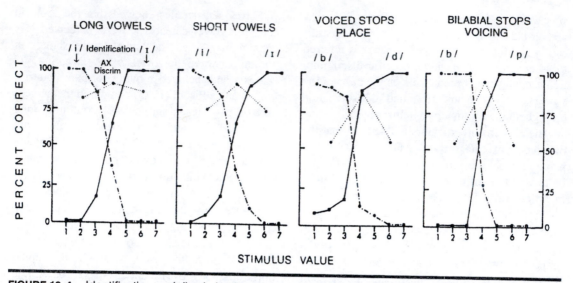

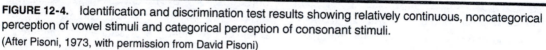

STIMULUS VALUE

FIGURE 12-4. Identification and discrimination test results showing relatively continuous, noncategorical perception of vowel stimuli and categorical perception of consonant stimuli.
(After Pisoni, 1973, with permission from David Pisoni)

perceived more continuously, especially when the steady-state vowels were long in duration.

Pisoni also demonstrated that discrimination of vowels became more categorical when the interstimulus interval (ISI) of AX comparison pairs was longer. While discrimination of cross-category pairs remained very accurate even for the longest ISI, discrimination of within-category pairs got worse as the ISI changed from 250 ms to 2000 ms. However, for the stop consonant continua, ISI appeared to have little effect on discrimination; within-category discrimination was poor for all ISI durations.

To summarize so far, Categorical Perception (hereafter CP) refers to the fact that perception of an acoustic cue that varies along a continuum of equal steps is discontinuous and that the discontinuities correspond to the boundaries between phoneme categories. CP is evidenced by correlated identification and discrimination according to four criteria:

1. Phoneme identification of equal interval steps along an acoustic cue continuum shows a steep slope, a rapid change in identification, in the vicinity of the phonetic category boundary. For acoustic cue values intermediate between the

boundaries, identification of the extant phoneme persists at a high level.

2. Accurate discrimination of equal-interval comparison pairs occurs only at category boundaries (i.e., discrimination is most accurate for cross-category comparisons).

3. Discrimination of within-category comparisons pairs is at or near chance.

4. Discrimination at each point on the continuum is highly predictable from phoneme identification performance. That is, the location and height of discrimination peaks and troughs can be predicted from performance in phoneme identification.[5]

In order to explore the extent of CP phenomena in speech psychoacoustics, dozens of studies were conducted with acoustic continua that var-

---

[5] To determine whether discrimination along a continuum meets the last criterion, "predicted" discrimination values are computed from subjects' identification scores under the assumption that discrimination would be no better than identification, and compared with discrimination scores "obtained" from the actual discrimination tests. If the two arrays of discrimination scores, predicted versus obtained, are not significantly different from each other statistically, then criterion 4 has been met.

ied the cues for place, voicing, and manner contrasts among consonants in a variety of vowel and syllable contexts. (See Repp, 1984, for a comprehensive review.) In general, they have shown that the pattern of identification and discrimination performance almost always satisfies the first two criteria listed above, but sometimes falls short of fulfilling the third and fourth criteria of chance discrimination between different stimuli within a phoneme category, and predictability of discrimination from identification. In those

cases, discrimination shows peaks across phoneme boundaries and troughs for within-category comparisons; however, discrimination of within-category pairs is significantly above chance, although still significantly *below* that of cross-category pairs. This pattern of performance is referred to as showing a *Phoneme Boundary Effect* (PBE). Although not meeting the strict criteria for CP described above, the PBE pattern nevertheless indicates that discrimination of acoustic continua underlying distinctions among con-

TABLE 12-1. Results of CP experiments with synthetic continua contrasting consonants and vowels in different contexts.

ACOUSTIC CONTINUUM	PATTERN OF DISCRIMINATION		
	CP	PBE	Continuous
Voicing: Stops			
F1 cutback (initial)	X		
VOT (initial)	X		
Vowel duration (final)			X
Silence duration (medial)		X	
Place of Articulation: Stops			
F2/F3 transitions (initial)	X		
F2/F3 transitions (final)		X	
Place of Articulation: Glides			
F3 transitions /r-l/	X	X	
F2/F3 transitions /w-r/		X	
Place of Articulation: Fricatives			
Noise bandwidth /s-ʃ/		X	
Manner of Articulation			
Silence duration (medial)			
"say-stay"; "slit-split"	X	X	
"go shop"-"go chop"		X	
Amplitude Rise Time (initial)			
/ʃ-tʃ/	X		
Oral-nasal stops	X	X	
Transition duration /b-w/		X	
Vowel Contrasts			
F1/F2 frequencies		X	X
Duration			X

initial = initial position in syllable
medial = between vowels or in consonant clusters
final = final position in syllable

CP = Categorical Perception (all four criteria satisfied)
PBE = Phoneme Boundary Effect (first two criteria satisfied)
Continuous = Discrimination uniform throughout continuum

sonants (and vowels in some cases) is highly constrained but not totally determined by the phonemic significance of the acoustic parameters.

Table 12-1 lists several synthetic speech continua that have been examined using the CP experimental paradigm. As the table indicates, discrimination of many acoustic cues for contrasts in voicing, place, and manner of articulation has been found to be discontinuous, evidencing either CP in the strict sense or a PBE. The exception is the cue of vowel duration, which serves as a cue for voicing of final stops and vowel identity. It can also be seen that the particular acoustic cue for a phonetic contrast and the syllable context in which it occurs can affect the categoriality of performance. For instance, VOT (the cue at release for voicing of initial stops) is highly categorical (Abramson & Lisker, 1967), while the stop duration (which is one cue for voicing in medial position) is perceived less categorically, showing a PBE but above chance discrimination of within-category comparisons. The perception of F2/F3 cues for place of articulation in stops is highly categorical in syllable-initial context, but somewhat less categorical (although still evidencing a PBE) when the same acoustic cue is in syllable-final position (Mattingly, Liberman, Syrdal, & Halwes, 1971).

PERCEPTION OF NONSPEECH ANALOGS

The finding that almost all of the acoustic continua that distinguish consonants were perceived categorically was interpreted by the Haskins researchers as reflecting a special "speech mode" of perception that was different from general auditory perception. They claimed that humans had evolved special perceptual mechanisms to "decode" the complex, context-dependent acoustic patterns that carry the phonetic message in speech (Liberman, Cooper, Shankweiler, & Studdert-Kennedy, 1967). Evidence that this unique mode of perception was "linguistic" (i.e., specialized for the perception of "encoded" speech signals) came from studies that examined listeners' discrimination of related *nonspeech* continua. In these experiments, the same

acoustic cues were varied as in speech continua, but the patterns were presented in acoustic isolation without their speech context. These isolated acoustic events are referred to as *nonspeech analogs*.

If the categoriality of acoustic cues in consonant perception was dictated simply by categorizing tendencies of hearing, then nonspeech analogs bearing the same critical changes as seen in the speech cues, but that do not sound like speech, should show categoriality and boundary effects similar to those seen in their speech counterparts. Many experiments were made to test this hypothesis. A study by McGovern and Strange (1977) serves as an example. They investigated the perception of variations in F3 transitions (the primary cue for the /r-l/ contrast) in four sets of synthetic stimuli. The two Speech continua consisted of a three-formant [ri] to [li] series and a three-formant [ir] to [il] series, in which only the F3 patterns varied as shown in Figure 12-5.

F3 onsets (offsets) varied from low to high frequency; transitions varied from rising (falling) to straight. The first and second formant patterns were constant across all stimuli of each continuum. In addition, two Nonspeech continua were tested; these stimuli consisted of the F3 patterns *presented in isolation* (i.e., with the F1 and F2 components deleted). These patterns sounded like bird chirps or musical tones with changing pitch (glissandi). The *differences* in F3 patterns within both Speech and Nonspeech continua were identical. However, when F3 patterns were combined with F1 and F2 components, the stimuli were heard as speech; when presented alone, the F3 patterns were heard as nonspeech auditory signals.

Figure 12-6 presents the results of Oddity Discrimination tests for Speech (dashed curves) and Nonspeech (solid curves) stimuli. The phoneme boundaries (derived from Identification tests of the Speech stimuli) are also indicated in the graphs by the vertical dotted lines labeled B. Notice first that for both syllable-initial and syllable-final speech stimuli, discrimination was most accurate in comparisons of cross-category stimuli, while discrimination for within-category comparisons was near

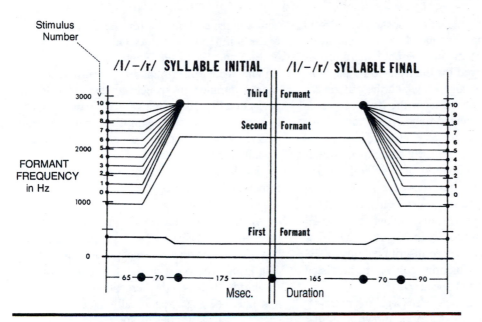

FIGURE 12-5. Stimulus formant tracks for constructing continua of stimuli to test the categoriality of perception of speech stimuli compared with perception of a nonspeech component, the F3 transition.

(From McGovern & Strange, The perception of /r/; and /l/ in syllable-initial and syllable-final position. *Perception and Psychophysics, 21,* 162-170, 1977. Adapted by permission of Psychonomic Society, Inc.)

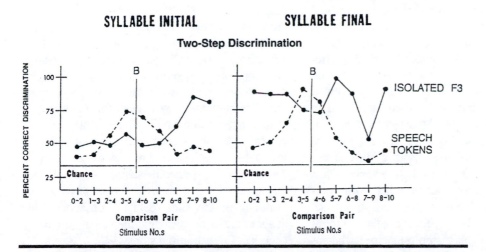

FIGURE 12-6. Results of tests comparing perceptual categoriality of speech and nonspeech stimuli. Discrimination was tested between members of pairs of stimuli, numbered on the horizontal axis according to the stimulus numbers of the preceding Figure. See text for discussion and conclusions.

(From McGovern & Strange, The perception of /r/; and /l/ in syllable-initial and syllable-final position. *Perception and Psychophysics, 21,* 162-170, 1977. Adapted by permission of Psychonomic Society, Inc.)

chance. That is, F3 transition cues were perceived categorically when presented in the context of speech patterns. A much different pattern of discrimination emerged for the isolated F3 patterns. Syllable-initial analogs, in which the differences between stimuli occurred in the beginning portion, were discriminated quite poorly (except for pairs 7–9 and 8–10, which contrasted rising transitions with straight or nearly straight transitions of F3). Nonspeech analogs of syllable-final patterns, in which the differences occurred in the end portion, were perceived much better (except for pair 7–9). In both cases, discrimination of the F3 patterns differed markedly in Speech versus Nonspeech contexts. Relative discriminability of F3 analog patterns in isolation could *not* be predicted from identification of speech patterns.

Studies of nonspeech analogs of place-of-articulation cues in stops have shown a similar pattern of results. (See Repp, 1984 for a review.) In one study, 40 ms F2 transitions distinguishing /b-d-g/ in initial and final position were presented in isolation, with all of F1 and the steady-state part of F2 absent (Mattingly et al., 1971). Discrimination was uniformly poor for initial transitions (which began at different frequencies and ended at the same frequency); discrimination was much better for final transitions (which started at the same frequency and ended at different frequencies). In neither case were there discrimination peaks for isolated F2 patterns that constituted cross-category comparisons when embedded in speech context. Thus, discrimination of these nonspeech analogs appeared to be governed by the auditory salience of the acoustic differences, rather than by their phonetic relevance when embedded in speech signals. In other words, perception of F2 transitions in a stop-consonant-like context seems to be especially adapted to or aimed at distinguishing stop phonemes whereas isolated F2 transitions are uniformly undistinctive (poorly distinguished).

Studies of nonspeech analogs of closure duration cues for voicing (as in "rapid" versus "rabid") and for the presence versus absence of a stop (as in "stay" versus "say") have shown differences in the perception of silence duration in speech

versus nonspeech modes (cf., Best, Morrongiello, & Robson, 1981; Liberman, Harris, Eimas, Lisker, & Bastian, 1961; see Repp, 1984 for review). Again, while discrimination of differences in silence duration in speech contexts reveals evidence of a PBE, discrimination of silence duration in nonspeech contexts exhibited a very different pattern: Discrimination was either continuously low throughout the continuum, or the peaks of better discrimination did not appear in locations corresponding to the phoneme category boundaries seen in speech context.

All the above studies showing differences in perception of speech and nonspeech analogs support the notion that speech perception is "special." However, other studies have demonstrated similarities between the perception of speech and nonspeech analogs. Specifically, studies with nonspeech analogs of cues to voicing in initial stops have produced categorical-like results. In one study (Pisoni, 1977) a Tone Onset Time (TOT) continuum was generated in which the onset of a low tone was delayed relative to the onset of a higher tone, analogously to the F1 cutback seen in voiceless stops. In another study (Miller, Wier, Pastore, Kelly, & Dooling, 1976) the relative onset times of two sounds (a periodic "buzz" and an aperiodic "noise") were varied analogously to VOT. Both TOT and Noise-Buzz continua yielded discontinuous discrimination functions resembling those found for continua testing stop voicing. Discrimination was best for comparisons spanning the +20 ms point on the continuum that corresponded to the phoneme boundary in English between voiced and voiceless labial stops. The authors interpreted these findings as evidence that there was a psychophysical boundary between "simultaneous" versus "delayed" onset occurring at about the same place that the voicing boundary occurs in English initial stops.

In summary, then, studies of nonspeech analogs of acoustic cues for several place, manner, and voicing contrasts have shown that, in general, discrimination of isolated acoustic components differs markedly from perception of the same acoustic components when they are embedded in a speech context. Subjects do not hear these isolated components *as speech*, nor do their discrimination functions show Phoneme Boundary Effects. Relative discriminability of these non-speech signals appears to be determined by the auditory salience of acoustic parameters, rather than by their phonetic relevance. Thus, we can conclude that categorical perception of *speech* continua reflects processes specialized for the decoding of speech signals, that is, perception in a "linguistic mode." (A more detailed discussion of the nature of these specialized perceptual mechanisms is presented in Chapters Thirteen and Fourteen). However, peaks in discrimination functions for some speech continua such as VOT may be due in part to the presence of "natural" psychophysical boundaries that would apply to perception of all sounds and are not special for speech.

PERCEPTUAL INTEGRATION OF ACOUSTIC CUES

Thus far we have seen how perception of the acoustic cues for consonants has been investigated using synthetic continua in which only one or two acoustic parameters were varied together, while other cues to the contrast were held constant or were absent. We know, however, that in real speech, most consonantal contrasts are distinguished by several acoustic features: Stop voicing, for example, may be signaled by both aspiration and F1 onset frequency. Furthermore, the relative salience and consistency of occurrence of the acoustic features vary depending on the phonemic and prosodic context and the talker's dialect, speaking rate, and style of speech. Thus, while a single acoustic cue may be *sufficient* to differentiate phonetic categories under restricted experimental conditions, important questions remain about how listeners utilize the multiple acoustic cues normally available in natural speech to identify the phonemes.

How do changes in a secondary acoustic cue affect the location of perceptual boundaries along a primary acoustic continuum that, by itself, is sufficient to distinguish the phoneme categories. Fitch and colleagues at Haskins found that phoneme boundaries shifted systematically as secondary acoustic cues were varied (Fitch, Halwes, Erickson, & Liberman, 1980). Two "slit"-"split" synthetic continua were generated that varied the duration of the [p]-silence between the frication noise [s] and the following part of the syllable, from 8 ms to 160 ms, in 8 ms steps. For one continuum, the following portion simulated the syllable [lɪt] as shown in Figure 12-7 (left); for the other continuum the following portion resembled

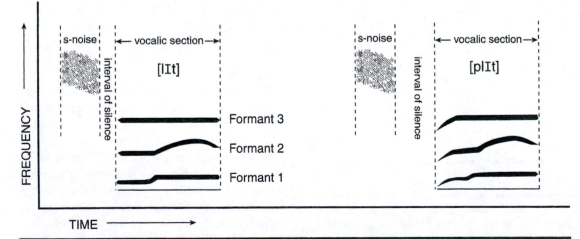

FIGURE 12-7. Schematic spectrograms of the stimulus patterns used to synthesize stimuli to test integration of a secondary consonant cue, silence, with formant transition cues to the consonant [l]. (From Fitch et al., 1980, with permission)

the syllable [plɪt] (right hand side of Figure 12-7). The only difference between these two patterns was that for [plɪt], F1, F2, and F3 began lower and contained rapid upward transitions (an acoustic cue for a preceding stop consonant), while for [lɪt], formants started higher and had no initial transitions.

Listeners consistently identified the stimuli of each silence duration continuum as either "slit" or "split," as shown in Figure 12-8. Stimuli with long silence durations (the primary cue for a stop) were labeled "split." However, as we see in the figure, the location of the phoneme boundary differed between the two continua. Stimuli in the mid-range, with 48 ms to 112 ms of silence, were identified as "split" more often when they contained rising formants than when they contained straight initial formants. That is, shorter silent intervals (indicating no stop) could be *offset* by the presence of formant transitions (indicating a stop) and vice versa. This reciprocal relationship between two cues for a phoneme contrast is called a *phonetic trading relation* (Repp, 1982). The shift in the phoneme boundary on one acoustic

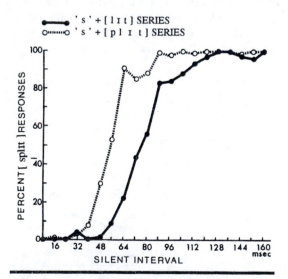

FIGURE 12-8. Identification of [splɪt] versus [slɪt] depending on the duration of the silent interval following [s] in the stimuli described in the previous figure.

(From Fitch et al., 1980, with permission)

continuum as a function of offsetting changes in another acoustic feature suggests that *both acoustic cues are integrated by the listener into a unitary phoneme percept.*

Interesting phonetic trading relations occur among the multiple cues for voicing contrasts between consonants. Summerfield and Haggard (1975) demonstrated that F1 onset frequency "traded" with VOT cues for voicing. Stimuli with low F1 onset (a cue for voiced stops) required longer VOT values to be identified as voiceless stops than stimuli with higher F1 onset. Likewise, the presence versus absence of "closure murmur" traded with silence and vowel duration cues for voicing in medial stops (Lisker, 1978). Vowel duration, frication noise duration, and F0 cues to fricative voicing have also been shown to trade off (cf., Soli, 1982).

Cues for place of articulation also enter into phonetic trading relations. The phoneme category boundaries on [r-l] continua differing in F3 onset and transition (the primary spectral cue) were shifted as a function of the duration of F1 initial steady-state and transition (a secondary temporal cue). Stimuli with longer steady-states and more abrupt ("l"-like) F1 transitions required lower F3 onsets to be identified as [r] than stimuli with shorter steady-states and more gradual ("r"-like) F1 transitions (Polka & Strange, 1985). Bailey and Summerfield (1980) demonstrated phonetic trading relations among stop place cues in [s] + stop + vowel syllables including (1) fricative offset spectrum cues, (2) closure duration cues, and (3) formant onset cues.

The ubiquity of cue-trading in consonant perception suggested that the multiple spectral and temporal features associated with distinctive articulatory gestures are integrated into a unitary phoneme percept by the listener. Thus, different combinations of cue-values along relevant acoustic continua can result in perceptually equivalent instances of a phoneme despite differences in acoustic pattern. Fitch and co-workers (1980) further demonstrated that variable combinations of acoustic features give rise to equivalent perceptual categories using discrimination tests of synthetic stimuli that independently varied multiple acoustic cues. The discrimination of three types of stimulus pairs was compared. The types differed in the number of cues varied (one versus two) and how variations in two acoustic parameters (silence duration and formant onsets) were combined.

One Cue pairs consisted of stimuli in which only formants onsets differed; silence duration was the same within pairs. *Two Cooperating Cue* pairs combined stimuli in which both silence duration and formant onsets differed. In each pair, one stimulus had a shorter silence (no stop) and higher formant onsets (no stop) while the other stimulus had longer silence (stop) and lower formant onsets (stop). Finally, the *Two Conflicting Cue* pairs also differed in both silence duration and formant onsets, but in reverse combination: shorter duration (no stop) with lower formant onsets (stop) versus longer duration (stop) with higher formant onsets (no stop).

Figure 12-9 presents the results of Oddity Discrimination tests. As expected, for stimuli with silent durations between 48 ms and 112 ms (where trading relations occurred), discrimination was best for Two Cooperating Cue pairs, and poorest for Two Conflicting Cue pairs. That is, the ability to discriminate stimuli that differed on two cue dimensions, silence duration and formant onset transition, was dependent on the phonetic relevance of those differences *in combination*. Two Conflicting Cue pairs were harder to discriminate even than One Cue pairs, because the perceiver responded on the basis of the integrated percepts, rather than on the basis of differences in individual acoustic features. That is, the Two Conflicting Cue pairs were not perceptually distinct, since *both* stimuli of each pair contained conflicting cues for stop and no stop categories. On the other hand, Two Cooperating Cue pairs were discriminated better than One Cue pairs, because *both* acoustic cues for the contrast differentiated each pair in a consistent manner.

Further studies have shown perceptual equivalence using combinations of other types of consonant cues (cf., Best et al., 1981; Polka & Strange, 1985; Repp, Liberman, Eccardt, & Pesetsky,

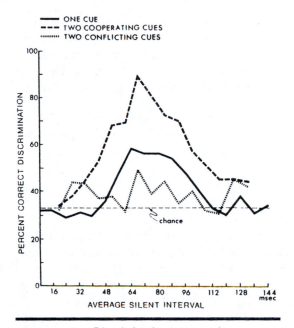

FIGURE 12-9.   Discrimination test results demonstrating integration of cues.

(Adapted from Fitch et al., 1980, with permission)

1978). In each case, when two acoustic cues were combined in ways that were *phonetically offsetting*, discrimination was poorer than when only one of the cues was varied, or when the two cues were combined in cooperating ways. This shows that listeners base their discrimination responses on integrated phoneme percepts. When spectral and temporal cues for the same articulatory gesture are manipulated in ways that give rise to phonetic trading relations, acoustically different stimuli are heard as perceptually equivalent.

CONTEXT AND RATE EFFECTS ON PHONETIC CATEGORY BOUNDARIES

We have seen how multiple acoustic cues for consonants, including acoustically diverse cues that occur sequentially (e.g., silence and subsequent formant patterns), can interact in complementary ways to determine phoneme category boundaries. Phoneme boundaries also shift as a function of the phonetic context in which consonants occur (i.e., the preceding and following phonemes) and as a function of changes in speaking rate. These contextual effects also demonstrate that listeners integrate into a consonant perception acoustic information that is spread over time intervals beyond the scope of the constriction gesture of the immediate consonant.

First, let us consider the effects of preceding and following phoneme context on perception of acoustic cues for consonants. As in the study of phonetic trading relations, synthetic speech continua have been employed to investigate shifts in the location of phonetic category boundaries with changes in context. For instance, one study explored the perception of a [ʃ-s] continuum in which the bandwidth of the fricative noise was varied from a wide band for [ʃ] to a narrow band for [s] by raising the lower cutoff frequency in equal steps across a 9-step continuum (Mann & Repp, 1980).

Two continua were presented to subjects in identification tests: a [ʃ-s] + [i] continuum and a [ʃ-s] +[u] continuum. They differed only in the vocalic portion; the noise bandwidths varied over the continuum in exactly the same way in both series. Identification functions showed that when these noises were followed by [i], more of the intermediate bandwidth stimuli were heard as [ʃ] than when the noises were followed by the vowel [u]. This reflects the fact that in natural speech, the lip rounding associated with [u] acts to lower the resonance frequencies of the vocal tract. Thus, anticipatory lip rounding during the consonant constriction results in wider bandwidths of noise for [s] in this context than in unrounded vowel contexts. Listeners "compensated" for the effects of anticipatory coarticulation on the fricative noises when assigning labels to the synthetic stimuli. The same (intermediate bandwidth) fricative noises were identified as [ʃ] when followed by [i] and as [s] when followed by [u].

In another study, Mann (1980) demonstrated that *preceding* context could also influence the location of phonetic boundaries. She tested identification of a [dɑ-gɑ] continuum when the stimuli were preceded by the syllable [ɑr] and when they were preceded by the syllable [ɑl]. The

[dɑ-gɑ] series of stimuli varied only in F3 transition cues; F2 transitions remained constant. As predicted, more of the intermediate stimuli were identified as [g] when preceded by [ɑl] than when preceded by [ɑr].

Again, this shift in phoneme boundary corresponds well with coarticulatory influences during the production of these two-syllable words. Acoustical analysis of natural [ɑrdɑ], [ɑrgɑ], [ɑldɑ], and [ɑlgɑ] stimuli showed that the velar stops following [l] had higher F3 onsets than velar stops following [r]. Alveolar stops following [l] also showed much higher F3 onsets. The perceptual results indicated that the phoneme category boundary also shifted to higher F3 values. In other words, perceptual category boundaries shift in ways that take into account articulatory and acoustic variations in the realization of phonetic segments in different contexts. This allows the perceiver to extract an invariant message from highly variable acoustic patterns.

Studies of the effects of speaking rate on the perception of phonetic categories also suggest complex compensatory perceptual processes that enable the listener to "decode" the phonetic message even though acoustic patterns vary as speakers speed up and slow down their rate of speech (cf, Miller, 1981, for a review of this literature). This can be seen in studies that examine how phonetic category boundaries on temporal cue dimensions shift with changes in speaking rate.

A study by Miller and Liberman (1979) demonstrated that the perceived rate of speech of the target syllable itself affects the perception of a temporal cue for manner of articulation. These researchers examined the perception of a [b-w] continuum in which the duration and rate of initial formant transitions varied from short, rapid transitions typical of stops to long, gradual transitions typical of glides. Five such continua were constructed that differed only in the duration of the steady-state vowel portion of the syllables (80 ms, 116 ms, 152 ms, 224 ms, and 296 ms, respectively). Thus, vowel duration was used to indicate speaking rate, since speech at slower rates contains longer vowels.

Figure 12-10 presents the results of identification tests on the five continua. As you can see, the [b-w] phoneme boundary shifted systematically toward longer, more gradual transitions as the duration of the following vowel increased. Transition durations between 28 ms and 52 ms were identified as [b] more often as vowel duration increased. Thus, listeners appeared to compensate for the fact that consonant transitions (as well as vowel durations) tend to be longer in slow speech than in rapid speech.

Several experiments by Quentin Summerfield (1981) demonstrated shifts in perception of VOT cues for stop voicing with changes in the speaking rate of a preceding carrier sentence. As predicted, when the preceding carrier sentence rate was slow, the phonetic boundary was located at longer VOT values than when the sentence was fast. That is, stimuli with intermediate VOTs were

heard as voiceless in "rapid" speech and voiced in "slow" speech. Further experiments demonstrated that the duration of the word immediately preceding the test syllables had the greatest effect on VOT perception. That is, perceptual boundaries shifted primarily as a function of the relative durations of immediately adjacent syllables.

These and other studies of the effects of speaking rate on the perception of temporal cues (Fitch, Halwes, Erickson, & Liberman, 1981; Miller & Grosjean, 1981) indicate that listeners "interpret" the multiple cues for phonetic contrasts within the context of a stretch of speech sometimes spanning several syllables. Coarticulatory and speech timing influences on the location of perceptual boundaries show that listeners integrate acoustic information spanning several adjacent phonetic segments in the course of "decoding" the intended phonetic message, taking into account the rate of utterance indicated by the segment durations (for a review see Pickett et al., 1995).

Perceivers appear to be sensitive to coarticulatory and timing influences that alter the articulatory patterns and thus the acoustic structure of speech signals. The finding that listeners appear to base their perceptual judgments *not* on the acoustic patterns *per se*, but rather on the underlying articulatory gestures that gave rise to those acoustic patterns reinforces the claims of several researchers that humans possess special perceptual mechanisms uniquely suited to the recovery of the linguistic message carried by the acoustic patterns of speech. These "articulatory theories" of speech perception are presented in Chapter Fourteen, as motor theories of phoneme perception.

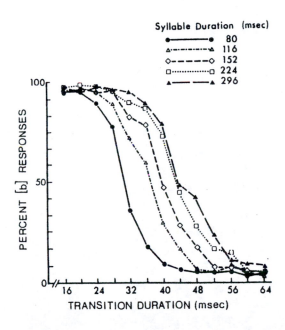

FIGURE 12-10. Identification of [b] versus [w] as a function of transition speed depends on the rate of utterance of the context, which is inversely proportional to the parameter syllable duration.
(Adpated from Miller & Liberman, 1979, with permission)

SUMMARY

In this chapter, we have described how acoustic cues for consonants are perceived. The research utilized synthetic speech stimuli in which the acoustic cues were varied systematically, either one at a time, or in combination. Studies of acoustic cues for contrasts of voicing, place, and manner of articulation revealed sharply defined boundaries between consonant categories as a cue is changed along a continuum of values. While discrimination of very small acoustic differences that distinguish these phonetic categories is highly accurate, discrimination within a phoneme category of the same acoustic variation is relatively poor. This *Categorical Perception* of acoustic continua appears to be restricted primarily to perception of speech patterns. Nonspeech analogs of most consonant contrasts, in which an acoustic cue component is presented as an isolated auditory signal, are not perceived categorically. That is, there is no correlation between discrimination accuracy and category boundary location on the acoustic cue continuum when it is presented in isolation.

The CP paradigm has been extended to investigate the perception of multiple acoustic cues. Results have shown that primary and secondary cues for consonantal contrasts enter into *phonetic trading relations*. Thus, acoustic patterns containing different values of combined acoustic cues are *perceptually equivalent* and cannot be easily discriminated. These complex interactions among acoustic cues that determine how speech sounds are identified and discriminated have led researchers to conclude that listeners integrate the multiple acoustic cues for a phoneme contrast and respond on the basis of a unitary phoneme percept.

The phenomena of the categorical and integral processing of widely varied acoustic cues are consistent with the theoretical view that phoneme perception takes place via special speech-specific processes, by reference to the underlying speech gestures rather than by general auditory discrimination/identification. This view, the Motor Theory, is further described and compared to competing theories in Chapter Fourteen.

CHAPTER THIRTEEN.

AUDITORY CAPACITIES AND PHONOLOGICAL DEVELOPMENT: ANIMAL, BABY, AND FOREIGN LISTENERS

SARAH HAWKINS

Here we begin our study of some fascinating theories about how the phonetic units of speech are perceived. First, in this chapter we look at phonetic perception by babies to examine the innate base of auditory capacities that are available for the perception process. We find that, at birth, babies possess acute auditory discrimination for the acoustic cue differences used to differentiate phonemes of all languages. Then, during the first few months' experience hearing the native home language, sharp cue discrimination becomes limited to the differences of the phonemic contrasts of the native language and the non-native contrasts are no longer easily detectable by the baby. As a result the very young child is perceptually ready for easy acquisition of the first words. Turning to perception theory in Chapter Fourteen, we present the two "classical" theories of phoneme perception that have stimulated the most research and controversy: the Motor Theory of Haskins Laboratories and the Quantal Theory developed at MIT. In Chapter Fifteen we expand the domain of perception theory from perceiving phonemes to word-recognition, leading to computer-like models of lexical access.

BACKGROUND: DOES PHONOLOGICAL PERCEPTION USE SPECIAL AUDITORY PROCESSES?

Any model of human behavior must take a position on how much its characteristics are one manifesta-

tion of a general ability and how much they are specific to that particular behavior. The question of how much speech perception is like other forms of auditory perception has been central for theorists. To what extent are the processes of perception based on general auditory properties and to what extent is there an independent phonetic mode of perception that is special to speech? A related question is how linguistic experience shapes perception. This section considers data that are relevant to these questions, namely babies' perception of speech, and cross-linguistic studies of adults' speech perception. We shall focus mainly on the perception of phonemic contrasts.

Young babies and nonhuman animals have in common that they have no linguistic system, including no system of phonological contrasts, so logic dictates that their responses to sounds from contrasting phonological categories of a language reflect relatively general auditory processes. When their responses are the same as those of adults who speak that language and respond in terms of its phonology, then there is a good chance that the phonological contrasts in question are also based on general auditory processes. Additionally, phonological knowledge develops rather gradually during infancy and early childhood, and the child's emerging linguistic structure will begin to influence his or her perception in ways that we are only just beginning to understand. Cross-linguistic studies of adults are different from those with babies and nonhuman animals in that the adults do have a system of phonological contrasts as part of their linguistic knowledge. But their own system will presumably influence their responses to foreign contrasts when they try to discriminate between sounds that are not contrastive in their native language. Unlike a newborn baby or an animal, a normal adult's response cannot be made in the *absence* of a phonological system: The fact that the person has had any linguistic experience must shape his or her responses in some way, unless (and this is possible under some circumstances) the unfamiliar sounds are responded to as if they were not speech. However, the nature and degree of the influence from the existing phonological system may depend on a number of factors, as we shall see.

TECHNIQUES FOR STUDYING BABIES' SPEECH PERCEPTION

Our knowledge about babies' perception is relatively new, because until the early 1970s there were no techniques for studying them. The trick was to find a method that would (1) hold a baby's interest for long enough that enough responses could be collected for the data to be reliable and suitable for statistical analysis, and (2) use a task that a baby understood and a response that it could do. The second requirement was the most elusive: Small babies cannot "do" very much. However, a number of techniques were developed that were suitable either for babies aged between about 1 and 4 months of age or from about 5 to 12 months of age. We still have no really good techniques for testing the speech perception of children aged between 12 months and 3 years: This is the time when speech and language are developing fastest, but the child is not easily persuaded to sit still and listen, much less respond systematically! Perceptual data for this age group are therefore sparse and fairly unreliable.

The methods for the youngest babies exploit either the baby's enjoyment of sucking, or else physiological "orienting" responses such as a change in heart rate to a novel stimulus. The principle is the same in both cases. A speech sound

such as a CV syllable is played over and over to the baby until he or she becomes used to the sound and stops behaving as if it is interesting— that is, until the baby acts as if it is bored by the sound. Then the stimulus is changed. If the baby's behavior also changes in a way that suggests it is interested again, then it is assumed that the baby has noticed that the new stimulus is different. If the baby responds in the same way to the new stimulus as to the old, boring stimulus, then it is assumed that the baby has not noticed any change in the stimuli.

If the method used is the "High-Amplitude Sucking" (HAS) technique, then first of all the baby's "base rate" or boredom-level of sucking is estimated by measuring how often it sucks strongly when nothing happens as a consequence. It is important to know the base rate, because the baby enjoys sucking for its own sake, and will occasionally give a good strong suck to relieve the boredom of nothing at all happening in the laboratory. Then the experiment proper begins. Each time the baby sucks sufficiently strongly, it will hear the stimulus once. When it is interested, it will suck quite often; gradually it loses interest because the stimulus is always the same, and eventually it will only suck at about its base rate, suggesting that this sound has become boring. When the rate of sucking is close to the base rate or boredom level, the experimenter changes the stimulus that follows the next suck. If the baby notices that the stimulus is different, it normally becomes interested and will suck more frequently for a while until the new stimulus also becomes too familiar to make hard sucking worthwhile. (A strong suck is required to make sure that the baby really intended it.) The change in rate of sucking between the base rate and the introduction of the new stimulus is the measure of whether the baby can discriminate between the two stimuli. Figure 13-1 shows typical patterns of sucking for two experimental conditions, one in which the baby hears no difference in the stimuli, and one in which it notices a change.

When heart rate is measured, the method is much the same except that the baby does not itself

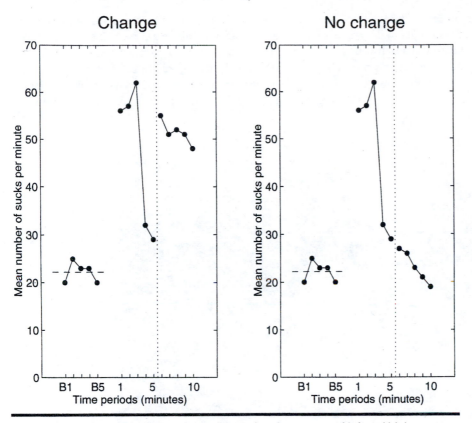

FIGURE 13-1. Simplified fictional data illustrating the pattern of infants' high-amplitude sucking responses. At the left of each panel are the mean number of sucks per minute for 5 minutes, B1 through B5, during which no stimuli are heard. The horizontal dashed line through these 5 points shows the average number of sucks during this period, called the base rate. The other data points in each panel represent mean sucking responses per minute when each high-amplitude suck produces a sound. In the "Change" panel (left), the stimulus changed at the point shown by the vertical dotted line. In the "No change" panel (right), the babies always heard the same stimulus, and the vertical dotted line shows where the stimulus would have changed. The experimenter measures the difference in mean sucking rate between the two points that straddle the vertical dotted line. The large increase in sucking rate in the Change condition indicates that the two stimuli sounded different, whereas the small decrease in sucking rate in the No change condition indicates that the babies (correctly) heard no differences and continued to lose interest in the sound.

control the rate of stimulus presentation. The heart rate is slower when the stimulus is novel and then increases to its normal level as the stimulus becomes familiar. When the experimenter introduces a new stimulus, the heart rate will decel-erate (fall) again if the baby can discriminate the difference between the two.

Older babies need a different technique because they do not naturally stay so still, nor so quiet, as newborns. The general method for these older babies relies on a "conditioned head-turn" to a new stimulus and is similar to the way audiologists test babies' hearing, though usually more stringently controlled. The general procedure is that the baby, sitting on its caretaker's lap, is entertained by a silent experimenter showing it toys, while a stimulus such as a CV syllable plays at regular intervals (e.g., every 2 s) from a loudspeaker set off in a poorly lit area to one side, as illustrated in Figure 13-2. The silent experimenter's job is to keep the baby looking straight ahead. A second experimenter, who can see what

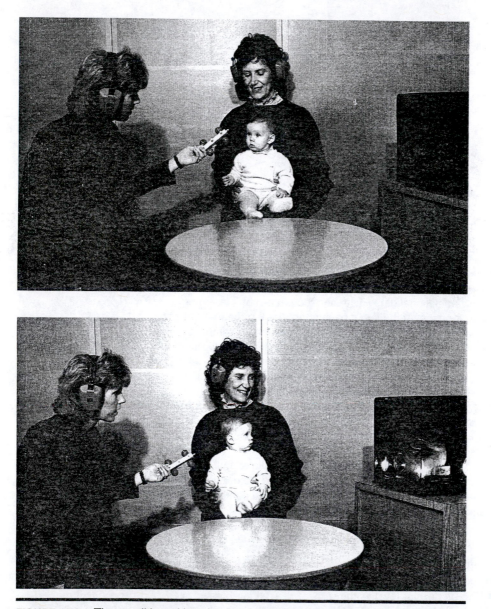

FIGURE 13-2.   The conditioned head turn technique used to study the auditory categorization abilities of babies aged between about 6 and 10 months.

is happening but is unseen by anyone else, judges when the baby is consistently looking straight ahead, and changes the auditory stimulus at this time. If the baby turns its head to look towards the source of the new sound, it is rewarded by seeing and hearing something interesting for a few seconds. For example, a normally dark (and thus almost invisible) transparent box on the loudspeaker will light up to show a toy monkey inside it banging a drum. Six- to twelve-month-olds love this, and very soon learn to look towards the box only when the stimulus changes: Looking at the box when the stimulus has not changed is not rewarded, so at these times, watching the silent experimenter's toys is more interesting. The "change" stimulus is only played two or three times before the original "background" stimulus is reintroduced and the baby is required to look straight ahead again before the next trial can begin. Half the trials involve a new stimulus, when the baby is "right" if it turns its head, and the other half involve no change of stimulus, so on these trials the baby is "right" if it does not turn its head. To be considered to have successfully discriminated between two stimuli, stringent criteria are used, typically 9 out of 10 consecutive trials correct. This technique is made experimentally sound by a number of other precautions (see for example, Kuhl, 1980). For example, the silent experimenter and the baby's caretaker listen to music through headphones so they cannot influence the baby's responses because they cannot hear what it is hearing.

Prior to the development of these techniques, speech researchers tended to assume that babies had to learn to discriminate the sounds of speech and that this learning took place at least up to when the baby began to speak, and probably, for some contrasts, for some time thereafter. This assumption was very different from what people who look after babies tend to observe—for example, that babies prefer (and can thus recognize) familiar voices, that they attend closely to speaking faces, and that most can recognize important words, like their own names, from 6 or 7 months of age. These laypeople's observations do not suggest that a baby's world is quite the "blooming, buzzing confusion" it was thought to be by laboratory scientists. Nevertheless, because experimental data were unavailable, scientists seemed to feel they should assume that babies bring only the most general and basic discriminatory abilities into the world.

CATEGORICAL PERCEPTION BY BABIES

Once techniques for examining babies' speech perception were available, it was soon found that babies can discriminate many sounds that function as phonological contrasts in a wide range of languages, and that their response patterns are much the same as those of adults who speak the languages concerned. In particular, babies seem to hear encoded sounds like stop consonants categorically, as do adults. (Encoded sounds are described in Chapter Fourteen, The Motor Theory.)

The first demonstration of babies' categorical perception of stops took the speech world by surprise. Eimas, Siqueland, Jusczyk and Vigorito (1971) used the HAS technique described above to test whether 4-week-old babies could discriminate a difference in voicing between stop consonants. They synthesized a set of syllables that varied only in VOT, from –20 ms at one extreme to +80 ms at the other, in 10 ms steps. These syllables did not sound very natural to adults, but most native speakers of English had no trouble hearing the extremes as /bɑ/ and /pɑ/ respectively. Adults' responses to the stimuli in identification and discrimination tests showed that they perceived them categorically: There was an abrupt crossover from /b/ to /p/ responses at about +25 ms VOT, and a peak in discrimination between pairs of stimuli at about this point as well.

What Eimas and co-workers (1971) showed was that, when 4-week-olds were tested on pairs of these stimuli, they behaved in much the same way as adults. They too could discriminate between pairs of synthetic syllables differing by only 20 ms if one came from the adults' /b/ category and the other from the adults' /p/ category, and they did not discriminate between such pairs of syllables when both came from within either the /b/ category or the /p/ category. In other words, the discrimination function for these newborn babies had a peak at about +30 ms VOT, just like the adults' function. As with all such discrimination experiments, there was always the same absolute difference in VOT between the two stimuli within a pair, so the peak in performance was presumably due to heightened discrimination at the category boundary and/or to reduced discrimination within a category. This pattern of response was interpreted as indicating that young babies hear phonetically relevant acoustic information in terms of the phonemic categories of the adult language.

Other work in a number of different laboratories soon followed showing that young babies' discriminatory abilities are very much in line with adults' on all the distinctions tested, including many syllable-initial and some syllable-final consonantal contrasts, syllables differing in pitch contour, and polysyllabic stimuli differing in the location of syllable stress. Phonetic contrasts that are difficult for babies are also difficult for adult native speakers of the same language, presumably because the acoustic differences are small. An example is English /f/ versus /θ/. For an early review, see Eilers (1980); for others, see Jusczyk (1994, 1986a, 1986b) and Kuhl (1986, 1987).

Notice that these types of data do not tell us that the infant is behaving linguistically: Babies cannot be asked to give linguistic labels to their responses. More importantly, babies do not know the phonology of any language. Phonological awareness for segments is thought to begin to develop around the end of the first year of life, when the child begins to understand and use more than just a few words, but it does not begin suddenly, and it is not adult-like until some years later (e.g., Ferguson 1986; for a discussion relevant to speech perception, see Werker & Pegg 1992). If the baby has no phonological contrasts, then it cannot be said to be discriminating phonemes, which are essentially contrastive. Nor do

these types of experiments with simple stimuli presented in isolation and in good listening conditions tell us that babies can discriminate these sounds in natural running speech. But they do suggest that the baby is equipped from birth or shortly thereafter to make the types of discriminations that will form the basis for phonetic categories later on. Thus, they do not support the claim that one must be able to make a particular sound before one can hear it as different from other sounds, because young babies can very definitely not produce the sound distinctions that we now know they can discriminate. A large number of perceptual abilities relevant to understanding speech precede the ability to produce those speech sounds.

SPEECH SOUND CLASSIFICATION BY BABIES: PROTOTYPES AND THE "PERCEPTUAL MAGNET EFFECT"

There are two ways in which categories of objects may be distinguished: by the clarity of the boundaries between categories and by the degree of similarity between most of the members within a category. Ideally, most members of a given category will be quite similar to each other, and the category boundaries will be quite clear-cut. Most natural classes do not have clear-cut boundaries however. Most birds fly and all have feathers; but penguins are birds, although they do not fly and their feathers are small and scale-like, different from those of other birds. Among a group of humans encompassing the entire age range, there are only fuzzy boundaries between babies and young children, children and adolescents, adolescents and young adults, and so on. The difference between babies and adults is indeed clear, but only when intermediate age groups have been excluded. The same is even true for anatomical signs of gender: There is a range of hermaphrodite states that blurs the boundaries between male and female (although in the West it is normal nowadays to "correct" such conditions so each person grows up clearly male or female physically.)

Even though the boundaries of most natural classes are normally unclear, the majority of members of such classes do not fall near the boundary, and so some members of the category are more typical of that category than others. A good example of the category bird is a robin, or perhaps an eagle, and not an ostrich or a penguin. Robins, eagles, and even ducks have more in common with each other than with ostriches or penguins. Bony fish-like herrings and mackerels are good examples of fish, whereas eels and flat-fish are not. Most people are born either clearly male or clearly female, and so represent good examples of one gender or the other. In more technical words, for many natural classes, the statistical probability of falling near the ideal of the category is greater than the probability of falling near the boundaries. People seem to use this statistical information to form conceptual categories that are represented by "typical" instances: a robin rather than an ostrich or penguin for the category bird; a herring rather than a flounder (flat-fish) for the category fish, and so on. People from the same culture have very similar views on what constitute good examples of many natural categories. For obvious reasons, typical examples of many categories are found in children's picture books.

In cognitive science, a good example of a category is often called a prototype. This term is taken from Rosch's (1975) theory of how we categorize sensory information. A prototype is the most representative instance of a category. It shares the most similarities with other members of its own category and has the most differences with members of other categories. According to Rosch's theory, a prototype is an abstraction; it develops from the statistical distribution of instances of the category, and it need not actually exist. It is also possible to define a prototype simply as a good instance of a category. This second definition makes fewer assumptions about the way the prototype is represented in the brain. Regardless of how they are mentally represented, experiments have shown that when a stimulus is a good, or

prototypical, example of a category, it has special status in perception. It is easier to classify, easier to remember, and preferred over other members of that category (e.g., Rosch, 1977).

The studies of categorical perception for speech discussed so far in this book focus on the boundaries between categories, and how humans (and sometimes nonhuman animals, see below) seem to have enhanced discrimination between items that straddle those boundaries but that are physically quite similar to each other. In other words, the focus of interest in categorical perception studies is on listeners' responses to ambiguous-sounding, poor examples of phonological categories.

Another way of looking at the organization of phonetic or phonological categories is to see how people respond to good examples of a category, using the concept of prototypes. In a series of experiments, Patricia Kuhl and her colleagues showed that adults can identify a "phonetic prototype" for the American English /i/, that is, they can identify a best instance of the phonemic category /i/ heard in isolation. Crucially, Kuhl also demonstrated that neither adults nor 6-month-old babies discriminate well between vowels that are auditorily close to the adults' prototype /i/. This was demonstrated by giving adults and 6-month-olds similar tasks in which they had to discriminate between pairs of synthetic vowels, divided into two sets. In one set, the comparison vowel was always the prototype, or best, /i/, and in the other set the comparison vowel was always a "nonprototype," or poor exemplar, of /i/. All vowels sounded like /i/, and the auditory-acoustic distance between pairs of vowels was the same in both sets. Accuracy of discrimination was significantly better for comparisons in the set with a nonprototype than in the set with a prototype, for both adults and 6-month-olds (Kuhl & Iverson, 1995).

Kuhl calls this decreased discriminability between exemplars close to the prototype the "perceptual magnet effect." This is a metaphorical phrase: The prototype is said to "pull" acoustically similar sounds towards itself much as a magnet attracts iron. She suggests that the brain works in such a way that the most typical members of a phonetic category become less discriminable from one another. Similarities between good category exemplars are emphasized (or conversely, differences between them are perceptually decreased). The process originates in perception—the brain imposes this structural organization on the phonetic category. In effect, when a phonetic category is formed, perceptual (or psychological) space is distorted so that the perceptual space around the best instances of the category functions as if it is smaller than it really is physically or psychoacoustically. There is no magnet effect near the category boundaries, where the poor exemplars of the category are found. Figure 13-3 illustrates the

principle. By the age of 6 months, babies have learned an adult-like /i/ category, manifested by both a prototype "similarity effect" and an across-boundary "dissimilarity effect."

The perceptual magnet effect offers an interestingly different point of view from that of categorical perception studies. Categorical perception demonstrations suggest that boundaries *between categories* are emphasized. Peaks in discrimination functions arise between stimuli that straddle the boundary between two phonetic categories: The two stimuli will be given different labels in identification tests. But in demonstrations of the perceptual magnet effect, listeners give the same phonetic label to all the stimuli. What we are seeing is not the accentuation of differences across a category boundary, but the reduction of differ-

Psychoacoustic space with no phonetic category: no magnet effect

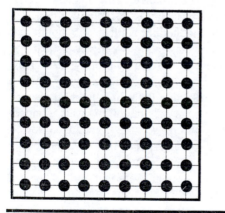

Psychoacoustic space with a phonetic category: perceptual magnet effect

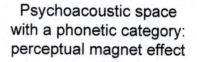

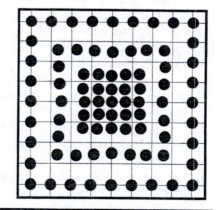

FIGURE 13-3. Schematic illustration of two types of perceptual space, showing the absence (left panel) and presence (right panel) of the perceptual magnet effect. The grids represent equal psychoacoustic steps along each dimension. Each circle represents a stimulus. All adjacent pairs of stimuli in the left panel are equally distinct psychoacoustically. Stimuli in the right panel are rearranged in psychoacoustic space, with those nearer to the black stimulus being heard as more similar to one another than those further away from it. The left panel represents the perceptual space of a person who does not have a phonetic category in this auditory region, whereas the right panel represents the perceptual space of someone who does. In the right panel, the black stimulus represents the prototype (ideal) for this phonetic category; the outermost ring of stimuli could be at or near the category boundary.

ences in the center of the category. There may also be an exaggeration of differences near the category boundary, and this might contribute to enhanced discriminability across it.

Details of the experiments that led to these conclusions have not been given here, mainly because early experiments by Kuhl have been criticized on a number of methodological grounds, for example, by Sussman and Lauckner-Morano (1995). However, later work (Iverson & Kuhl 1995; Sussman & Lauckner-Morano, 1995) indicates that while details of Kuhl's early work may be in error, her general observations about the perceptual magnet effect are not. Nevertheless, generalizations from these data must be cautious. The effect has been well documented only for the vowel /i/, and there are some problems of interpretation that remain to be resolved. Some of these problems are discussed further below, in the context of Kuhl's Natural Language Magnet (NLM) model of speech perception.

Our summary of this introduction to the perceptual magnet effect is that, in addition to being able to discriminate *between* phonetic categories, 6-month-old babies show evidence of structure *within* phonetic categories, at least for vowels, in that the perceptual space is compressed near the phonetic prototype. In the following sections, we shall see that animals are said not to have magnet effects and that the magnet effect seems to require linguistic experience to develop. These observations have interesting theoretical consequences.

SPEECH SOUND CLASSIFICATION BY BABIES: PERCEPTUAL CONSTANCY

One way to show that these discriminatory abilities of babies are relevant to the perception of natural speech is to ask whether babies can make distinctions between segmental-phonetic categories when the stimuli vary in other natural ways, such as when the same syllables are spoken by different people. The test is how the listener classes two signals that belong to the same phonetic class yet are very definitely different from one another, as when two instances of the vowel

/i/ are spoken by two different people. Adults have no trouble with this. If the babies respond to a phonemic contrast even when the stimuli also vary in a number of other acoustic properties, at least some of which *could* be the contrast the experimenter is interested in, then we can be reasonably sure that the babies categorize speech sounds in phonetically appropriate classes. Such categorization of acoustically very different stimuli into classes based on phonemic contrasts of the adult language has been called "perceptual constancy" for speech-sound categories.

Patricia Kuhl pioneered work on babies' perceptual constancy for phonemic contrasts. In one experiment (Kuhl, 1979), she trained 6-month-old babies to turn their heads to see a visual display whenever the repeating background sound changed from [ɑ] to [i] (or vice versa, for a second group of babies). The babies were first trained on a pair of synthetic vowels from a single "male talker." After they had mastered this task, more [ɑ] and [i] tokens in a female and a child voice, both synthetic, were added to both the background and the change stimuli. In addition, the pitch contour varied: It might be either rising or falling. The babies continued to turn for the vowel class ([ɑ] or [i] depending on which they had been trained for), despite the fact that they were now hearing a large number of vowels spoken by different "people." In other words, the babies tracked the vowel category, and not the particular spectral shape of the first vowel that they had learned to turn their heads for.

Other experiments showed similar category-specific responses for complicated contrasts in which there were irrelevant changes in pitch contour as well as segmental category and gender or age of talkers. Kuhl (1980) describes an experiment in which babies were trained to respond only to one or other of the consonants [ʃ] and [s] in the syllables [ʃi ʃɑ ʃu si sɑ su], each spoken by four different people. Kuhl (1983) trained babies to discriminate between [ɑ] and [ɔ], even though the inclusion of different talkers resulted in considerable spectral similarity between tokens of vowels from the two different categories.

Perceptual constancy (for speech) is almost certainly a speech-relevant process, and not just the result of a general auditory response learned to a single, simple acoustic property in the particular stimuli used in an experiment. Indeed, there is sometimes a tendency to assume that evidence for perceptual constancy for speech sound categories by babies demonstrates that babies have adult-like speech perception for these categories. This, however, is no more than an assumption: If the response is the same, then it is very possible that the decisions leading to the response are made in the same way. But it is also possible that those decisions are made in different ways, just as an adult and an 8-month-old baby may both cross a room, but the adult would probably walk while the baby would probably crawl. Whether the important thing is *that* the room was crossed or *how* it was crossed depends on your point of view. It is worth bearing this point in mind in evaluating data on babies' perceptual abilities.

SPEECH SOUND DISCRIMINATION BY ANIMALS

One question that arises naturally from the above data on babies' categorical perception, perceptual magnet effects, and perceptual constancy is how species-specific the babies' abilities are. Experiments using various speech-like stimulus series with several quite disparate species of animals have elicited response patterns that look as if these animals, too, are perceiving categorically. The first demonstration was by Kuhl and Miller (1975), who tested chinchillas' discrimination between /Ca/ syllables containing alveolar stops that varied along a VOT continuum (0 ms, heard as English /d/, at one end, and +80 ms, heard as English /t/, at the other). In the training phase of the experiment, the chinchillas were divided into two groups. One group learned to respond to the 0 ms stimulus by crossing a barrier into the other side of the cage, and not to cross the barrier in response to the +80 ms stimulus. When they responded correctly to the /da/ stimulus, they avoided a mild electric shock and a buzzer sound-

ing. When they responded correctly to the /ta/ stimulus, they were rewarded with a drink of water. The other group was trained in the same way, except that the /ta/ stimulus was the signal to cross the barrier to avoid the shock and buzzer, and the /da/ stimulus was the signal not to cross, rewarded with water for correct responses.

When the animals' responses to the two endpoint stimuli were nearly perfect, they were then presented with stimuli from the entire stimulus series, in random order. Responses to the two endpoint stimuli were still rewarded or punished as before, but responses to the intermediate stimuli were always rewarded: The animal was always right for these stimuli, no matter what its response.

This design elicited behavior from the chinchillas that comes close to the identification test of standard categorical perception experiments with adult humans. There are two different responses, and the task is to choose which response to make, for each stimulus of the acoustic series. In this way, it was possible to estimate where the perceptual boundary between /da/ and /ta/ lay for these chinchillas.

The chinchillas' response function was remarkably close to that of a group of adult native speakers of English to the same stimuli: The boundary values (50% crossover points) were 33 ms for the chinchillas, and 35 ms for the humans. Moreover, Kuhl and Miller (1978) went on to show that chinchillas' VOT boundaries change with place of articulation to mirror patterns found in speech production, just as do adult humans'. The boundary for a bilabial series, /ba-pa/, was at about 25 ms for animals and adult humans, and that for a velar series, /ga-ka/, was at 42 ms for both groups.

Other experiments compared animals' and adult humans' discrimination of pairs of stimuli in various synthetic stimulus series. For example, Kuhl and Padden (1983) showed that macaque monkeys and adult humans had the same pattern of peaks and troughs in discrimination functions for a 15-stimulus series of 2-formant syllables ranging from /ba/ through /da/ to /ga/, in which only the starting frequency of F2 varied. (Kuhl, 1987, discusses these and other experiments.)

Dooling, Okanoya, and Brown (1989) showed results very like that of Kuhl and Miller (1978) for budgerigars' response to stimuli varying in VOT. The birds not only showed evidence for categorical sensitivity to VOT, but, like Kuhl and Miller's chinchillas and humans, their category boundaries reflected the patterns of natural speech: shortest for bilabials and longest for velars.

How far do these parallels between human and nonhuman responses to speech-like stimuli extend? This is an important question because it bears on how far theories of speech perception should invoke general auditory processes, independent of processes special to speech. The most telling comparisons are probably those for which humans, and especially babies, show evidence of complex equivalences in their assignment of stimuli to phonetic categories: evidence of phonetic trading relations, perceptual magnet effects, perceptual constancy, and cross-modal equivalences. It is in these areas that we might expect differences between animal and human abilities that could indicate whether, and if so in what ways, speech perception demands special processing. In Kuhl's words, "What can human infants do that animals can't?" (Kuhl, 1987:376).

Trading relations were discussed in Chapter Twelve. When two or more acoustic properties cue a perceptual category, they often enter into trading relations with one another: Different combinations of cue values can result in perceptually equivalent instances of a phonetic category, despite differences in acoustic pattern. Trading relations in humans have been demonstrated mainly for complex consonants like stops, and although theoreticians suggest very different mechanisms as governing them, it is agreed that at least some of them provide evidence for integration of acoustic properties at some higher level of perception than when the signal is first processed (Kingston & Diehl, 1994; Parker, Diehl, & Kluender 1986; Repp, 1982, 1984). If basic auditory processes are the primary determinants of phonological categories, then we would expect animals to show at least some trading relations. And if animals did show trading relations for speech contrasts, it

could have profound implications for theories of speech perception. Few experiments have yet addressed this issue. However, work by Kluender and colleagues suggests that Japanese quail show trading relations for the voicing distinction in stops, according to patterns that are very similar to those of human adults. Both humans and birds hear more voiceless stops in a series of stimuli varying in VOT when the starting frequency for F1 is higher (Kluender, 1991, Kluender & Lotto, 1994).

As we noted above, the perceptual magnet effect describes an apparent compressing of perceptual space in the vicinity of the best exemplars of phonemic categories. It is a language-specific phenomenon that is in place for at least some vowels by 6 months of age. If perceptual magnet effects reflect the beginnings of linguistic structure, then nonhuman animals may fail to show magnet effects.

Unlike normal humans, animals neither learn to speak nor to understand anything but the simplest speech at best. The implication of these experiments with nonhuman species, then, is that at least some of the contrasts fundamental to speech perception are based on general auditory processes. In the case of VOT, for example, it might be the detection of two events rather than one, as discussed in Chapter Twelve. This would suggest that the English VOT boundary capitalizes on this basic auditory process. (See Ehret, 1987, for a thoughtful development and critique of this area.) However, we have yet to explain why so many languages do not take advantage of the "English" boundary if it is so natural: Many languages (e.g., French, Spanish, Thai) divide the VOT continuum at different places (Ladefoged & Maddieson, 1996; Lisker & Abramson, 1964). Nor does this explanation account for why chinchillas and other nonhuman species might be sensitive to differences in VOT due to place of articulation. Since suggestions that have been advanced are not theory-neutral, we will discuss them under the relevant theories below. Our theory-neutral interim summary must be that we are still far from knowing how much nonhuman species' perceptual processes mirror those of humans; there is clearly much left to be done in this area.

THE EFFECT OF EXPERIENCE ON SPEECH SOUND DISCRIMINATION

Natural Linguistic Experience: Perception of Non-Native Contrasts by Babies and Adults

Another question that arises naturally from the studies of categorical perception of speech by babies is how language-specific their abilities are. The answers to this and related questions are not just important to our understanding of how language develops, but are central to evaluating theories of speech perception. In the past, research on adult speech and language tended to ignore developmental studies. But speech-language development is now receiving increasingly widespread attention because it has been recognized that the way speech-language develops has implications for the way it is structured in the adult brain. This new interest in linking ideas on babies', children's, and adults' speech processing rests partly on the fact that theory and experimental techniques have become more sophisticated in all three areas. The questions that are now being asked have demystified some of the puzzles thrown up by the earliest studies and made the links more obvious, partly because newer studies are looking at wider and more subtle aspects of speech, such as the perceptual information in allophonic variation, links between prosodic and phonemic perception, phonotactic knowledge, and the relationship with the lexicon (e.g., Jusczyk, 1994; Jusczyk, Hohne, & Mandel, 1995).

Current knowledge on the development of language specificity in babies' perceptual abilities has been succinctly summarized in four points by Werker and Pegg as follows. "Young infants can discriminate nearly every phonetic contrast on which they have been tested—including those that do not occur in their language-learning environment. . . . There is a profound change across age in the ease with which people discriminate some non-native contrasts . . . although this devel-

opmental change does not apply to every non-native contrast. . . . This developmental change is evident within the first year of life. . . . The change involves a reorganization in perceptual biases rather than a loss of initial auditory capabilities" (Werker & Pegg, 1992: 285–286). Each of these points is considered below.

It was first demonstrated about twenty years ago that young babies can discriminate between phonetic contrasts that are not phonemic in their own language environment (e.g., Lasky, Syrdal-Lasky, & Klein, 1975; Trehub, 1976). Since then, contrasts from a wide range of languages have been examined. Babies can distinguish, apparently categorically, nearly every phonetic contrast that they have been tested on, whether or not that contrast is phonemic in the language(s) they hear around them (see Werker and Pegg, 1992). There are some exceptions, but they are few (e.g., Eilers, Gavin, & Oller 1982).

In summary, adults are adept at discriminating between phonemic categories of their native language, but their discrimination of phonemic contrasts from foreign languages is more variable, being influenced both by the listeners' native phonological classes and by the acoustic distinctiveness of the sounds being contrasted. When the two sounds representing the foreign contrast can be assimilated into two different phonemic classes in the listeners' native language, then they will be easily discriminable. When the two sounds of the foreign language fall into a single phonemic class in the listeners' native language, then they are less likely to be readily distinguishable from each other. If the two sounds are acoustically distinctive and one or neither fits into any phonemic class of the listener's native language, then they too are likely to be readily discriminable. Unlike adults, young babies can typically distinguish all sounds that contrast phonemically in any language, whether they have heard that language before or not. Contrasts that babies have more difficulty with, like English /f/ versus /θ/, tend also to be relatively poorly discriminated by adult native speakers of the language in which they are contrastive. Usually, these contrasts are acoustically more similar to each other than easily discriminated contrasts.

Natural Linguistic Experience: Age-Related Changes in Babies' Perception of Native Contrasts

The burning question was, of course, at what age do people stop discriminating between sounds that are not phonemic in their own language? Werker and Tees (1984) showed that it is at about 10 to 12 months of age. This is interesting because 10 months is about the earliest age that babies begin to use their first words meaningfully. Furthermore, by about 9 months of age, babies have learned a lot about the phonetic structure of their native language and show many signs of preferring to listen to their own language rather than to foreign languages. Indeed, Jusczyk, Hohne, and Mandel (1995) discuss evidence, most of it recent, that babies discover many of the most fundamental properties of their to-be-native language in the first nine months of life. This knowledge should make it easier to learn the phonology, morphology, and grammar of the language and to identify words in connected speech.

The most global properties of the baby's to-be-native language are prosodic, and some of these may even be learned at or before birth. Rhythm and pitch patterns can be heard in utero, since they are what is left in the signal when the mother's voice reaches the uterus, low-pass filtered through her body. Both rhythm and pitch are patterned quite differently in different languages (though there are also similarities between some languages, of course). In one study cited by Jusczyk and co-workers (1995), 4-day-old babies could distinguish between utterances spoken in their mother's native language and those spoken in a foreign language; however, they showed no sign of distinguishing between utterances spoken in two different foreign languages. Their response patterns were the same regardless of whether the speech was heard unfiltered, or low-pass filtered so that only the prosodic information remained. Newborns, then, seem already to recognize and

give preferential attention to the language of their mothers. Other evidence suggests that babies are sensitive to the language-specific prosodic properties that cue clause boundaries by about 6 months of age and to those marking phrasal boundaries by 9 months. It seems reasonable to assume that these and other sensitivities discussed by Jusczyk and co-workers (1995) provide the first tools for learning (or "bootstrapping") grammar from speech.

By 9 months, the baby also knows a significant amount about other phonological regularities in its native language. Jusczyk and co-workers (1995) discuss evidence that by 9 months American babies learning English recognize and prefer sound sequences that obey English rather than foreign phonotactic rules, and that they prefer more common sound sequences of English over less common ones. (Phonotactic rules specify the permissible combinations of sounds within a single syllable in a given language. For example, English can have at most three consonants syllable-initially; if there are three, the first must be /s/, the second a voiceless stop, and the third an approximant; some approximants cannot co-occur with some stops.) Nine-month-olds also seem to be aware that English words are most commonly stressed on the first syllable. Such knowledge about word and syllable structure is presumably used, among other things, to segment words from the stream of connected speech. Word segmentation is necessary for the child to begin saying words, as well as to understand them.

Finally, 6-month-old American babies show a perceptual magnet effect for American English /i/, but not for Swedish /y/, whereas 6-month-old Swedish babies (tested in Sweden with the same equipment and conditions as the American babies) show the opposite pattern: They had a perceptual magnet effect for Swedish /y/, and not for American English /i/ (Kuhl, Williams, Lacerda, Stevens, & Lindblom, 1992; see also Kuhl & Iverson, 1995). By 6 months, then, although the baby can still discriminate between contrasting phonetic categories that it has never heard before, it has also formed distinct perceptual categories for (presumably) most vowels of the language it hears daily, and it knows what sounds represent good instances of one of those categories. It has no such structured categories for foreign sounds.

In summary, we have seen that although babies know a great deal about the phonetic properties of their native language at 9 or 10 months of age, that knowledge is not all learned suddenly when the baby is 9 months old but is learned over the entire period from (or even before) birth. The failure to discriminate between foreign phonemic contrasts at 10 to 12 months may not represent a sudden change in the baby's behavior, then. It may be better viewed as just one more manifestation of the process of sorting out the salient properties of the native language, a process that has been going on steadily since birth. On the other hand, much of the linguistic-phonetic knowledge that the baby acquires in its first nine months is fairly general and may be due to general abilities to discriminate patterns rather than to the development of linguistic structure. If one takes this second view, then what the baby learns in its first nine months is probably best seen as providing a solid platform from which to begin linguistic development. Each of these two views has merits, and to some extent the one you prefer will depend upon the theory of speech perception that you espouse. Even if the first view is preferred, however, the change in babies' ability to discriminate between foreign phonemic contrasts must be seen as representing one of the most significant steps towards becoming a native speaker-hearer of a particular language.

DEVELOPMENTAL LOSS OR SELECTIVE ATTENTION? THE EFFECT OF RETRAINING

Why should there be such a profound reorganization of speech perception at 10 months of age? And what form does it take? A number of views have been expressed. It seems clear that there is no significant loss in auditory acuity or in discriminative ability itself, because adults can be retrained to hear the foreign distinctions. We know this from phonetics classes, in which students throughout the world learn to accurately hear and produce distinctions from many other

languages. There is also experimental confirmation that adults can be successfully retrained in a relatively short period, given an appropriate method (for a review, see Pisoni, Lively, & Logan, 1994). Pisoni and co-workers suggest that both loss and subsequent regaining of discriminatory powers is due to changes in selective attention, based on experience of what is important. Criterial attributes of the signal become perceptually more distinctive, and noncriterial attributes become less distinctive. This is the standard view of category formation in all aspects of cognition. In effect, the experienced listener learns to exaggerate the important differences, and to deemphasize unimportant ones. So, for example, a native-speaker of English who is learning Hindi must learn to pay attention to whether the voicing at the beginning of the vowel following a voiced stop is breathy or not; this makes for a phonemic contrast between /d/ and /dh/ in Hindi, but it is irrelevant in English. Conversely, the native-speaker of Hindi who is learning English must learn to ignore this difference. A native speaker of French must learn to group nasalized and non-nasalized vowels in the same phonemic class when listening to English. Notice that the perceptual magnet effect described above could underlie all or part of this restructuring of the perceptual space.

Pisoni and co-workers (1994) describe experiments that show it is easier to form robust categories if one has heard a wide range of instances of each category, presumably because the variability thus experienced helps to define each category. Other experiments show that training involving labeling is more effective than that involving just discrimination. This is, of course, exactly what happens in phonetics classes. The IPA alphabet provides the category labels. And the most effective teaching is not from tapes, or even videos with their added visual information, but from a skilled teacher interacting with the students. A good teacher provides at least three things that audio and video tapes don't: a comparatively unlimited number of instances of the category, each slightly different from the others yet still a member of the class being demonstrated;

contrasts with other categories that students have particular difficulty with; and immediate feedback about whether the student is right or not. Pisoni and co-workers (1994) cite data showing that each of these factors improves performance on foreign phonetic contrasts.

Pisoni and co-workers (1994) also note that distinctions are easier to learn in some phonetic contexts than in others, another thing taken advantage of by phonetics teachers. A good teacher will introduce gradation in clarity of any given contrast by intelligent use of phonetic context and by the degree of exaggeration of salient features. The reason that phonetic context is a factor to consider in developing effective training techniques has been discussed in the previous section: Success in discriminating phonetic distinctions depends partly on the type of contrast and its role in the native language of the listener. Both the acoustic distinctiveness of the sounds to be discriminated and the extent to which they can be assimilated into phonemic categories of the listener affect how successfully they will be distinguished one from another (see Best, 1994; Werker & Pegg, 1992).

The point to be taken, then, is that we do not lose our ability to distinguish phonetic categories at around the first year of life. Instead, by that age, we have learned enough about our native language to allow us, in effect, to attend mainly to its more salient aspects, and to ignore, or to respond to in a different way, variation that does not distinguish words.

SUMMARY

Babies younger than 10 to 12 months can discriminate between most phonemic contrasts on which they have been tested, regardless of whether the contrast is phonemic in the language-environment the baby is living in, or only in languages the baby has never heard. The response functions of young babies to these contrasts suggest that they hear the sounds in much the same way as adult native speakers of the languages in which the contrast is phonemic. In particular, they seem to perceive consonants categorically where

native-speaker adults do. In at least their own language, they are also sensitive to trading relations and demonstrate perceptual equivalence (or constancy), for example, for phonemic categories in the context of variations in voice quality and intonation. Adults, on the other hand, can discriminate only some phonemic contrasts from languages other than their own.

The change between young babies' and adults' abilities to discriminate foreign contrasts occurs at about 10 to 12 months of age, and appears to be a reorganization rather than a loss of ability, because adults can be retrained to discriminate between distinctions that are phonemic in some languages, though not their own.

During the time that babies can still discriminate foreign phonemic contrasts with ease—in the first nine months of life—they are nevertheless learning a great deal about their own language. By 9 months, English-learning babies prefer to listen to speech in their own language rather than in an unknown one, can recognize whether pauses are prosodically appropriate in both clauses and phrases of English, and prefer common rather than rarer phoneme sequences in English. By 6 months, babies can recognize good instances of (at least some) vowel categories in their own to-be-native language, but not in foreign languages. The pattern of their discriminative responses between vowels is consistent with the interpretation that, by 6 months, native-language vowels are represented as prototypes that exert perceptual magnet effects. This is not the case for foreign-language vowels.

These data can be interpreted in different ways. Major differences of interpretation include to what extent speech perception is based on special processes rather than general auditory ones (for which animals' perception of speech is of interest), and what linguistic units are normally used in speech perception. On these issues, the verdict is not yet in. What does seem clear though, is that during the first year of life, the baby uses the speech it hears to gradually enrich its linguistically relevant knowledge. By the end of the first year, it seems to have done enough to start to become a proficient user of language: that is, a true native speaker-hearer.

CHAPTER FOURTEEN

LOOKING FOR INVARIANT CORRELATES OF LINGUISTIC UNITS: TWO CLASSICAL THEORIES OF SPEECH PERCEPTION

SARAH HAWKINS

DEFINING THE TASK OF SPEECH PERCEPTION

Before we consider theories of speech perception, we should define what such a theory is expected to explain. This entails defining what we mean by the process, or task, of speech perception. As we've seen in our earlier chapters, most research on perception has studied the listener's identification of phonemes in simple syllables, often isolated from further context. This narrow approach sacrifices realism for the sake of experimental control: The number of variables to be manipulated is reduced, but it is usually difficult to generalize the findings to speech perception in real-life situations. Most utterances in real life consist of several syllables, so that listeners normally have to deal with coarticulatory and connected-speech processes that never arise when syllables are spoken in isolation. Furthermore, spoken messages normally make sense, and listeners' interpretations of what they hear are affected by what they expect to hear. A narrow definition of speech perception that fails to take these real-life considerations into account constrains the questions that tend to be asked and so the types of theories that are likely to be developed.

A more realistic view of speech perception is that the listener's task is to understand the meaning of what someone else has said. That is, the task is to extract meaning from the speaker's acoustic signal. Although this definition is realistic about the nature of the task, it is too broad for a single discipline to cope with at present, for it demands that we should examine not only the acoustic cues to speech perception, but also how they interact with higher-order linguistic functions such as grammar and the choice of words, as well as with more intangible influences like speaker's and listener's expectations, which are affected by their shared culture. This comprehensive definition of speech perception, then, acknowledges that speech cannot be separated from language. There are currently no such comprehensive theories, nor are any feasible in the near future.

The approach taken here lies between these two extremes. We will define the task of speech perception as identifying words, meaningful or not. Psychologists call this task *lexical access* (see, e.g., Frauenfelder & Tyler, 1987). Our aim in broadening the scope of traditional acoustic-phonetic theories of speech perception to include lexical access is to force consideration of the phonetic structure of whole utterances. By doing this, we undertake to study what people do to understand natural speech in normal, everyday conversations, as well as in highly controlled laboratory conditions using synthetic speech. This might seem an obvious thing to want to do, but we will see that, while some of the original theories of speech perception are still the best researched and most influential, none of them satisfactorily addresses how we identify words in conversational speech.

OVERVIEW OF ACOUSTIC-PHONETIC THEORIES OF SPEECH PERCEPTION

The preceding chapters have shown us that the speech signal contains a wide variety of acoustic properties. In the right circumstances, most if not all of these properties can function as perceptual cues to the identity of some sound or feature, and many of them contribute to more than one linguistic sound or feature. This variety, or redundancy, is one of the greatest strengths of natural speech because it makes it robust, yet it has also been one of the greatest enigmas in the history of speech perception research.

Speech sounds are represented redundantly in the acoustic signal, so people can and do use a number of different acoustic properties to identify them. One consequence is that speech is, for example, robust in noise: If one acoustic property is missing or obliterated by an extraneous noise, there are usually others that can be used instead, and perception does not suffer. On the other hand, the redundancy means that the acoustic correlates of linguistic units are typically complex, simultaneously contribute to more than one linguistic unit, and do not cluster into discrete bundles. Moreover, although some crucially important perceptual cues are concentrated in just 10 or 20 ms stretches, others can extend over long sections of the signal.

The preceding chapters have also shown that the crucial thing for speech to be perceived normally is that its acoustic properties are in particular relationships with each other. They must form particular patterns in the spectrum, the sound source, or the time course of the signal. The presence of "simple" things like a single formant frequency or its transition, or the absolute duration of the transition or the steady state of a vowel, is not by itself enough for the signal to be heard as speech. Whether a particular property of the signal functions as a perceptual cue depends partly

on its context. In other words, perceptual cues are defined in relational terms. For example, loosely speaking, the crucial thing about an /i/ is that the second formant frequency should be high (far removed from F1) and close to F3; its exact frequency does not matter so much. Indeed, Chapter Eleven points out that vowels' "target" frequencies need not even be achieved as long as the formant transitions have the right overall pattern. Similarly, whether a bilabial transition in a synthetic syllable is heard as /b/ or /w/ depends, within fairly wide limits, on the duration of the vowel that follows. Chapter Twelve makes this point for a wide range of consonants.

Research into speech perception is still in the early stages, and although over the last forty or fifty years we have learned a great deal, we still have more questions than answers. One thing we shall see is that those theories that stress abstract referents—that conceptualize the process of speech perception as one of filtering out an invariant "signal" from irrelevant "noise"—are to a large extent untestable in a rigorous way, and are perhaps best thought of as philosophies rather than as empirically grounded theories or models. The fact that many of our theories are as much or more philosophies than empirically testable models does not mean that they are necessarily either wrong or unhelpful (although they cannot all be right!). Polarization of theoretical viewpoints provides one source of lively debate in the field that can generate new findings that increase our understanding.

The fact that the classical acoustic-phonetic theories have tended to assume a fairly simple, rigid and narrow process of speech decoding is no bad thing. When a complex field is only just being opened up to research, it is usually necessary to make simple assumptions and to ask simple questions. When the answers to these questions begin to contradict one another, we ask why, and so gradually make our questions more appropriate. For better or worse, it is human nature to learn mainly from our mistakes! The early to mid-1990s may prove to be a significant turning point in the history of speech perception in that theories are beginning to be more comprehensive and sophisticated. They have become so because of what we have learned from experiments conceived within the early theoretical approaches.

INTRODUCTION TO TWO CLASSICAL THEORIES OF SPEECH PERCEPTION

Some of the earliest theories of speech perception are still the most influential, and they have led to lively debate and a wide range of often ingenious experimental designs. In this chapter, we focus on the two most influential classical theories, which reflect the two main opposing schools of thought: the Motor Theory[1] developed mainly by Alvin Liberman and other psychologists at the Haskins Laboratories, and quantal theory and its developments, which may be termed the theory of acoustic invariance, developed mainly by Kenneth Stevens, an engineer at the Massachusetts Institute of Technology.

These two theories are distinguished more by details of the mechanisms or processes that they assume underlie the perception of speech than by the empirical findings they try to account for. They are similar in that each tries to account for categorical perception (see Chapter Twelve), and each looks for invariant properties in, or derivable from, the speech signal: Their goal is to map linguistic units, namely phonemes, directly onto properties of the acoustic signal. That is, each assumes processes that "simplify" the signal by making it as abstract as possible (like a phonemic transcription) as soon as possible, with information that is irrelevant to the linguistic message being stripped off en route. What differs between them is what the invariant is. As their names suggest, the Motor Theory assumes that the invariant referents, the phonemes, are associated with the movements that produce speech, while the theory of acoustic invariance suggests they are in the acoustic signal itself, or its auditory transforms.

THE MOTOR THEORY OF SPEECH PERCEPTION

1. We perceive the speaker's intended phonetic gestures; these are the invariants.
2. Speech perception is automatically mediated by an innate, specialized speech module to which we have no conscious access and whose properties are unique.
3. Speech production and perception share a common link and a common processing strategy.

The essence of early Motor Theory was that listeners interpret the acoustic signal in terms of the articulatory patterns that would produce auditory patterns like those being heard in the signal. In the earliest version of the Motor Theory (Liberman, Cooper, Shankweiler, & Studdert-Kennedy, 1967), it was the vocal tract movements themselves that were thought to be reconstructed when the auditory patterns were decoded. In the most recent version, called the revised Motor Theory (Liberman & Mattingly, 1985), listeners are said to reconstruct the talker's *intended gestures* for phonetic categories such as tongue backing, lip rounding, and jaw/tongue raising. These intended gestures can be thought of as abstract control units that can give rise to linguistically relevant vocal tract movements; they are not the movements themselves. Thus, in the current version of the theory, the listener perceives the articulatory plans that control the vocal tract movements that would produce a perfect rendition of the talker's intended utterance.

Each intended gesture, or plan, contributes to part of a "pure" phoneme. For Motor Theorists, coarticulation between adjacent phonemes occurs during the execution of movements. Thus, coarticulation is not essential to the linguistic structure of the signal and is not represented at the

---

[1]In this and the next chapter, capital letters are used for the Motor Theory of Liberman et al. to distinguish it from other theories that are also motor theories. All the other theories discussed in these two chapters have distinctive names, so there is unlikely to be confusion between any other specific theory and a general class of such theories. The names of these other theories are not capitalized, therefore.

level of abstract gestures. It is seen largely as a smoothing process between successive gestures that occurs inevitably during the execution of movement, because the nature of the vocal tract means that there must be movement between successive targets, and those movements must be relatively smooth. In this view, coarticulation destroys the purity of the underlying phoneme string: It produces variability that makes the acoustic signal itself contain no invariant properties that can be related to linguistic units.

Coarticulation is seen as having as important a role in speech perception as in production. First, it is seen as increasing the efficiency of speech production by speeding up the rate at which phonemes can be transmitted, and it plays a parallel role in perception. Since information about more than one phoneme is normally transmitted simultaneously, each articulation effectively lasts longer than the acoustic segment most closely associated with the "pure" phoneme. In consequence, listeners have more time to decode each separate gesture. Since it was originally thought that the rate at which phonemes can be transmitted in normal speech (up to about 30 phonemes per second) was too fast for a listener to process, this extra time was seen as necessary, and it is probably helpful. However, it may not be essential, because listeners can identify brief sequences of sounds at rates of up to 100 per second (one every 10 ms), although at these short durations it seems that the listeners learn the overall sound pattern rather than perceiving each item separately (Moore, 1997). The significance of this point for speech perception will become clear in the next chapter.

The other role attributed to coarticulation is that of guiding listeners toward uncovering the underlying gestures. Although the theory is not explicit about how this is done, listeners are thought to "know about" coarticulation, and to somehow filter out its acoustic effects in the process of reconstructing the phonemic intentions of the speaker. Chapter Twelve describes an experiment by Mann and Repp (1980) that nicely illustrates this point. They made two sets of stimuli by appending naturally spoken /u/ or /ɑ/ vowels to

synthetic fricative noises that formed a series ranging from /s/ to /ʃ/. When the vowel of the resulting CV syllable was /u/, listeners heard more /s/ and fewer /ʃ/ sounds than when the vowel was /ɑ/. In naturally spoken English, the rounding of the lips for /u/ typically "spreads" onto a preceding /s/, and this often results in the fricative having high-amplitude energy at lower frequencies than when the lips are spread, as when the following vowel is /ɑ/. Listeners know this and allow for it when deciding whether a syllable is /su/ or /ʃu/; thus, they divide the /s~ʃ/ series of stimuli in different places depending on whether the vowel of the syllable is rounded or not. The intended gesture for the underlying pure phoneme is retrieved from the variable acoustic signal by compensating for the coarticulatory effects. This is the standard Motor-Theoretic viewpoint; later, we shall discuss an alternative interpretation of these data (see acoustic invariance).

The revised Motor Theory (Liberman & Mattingly, 1985) suggests that this reconstruction of the speaker's intended abstract gestures takes place in a specialized phonetic module in the brain and is an innate, automatic process to which the listener has no conscious access. Once the phonetic module is active, the auditory properties that initiate its activity are not accessible to other modules in the listener's brain, so that the same stimulus cannot normally be heard both as speech and as nonspeech simultaneously. In a sense, the phonetic module is in competition with a general auditory module. Following more general ideas on mental modules (cf., Fodor 1983), Motor Theorists also suggest the existence of other modules for speech and language, including ones for phonology and for syntax, but they do not discuss how they work together. Nor do they suggest how the translation from the acoustic signal to the phonetic gestures is done: They say only that it is direct and automatic—the listener has no choices within the phonetic mode.

The intended gestures are seen as the only invariant property that unites the phonemic message through differences in rate of speech, talker, and so on. They are therefore the only invariant

202 PART TWO SPEECH DECODING BY HUMAN AND MACHINE: FROM SOUND STREAM TO WORDS

property the child can pick up from the signal. Gestural information is linguistic, because it is phonetic, even for a baby, but it is not connected with the phonological module until later infancy or beyond.

Summary

Motor Theorists hold that speech is translated into linguistic units by a special phonetic module rather than by general auditory processes. The linguistic units are said to be abstract gestures that would produce particular constrictions in the vocal tract, each constriction being appropriate for a specific phonetic place and manner of articulation. In this way, coarticulation is not part of speech representation. The perception of speech is thus "nonhomomorphic" with the auditory signal: The percept is entirely different from the signal. Motor Theorists believe that perceiving intended vocal-tract gestures makes speech perception special. They argue that, whereas the speech percept is non-homomorphic with the auditory signal, perception of nonspeech auditory signals is homomorphic with the signal (that is, the percept has the same form as the signal; it varies as the signal varies). Thus, the two forms of perception are quite unlike one another. The speech percept has a motor character, rather than being homomorphic with the acoustic signal, because we use our innate knowledge of how to make sounds when we understand speech.

The Motor Theorists' position on the relationship between speech production and perception is consistent with the precedence they give to the motoric gesture. They believe that the human vocal tract evolved to its present state partly to make speech possible, and that the brain's perceptual abilities developed in tandem with, and in response to, its productive abilities, but never before them. The consequence is that perception and production are unified within the phonetic module, because all the module's processes take place with reference to perceived, intended production.

The arguments and evidence that led to the current position are complicated and are based on

some of the most intriguing and wide-ranging work in the literature of speech perception. In order to understand them, it is helpful to go back to work that was done to test the original (pre-1985) Motor Theory, for it was some of that work, of course, that led to the current theory. The following sections, then, are a critical discussion of the Motor Theory from a historical as well as a current perspective.

Evaluation of the Motor Theory's Propositions: Empirical Work and its Interpretation

The Motor Theory of speech perception developed in response to the early, and unexpected, observation that there is no simple relationship between the acoustic signal and the perceived phoneme. Before spectrograms became available, it was expected that the acoustic signal would reveal a reasonably clear correspondence between acoustic segments and linguistic segments, namely phones or phonemes. When speech could be examined spectrographically, researchers were unable to locate phones unambiguously in the signal, and those at Haskins Laboratories described much of the speech signal as *encoded*: Acoustic cues to phonemes overlap one another rather than being individually identifiable as discrete elements. If a signal is encoded, then it needs decoding in order to be understood. The challenge was to work out how this decoding takes place. Work was begun that soon led to the discovery that very different acoustic signals can lead to the same, unitary percept of a particular phoneme, whereas the same acoustic signal can be heard as different phonemes if presented in suitably different contexts. Viewed in this light, the common factor was taken to be not the pattern of cueing properties in the acoustic signal, but the articulation that produced them.

For example, Figure 14-1B shows two-formant schematic spectrograms (as used for the Haskins Pattern Playback synthesizer) that are heard as the syllables /di/ and /du/. The initial consonant is always heard simply as /d/ rather than as two dif-

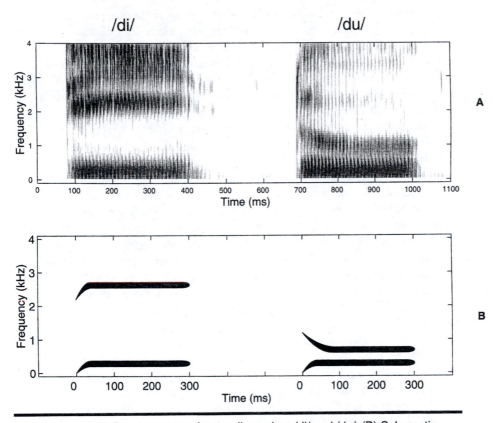

FIGURE 14-1.   (A) Spectrograms of naturally spoken /di/ and /du/. (B) Schematic spectrograms of two-formant stimuli sufficient to be heard as /di/ and /du/, as in the experiment of Liberman et al. (1967). In the schematic spectrograms, the F1 transitions are identical for both syllables, but F2 transitions differ in direction, following roughly the same patterns as in the natural speech.

ferent sounds, yet the F2 transition rises in the case of /di/, but falls in the case of /du/. The F2 transition is the only property that distinguishes the two syllables in this example, so it is interesting that such different patterns are heard as the same consonant.[2] Not surprisingly, these very simplified synthetic stimuli do not sound as con-

vincing as natural speech, because they omit a great deal of information, as you can see by comparing them with the spectrograms of natural /di/ and /du/ in Figure 14-1A. Nevertheless, people are able to report consistent speech-like percepts, and most researchers believe that listeners respond to them in much the same way as they respond to natural speech.

The perception of the same consonant for different formant transitions is an example of perceptual invariance, a phenomenon characteristic of sensory perception in general. For example, when we look at an object, the object is perceived as constant, or invariant, despite changes in distance and point of view that change the pattern of

---

[2]At the time this work was done, F2 was seen as crucial to the distinction between bilabial, alveolar, and velar places of articulation, and it is often set up to be the deciding factor in synthetic speech stimuli for perceptual research; however, subsequent work with natural speech has shown that F2 transitions often do not pattern in the reliable way that they should if they are in fact a principal acoustic property for cueing place of articulation (Kewley-Port, 1982).

stimulation on the retina of the eye. This is visual invariance. In consonant perception by ear, the object perceived is the consonant articulation, despite changes in the sound pattern because of different adjacent sounds.

In contrast with the example of /di/ and /du/, in which different F2 transitions lead to a percept of the same consonant phoneme, in other conditions the same F2 transition leads to a percept of different phonemes. Cooper, Delattre, Liberman, Borst, and Gerstman (1952) showed that the same synthetic stop burst could be heard as /p/ before front and high back vowels, but /k/ before low vowels. So, for example, one could create "peekapoo" by alternating a stop burst whose main spectral prominence was between about 1400–1900 Hz, with steady state formant frequencies appropriate for /i/, then /ɑ/, then /u/.

The articulation of bilabial versus alveolar versus velar stop differs mainly in the place of constriction, but the movements to and from a given constriction are different depending on what tongue configuration is necessary for the following vowel. Differences in the changing shape of the vocal tract give rise to different patterns of formant transition. The argument is that somehow the perceptual system seems to "know" this and immediately, automatically, hears these acoustic patterns as different consonants when they reflect changes in vocal tract shape that involve different places of articulation, and as the same consonant sound when they reflect changes in vocal tract shape that involve the same place of articulation.

This type of argument is used to explain categorical perception of consonants. Motor Theorists appeal to articulation as the unifying factor: Sounds that could come from a single type of articulatory constriction are responded to as functionally equivalent—that is, the listener gives them the same label, such as /b/ or /d/, and does not hear that they are different. Motor Theorists suggest that there is no other basis for making a single category out of very different acoustic signals. At first, it was thought that the invariant property was the muscle contractions for particular articu-

lations. However, work done mainly at Haskins Laboratories soon made it clear that invariance was no more to be found in the movements of individual speech organs or their component muscles than it was in the acoustic patterns. Electromyographic studies, for example, showed just as much variability in muscle activity between contexts and between individuals (cf., Harris 1974; MacNeilage & deClerk 1969).

In response to this evidence, the revised Motor Theory proposed that the invariants are more abstract than that of actual movement: that the listener perceives the speaker's planned, intended gestures for phones. Alternative approaches would be to look further for invariants in the acoustic signal by using different methods of analysis, or to place less emphasis on the search for one-to-one correspondences between properties of the signal and phones. Other researchers have adopted these alternative approaches, and their views are discussed below, but Motor Theorists instead sought new evidence to support their main tenet, of the primacy of reference to the motor control plan of speech, with minimal modifications. For example, the term *gesture*, and the abstract level at which it is conceived, was developed in tandem with but independently of revision to the Motor Theory. The term comes from a large body of research on nonspeech as well as speech movement (see Hawkins, 1992, for a description relevant to speech) and has been used in a number of other theoretical approaches to both speech production and perception (e.g., Browman & Goldstein, 1986, 1992; Fowler, 1986). A gesture is one of a family of movement patterns that all achieve the same goal, such as a particular constriction in the vocal tract—for example, bilabial closure. Gestures for speech can be thought of as the basic units of speech production, which control and coordinate the cooperative activity of the articulators. To suggest that gestures are also the basic units of speech perception is appealing in terms of elegance and economy of theoretical constructs. And to employ concepts that are independently motivated from other research areas strengthens the theoretical approach.

Evidence from Cross-Linguistic Studies of Adults' Perception   What empirical evidence is there that categorical perception arises because we perceive by reference to speech movements? One source of support could be the difficulty that adults have in distinguishing between sounds that are not phonemic in their native language. Earlier, we reviewed data showing that we cannot make general statements about adults' perceptual abilities with non-native contrasts. Adults can discriminate between foreign sounds quite well when those sounds are acoustically distinctive, and/or when they are acoustically most similar to sounds from different phonemic categories of the listeners' native language (Best, 1995; Werker, Gilbert, Humphrey, & Tees, 1981). Listeners are much less able to distinguish between two foreign sounds that both fall within the same phonemic category of their own native language. However, we have also seen that adults can be taught such new discriminations.

The question is, what are these adults learning? The revised Motor Theory does not require that all such learning necessarily includes retraining listeners' own speech production systems, because perception is done with respect to the *speaker's* intended gestures. The revised Motor Theory accounts for this learning in terms of some type of reactivation of innate knowledge that has been reorganized in early childhood. But there is as yet no evidence that clearly shows that we relearn motoric gestures, rather than reattune auditory categories. The Motor Theorists' claim is consistent with their general claim that the common element that explains categorical perception for varying acoustic signals is the motoric gesture, but it is no more than that.

Evidence from Animals' Perceptual Abilities   For some researchers, the fact that animals make apparently categorical discriminations in some acoustic series is a major mark against the Motor Theory. To Motor Theorists, it is not. Liberman and Mattingly (1985) argue that all the data taken together logically point to the priority of production over perception and to the modularity of the

speech perception process. They further argue that proponents of auditory-based theories must logically take the position that speech production evolved to its present state in order to satisfy the processing demands of the auditory system. This applies particularly to those who stress that basic speech perception is for the most part not special, which includes most animal researchers. Liberman and Mattingly imply that this position is untenable because it entails that speech production, as well as speech perception, is governed by general auditory principles.

We may never be able to resolve this argument about whether the evolution of production preceded that of perception, or vice versa, because we have no access to really reliable data on the evolution of speech. One possibility that Liberman and Mattingly (1985) seem not to entertain seriously is that production and perception evolved in tandem with one another. Another possibility is that, regardless of whether one preceded the other during evolutionary development or whether they evolved in tandem, the central processing of speech takes place in some neutral way that makes direct reference to neither production nor perception. And a third possibility is that both auditory and motoric referents are available, and each will be used as the situation demands.

Evidence from Trading Relations   Trading relations between different acoustic cues to the same phoneme have been described in Chapter Twelve and admirably reviewed by Repp (1982). Most trading relations have been discovered since the original Motor Theory was proposed. The revised theory argues that the number of cues that enter into trading relations is too vast and too disparate to be accounted for elegantly by a theory based on the acoustic signal: There are more potential cues, of very different acoustic properties, than potential acoustic features. In contrast, Motor Theorists argue that referring perception to an invariant motoric gesture accounts simply and elegantly for many of these cues.

The number and varied nature of cues that enter into trading relations with one another does pose a problem for non-motor theories, but it is not clear that the Motor Theory is right in claiming that motoric underpinnings must account for all of them. One reason is that cues can enter into trading relations for different reasons. One group of trading relations arises when the same vocal-tract behavior has a number of acoustic conse-quences. This type of trading relation was among the earliest found, because it applies to several of those for stops, such as VOT with aspiration amplitude, short-term f0 perturbation, burst ampli-tude, and F1 cutback (cf., Chapter Twelve). All of these disparate acoustic properties are thought to pattern as they do as a consequence of the laryn-geal adjustment required to produce short-lag versus long-lag VOT. Perception of the motoric (laryngeal) gesture is a more elegant explanation than perception of the several acoustic cues inde-pendently.

Very similar response patterns to those found in trading relations experiments also arise from stimulus variation of a very different kind. When one end of a continuum that could be used to demonstrate categorical perception is a real word and the other end is a nonsense word, listeners report more instances of the consonant that makes the real word than of the contrasting consonant that makes the nonsense word. This effect is usu-ally called the Ganong effect, after a researcher who gave one of the first demonstrations of it (Ganong, 1980). Ganong made series of stimuli that varied in equal acoustic steps along a VOT continuum. In one set, the end stimuli were *deak* and *teak*, and in another they were *deep* and *teep*. Listeners asked to identify the first consonants as /d/ or /t/ gave more /d/ responses to the *deep-teep* series and more /t/ responses to the *deak-teak* series.

The explanation of the Ganong effect is that we hear real words in preference to nonsense words whenever possible, and that perception is influenced by our knowledge of the world, includ-ing linguistic knowledge such as whether a sylla-ble is a word or not. It is obvious that the Ganong effect does not involve interpretation in terms of motoric gestures, and no Motor Theorist would

claim that it does. However, the *pattern* of response is the same. It is worth considering, therefore, whether there might be a more general explanation even for trading relations that are neatly explained in terms of the Motor Theory.

We are left with an impasse: It is theoretically simpler and more elegant, and hence preferable, to explain all cue trading in the same terms. But while responses to some properties, notably those associated with VOT, are most simply explained by reference to unitary underlying motoric causes, responses to others are not, and some responses, such as the Ganong effect, are clearly the result of interactions between acoustic-phonetic responses and other knowledge, in this case lexical. The simplest explanation may therefore be that listen-ers learn patterns of co-occurrences in the signal, and their responses are influenced by all relevant information, which would include these co-occurrence patterns and whether a real word can be fit to the stimulus if the acoustic information is at all unclear. But this explanation tells us nothing about how listeners learn these patterns: They could be motoric, or they could be acoustic/auditory. We return to this point when we consider the Motor Theory's claim that speech is special.

"Speech Is Special," Processed within an Inde-pendent Module   One of the strongest claims of the Motor Theory is that speech is special, in that it is processed in a separate brain module in a dif-ferent way from any other type of processing. Much of the evidence brought in support of this position comes from the same types of experi-ments that contribute to the basic Motor Theory position that the invariant in the speech signal is the intended gesture of the speaker. The intended gesture transcends, or cuts through, the acoustic variability. But now we are considering not what provides the simplest explanation *within* the speech modality, but the extent to which the per-ception of speech sounds is mirrored by percep-tion of nonspeech sounds. Studies of this type usually concern categorical perception, either directly using nonspeech analogs of simple pho-netic contrasts, or more indirectly by looking at complex combinations of properties, including trading relations for nonspeech sounds and the phenomenon of duplex perception.

Trading Relations for Nonspeech Sounds   Trading relations do occur for some nonspeech sounds, although they seem to be more common for speech sounds. For example, interaural time differences can be traded for interaural level differences in sound localization (Moore, 1997, Chapter 6).

Some of the most interesting work on trading relations concerns experiments in which different patterns of responses are obtained depending on whether the listeners hear the sounds as speech or as nonspeech. These experiments are fundamental to deciding whether trading relations operate at an auditory or a phonetic ("special") level of perception. Best, Morrongiello, and Robson (1981) used synthetic nonspeech stimuli to test trading relations between two cues that can distinguish *stay* from *say*: the duration of silence between the fricative and the vowel and the starting frequency of F1 at the beginning of the vowel. The best *say* stimulus had an /s/-like portion made by reshaping the amplitude of a naturally spoken /s/ so that it sounded like a hiss, and a sine-wave analog of a "diphthong" /eɪ/ made with three sinusoidal tones corresponding to the first three formants. The "diphthong" included initial tone transitions like formant transitions suitable for movement out of an alveolar consonant, so that the whole syllable sounded coherent. The starting frequency for the tone that corresponded to F1 was relatively high (430 Hz). The best *stay* analog was the same as the best *say* analog except that it had a 96 ms silence between the /s/-like and diphthong-like portions, appropriate for the closure duration of /t/, and a low F1 starting frequency (230 Hz). The lower F1 starting frequency is typical after a stop.

From these two stimuli, Best and co-workers synthesized two series of intermediate stimuli whose silent intervals varied in equal steps between 0 ms and 96 ms. By this various combinations of silent intervals and F1 starting frequency, Best and co-workers were able to test how these two acoustic properties influenced the perception of the two words. They used an AXB identification test in which A was the clear analog of *say* and B was the clear analog of *stay*. X was either one of the intermediate stimuli, or stimulus A or B. Listeners were asked to say whether X sounded more like A or B. They also tested listeners' discrimination using a three-way oddity test.

The results are reproduced in Figure 14-2. The listeners could be divided into groups on the basis of how they heard the stimuli: those who heard the stimuli as the words *say* or *stay* and those who did not. This latter group reported either various nonspeech sounds or other speech sounds. The four people who heard the words as *say* and *stay* showed evidence of trading relations between the duration of silence and the frequency of F1 onset, shown in panel (a) of Figure 14-2. That is, at intermediate durations of silence, a lower F1 starting frequency (the solid lines with closed circles) was perceptually equivalent to more silence for these listeners. The listeners who did not hear the stimuli as speech attended to only one or other of the two available cues, rather than both. Of these, five listeners reported attending to the durational cues, and their responses are shown in panel (b) of the figure. These "temporal" listeners showed no trading relations with the spectral cues of F1 onset: They treated the two variables as perceptually nonequivalent, as demonstrated by the overlapping curves in panel (b). The other five listeners in the nonspeech group indirectly reported attending to the spectral cues (e.g., they listened for different sounds of water dripping), and their response curves, shown in panel (c), suggest that they were indeed focusing on the spectral cues of F1 onset frequency. Stimuli with a low F1 onset frequency were almost all heard as more like *stay* than *say* at better than chance level, while almost all stimuli with a high F1 onset were heard as more like *say* at better than chance level. In consequence, the two functions (one for the stimuli with low F1 onset, the other for the stimuli with high F1 onset) were very separate throughout the entire range of durations. The duration of silence did affect the responses systematically, in that longer silent intervals

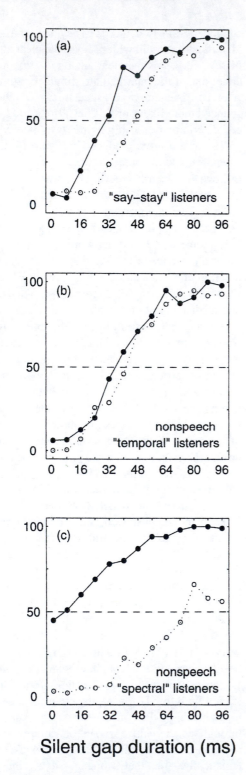

increased the number of *stay* responses for all stimuli (the curves slope up from left to right), but it was much less important than F1 onset frequency. In other words, there was no evidence of perceptual equivalence: Lengthening the silence never completely compensated for a high F1 onset and removing it never completely compensated for a low F1 onset. This was not the case when the stimuli were heard as speech, where the two response functions overlap at the extremes of the stimulus series (panel a).

Best and co-workers interpreted their data as indicating that speech is perceived in a special phonetic mode, because the pattern of trading relations and discrimination for those listeners who heard the sine-wave analogs as speech was like that of subjects hearing more natural speech stimuli varying between *say* and *stay* along the same parameters. These listeners demonstrated perceptual equivalence for the sine-wave stimuli. In contrast, those listeners who heard the stimuli as nonspeech either showed no trading relations or a pattern of influence that was quite different from that of speech-like stimuli. In particular, there was no evidence of the perceptual equiva-

FIGURE 14-2. AXB identification functions for sine-wave stimuli where A is the most like *say*, B is the most like *stay*, and X is another stimulus. Solid lines with closed circles represent responses to stimuli with a low F1 onset; dotted lines with open circles represent high F1 onset. The curves show the percentage of B responses (judged most like the "ideal *stay*") for three groups: (a) listeners who heard the sounds as words, *say* or *stay*; (b) listeners who heard them as nonspeech and attended mainly to the duration of the silent gap; (c) listeners who heard them as nonspeech and attended mainly to spectral differences (F1 onset frequency).

(Adapted from Best et al., *Perception and Psychophysics, 29* (1981) 191–211, Figures 9–11. Reprinted by permission of Psychonomic Society, Inc. and the author)

lences found in speech. Best and co-workers' discussion is couched in phonetic versus auditory modes of perception and a strong interpretation in favor of the Motor Theory is avoided. Consistent with the discussion in the section above, they stress that perception is influenced more by what the listener perceives the stimuli to be—and hence by the type of information that he or she focuses on—than by the detailed physical properties of the stimuli.

However, Parker, Diehl, and Kluender (1986) question Best and co-workers' conclusions. They ask whether the data from the five "spectral" listeners (panel c) should be dismissed as not indicative of trading relations. Because the identification functions never overlap, they conclude that these listeners showed trading relations for duration and spectral properties that were much greater than those seen in speech or in the sinewave analogs heard as speech. They question whether it is reasonable to argue for distinct perceptual mechanisms from differences in the magnitude of an effect and suggest instead that a common auditory basis for the observed effects should be sought. Parker and colleagues also point out that there are three response patterns in the data (one for speech mode listeners and two for the two nonspeech mode listeners) but only two interpretations (phonetic and auditory).

The first argument rests partly on differences in definition. Best and colleagues consider that phonetic perception is demonstrated only when two acoustic cues show perceptual equivalence: They enter into trading relations with one another so completely that their respective effects are phonetically indistinguishable from one another. They would thus argue that it is reasonable to distinguish between quantitatively different as well as qualitatively different effects, partly because there was complete compensation between the two acoustic cues in the speech stimuli and for the sine wave analogs heard as speech, whereas there was only a small influence of duration for the sinewaves analogs whose spectral properties were attended to.

Parker and colleagues' second argument may be unimportant, as they themselves suggest. Best and co-workers' two-way distinction is logical if they simply mean that phonetic perception involves knowing where to listen for critical information in stimuli perceived as speech. It is less logical if they meant that phonetic perception is specialized and auditory perception is not. More recently, Best placed her work within the context of direct realism, which is a logical extension of the argument she used in 1981 and in this respect compatible with Parker and colleagues' point of view.

Like the arguments around categorical perception of nonspeech sounds, the general conclusion must be that trading relations take place within a context, or meaningful system of contrasts, as pointed out by both Best and colleagues (1981) and by Parker and co-workers (1986). Nonspeech stimuli whose properties show trading relations also tend to be part of a system that the listener understands well. The example of sound localization above is one such case. Equally, it is reasonable that trading relations are rare for stimuli made by manipulating the spectrum in ways that do not occur in the natural world. Different stimuli will be perceptually equivalent insofar as they conform to the system the listener believes they are part of. To this extent, speech is special, and phonetic trading relations are special to speech. But whether perception is related directly to the motoric system is still a matter of personal belief rather than of incontrovertible evidence.

Duplex Perception   Duplex perception, first described by Rand (1974), has been investigated extensively by Motor Theorists (e.g., Liberman 1979, Whalen & Liberman 1987) because it provides strong evidence that speech is processed in a special phonetic module. In a duplex perception experiment, an isolated, synthetic formant transition is presented to one ear while the other ear simultaneously receives a "base" stimulus that comprises all the remaining material necessary to hear a simple syllable like /dɑ/. This design is illustrated in Figure 14-3. Figure 14-3a shows a schematic spectrogram of a three-formant synthetic stimulus that would typically be heard as /dɑ/. In a duplex perception experiment, the syllable is divided into two parts, illustrated in Figures 14-3b and 14-3c. The base (shown in Figure 14-3c), comprising all of F1 and F2 together with the steady state of F3, is presented to one ear. Simultaneously, the F3 transition (as in Figure 14-3b) is presented in isolation to the other ear.

Listeners report hearing two sounds simultaneously. They hear the complete syllable, /dɑ/, at the ear that received the base syllable. And they also hear a nonspeech "chirp" at the ear that received only the F3 transition. They do not hear the base syllable alone, which, when it is heard alone, sounds like a stop-vowel syllable whose stop has an indeterminate place of articulation.

Two general properties of duplex perception are especially important to its role as a principal proof of the modularity of speech perception. First, duplex perception only occurs when the stimulus that is not the base is short and extremely unspeechlike. For example, duplex perception

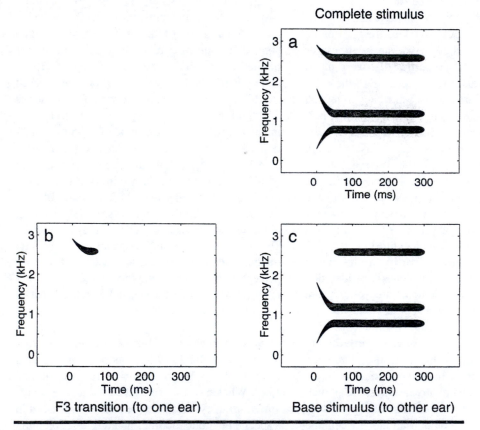

FIGURE 14-3. Schematic spectrograms of stimuli used to demonstrate duplex perception. Panel (a) shows a three-formant synthetic stimulus sufficient to hear the syllable /dɑ/. The lower two panels, (b) and (c), show this stimulus separated into two parts. Each part is presented to a different ear. Thus, one ear receives only the third-formant transition as shown in (b), while the other ear receives the "base," comprising the first and second formant transitions and steady states, together with the steady state of the third formant, as shown in (c).

will not occur when the base stimulus consists of the first two formants and the other stimulus is the entire third formant. Under these conditions, a single, coherent syllable is heard, suggesting that the two stimuli are perceptually fused centrally, but no more than that. Second, only two, rather than three percepts are heard: the entire syllable, and the chirp. The base stimulus is not heard as a separate entity. Thus, Liberman and Mattingly (1985) stress that duplex percepts do not simply reflect the ability of the auditory system to fuse input from the two ears into something meaningful. If that were all that was happening, they suggest the percept should be "triplex": a chirp, an ambiguous stop-vowel syllable, and a /dɑ/ syllable. Instead, only the isolated F3 transition is heard concurrently both as speech and as nonspeech.

Further support for the specialized module for speech comes from an experiment by Mann and Liberman (1983). They used the duplex perception paradigm to present listeners with a series of stimuli with various falling or rising F3 transitions ranging from /dɑ/ to /gɑ/. When listeners were asked to attend to the speech percept, they showed evidence of categorical perception: They discriminated better between stimuli that spanned the phoneme boundary than between stimuli that were given the same phonemic label. When listeners attended to the nonspeech chirp, however, they had no such peaks in their discrimination functions and thus showed no sign of categorical perception. Other experiments, reviewed by Repp (1982), show that the two percepts are independent. For example, when the intensity of the isolated transition is increased, the chirp sounds louder, but the speech percept is unchanged.

Duplex perception thus provides strong evidence for Motor Theorists that speech is processed in a special module. It violates the psychoacoustic principle of "disjoint allocation," which states that we can assign an element in a sound to only one source at a time (see Moore, 1997). In duplex perception, the same sound is heard in two ways: it contributes to a speech source, and it functions as a "chirp source" in its own right. If we assume that the principle of disjoint allocation operates

within, but not between modules, then the phenomenon of duplex perception nicely illustrates that speech and nonspeech sounds are processed in independent modules.

However, there are alternative explanations to that of the Motor Theorists (cf., Bregman, 1987; Darwin, 1991; Repp, 1991), and Moore (1997) also notes that the principle of disjoint allocation is sometimes violated for nonspeech sounds too. For example, when a single harmonic in a complex tone is mistuned in frequency it can contribute to the overall percept of the complex tone and at the same time be heard as a pure tone. Similar violations occur for visual stimuli. Moore suggests that violations of the principle seem to be more common for speech than for other types of stimuli. One conclusion could be that the Motor Theory has identified in modularity an important and somewhat distinctive property of speech processing, but that its uniqueness to speech may have been exaggerated.

Listening in a special speech, or phonetic, mode undoubtedly takes place, and it seems to be an automatically triggered process over which the listener has little or no control, although suggestion also plays a part. Most people are more likely to hear ambiguous sounds as speech if they expect to hear speech. As Moore (1997) points out, listening in a specific perceptual mode is not specific to speech, but the speech mode is unusual in that it applies to a wide range of complex and varied sounds whose main common feature is that they come from a vocal tract. Nevertheless, real speech sounds can be misperceived as nonspeech, as the click and chant examples illustrate. The unifying factor, then, may not be that the sounds come from a vocal tract, but rather that they conform to a system that the listener knows and only incidentally come from a vocal tract. Perception within a particular meaningful system may form the basis of modularity in perception. That fewer trading relations have been shown for nonspeech stimuli than for speech stimuli may simply be because the nonspeech stimuli of psychoacoustic experiments fit less often into meaningful systems of everyday auditory life. In other words, if speech has its module, every meaningful sensory system may have one, too. If this is right, there will be no general auditory module in simple contrast with a phonetic module, but rather a module for every type of auditory signal that the listener recognizes as part of a larger system.

Innate Knowledge of Gestures as Phonetic Motor Plan   When the original Motor Theory was developed, nothing was known about babies' perception of speech sounds because there were no techniques for studying them. As mentioned in Chapter Thirteen, most researchers tended to assume that babies take a long time to learn to discriminate the sound contrasts of their native language in a process that continues beyond when they begin to speak. Given these beliefs, together with contemporary views within behaviorist psychology, it is understandable that early Motor Theorists assumed "that the connection between perception and production was formed as a wholly learned association, and that perceiving the gesture was a matter of picking up the sensory consequences of covert mimicry" (Liberman & Mattingly 1985: 23). In other words, the early Motor Theory did not need to account for babies' speech discrimination, because it was assumed that the baby first learned the connections between movement and sound from its own sound play and then learned to discriminate sounds in other people's speech by referring them to, or reconstructing, the motoric gestures that would be needed to make those sounds. In this view, accurate perception of other people's speech followed the development of the baby's own abilities.

There are some logical difficulties to this position, such as the fact that babies' vocal tracts are very different from those of adults and older children, so that it is unlikely that babies could "know about" real movements that older humans produce. This problem is part of what is called the "vocal tract normalization" problem, and even today we do not fully understand how humans instantly adjust to the idiosyncrasies of a new speaker of the same language and accent (see Chapters Three and Eleven). But these difficulties

were not given much attention by early Motor Theorists, who, like most speech researchers, tended to disregard developmental issues and to put vocal tract normalization aside as intractable. Others saw these difficulties as serious problems for the theory (see, e.g., Lane, 1965).

The Motor Theory's position that sound categories are not "properly" perceived until after they can be produced was very soon thrown into question, initially by the demonstration by Eimas and co-workers (1971) that babies perceive VOT categorically, and thereafter by the increasing body of evidence that babies' perception of basic phonetic contrasts is in some ways better than it will ever be again. These data have been discussed in the previous chapter. They do not support the idea that perception *follows* production, because babies can very definitely not make the sounds and the sound distinctions that we now know they can discriminate. Quite a range of perceptual abilities for speech seem to precede the ability to make most of the movements for speech. This was a problem for the early Motor Theory.

Motor Theorists answered this problem by revising the theory to its present position. These and other data from babies (as, for example, that discussed above) were one of the major reasons why they developed the notions that speech is perceived by reference to innate knowledge of intended gestures. The beginnings of this idea had been expressed much earlier—for example, by Studdert-Kennedy (1976:244)—who noted that the translation of the speech signal into a motoric referent means that the phonetic category automatically "names itself."

Innateness also offers an account of why babies process speech in a linguistic (phonetic) way rather than a general auditory one right from the start. The phonetic module is innate, and auditory information with the right properties is automatically processed by the phonetic module. No knowledge is required, and the baby has no choice. In a sense, the development of phonology is given a kick start because the baby does not have the initial task of sorting out what is linguistically relevant from what is not.

These ideas are neat and attractive, and it seems clear that a great deal of our linguistically relevant auditory sensitivities are inborn. There is a danger in couching explanations in terms of innateness, however. There has been a tendency for the term to eventually become a meaningless ragbag for everything for which we have not yet found another explanation. This is not a reason to avoid using the term, but it does underline the need to use it with caution and to continue to search for other explanations.

Similar conclusions can be reached from data on second language learning and retraining non-native phonemic discriminations. Recall that a non-native discrimination is more likely to be learned easily if it is inherently acoustically distinctive and/or engages (is assimilable to) contrasting phonemic categories of the listener's native language. Although the data can be interpreted in terms of the Motor Theory, non-motoric interpretations are at least as compatible with the observed (and unsurprising) interactions between the acoustic distinctiveness of the contrasts and their relationship with the phonemic categories of the listeners' native language.

Finally, evidence that animals perceive some aspects of speech as humans do, while not negating the Motor Theory, does weaken its arguments for innate human mechanisms specific to speech.

The Motor Theory must argue that phonetic gestural referents are innate because babies can discriminate a large number of phonetic contrasts long before they can speak, and because people who cannot speak from birth but whose hearing is normal can nevertheless perceive apparently normally. If the units of speech perception are linguistic and motoric, then we must be innately endowed with this referent system in order to discriminate between sounds before we can produce them. The theory suggests that language-specific parameter values are reset towards the end of the first year of life, corresponding to the time when babies' discrimination of phonetic contrasts becomes strongly influenced by their native language. That broad discriminatory skills are innate seems undeniable; but the Motor Theory will need substantial refinement before it can explain an increasing number of facts of infant speech perception, most of which have been discovered since the revised theory appeared in 1985.

General Summary of the Motor Theory

The Motor Theory's main tenets are as follows. A lack of invariance in the acoustic signal, coupled with evidence that different acoustic signals give rise to percepts of the same phoneme, made by the same articulator, led to the idea that listeners perceive speech by reference to phonetic gestures. A gesture is an abstract representation of a vocal-tract constriction, defined as that part of a vocal-tract configuration that produces the most salient property(ies) of a phoneme. The percept takes place by way of the speaker's plan for gestures because coarticulation is seen as preventing invariant phonemic units from being produced. The perceived intended gestures are therefore the invariants of speech perception. Perceiving gestures makes speech perception special, because Motor Theorists believe that perception of nonspeech sounds is closely tied to the properties of the acoustic signal itself, whereas perception of speech sounds often is not. Phonetic perception takes place in a specialized module that operates independently of other linguistic modules and in competition with a general auditory module. The parameters in the module are innate, although their values are recalibrated in response to exposure to the native language.

The Motor Theory is appealing because it offers a unified explanation of a great diversity of data within speech perception. Moreover, it is clear that articulatory reference does influence perception, and we will take this point further in later sections. Likewise, some influences on the way the speech signal is processed are different from nonspeech signals. For example, phonemic categories often dominate responses to many speech stimuli; categorical responses to nonspeech stimuli are rarer.

However, the Motor Theory can be criticized for interpretations that effectively define traditional problems out of existence. For example, coarticulation does not need to be dealt with because it is not processed by the phonetic module; (non)invariance in the signal is redefined as coproduction of overlapping, invariant abstract gestures; the problem of how we segment the speech signal into phone-sized units is redefined as direct perception of individual gestures (or gesture plans); the control of timing and time-dependent effects does not need to be represented, because the effects are automatically taken care of in the gestural control structure; and the perceptual abilities of babies and people who are congenitally unable to speak, vocal tract normalization, and invariant percepts over changes in speaking rate are accounted for in terms of innate transforms between the acoustic signal and the gestures.

One difficulty with these redefinitions is that, while there is a unifying logic, there is little or no empirical support for the claims, because the Motor Theory is more a philosophical guide than an empirically testable theory. When aspects of the theory can be tested, there is usually more than one way to interpret the results (cf., Lindblom, 1996), and many of the important beliefs are not testable. For example, there is no explanation of what in the signal allows perception of intended gestures. There is no explanation of how the acoustic-motor transformation is done, and current analytic techniques cannot do it. Some critics believe there is often nothing in what is postulated that demands an explanation tied to articulation rather than acoustics, and that the transformation to articulatory parameters is an unnecessary extra step. Some of the claims for special processes in speech perception do also occur with nonspeech stimuli, although it is usually true that many such processes are more common for speech than nonspeech sounds. It is arguable that at least some phonemic categories depend on general acoustic properties rather than being unique to speech. One possibility is that the modular portrayal of speech perception is correct, inasmuch as speech provides a well-known and highly structured system that governs responses

more closely than that of many other domains. But this is a looser definition of modularity than Motor Theorists adopt. They counter the general auditory theorists (Chapter Fifteen) with arguments that it is highly implausible that the general auditory and cognitive processes can untangle the articulatorily encrypted complexities and deal parsimoniously with the well-known speed and adaptability of phonetic perception (Liberman, 1996:28-41).

Because Motor Theory is couched in somewhat abstract terms, it runs the risk of assigning too much to the unanalyzable module—a black box. More importantly, it fails to address a number of phonetic issues. For example, there is no detailed discussion of how phonetic knowledge is linked with other linguistic knowledge, of the significance of allophonic information to the identification of words, and of the complexities of perceiving connected speech compared with single syllables and isolated words. It is important to bear in mind that many of these weaknesses (especially those connected with narrowness of interpretation and phonetic oversimplification) are true for several, if not most other theories of speech perception, especially of this era. Narrowness and oversimplification can be advantageous at the beginning of an investigation.

ACOUSTICAL INVARIANTS: THE QUANTAL THEORY OF SPEECH, RELATIONAL ACOUSTIC INVARIANCE, AND LEXICAL ACCESS FROM FEATURES (LAFF)

Developing from about the same time as the Motor Theory is the idea that invariants are either directly in the signal, or else arise during the transformations that the signal automatically undergoes as it is processed by the specialized nerve cells of the inner ear and the brain on its way through the auditory system to the cerebral cortex of the brain. Of the theories that fall into this category, the most consistent and longstanding body of work is that of Stevens of MIT, who proposed quantal theory and its development into "acoustic invariance theory" and a model of speech perception known as LAFF (Lexical Access from Features).

The Quantal Theory of Speech

1. Vocal-tract configuration and acoustic output have a nonlinear relationship that favors the establishment of categories of sound: As the shape of the vocal tract changes continuously along some dimension, the resulting change in sound will at times be large, and at other times very small. The auditory system is predisposed to respond distinctively to these quantal changes.

2. The auditory system itself responds with similar patterns of change and stability to steadily changing acoustic parameters.

3. The inventory of sounds of each language is chosen from these regions of acoustic or auditory stability.

Two major questions motivated Stevens' development of the quantal theory (1972, 1989): Why are some sounds common to most languages, and others found only in a few? Why does the great range of sounds that people produce resolve into a small number of classes in our minds? The first question addresses one of the most fascinating phenomena of linguistics, and the second, of course, concerns categorical perception. Stevens used principles of aerodynamics and acoustics to show that the relationship between articulatory configuration and the resultant sound output could account for linguistic structures and phonetic perception. He pointed out that acoustic theory predicts that, for a given articulatory parameter, there will be some regions in which a small articulatory change leads to a significant change in the acoustic output, and other regions where an equally small articulatory change produces no appreciable acoustic change. This principle is illustrated in Figure 14-4.

Consider just the axes labeled (a) (nonitalic text) in Figure 14-4. For these axes, the curve rep-

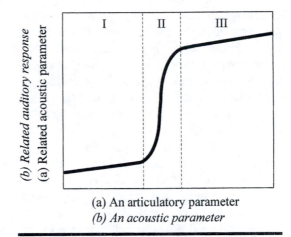

(a) An articulatory parameter
(b) An acoustic parameter

FIGURE 14-4. Curve illustrating schematically the basic principle of the quantal theory of speech. The plain axes, labeled (a), show changes in a relevant acoustic parameter as an articulatory parameter steadily changes. The italicized axes, labeled (b), show changes in the relevant human auditory response as an acoustic parameter steadily changes. The pattern of response is the same in both cases. See text for further explanation.

resents the acoustic output of the vocal tract for each value of the articulatory parameter represented along the horizontal axis. If the articulatory parameter were distance of a constriction from the glottis, then the acoustic parameter on the vertical axis would reflect place of articulation (it might be the frequency of F2, for example); if lip aperture were the articulatory parameter, then the acoustic parameter would represent manner of articulation (vowel-fricative).

The crucial principle being illustrated is that the curve is nonlinear: It is somewhat s-shaped rather than a straight line. You can think of it as representing a "quantal jump" between two different states, each of which is relatively stable. As long as you are in the Part I region, changes in the articulatory parameter produce negligible acoustic changes (the curve is almost flat as you step along the horizontal axis). But when you change the articulatory parameter at values that fall within its

Part II region, there will be huge changes in the acoustic output. Once past the Part II region and into the Part III region, however, the acoustic output is again insensitive to articulatory changes, although the acoustic response is quite different from what it was in the Part I region. If the articulatory parameter were lip aperture, then all articulations within the Part I region might produce vowels, while all those within the Part III region might produce fricatives. Lip apertures in the Part II region would produce sounds that were unstable between vowels and fricatives: They would have some sonorant qualities, but also some turbulence noise and would probably be avoided by most languages.

Stevens suggested that these regions of acoustic stability, as in Parts I and III of Figure 14-4, form the basis for the sound inventory of languages. They provide, as it were, the "first cut" along which languages begin to divide up the sound space into contrasts. Regions of stability, Stevens suggested, allow an articulator to move smoothly towards and then away from an articulatory target while the acoustic result remains relatively steady. In this way, the signal that the listener receives will be relatively stable, while the talker has some flexibility in the particular articulatory movements used. This is the sort of relationship between tongue/jaw height and acoustics that we see for vowels, for example, and for some consonants like fricatives.

These ideas have been carefully worked out for many aspects of speech production and have generated a lot of research (for details, see Hawkins, 1994, and then Stevens, 1989). The aspect of quantal theory that addresses speech perception is represented as the italicized parameters of Figure 14-4, labeled (b). Here, the same nonlinear relationship is schematized as representing an acoustic parameter along the horizontal axis and a related auditory response on the vertical axis. What the curve represents, then, is presumed changes in the auditory system's response to changes in an acoustic parameter. Just as with speech production, the claim is that equal changes in the acoustic parameter will not always

lead to the same degree of change in the auditory response: Some acoustic changes produce very little difference in the auditory response, while others produce huge changes.

Categorical perception, of course, is ideally described by this nonlinear curve. If the acoustic parameter represented increasing values of VOT (cf., Chapters Eight and Twelve), then Part I of the curve would describe voiced sounds and Part III voiceless sounds, while Part II represents the division between the two contrastive categories.

Stevens hypothesizes that the acoustic-auditory relationship represented by this type of curve could also underlie the set of phonological distinctive features. (For a description of features, see Chapter One, Table 1-1, and Chapter Six, Table 6-1.) He does not claim that a simple auditory property detector underlies each distinctive feature, but he maintains a strong interest in neurophysiological research that could lead to the discovery of such simple response systems. For example, Hawkins and Stevens (1985) suggested such a potential system might underlie the distinction between non-nasal and nasalized vowels. When a vowel is nasalized, the spectrum in the vicinity of the first formant is broader and less prominent (lower in amplitude) than when the same vowel is not nasalized, as we noted in Chapter Four. Neurophysiological work (Sachs & Young, 1980) shows that frequency-sensitive cells in the cat's auditory nerve fire in qualitatively different ways when a spectral peak has a broad bandwidth and low amplitude, compared with when it has a narrow bandwidth and high amplitude. Hawkins and Stevens (1985) suggested that these different response patterns might underlie the nasal-nonnasal distinction for vowels.

However, it is important to realize that the auditory pathway is complex. Transformations to the signal that occur in the auditory nerve are not necessarily preserved in the same relationship until they reach the part of the brain where the signal is understood as speech. Thus, the acoustic-auditory work is more speculative than the work on articulatory-acoustic relationships. While the latter is rooted strongly in acoustic theory, much of it Stevens' own, the former is based on neurophysiological studies of nonhuman animals in the literature, or on inferences from behavioral changes in humans in response to acoustic stimuli. Speculations about neural processes made from quantal theory, though interesting, must be treated cautiously.

Invariant Acoustic Correlates of Distinctive Features and Speech Perception

1. For every phonological distinctive feature, there is an invariant property or pattern that the auditory system is sensitive to. Some of these properties are present in the acoustic signal itself; others arise in the auditory system as the signal is processed. Invariant properties reflect short-term states of the vocal tract or changes in its behavior at critical times.
2. Presence of an invariant property signals a positive value of a distinctive feature; absence signals a negative value.
3. Under ideal conditions, the perceptual system responds in an all-or-nothing way to the presence or absence of each property, so its output is in terms of binary values of features, ready to feed directly into the listener's phonological system.
4. Words are stored in terms of bundles of distinctive features rather than phonemes. Mapping between auditory responses to the signal and the lexicon is thus comparatively direct. Phonemes are not involved in word identification. Under some speaking or listening conditions, values of invariant properties may not be binary.

Quantal theory holds that at certain times in an utterance the speech signal is especially rich in linguistically relevant information. This information is invariant, either due to the quantal properties of the articulatory-acoustic relationships of speech or to quantal responses of the auditory system to particular types of acoustic property. A natural extension of this thinking is that there will be an invariant property of the signal to which the auditory system is especially sensitive for every linguistic unit. Stevens has looked systematically for such invariant properties over a wide range of linguistic contrasts. Much of this thinking is summarized in his exposition of quantal theory (Stevens, 1989), but he has also treated them separately, as the theory of acoustic invariance.

Stevens' approach is like that of the Motor Theorists in that it assumes that invariant properties can be directly linked to linguistic units. It differs from Motor Theory in two main ways. First, it assumes the invariants are part of the signal itself or of an early stage in the auditory pathway's response to the acoustic signal. Second, it is quite explicit in assuming the linguistic units are smaller than phones or phonemes, namely the distinctive features of phonology. Thus, Stevens set himself the task of searching for invariant properties of the acoustic signal that are acoustic or auditory correlates of phonological distinctive features.

As discussed in Chapter Six, distinctive feature systems use a small set of labels (or categories) to describe acoustic or articulatory attributes of sounds that capture relationships between classes of sounds such as voicing, nasality, and place of articulation. Combined appropriately, distinctive features specify phonemic contrasts between languages and within a language. Distinctive feature systems appeal to theorists looking for a simple yet principled approach to speech perception. For example, they are speaker-independent; they have acoustic and/or articulatory descriptions yet account for phonological (phonemic) contrasts; most are binary, meaning that the feature is classed as either present or absent (but not partly present), which makes it easy to come up with clear contrasting categories; they are intended to be universal—to account for all phonemic contrasts in all languages of the world; and there are only a few of them, normally about 20.

Distinctive features also offer a number of other advantages. For example, each phoneme is composed of a group (or "bundle") of distinctive features, but the features themselves do not have to start and stop at exactly the same time. So the feature *nasal* can start before the feature *consonantal*, thus describing anticipatory coarticulation of nasality onto a preceding vowel. Thus, when the distinctive feature is taken as the basic linguistic unit, there need be no assumptions that the signal must segment into "vertical time slices" corresponding to phones or phonemes. Indeed, there is no longer any requirement for a phonemic level of analysis at all.

A major strength is that distinctive feature systems have been a central tool of phonology for at least half a century. (Chapter One describes phonology and its important uses in linguistics). Since phonology describes the sound patterns of languages, these systems potentially offer a neat link between the acoustic signal and the linguistic systems that the output of the speech perception mechanism must feed into. That the phonologies come from another discipline also gives acoustic distinctive features an independent credibility.

In accordance with these ideas, Stevens turned away from the traditional reliance on spectrograms in searching for cues for different phonemes. Instead, he used other types of analysis, usually spectra. As they are typically used, spectra show less temporal information than spectrograms, but they give a clearer picture of the amplitude of the acoustic signal at particular frequencies. By comparing spectra made at the boundary between two adjacent acoustic segments, or just before and just after it, Stevens tried to identify acoustic properties that are always present as the vocal tract moves from one manner of articulation to another, or from one particular place of articulation to another.

Stevens used Chomsky and Halle's (1968) articulatory feature system. He reasoned that each articulatory feature must have an acoustic correlate, because each articulatory configuration has a predictable acoustic consequence. He and a colleague, Sheila Blumstein, worked at first on invariant acoustic correlates for place of articulation for stops, the class of sounds that are basic to speech yet are very difficult to describe simply. They first proposed that spectra of the early part of stop consonant releases (the transient and beginning of the

transitions taken together) are of very invariant form, depending mainly on the place of release and independent of the variation in tongue configurations that results from anticipation of different following vowels. Thus they viewed an invariant property as static: a spectral shape that conformed to a very simple "template" (Blumstein & Stevens, 1979; Stevens & Blumstein, 1978). This mirrored the traditional interpretation of distinctive features as describing static articulatory or acoustic states.

These first ideas about acoustic invariance are illustrated in Figure 14-5. The top left panel shows the spectrum of about 26 ms taken from the burst and vowel onset of a /b/, as shown in the waveform below it. Notice that the spectrum is relatively flat and falling (its amplitude is greater at low frequencies than at high ones). All the peaks of this spectrum lie between the two parallel dashed lines that also slope downwards across the spectrum from low to high frequencies. Stevens and Blumstein suggested that any burst spectrum whose peaks lie within these two parallel lines would be identified as bilabial. The dashed lines represent the "bilabial template."

The middle and right-hand panels of Figure 14-5 show the same principles for, respectively, alveolar and velar stop bursts and vocalic onsets. The alveolar template in the top middle panel is like the bilabial one in that it consists of two parallel lines, but it slopes upwards with increasing frequency rather than downwards. The peaks of the spectrum of the example alveolar burst all fall within the areas enclosed by the two dashed lines. The velar template has a single hump in the middle frequencies, and the spectrum from around the natural velar burst also has a peak within this region. In Blumstein and Stevens' (1979) database of several hundred stops in isolated CV and VC syllables, the spectral peaks of more than 80% of the syllable-initial bursts and vowel onsets and syllable-final bursts were accepted by the correct template and rejected by the other two.

The shapes of these templates are not arbitrary; nor are they derived solely from measurement of the spectra of stops. They reflect the main acoustic

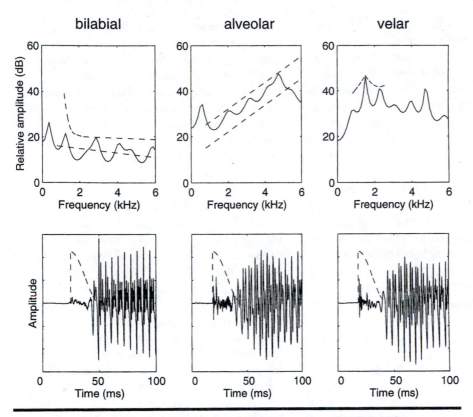

FIGURE 14-5. Spectral templates proposed by Stevens and Blumstein for determining place of articulation of stops. In the top leftmost panel, the dashed lines form the template for bilabial stops. The solid line shows the lpc spectrum of the burst and vowel onset of the syllable /bɑ/ spoken by a woman. The spectrum was made using a 26 ms window centered on the stop burst and shown as a dashed line in the waveform of the syllable onset in the lower leftmost panel. The spectral peaks fall within the slightly falling dashed lines of the template, and thus this stop would be correctly identified as bilabial. If the maximum amplitude of a spectral peak within the frequency-range of the template fell outside the dashed lines, the syllable would be classed as not bilabial. The upper middle panel shows the alveolar template (dashed lines) and the lpc spectrum of the burst of a "good" /dɑ/ from the same speaker: The amplitudes of the peaks within the frequency range of the template all fall within its upper and lower limits. The lower middle panel shows the waveform and spectral window from which the spectrum was taken. The rightmost panels show the velar template and a "good" /gɑ/ from the same speaker. The velar template has no lower limit—it requires only that mid-frequency spectral peaks do not rise above the outlines of the dashed line, which gets broader as the frequency of the most prominent peak rises. Only one such template is shown here, suitable for the frequency of the spectral prominence with greatest amplitude in this particular syllable.

properties associated with the shape of the vocal tract at the moment of release of a stop. The bilabial template slopes downwards with increasing frequency because a sound source at the lips, as for /b, p, f, v/, is at the end of the vocal tract, with no resonating cavity in front of it to shape the sound with its own natural frequencies. The sound escapes immediately into the air. The upward sloping alveolar template captures the fact that higher frequencies are excited more than lower frequencies, mainly because the sound source created in the vicinity of an alveolar constriction mostly excites the the short cavity in front of the constriction, between the alveolar ridge and the lips. The single, mid-frequency hump of the velar template mainly reflects two things. First, when the constriction that makes the sound source is in the velar region, a resonance associated with the front cavity has a very similar frequency to one of the resonances of the back cavity, and so this back cavity resonance is excited in sympathy with the front cavity resonance, even though the sound source is in front of it. Second, the constriction is relatively far back in the mouth, so the front cavity is quite long, with correspondingly low-frequency formants.

Blumstein and Stevens (1980) went on to show that listeners can identify both stops and vowels quite well from short synthetic stimuli whose onset or offset spectra conformed to the patterns specified by acoustic theory. They interpreted their data as confirming a theory of speech perception in which place of articulation is cued by invariant properties of the spectrum over a very short section of a syllable, for example, the release bursts of Figure 14-5.

These ideas were very appealing. However, although the templates accounted reasonably well for a majority of stops in clearly spoken syllables, they accounted for too few to make them the sole basis of speech perception. Kewley-Port (1983) showed that better identification of CVs was obtained using a series of spectra made at 5 ms intervals over the first 40 ms from the release of the stop. These are illustrated in Figure 14-6. The criteria she suggested are similar to Blumstein and Stevens' (1979) templates, but they separate the burst and vocalic onset spectra and add more information such as place-dependent differences in VOT. See also Figures 9-2 and 9-3, pp. 135–136.

Kewley-Port had demonstrated that dynamic information reflecting changes in vocal tract con-

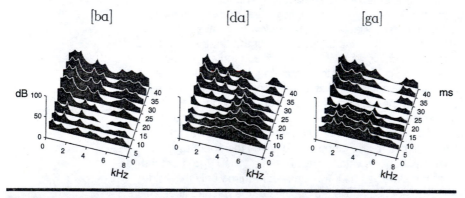

FIGURE 14-6. The burst and vowel onset from each of the stimuli in Figure 14-5, shown here as 8 lpc spectra (with a 26 ms Hanning window) taken at 5 ms intervals over the first 40 ms of each syllable. The first spectrum is centered on the stop burst, and the last ones include much of the vocalic transitions. These "waterfall" spectra illustrate the principles that Kewley-Port (1983) proposed as better than the simple templates of Stevens and Blumstein for distinguishing place of articulation of syllable-initial stops.

figuration must be included in descriptions of potential acoustic invariants. Stevens and Blumstein's later work also incorporated explicit dynamic information, though again the emphasis was on maximal simplicity. For example, instead of Kewley-Port's series of spectra from the burst through the transitions into the vowel, Lahiri, Gewirth, and Blumstein (1984) proposed that place of articulation could be identified from the relationship between just two spectra, one made at the release transient and the other being the average of the first three voiced periods following the release. (The stops they measured, including from Malayalam and French, had short VOTs, so voicing began very soon after the release.) This approach incorporates the principle that invariants should reflect changes *across* acoustic segment boundaries and are thus *relational* rather than based on static templates.

Later work followed this same principle of describing potential relational invariants in terms of just two or three spectra, one on either side of an acoustic segment boundary, and began to search for an invariant relational acoustic property for each of Chomsky and Halle's (1968) distinctive features. Although Stevens and colleagues have proposed invariants for most features in Chomsky and Halle's system, only some are published in detail (e.g., Kurowski & Blumstein 1987, Lahiri et al., 1984; Stevens 1980, 1985; Stevens & Blumstein, 1981). Summaries are in Stevens (1983, 1989). Here, we give just two examples of proposed relational acoustic invariants for consonantal distinctive features: *consonantal* and *strident*.

As its name suggests, the feature *consonantal* distinguishes oral and nasal stops, fricatives, affricates (and also prevocalic [l ɹ]) from nonconsonantal sounds, which include vowels and [h, w, j]. Sounds that are consonantal have a narrow constriction in the midline of the vocal tract. The acoustic consequence of such a narrow constriction is that there is a rapid change in the shape or the amplitude of the spectrum as the constriction is made and then released. Sounds that are nonconsonantal have a less narrow constriction, and in consequence less abrupt changes in

spectral shape and amplitude. Figure 14-7 illustrates this for the sounds [b] and [w] in the syllables *bet* and *wet*: [bɛt] and [wɛt].

The left-hand side of Figure 14-7 shows a spectrogram of [bɛt] at the top, and three superimposed 26 ms spectra below. The spectrum labeled 0 ms is taken from the release burst of the stop, and the other two are taken respectively 10 ms and 20 ms later. The vertical arrows on the spectrogram show where the spectra were taken from. On the right-hand side of the figure, the same data are given for [wɛt], the spectra being made from where the formant frequencies change most rapidly as the approximant gives way to the vowel. There is much more difference in both shape and overall amplitude between the three spectra from [b] than between the three from [w]. The differences between the spectra from [bɛt] indicate a consonantal sound, while the similarities between the spectra from [wɛt] indicate a non-consonantal sound.

Figure 14-8 illustrates the difference between the strident [s] and the nonstrident [θ] in *sing* and *thing*. Strident consonants are a subgroup of the fricatives and affricates—roughly, the sibilant or "hissy" ones, [s, ʃ, z, ʒ, ʧ, ʤ]. All other sounds are nonstrident, so the feature strident subdivides the fricatives and affricates into two sets and distinguishes the strident set from every other sound. A strident consonant results from a rapid airstream being directed against an obstacle such as the teeth. When the air hits the teeth, the amplitude of the noise increases greatly in the high frequencies. Because the spectrum of a strident sound slopes upwards as frequency increases, the amplitude of the spectrum at high frequencies is greater in strident consonants than in a following vowel. Nonstrident consonants have lower-amplitude energy at high frequencies than in the following vowel. The spectrograms at the top of Figure 14-8 show this difference, but it is easier to see in the spectra beneath them.

In summary, invariance theory proposes a distinct acoustic or auditory correlate of every distinctive feature in the Chomsky and Halle (1968) system. An invariant is either present in the signal

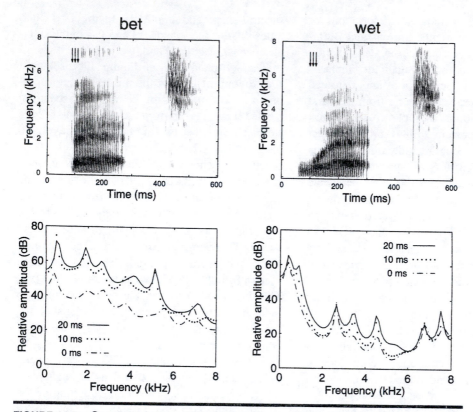

FIGURE 14-7. Spectrograms and 26 ms lpc spectra illustrating Stevens' suggested acoustic invariants for the feature *consonantal*. The top left panel shows a spectrogram of the word *bet*. The three arrows at the consonantal release are spaced at 10 ms intervals and indicate where the three superimposed spectra in the lower left panel were centered: 0 ms was centered on the stop release burst, and the other two were centered respectively 10 ms and 20 ms later. The top right panel shows a spectrogram of *wet*, and the three arrows, also at 10 ms intervals, show where the three spectra in the lower right panel were centered: in the region of fastest change between the approximant and the vowel. Both words were spoken by a woman. The /b/ of *bet* is consonantal because there are large differences between successive spectra at its release. The /w/ of *wet* is nonconsonantal because successive spectra at the release of the /w/ are very similar to one another.

itself or in the auditory transform of the signal. These invariant correlates of phonological distinctive features reflect the way the signal changes as the vocal tract moves, so they are relational, exploit quantal relationships, and are found in short (10–40 ms) sections at the boundaries of acoustic segments. Since the only acoustic consistencies are due to articulatory consistencies, perceptual responses naturally must reflect the articulatory sources, but no articulatory representation is necessary to the perceptual process nor to its aquisition by the child.

Lexical Access from Features (The LAFF Model of Speech Perception)

The Lexical Access from Features (LAFF) model of speech perception is Stevens' (1986, 1988;

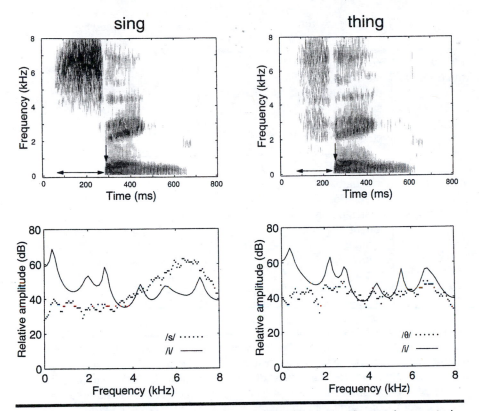

FIGURE 14-8.   Spectrograms and 26 ms lpc spectra illustrating Stevens' suggested acoustic invariants for the feature *strident*. The speaker and layout are the same as for Figure 14-7, but only two spectra were made for each word: The fricative spectra (dots) are average dft spectra calculated over the range indicated by the horizontal arrow in each upper panel, and the vocalic onsets (solid lines) are 26 ms lpc spectra centered at the point indicated by the vertical arrow in each upper panel. The /s/ of *sing* is strident because the amplitude of its spectrum at high frequencies (4–6 kHz) is greater than that of the following vowel onset. The /θ/ of *thing* is nonstrident because the amplitude of its high-frequency spectrum is less than that of the following vowel.

Stevens, Manuel, Shattuck-Hufnagel, & Liu, 1992) model of how words are identified from the acoustic signal. In this model, words are stored in the brain as patterns of distinctive features. There are no phonemes. There are some important differences from the standard way of representing features, illustrated in Figure 14-9 for the word *tan*. Temporal sequencing of the features is roughly indicated by whether the feature (or acoustic/auditory event, a relational invariant) occurs at the beginning, middle, or end of the standard acoustic

segment for that phone, or sound. So in Figure 14-9 the + for the nasal feature occurs before the other attributes of /n/, indicating anticipatory coarticulation of nasality. For any given word, each feature is marked in one of three possible ways. It may have either a plus or minus if its value is crucial to the sound in that word, or no specification if the value of the feature is irrelevant, is predictable from the values of other features, or can vary freely, or it may have a tag [M] to show the feature can be modified in some circumstances,

Type of feature	Specific feature	Lexical specification		
		t	æ	n
Articulator-free: Landmark (Mainly manner of articulation)	consonantal	+	−	+
	sonorant	−	+	
	continuant	−		−
	syllabic		+	
	lateral			−
	strident			−
Articulator-bound 1 (Place of articulation)	lips round			
	tongue blade	+		+M
	anterior	+		+M
	distributed	−		−M
	tongue dorsum		+	
	high		−	
	low		+	
	back		−	
Articulator-bound 2	voiced	−	+	
	nasal	−	+	

FIGURE 14-9.   General form of the lexical representation of the word *tan* according to LAFF. Positive values of features are shown by +, and negative values by −. M next to a feature value shows that the feature may be modified in different contexts. The vertical displacement of the features with respect to one another and to phone boundaries shows the relative time of occurrence of each featural "event" during the perception of the word. Consistent with an approach stressing economy of information and the emphasis on short-time acoustic or auditory "events," the value of a feature is noted only when it changes. The list of features shown is partial, and Stevens' use of these particular features is tentative.

for example in connected speech processes. In Figure 14-9 the place of articulation features for the /n/ of *tan* are marked M because alveolar nasals at the ends of words can be assimilated to the place of articulation of the following phone.

The features are organized into categories or tiers, rather as in autosegmental phonology (Goldsmith, 1990, or see any recent phonology textbook). One category, the "landmark" features, describes manner of articulation (the degree of constriction) and so distinguishes between the syllable nucleus and its margins. Features in this category include consonantal and sonorant, and are "articulator-free" inasmuch as they are specified independently of particular articulators. A second category shows place of articulation (the major articulator involved in the constriction).

These include features that describe lip, tongue blade, and tongue body position. A third category shows values for additional articulators that are involved—for example, the spread glottis to produce aspiration upon release of an initial voiceless stop, and the position of the velum that determines whether an alveolar stop is oral or nasal.

Landmarks for consonants are a boundary between two acoustic segments, as described above. For vowels, they are where the vocal tract is maximally open between two consonants, and hence approximately at the center of a vowel steady state, identified as the point between two consonantal landmarks where F1 is highest in frequency and low-frequency amplitude is greatest.

Word identification takes place as follows. The speech signal is perceived as a series of relational acoustic or auditory correlates of distinctive features. These are identified in a particular order that increases the efficiency of identification. First, landmark features that define manner of articulation and hence syllable structure are identified. Next, the region around each landmark feature is examined for evidence of features for place of articulation. Only place features appropriate for the particular landmark features are evaluated, and the particular place in the signal that is evaluated depends on what manners of articulation have been identified. This series of invariant correlates is matched directly against the feature matrix for each word in the mental lexicon, without reference to phonemes.

The LAFF model includes two interesting and important departures from Stevens' earlier assumptions about acoustic invariance and emphasis on binarity. First, features can be represented with different degrees of strength (or certainty), which reflects the fact that the signal is clearer at some times or in some circumstances than at others. At the time of writing, however, Stevens does not espouse this position (personal communication). Second, each specified feature in a lexical item includes information about its relative importance in the word. In effect, the first point allows so-called invariants to be rather variable, and the second could introduce probability weightings against each expected binary value of a feature. This means that although features in the lexicon are binary, the listener's responses can vary more continuously. Both principles acknowledge the need to allow for variation in the way words are pronounced, and may represent a movement away from a strict interpretation of acoustic correlates of distinctive features as invariant.

As Stevens acknowledges, more work is needed in several areas, for example, to show how words are identified in connected speech, but this model is promising in that it is based on solid theoretical principles and has been partially implemented as a computer program (Stevens, Blumstein, Glicksman, Burton, & Kurowski, 1992).

In summary, the quantal theory of speech and more particularly its development, acoustic invariance theory, posit that each place or manner of articulation always results in the same (invariant) acoustic or auditory response. Invariance theory assumes that the output of the perceptual system is in terms of binary (plus or minus) values for phonological distinctive features. The LAFF model of speech perception proposes that the lexicon is stored in terms of distinctive features; the auditory system's responses to the invariant acoustic correlates of distinctive features in the acoustic signal are mapped directly onto the binary feature maps that comprise the lexicon, with some allowance made for variation in the clarity with which invariants are present in the signal. Phonemes are not identified before words are identified.

Evaluation of the Quantal Theory of Speech, Relational Invariance, and LAFF

There have been fewer experimental tests of Stevens' theory than of the Motor Theory of speech perception, and more evaluations of quantal theory concern speech production than perception. Since "quantal regions" in the acoustic output provide one form of acoustic invariance, we will discuss evidence from production as well as perception, although we will give more attention to issues that directly concern perception.

Quantal Theory   We consider first the view that quantal theory is fundamentally wrong. Some experiments have compared the degree of acoustic or articulatory variation in various "quantal" sounds with that in "nonquantal" sounds, or observed whether steady changes in one parameter cause quantal changes in output. Several of these studies suffer from the same flaw as the theory itself: It is difficult to define "precision" and how much variation in, say, formant frequencies, constitutes "no difference." Making comparisons between vocal-tract parameters can be like comparing apples with oranges: Different articulators can be controlled with different degrees of precision, a change of 50 Hz may be noticeable at 800 Hz, but not at 2000 Hz, and so on. Additionally, many vocal-tract parameters interact because of the way the vocal tract works. In consequence, it is hard to test the claim that a particular quantal effect results from a change in a single parameter, and even harder to assess whether, if true, the effect is reliable enough in real speech to be a plausible basis for distinguishing between two sound categories.

Although some tests of quantal theory have been negative (e.g., Pisoni, 1980), sophisticated studies of movement together with acoustics give cautious support to quantal theory. Perkell and Nelson (1985) and Beckman and colleagues (Beckman, Jung, Lee, de Jong, Krishamurthy, Ahalt, Cohen, & Collins, 1995), for example, measured the location and degree of constriction made by the tongue for peripheral (i.e., noncentral) vowels and correlated these with their formant frequencies. Consistent with quantal theory, they found more variation in articulation along the front-back axis of the vocal tract (in constriction location) than variation perpendicular to the vocal tract midline (in constriction degree). That is, within the range of articulations appropriate for a given vowel, speakers in these studies seemed to exercise less precision over a constriction's location than over its degree. This is important because (within the specified range) formant frequencies reflected the degree of the constriction more closely than its location.

As we noted for the Motor Theory, a theory need not be wrong because it is hard to verify empirically. One of the most important strengths of quantal theory is that it is rooted in acoustical theory. To the extent that the acoustical theory of speech production is valid, the observations of quantal theory will be valid. For production, this is a major strength. It is less obviously an advantage for perception because the generalizations to perception are more speculative. However, the emphasis on links between production and perception is appealing.

Among the most serious criticisms of quantal theory is that it cannot explain details of sounds that distinguish many aspects of variation between languages and accents. Ladefoged and Bhaskararao (1983) present x-rays showing that although retroflex is a "quantal" sound, it is produced in quite different ways by speakers of different languages of India. This criticism limits the generality of quantal theory: A comprehensive theory must explain why languages and accents differ so much in the details of basically similar sounds, and why speakers learn exactly the right details for their accent. On the other hand, it is most unlikely that the complex and redundant speech production-perception system can be explained by a single simple system, and quantal theory could be used as an elegant partial explanation, especially of the production and perception of many of the basic sound categories of speech.

This argument brings us to the next criticism, that quantal theory is too narrow. According to this view, the general approach has merit, but it stresses some factors while ignoring others that may be just as important. It is narrow in two ways: It is not clear how closely it applies to connected or fluent speech, and it ignores some important influences on the nature of speech. We consider these in turn.

The appeal of quantal theory lies partly in its simplicity, whereby a particular acoustic pattern is related to change in a single parameter. But this simplicity is gained at some cost. Consonants have been modeled in rather few contexts, and no attention has been given to changes due to prosody. In fluent speech, coarticulation and processes such as elision and assimilation modify places, lengths, and degrees of constrictions. If quantal relations hold for the simple situations of canonical CV syllables, they are unlikely to be so influential in a heavily coarticulated, casually spoken utterance. Yet people still understand these utterances.

The second accusation of narrowness brings us to one of the more serious criticisms of quantal theory as a model of speech production: Some sounds that it explains most easily are not those that are most common in languages of the world. For example, quantal theory accounts better for retroflex and pharyngeal consonants than alveolars. This is a problem because alveolars occur in most languages, whereas retroflexes and pharyngeals are rare. This type of criticism suggests that quantal theory alone is not enough to explain sound inventories. There must be other influencing factors besides articulatory or auditory precision, and nonlinearities between articulation and acoustics. In perception, these additional factors can be higher-order linguistic knowledge, and enough contrast of the right general sort rather than maximum consistent contrast. In production, some additional factors might be ease or naturalness of articulation, and sensory feedback. For example, in fluent, rapid speech it is easier to move the tip of the tongue to make alveolar and dental consonants than strongly retroflex consonants. Similarly, pharyngeal consonants are probably more difficult to make than lingual and labial consonants. There is also evidence that the most common articulation for an /i/ is a little further back in the mouth than that for the ideal "quantal" vowel; the more backed articulation involves greater contact between the tongue and the palate, and thus more sensory feedback.

Quantal theory looks for regions of acoustic stability and maximal contrasts between particular features such as place of articulation along the vocal tract, largely ignoring the structure of the system as a whole. Lindblom (1986) and Lindblom and Engstrand (1989) argue that sufficient rather than maximal contrast should be stressed. From computer models that implement the notion of sufficient perceptual and articulatory contrast to predict the particular sound contrasts a language will use given the total number of phonemes it has, he concludes that there is a tendency for each language to employ sufficiently distinctive contrasts, but not necessarily to seek maximal distinctiveness between its contrasts. So, for example, most languages that have five vowels have categories that correspond to /i, ɛ, a, o, u/. Quantal theory predicts /y/ instead of /ɛ/. Like /i/, /y/ has F3 close to F2 and so is stable in quantal terms and should be favored by languages, but it is in fact quite rare. In contrast, /ɛ/ is not a stable vowel in quantal terms because its formants are quite

widely spaced, so it should be rare, but it is in fact common. In other work, Lindblom (1990, 1996) suggests a larger number of principles that govern the sounds of language, how adult listeners perceive them, and how children learn them. These include ease of articulation and shared knowledge between speaker and hearer, and they are discussed further below. Quantal theory and invariance theory can contribute to Lindblom's models (cf., Diehl, 1989; Lindblom & Engstrand, 1989) but on their own they do not account for all the data.

Relational Invariance The theory of acoustic invariance has similar strengths to quantal theory, and is criticized in similar ways: It is claimed to be too simplistic, too narrow, or not to account for all the data. One problem is that convincing invariant properties have not been found for all features. For example, in practice it is hard to distinguish between *consonantal* and *continuant*, because both involve presence versus absence of rapid spectral change. (Fricatives and most approximants are distinguished from other consonants by being continuant.) Consonantal sounds involve a rapid change in spectral shape, which normally involves a change in spectral amplitude as well, but Stevens (1989) describes noncontinuant sounds as having an abrupt increase in amplitude in the mid or high frequencies. This definition also produces a rapid change in spectral shape, so the same acoustic property is associated with two features.

Setting aside definitional problems, which are always open to refinement and change, there are at least two reasons why invariance theory must be only partly correct at best. First, most invariants describe short-term events, yet the durations of segments are perceptually important. Many experiments on cue trading demonstrate this point. Vowel duration contributes to perceived vowel quality and to properties of other sounds, such as the voicing of consonants in final syllabic position; the duration and amplitude envelope of noise helps to distinguish between voiced and voiceless fricatives, between fricatives and affricates, and between stops and fricatives; the durations of formant transitions can distinguish between vowels and approximants, and there are strict limits on the possible range of durations of the transition in a diphthong. Similarly, rhythm, though acknowledged as important, is ignored, as it is by all phonetic theories of speech perception.

Second, most definitions of acoustic invariants apply mainly, or only, to CV and sometimes VC syllables, and even for these restricted contexts, there are sometimes problems, either in the definitions themselves, or because some syllables lack the properties identified as invariant yet are highly intelligible. As with quantal theory, consonants have been modeled in few contexts. Although some of the proposed invariants, such as strident consonants, are resilient to changes in segmental or prosodic context and style of speaking, others are not. Consider English velar stops, which are fronted before front vowels and backed before back vowels. The relational invariant for velars is the compact mid-frequency spectral peak described above for velars, together with the requirement that it should be continuous with F2 or F3 or lie between them. But this relationship is reliably found only with back vowels like /gɑ/ and /gu/ and much less with fronted syllables like /gi/, whose spectra can look more like alveolars than velars (for example, see Figures 9-4 and 9-5). The bursts and transitions of rounded alveolars like /du/, in contrast, often look like velars. (Although they have different temporal patterns and formant transitions, these properties have not been formalized in the theory of relational invariance).

A number of solutions have been applied to this problem. Stevens, Keyser, and Kawasaki (1986), reasoning from the facts that no language uses all the phonological distinctive features contrastively and that distinctive features often occur together, suggested a theory of "redundant features" and enhancement of properties. Redundancy is optional in that a language may or may not use it. One type of redundancy occurs when a feature that is not used distinctively in some phonemic contrast nevertheless contributes to it. Put another way, when a phonemic distinction is hard to perceive, it may be made easier by adding

another feature that enhances the acoustic contrast or that adds another acoustic property that helps make the distinction clearer. Examples are the secondary distinctions between alveolar and dental stops, and the redundant co-occurrence of rounding with back vowels in most languages.

In Malayalam, a language of India, dental stops are laminal (made with the blade of the tongue) and alveolar stops are apical (made with the tip of the tongue). In featural terms, laminal stops are distributed, and apical stops are not distributed. The acoustical difference between these stops is very subtle and hard to hear, mainly involving slightly faster release of the tongue tip than the tongue blade. Malayalam enhances the difference by introducing another feature, tongue fronting/backing. The body of the tongue is more fronted during the alveolar stop than the dental stop. Fronting the tongue body raises the frequency of F2, and the raised frequency presumably functions as an additional—or perhaps on occasion the primary—acoustic cue to the distinction. Interestingly, Donegal Irish has a different articulatory way of achieving the same pattern of enhancement: The low frequencies of apico-dentals are emphasized by velarizing or pharyngealizing them, while, as in Malayalam, their high frequencies of laminal postalveolars are emphasized by palatalization.

The co-occurrence of labialization (lip rounding) with back vowels is another example of enhancement. A tongue constriction towards the back of the mouth and a constriction at the lips both tend to lower formant frequencies, especially F2. So lip rounding can enhance the acoustic effect of backing the tongue. In English, theoretically back rounded vowels like /u/ are often produced either not very back or not very round; as long as one of the two features is present, listeners have no trouble perceiving the sound correctly.

This example with back rounded vowels demonstrates another aspect of redundancy: The sound system of a given language may be organized in such a way that some features do not need to be produced for a particular phonemic category to be recognized. Assimilations, discussed earlier, provide one example. As another example, consider English velar consonants. There are voiced and voiceless velar stops, /g, k/, but no velar fricatives or approximants. As long as the sound produced is back and consonantal, it does not have to be a stop: Some speakers of English usually say a voiced velar approximant or fricative rather than a stop for intervocalic /g/, and most people sometimes say them, especially in fast or casual speech. Thus, we find words like *legal* and *rugged* pronounced as [liɣəɫ] and [ɹʌɣəd]; listeners rarely notice. If enhancement through redundant features proves to be right, it may mean that the failure to find clear invariants for some features and their absence in some contexts does not hinder perception. This approach also has fascinating implications for phonology as well as perception.

Another solution to the problem that invariant correlates for some distinctive features have not been found for all contexts is to restrict the list of invariants. Stevens has not tried this, but Zue and his colleagues (e.g., Zue, 1985) identified a set of about seven "robust features" that provide very reliable cues to phonetic identity across many contexts, speakers, and speaking styles. Candidates for robust features are strong fricatives (the strident ones, like [s, z] and [ʃ, ʒ]), weak fricatives ([f, v, θ, ð]), nasal, voicing (periodicity in the spectrogram), silence, transient, and vowel. Among

vowels, high can normally be distinguished from low, and front from back. All these robust features are familiar from previous chapters, and they are very clear on spectrograms. You might like to identify them for yourself in the spectrogram in Figure 14-10, of "My family lives in Oxford" (Southern British accent). An advantage of robust features is that they are largely independent of one another. Although several robust features are described in terms of single acoustic segments rather than as changes across segmental boundaries, most could be described in terms of relational properties, like Stevens' relational invariants.

Robust features are not, of course, sufficient to allow words to be identified without other information. But they may offer a reliable core of invariant acoustic features from which to make preliminary decisions about what words were spoken, together with knowledge about the particular language (permissible sound sequences, the lexicon, grammar, and meaning). This makes them potentially very powerful, especially in poor listening conditions when the acoustic signal is of limited reliability. Zue's group has used this method successfully in systems for automatic speech recognition.

However, the evidence from babies' perception of speech suggests that robust features provide only one type of basic acoustic information. Distinctions between quite complex stimuli seem to

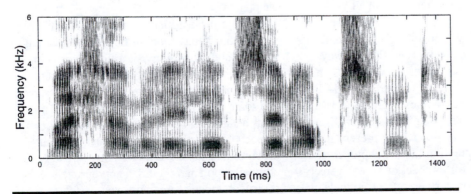

FIGURE 14-10. Spectrogram of the sentence *My family lives in Oxford* (male speaker, British accent).

be made from early infancy with no trouble at all, at least in good listening conditions. One might assume that evidence of babies' perceptual skills supports the idea of acoustic invariants. It is certainly easier to explain babies' perceptual abilities within a system that provides a small number of invariant units (like both the Motor Theory and quantal theory/acoustic invariance theory) than to assume that the baby is initially sensitive to all the variation in the speech signal and must learn to impose a relatively simple linguistic code on it. But the evidence points in both directions. Kuhl's demonstration of the perceptual magnet effect and Werker's of decreased ability to discriminate between non-native contrasts after about 10 months of age show that category formation is language-specific and develops throughout the first year of life at least. As with many aspects of speech, there seem to be several different types of influence at work.

The undoubted strengths of the relational invariance approach make it attractive despite its acknowledged problems. For example, phonetically, it represents a useful attempt to describe invariance "within" acoustic variability, and it is theoretically appealing because distinctive features are independently motivated from phonology. That is, they were developed for different reasons in a different discipline. (It is also true, however, that some of the features are slightly redefined from Chomsky and Halle's originals because they suit the acoustic data better. This is seen as a strength by some researchers, but not all.) As with quantal theory, the emphasis on simple properties is appealing and worthwhile. For example, it encouraged more innovative and flexible ways of looking at the acoustic signal, and, because it is simple, the approach is more easily tested—and refuted—than a more complex approach. It is also rather more testable than the Motor Theory because invariants are potentially present in the signal itself. The stress on relational properties is probably essential for a model of speech perception: Relational properties reflect articulatory gestures and reduce the problem for perception

of systematic variability due to factors that may be irrelevant to the meaning of the message itself, such as the size of the speaker's vocal tract, his or her speaking rate, and phonetic context. Finally, although it seems clear that relational invariants cannot be found at present for all distinctive features, it is also clear that when they are present in the signal, they provide powerful cues to important phonetic contrasts.

Evaluation of LAFF   Several aspects of LAFF need more work, as Stevens notes. Like the Motor Theory, LAFF is vague on how decisions are made and on how weightings on features are translated into binary values. Although the problem of allophonic variation at word boundaries is acknowledged by using the M feature, how this works is not yet explained. Prosodic effects need to be included, the most urgent being the durational properties of acoustic segments, which are at least as important as the spectral properties of speech. Representing durational properties as asynchronies between feature onsets is a start in the right direction, but only tells us about sequencing, and not about actual durations. Further testing will probably show that the model accounts for only some speech, and although it retains quite a lot of information about variability because it includes the relative strength of features and avoids translating features into phonemes, some researchers believe it may still throw away too much information, as we shall see in the next chapter.

Despite these criticisms, this model is impressive in that it has roots in both acoustical engineering and phonology, it offers a principled, systematic way of deriving a series of discrete linguistic units from the variable acoustic signal, and some of its main stages have been implemented as a successful computer program. Although it neglects some important areas, such as timing, it provides a testable set of ideas that can be gradually built upon and modified appropriately. Some statistical models are more successful at word identification, but they do not use so much information about the relationship between vocal tract behavior, acoustics, and linguistic structure. This alone makes LAFF valuable.

General Summary of Quantal Theory

Quantal theory is based on acoustic theory, so to the extent that acoustic theory is right, quantal theory may offer valid principles for both speech production and perception. But much of the work on auditory transforms is speculative, and there are serious problems in that canonical articulations are comparatively rare in natural speech, articulatory parameters interact in complex ways that quantal theory intentionally neglects, and connected speech processes are not accounted for. The issue of variation between languages in the details of sounds also needs to be addressed. Overall, the data suggest that quantal theory will not explain either speech production or perception by itself. Its main fault is that it is too narrow to explain as multifaceted a system as speech. Stevens is aware of these failings and keeps the approach narrow to allow more detailed testing of the very complicated articulatory-acoustical relationships he is interested in.

Quantal theory may, however, explain certain basic contrasts in speech sounds and perhaps contribute to how babies first divide up the sound space. Its emphasis on "properties" as holistic, production-based acoustic patterns, rather than on treating particular parts of the signal as separate perceptual "cues," means that it deals well with vocal tract normalization and some aspects of acoustic variability, and it could form part of a broader theory that also accounts for other influences on the speaking-hearing process. For many people, its explicit connections between articulation and perception are also a strength. Since the only acoustic consistencies are due to articulatory consistencies, perceptual responses naturally must reflect articulatory sources, but no articulatory representation is necessary to the perceptual process nor to its acquisition by the child. Thus vocal-tract dynamics are inherent in the acoustics.

The problem that there is variation in the strength of a feature in different signals has been dealt with in LAFF by removing the requirement for strict binarity. LAFF also deals well with departures from canonical articulations, but it is vague about how word boundaries are dealt with, and duration is not addressed. However, overall it is more explicit and more closely tied to the problems of natural connected speech than many phonetic theories of speech perception, and for this reason alone it is impressive. The departure from strict binarity makes LAFF more moderate than the form of acoustic invariance theory published before the mid-1980s, and this, if anything, makes the model more attractive. Speech may be better described by a flexible and redundant system than by any single rigid algorithm. This view is consistent with the suggestions of some other researchers (e.g., Lindblom) that Stevens' approach provides valuable guiding principles for incorporation into a broader theory. For the most-advanced version of quantal theory, see Stevens (in press).

A comparison of Motor and quantal theories with all other theories is made in Table 15-1 at the end of Chapter Fifteen.

REEVALUATING ASSUMPTIONS ABOUT SPEECH PERCEPTION: INTERACTIVE AND INTEGRATIVE THEORIES

SARAH HAWKINS

Viewing [extreme theoretical positions] from below, with a fuller appreciation of what might be and fewer postulates about what must be, may lead to a theory of phonological contrast that more closely resembles what is.
—Nearey, 1995

WHAT HAVE WE LEARNED FROM THE CLASSICAL THEORIES?

Research in the context of the Motor Theory and of quantal theory and its developments has failed to show convincing evidence of the consistent presence of invariant correlates of linguistic units. A minor objection to Motor Theory is that there has typically been little attempt among Motor Theorists to look for acoustic regularities that could explain perception without recourse to underlying motoric representations. More importantly, movements themselves are not invariant, and the abstract, intended gestures proposed as invariants by the revised Motor Theory are neither falsifiable nor directly supportable by empirical tests. Similar problems exist for quantal theory. Evidence for acoustic invariants has so far been found in only a small proportion of natural speech, and although invariant properties could arise in the signal as it proceeds through the auditory system, this argument is weakened at present by our ignorance of how the auditory system works.

Both approaches experience problems in that speech is more complex than either can easily account for. The Motor Theory's claim that phonetic processing takes place in a specialized module is one way of dealing with the complexity: Though the details have not been specified, it may be plausible and productive to assume that the module's attributes include the ability to deal with these complexities. Stevens' acoustically based theories try to answer the demands of complexity by the concepts of redundancy and enhancement and the departure from strict binarity of features in the LAFF model. But further modifications will be necessary, and it is possible, therefore, that any final model coming out of this approach will bear rather little resemblance to the current form.

What does research on these theories tell us? First, it suggests that the immediate units of speech perception, whatever their ultimate linguistic designation, are almost certainly relational in nature: They reflect dynamic changes in vocal-tract behavior rather than static "target states." Second, exclusive emphasis on invariance may be misguided. Third, but connected with the previous point, the importance of categorical perception in normal listening conditions may be exaggerated. Categorical perception may be something that can be produced in a laboratory but has little to do with perception of natural speech; or it may be only one of several modes of normal response, so that it plays a less crucial role in perception of natural speech than the older theories would suggest. A change in the emphasis placed on invariance and categorical perception highlights the fact that much variability in the signal is context-dependent, and because of this, it is systematic and so can provide potentially valuable information even if it is somewhat ambiguous. In particular, although coarticulatory effects can be seen as ambiguating the signal, they also contribute information, for example, that an upcoming consonant is nasal, or that a vowel will be lip-rounded. In conversational speech, such context-dependent information is often all that seems to be available to the listener; it needs closer scrutiny from a theoretical point of view. Fourth, it is probably misguided to represent speech perception as taking place in a single, particular sensory modality. Neither purely motoric nor purely acoustic information channels are appropriate. The rest of this chapter discusses more recent theoretical approaches to speech perception in the light of these points.

INVARIANCE IN THE PERCEPT BUT NOT THE OBJECT: THE THEORY OF DIRECT REALISM

Speech perception follows the same principles as all other types of sensory perception. When we perceive something, we experience the physical cause of a sensation, rather than the sensation itself. Vocal-tract gestures cause speech sounds, so listeners perceive vocal tract gestures directly, without mediation.

A General Theory of Perception

The direct realist theory of speech perception was developed from the 1980s (Fowler, 1986; Fowler & Rosenblum, 1991), partly from a wish to account for speech perception in the same theoretical framework as other aspects of perception, particularly vision, and partly from dissatisfaction with some (but not all) of the assumptions of the Motor Theory of speech perception. Unlike Motor Theorists, direct realists believe that speech is not special, but rather just another aspect of perception, governed by the laws that govern all perception. These laws are taken to be those of the direct realist school of perception developed by Eleanor and James Gibson (E. Gibson, 1991; J. Gibson, 1966) and also known as ecological psychology, or the ecological theory of perception. To understand these laws requires discussion at a very different level of analysis than most speech researchers use.

The philosophy behind direct realism is that we perceive objects and events "directly" as an immediate experience of the actual object in the environment. When either a pin or a finger presses into your skin, you do not perceive a small or a broad skin depression, but experience either a sharp or a blunt object pressing into you. You seem to perceive the object, not the sensory stimulation itself. This view contrasts sharply with that of most other theories of perception, which assume that the brain either interprets or (re)constructs the object or event from the sensory input by processing the patterns of sensation.

The direct realist philosophy stems from a functional, evolution-based view that, in order to survive, an animal must "know the world directly" not just interpret the world from indirect and partial information. Direct knowledge comes from a wide range of sources (it is polymodal) and includes information from the perceiver's own activities as well as from its sensory organs: Action and sensation interact so that their influences are indistinguishable in the percept.

Consider a child looking at a box of cookies. If the child knows what it is, has handled something like it before, and so on, it is experienced as a cookie box, as a complete object, knowing its shape even if not all of it can be seen from one position, knowing how much force to use to open it, and so on. If you have never seen a cookie box or its like before, you experience it differently: You may guess, but do not know what the shape of the invisible part is, you do not know how heavy it is, and so on. The inexperienced person has a different percept from the experienced person, even though exactly the same set of lines and colors strike both their retinas.

Direct realism makes no claims about what is innate and what is learned, but does assign an important role to learning. It claims that all perceptual systems take in sensory information such as patterns of light, or of sound waves, that are "caused" by environmental objects or events. It terms this sensory information the *proximal stimulus*. The proximal stimulus is only useful in terms of what it means about the actual physical environment, which is called the *distal object* or *distal stimulus*. In other words, the child directly perceives a box (the distal object) and not the set of lines, colors and shadows that comprise the proximal visual stimulus. The proximal visual stimulus is caused by the interaction of light on the actual object, but is in itself intrinsically meaningless: It is the physical box that is relevant to the child, and thus what is perceived.

One important property of perception is that, once you have perceived a stimulus as some particular thing, it is usually impossible, or nearly impossible, to perceive it any other way. As a perceiver, your knowledge about the environment gives meaning to the otherwise meaningless proximal stimulus; and once the proximal stimulus has been given meaning, you have no choice but to perceive the distal object—you cannot recover your earlier "unknowing" state. Most of us have this experience thing from time to time. For example, when you see a logo for the first time, or look at a picture from an unusual angle, it sometimes seems to be a meaningless jumble, but once you have recognized what it is (its structure), you can no longer see it as a jumble even if you try to.

These rules are obeyed even by ambiguous visual patterns that we see as continually alternating, such as the orientation of the Necker cube and the reversals of "figure" and "ground" that cause a picture to be experienced alternately, and uncontrollably, as two quite different things—for example, first as two faces, then as a vase. Although the observer sees these patterns alternating between two objects, it is "things" that are seen, and not unstructured jumbles. These interesting visual effects are discussed in Gregory (1970) and in many psychology textbooks.

The most important claim of direct realism, then, is that we apprehend (or experience) the perceptual object itself, rather than a representation of it, and that we actively "pick up" sensory information rather than waiting for it to come to us and then integrating it into something meaningful through a variety of mental processes.

Direct realism assumes there should be invariants in the signal. Some invariants are in the sensory signal (the proximal stimulus) because whatever causes the signal is an object or event that has predictable physical consequences. Other invariants are higher-order properties of the *distal* stimulus, the perceived object or event. They are thus not necessarily in the proximal or sensory stimulus itself, but they are available in the flow of complex stimulus information, rather than as products of mental processes or mental representation. For example, to an adult standing attentively at a busy roadside, danger is an important and invariant part of the percept of moving cars; danger is much less part of the percept for that same adult standing beside a stationary car in a driveway. Once the person has noticed that a situation is or is not dangerous, the level of danger felt is as much part of the percept as the sight and sound of the cars. It will change as the environment changes: if the cars slow down, if the person moves away from the side of the road, and so on. A small child needs to learn that danger is attached to the roadside but not normally to the driveway situation, so the same proximal stimuli provide different percepts to the child and the adult, and the child lacks access to one higher-order invariant, the roadside situation, that the adult has experienced together with the signal. Part of the process of perceptual learning involves increased "attunement" for detecting higher-order invariants in the stimulus.

Direct Realism Applied to Speech Perception

The sensory or proximal stimulus of speech is the acoustic signal and, secondarily, the sight and feel of the moving vocal tract. The distal object of speech is the cause of these things: the gestures, because it is gestures that cause significant acoustic or vocal-tract events, such as complete bilabial closure, partial alveolar closure, and moderate jaw lowering. For direct realists, it must be the speaker's actual motoric gestures that the listener perceives, because these gestures cause the structure in the acoustic signal, just as a physical chair (plus light) causes the patterns of light that form the proximal stimulus for the percept of a chair. For speech perception to follow the same biological principles as other modes of perception, gestures are the necessary perceptual "primitives," the basic elements upon which a theory is built and beyond which one does not need to analyze to explain, in this case, perceptions.

The gestures of the direct realist theory of speech perception are like those of articulatory phonology (Browman & Goldstein, 1992). They are the perceptually significant gestures, not the actual movements of the speaker, and for this reason direct realists prefer to use the term gestural phonology rather than articulatory phonology (e.g., Best, 1995), but the two mean the same thing. Gestures in this system refer to the place and degree of constriction of active articulators in the vocal tract. Best (1995) also suggests that listeners could pick up the overall shape and aerodynamic conditions of the vocal tract, as a higher-order invariant based on formant-frequency information. Vocal-tract shape is the distal stimulus, or object; formant frequencies are the proximal stimulus.

Notice the key difference between direct realism and the Motor Theory. The Motor Theory maintains that the perceptual primitives are the speaker's intended gestures. Direct realism sees the speaker's actual gestures as the perceptual primitives. This difference is important. The intended gestures of the Motor Theory are neuromotor commands that are specific to speech and therefore to humans. They are phonetic in character, invariant, and accessible only in the specialized phonetic module. They are invariants of the human mind. The gestures of direct realism are not speech- or language-specific. They are intrinsically nonlinguistic, so they are not necessarily specific even to humans: They are part of what humans and other animals learn about vocal tracts. Thus, direct realists assume that speech perception is not special, whereas Motor Theorists assume that it is. Moreover, unlike the Motor Theory, direct realism allows that invariance could be in the acoustic signal as well as in the percept, but is no more interested in acoustic invariance than in acoustic variability because the acoustic signal is not what is directly perceived. For a discussion of Fowler's views on acoustic invariance, see Fowler (1994).

How then are gestures related to language and meaning in direct realism? Best (1994, 1995) explains it as follows. The prelinguistic infant merely picks up the simple gestures: the closures and openings and their location in the vocal tract. With increasing exposure to a particular language, the baby becomes "attuned" to "complex coordinations among such simple gestures that correspond to language-specific phonological elements such as phonemes, syllables, and their constituents, and rhythmic units" (1995:182). Attunement to (or learning) these higher-order invariants involves learning to ignore the details of the proximal stimulus, such as the actual sounds, and focusing only on the linguistically significant higher-order percepts. In a sense, this describes a process of learning to be efficient at picking out the critical parts of the information flow. In speech-language, these critical parts form the phonetics, phonology and other higher-order linguistic units.

Direct realism's account of coarticulation is simple and elegant. Talkers produce gestures, one for each phoneme (or "phonetic segment"). Adjacent gestures are "coproduced": They overlap one another in time so that at any given point, the acoustic signal is likely to show influences of two or more phonetic gestures. Consequently, each gesture lasts for longer than the acoustic segment with which it is mainly associated, and acoustic information for that single gesture waxes and wanes over the gesture's duration. At first it is only weak, co-occurring with another stronger gesture, then it is the main information of the next acoustic segment, and finally its influence lessens, or wanes, in the following segment. Listeners "disentangle" the different influences from the signal, treating acoustic information about a given segment, b, that is present in a preceding segment, a, as information about b and not about a. In other words, overlapping gestures are not smeared together so that the original character of each is lost; each gesture remains separate and coherent, and its coherence is both reflected in the acoustic signal and perceived by the listener. It is as if you had three pieces of clay of different colors arranged in a line. When you smear the three together, you have a single larger piece of clay, but you can still see the component clays at the boundaries, and how they fit together, because each maintains its own color. Coarticulation thus provides part of the continuity that is necessary, in direct realism, for the signal to form a coherent percept of a single linguistic message, yet the perceptual system responds to the acoustic effects of two coarticulated gestures as if they are separate.

Fowler argues that the fact that listeners "factor out," "compensate for," or otherwise ignore coarticulatory information from other segments means that they are perceiving each segment independently of its coarticulatory context—hence the use of the term "disentangle." Her data come from two main sources. One is the literature on prosody. Recall that high vowels have a higher intrinsic pitch than low vowels, and that f0 tends to be higher immediately after a voiceless stop than after a voiced stop. Listeners' judgments of intonation contours seem to ignore these short-term perturbations in f0: Such lawful

increases in pitch are not noticed (whereas an f0 contour that failed to rise slightly during a high vowel might be heard as dipping in pitch). "Phonetic segmental perturbations of the fundamental frequency contour of an utterance, including those due to variation in vowel height and consonant voicing, serve as information for their causes, namely vowel height . . . and consonant voicing . . . respectively." (Fowler, Best, & McRoberts, 1990: 568).

The second line of argument concerns perception of coarticulatory effects. It comes most directly from work of Fowler and her colleagues themselves (Fowler, 1984; Fowler et al., 1990; Fowler & Smith, 1986) and is indirectly supported by other work (e.g., Krakow, Beddor, Goldstein, & Fowler, 1988; Martin & Bunnell, 1981). Briefly, these experiments show that even when listeners can *predict* an upcoming sound from coarticulatory influences on the preceding syllable, they cannot necessarily discriminate *between* pairs of such syllables that are the same phonemically, but have been taken from different phonetic contexts so that they differ in the coarticulatory information they contain that is irrelevant to the discrimination task. Although these experiments are interesting, ingenious, and carefully done, they are not described here because their message to direct realists is clear, yet proponents of other theories remain unconvinced. Some of the problems are methodological and others are interpretational. The debate, which has been long, complicated, and somewhat acrimonious, is technical and goes beyond the scope of this book. You can get a flavor of the type of argument by comparing the reasoning of the direct realists with that of Diehl's auditory enhancement theory described in the next section. For more, read Diehl and Kluender (1989a, 1989b), Fowler (1989, 1996a), and Ohala (1996).

Direct realism sees speech perception as obeying the same principles as all other types of sensory perception. Perception entails using a structured sensory signal as information about what caused it, rather than as information that must be interpreted before its environmental causes can be understood. The gesture is the phonological primitive, and this allows phonological primitives to structure the acoustic signal in the same way as a physical chair structures the light that falls onto the retina in the eye. Therefore, when we hear sounds, what we perceive is the gestures that structure those sounds phonologically: Overlapping, discrete gestures of the phonological system are what are produced and what are perceived.

Evaluation of the Direct Realism Theory of Speech Perception

As a theory of speech perception, direct realism is still quite young. Partly because researchers have been mainly concerned with establishing the validity of its basic tenets, it has not yet seriously addressed how higher-order linguistic structures beyond the phoneme develop (but see Best, 1994, 1995 for discussions at this level). The focus is almost entirely on gestures, which, following articulatory phonology, are taken to be the basic phonological units. Gestures seem to be very similar to phonemes, or perhaps to a sort of idealized allophone in syllabic structure, because each gesture is seen as independent of coarticulatory influences. For production, Fowler (1996b) proposes introducing linguistic structures by means of a specialized type of neural net, as discussed later in this chapter. By implication, because this is part of a direct realist model, the net should apply to perception as well. Indeed, Fowler (1984) likened the waxing and waning of coarticulated gestural information to the increase and decrease of probabilities associated with different phonemes in TRACE, a connectionist model (or neural net) discussed below. Notice that although direct realism demands that the net must be defined in terms of gestures, proponents of nonmotoric theories might propose nongestural units. Neural networks are themselves theory-neutral in this respect and need not depend on gestures.

Arguments against the direct realist theory of speech perception dispute its general philosophy and the interpretation of particular experiments. Fowler (e.g., 1996a) concedes that experimental evidence adduced to support the theory is not conclusive, but rather "converges" on the conclusion that listeners perceive vocal-tract gestures. No other theory, she suggests, can explain such a range of experimental findings so elegantly. Not surprisingly, this claim is controversial. One problem seems to be that the theory makes a lot of sense in its own terms, but many researchers can't help asking *how* the transformation from acoustic signal to percept is made. Direct realism does not explain this in a way that can satisfy proponents of other theories, nor researchers who are relatively theory-neutral. As noted above for the discussion of coarticulation, the arguments on both sides are complicated and cover a lot of data in a variety of experimental designs involving speech and nonspeech signals, the perceptual behavior of human adults and babies, and of animals. Neither side is convinced by the others' arguments, and at this time it seems unlikely that either side will ever manage to convince the other (cf., Diehl & Kluender, 1989a, 1989b, Fowler, 1989).

Much of the problem is that direct realism rests on a philosophy that has many merits and is couched in such a way that it is hard to disprove conclusively. However, a number of arguments have been made against it on general grounds. An example is that we can appreciate (or "understand") music without knowing how it is produced. We need not know how to play each instrument, nor need we be able to follow the sounds made by violins, oboes, trumpets, and so on in a symphony in order to recognize and enjoy it. Another example is that the sense of smell does not work like vision: We can recognize smells without knowing what causes them. If that is so, why should we assume that audition works like vision rather than like smell? These types of argument are made, for example, by Ohala (1996). Fowler (1996a) responds that listeners' knowledge about environmental causes need not always be perfect. It will be best for systems that are biologically important to the animal, and, since speech falls into this category, our implicit knowledge of vocal tract movement is good. We rely much less on music and our sense of smell.

Because support for direct perception of speech gestures is so much a matter of personal belief, it is not worthwhile examining in detail attempts to disprove the theory. Instead, we consider here direct realism's positive contributions to thinking about speech perception, and then move on to other theories, drawing connections with direct realism as appropriate.

Direct realism is neat and economical in placing speech perception in the context of a general theory of perception and also in its relation to speech production. The gestures that Fowler and her colleagues take to be the phonological primitives of speech production are also the primitives of speech perception. Direct realists call this symmetry "parity": in Fowler's definition (personal communication), parity is achieved when the message the speaker intends to send and does send is the same as the message received by the listener. Parity is valued because it offers economy. Fowler notes that most theories of phonology, speech production, and speech perception introduce constructs as they seem to be internally necessary, without necessarily aiming for parity. So the phonemes and phonetic segments of phonology, and the features they are composed of, are destroyed in the vocal tract, partly due to coarticulation. The coarticulated gestures of the vocal tract produce acoustic segments that must be reconverted into discrete phonetic units, sometimes via intermediate stages. Direct realism avoids this sequence of destruction and reconstruction by taking gestures as the units at all three stages, phonology, production, and perception.

Notice that direct realism is not the only theory that approaches some sort of parity. Stevens' work on quantal theory and acoustic invariance associated with distinctive features also aims, in a sense, for parity, although he does not use that word. The Motor Theorists also aim for parity.

However, claims about parity depend very much upon one's starting philosophy. To some extent, whether parity is thought to be achieved may depend on whether the units of the theory are seen as satisfactory. One problem with direct realists' gesture-based claim of parity is that it is not clear that gestures are "the right" units for models of either production or perception. For example, articulatory (gestural) phonology does not include all issues phonologists try to account for, such as vowel alternations and vowel harmony. More importantly, these gestures presuppose discrete linguistic units, largely at the level of the phoneme or of gross allophones. This in itself is a model resulting from a particular type of thinking, to which there are alternatives. If discrete consonant and vowel articulations were not taken as axiomatic (as they need not be), then there would be no value in discrete gestures (cf., Remez, 1994).

Another strength of direct realism is its "biological" approach. Following the principle that the more general the explanation the better, direct realism holds that speech is perceived according to the same laws as any other type of sensory perception. Any organism with an auditory system capable of detecting gestural structure in the acoustic signal will be able to discriminate between speech sounds like human adults do. So the fact that human babies, other mammals, and even birds such as quails discriminate between speech sounds the same as adult humans does not surprise direct realists. It simply means that these organisms have auditory systems that are similar to those of adult humans; there is no requirement that they can also produce the sounds. They will perceive the gestures, but perceive them nonlinguistically. As it grows older, the human baby's brain will register coincidences of occurrences in the signal, and from these it will gradually develop the higher-order invariants that are linguistically relevant gestures. This approach is appealing because it allows scope for individual differences and for errors in the system. Notice that there is no hope of parity in the baby's or animals' perceptual experiences. Presumably parity is irrelevant because these organisms are not communicating linguistically. More importantly, there is no discussion of why humans construct the higher-order units directly and other animals do not, even though the invariants are there to be noticed in the signal. Nevertheless, the open attitude to evolution, and to stages in evolutionary and ontological development, is a welcome variant amongst theories based on motoric behavior.

A third strength of direct realism is its emphasis on the listener trying to find the source of the sound. Many of the more recent experiments stress the importance of gestural coherence in phonetic decisions (cf., Fowler, Best, & McRoberts 1990): that listeners expect a single message to come from a single talker, so they actively seek a single source for a single message, and more than one source if several messages are occurring at the same time. The clarity of this view is relatively recent in the history of speech perception, and although it can be (and has been) stated in acoustic or multimodal rather than gestural terms, direct realism has contributed significantly to its formulation.

A connected strength is direct realism's emphasis on the contribution of partial proximal information and its attitude to multimodal sensory information. The listener seeks to "make sense of" the proximal information, not in terms of word meaning, but in that it is assumed that the signal, if it is coherent, must come from one talker. Proximal stimuli are perceived consistent with this need. Some of the complex arguments against auditory theories, in fact, are couched within the logic of a listener actively interacting with the proximal stimulus, as if looking for a coherent signal that could come from a single vocal tract.

In summary, many of the tenets of direct realism are probably true in some sense. It is appealing because it forms part of a wider theory of perception, with a biological perspective that allows similarities between humans and non-humans. The link between production and perception is attractive, as is the emphasis on distinguishing between particular qualities of information that have often been lumped together in the past. No other theory brings to the fore so effectively that what is perceived depends crucially on how the individual perceiver's experience and behavior interact with the stimuli in the environment. The stand on acoustic invariance

also gives welcome breadth to an otherwise motoric theory. And there is no doubt that, from infancy, humans are peculiarly sensitive to the correspondences between vocal-tract behavior and acoustics.

But direct realism is not explicit about how perception takes place. Prosody is barely addressed (apart from its contribution to phonemic identity), and there has been little discussion of how units higher than the gesture come to be organized into linguistic units. Because it focuses on vocal-tract gestures as the distal object, it has not systematically identified what in the sensory signal is normally important: what is relevant information, and what is not. Unlike in acoustic theories of speech perception, the proximal invariants are seen as uninteresting, as meaningless in themselves, because they are only properties that help to instigate the perception rather than being the stuff of the perception itself. This stand is an essential part of direct realism, but it can run the risk of leading to *post hoc* explanation, although Fowler and her colleagues make great efforts to avoid that. The undoubtedly valid point that the perceiver partly determines what is perceived is an added problem in this context, because it means that there will always be individual variation in how the same stimulus is responded to. Lastly, to direct realists, it is axiomatic, and therefore not open to question, that the object of perception is gestural, and that perception is direct, or unmediated. To others, neither of these principles is necessary. Some theorists take an extreme counterposition that perception is mediated entirely or almost entirely by general auditory processes, while others favor a multimodal or amodal approach. Almost all differ from direct realism in assuming some sort of mediation, or hypothesis-testing. These models are discussed in the next sections.

To conclude, this very elegant model is attractive in its generality to all perception, its attempt to account simply for speech production and perception, and its emphasis on interaction between an individual and its environment. But it is controversial, and will probably remain so, partly because it is hard either to prove or to disprove conclusively, and in particular in its insistence that discrete motoric gestures are the common units of phonology, speech production, and speech perception.

A GENERAL AUDITORY MODEL WITHOUT ACOUSTIC INVARIANCE: AUDITORY ENHANCEMENT THEORY

Background: Properties of General Auditory Theories

A number of models of speech perception contrast with all those discussed so far in that they suggest that much, if not all, of speech perception can be accounted for by general auditory processes working on the acoustic speech signal, without making strong assumptions about acoustic invariance. Although these theories place most emphasis on the acoustic signal, none would say that there is no influence from the motoric system, and indeed, some are increasingly looking for links between auditory and visual speech modalities. Therefore, their designation as auditory is mainly one of emphasis. The acoustic/auditory mode is primary, which is consistent with our being able to understand speech over the radio without trouble.

Apart from the obvious conflict about what are the primary data, or perceptual primitives, these general auditory theories differ from the Motor Theory in that speech perception is seen as not special. Speech is perceived through basic processes of the auditory system, although cognitive processes are also involved, usually with some form of mediation. Another difference from the Motor Theory is that the young listener learns auditory patterns that are gradually organized into linguistic structure, rather than being born with innate knowledge of linguistically significant intended gestures.

There are, on the whole, fewer points of conflict with direct realism, but the two viewpoints are nevertheless quite opposed to one another. As with the Motor Theory, one obvious conflict is in the perceptual primitives: Whereas for direct realism it is the distal motoric gestures, for general auditory theories it is the information in the acoustic signal itself—direct realism's proximal stimuli. So the actual perceptual mechanisms proposed stay close to known properties of the acoustic signal and the auditory system, without necessarily assuming acoustic invariance. Unlike direct realism, for which time can be implicit in gestures, most of these auditory theories are inexplicit about the role of time in perception; but this point of difference rests more in the conceptualization of the primitives than in the processes being better understood by direct realists than by auditorists.

Points of similarity between these acoustic theories and direct realism are that they both assume that processes used in speech perception are not specific to speech or to humans, and that babies' responses to speech are initially nonlinguistic and only gradually become linked with linguistic structure. But in direct realism the structure is directly perceived (by inexplicit processes) whereas in auditory theories some form of mental representation develops. Most auditory theories, implicitly or explicitly, take a somewhat statistical approach to perception: Speech is represented in the brain as some form of memory trace, a template (cf. Stevens' and Blumstein's model), or an ideal prototype, with which the incoming signal is compared to select which is more probable. This type of learning contrasts with tuning the speech module, as in the Motor Theory, and with attunement (sensitivity) to vocal-tract gestures, as in direct realism.

Auditory Enhancement Theory

1. To produce phonological contrasts, speakers control sets of articulations to limit energy expenditure or to produce complex, mutually enhancing acoustic effects that encourage the formation of distinct phonetic categories rather than continuous variation along each phonetic dimension.

2. Perception is seen in similar terms. Many acoustic properties typically combine to form

complex intermediate perceptual properties, which in turn combine to contribute in varying proportions to the identification of a distinctive feature.

3. The theory emphasizes the perceptual role of acoustic redundancy and maintains that perceptual needs determine articulatory patterns: Perception drives production.

An example of a strongly auditory approach is that of Diehl and his colleagues (now working in a number of institutions across the United States) and summarized, for example, by Diehl, Kluender, and Walsh (1990). This group has systematically sought counterevidence to motoric approaches to speech perception and so has mainly focused on the perception of sounds they believe cannot be explained within a gestural theory. In addition to the general position outlined above, the main argument of auditory enhancement theory is that perceptual needs determine articulatory patterns, and that speech articulation is controlled in such a way that phonological distinctions in a given language will be perceptually enhanced. Enhancement produces a range of redundant acoustic features that, when combined, either directly increase the chance of identifying a particular value of a distinctive feature, because more of that property is present in the signal, or indirectly increase its chances because a strong presence in one acoustic property changes perception of another towards a more extreme value, as in the cue-trading paradigm.

Auditory enhancement theorists start from the position that units of speech perception include distinctive features. Like Stevens and Blumstein, these researchers focus exclusively on how distinctive features are identified from evidence in the acoustic signal. Unlike Stevens, however, who has searched for a single, preferably simple, invariant acoustic or auditory correlate for each distinctive feature and only brought in redundant features when the simple approach clearly fails, Diehl's group gives primary emphasis to redundancy of acoustic-phonetic properties in specifying distinctive features.

They argue that although a single acoustic property *may* correspond to a single auditory property, it is more typical for a feature contrast to be conveyed by a number of different acoustic distinctions. They propose three types of "phonetic redundancy" (Kingston & Diehl, 1994): (1) Each acoustic property can correspond to an independent auditory property; (2) a number of acoustically independent properties can act as subproperties of a single auditory property; and (3) some of these subproperties may contribute to more than one independent auditory property. These independent auditory properties are not distinctive features, but *intermediate perceptual properties* (IPPs) that in turn contribute to the identification of one or more distinctive features. Thus, acoustic properties (normally combine to) form intermediate perceptual properties, a number of which normally combine to form a particular value of a distinctive feature. This process is schematized in Figure 15-1.

Figure 15-1a illustrates the relatively straightforward mapping of acoustic/auditory properties onto distinctive features as ideally conceptualized by Stevens and Blumstein (1981). Figure 15-1b illustrates the more complex model of Diehl's group. There are two crucial differences between the models. Most obviously, (a) has no IPPs. More significantly, however, the acoustic components comprising a single IPP (1) may come from very different parts of a syllable and (2) may contribute to more than one IPP. That is, they can be independently controllable.

Much of the evidence Diehl's group use to support auditory enhancement theory has already been described in Chapters Thirteen and Fourteen. It includes work showing that animals perceive some speech contrasts as humans do (e.g., Kluender, Diehl, & Killeen, 1987), and much work looking for general auditory explanations of trading relations in categorical perception of speech and nonspeech stimuli (e.g., Diehl & Kingston, 1991; Kingston & Diehl, 1994; Parker, Diehl, & Kluender, 1986). One part of the work on trading relations comprises trying to establish that properties that enter into trading relations are

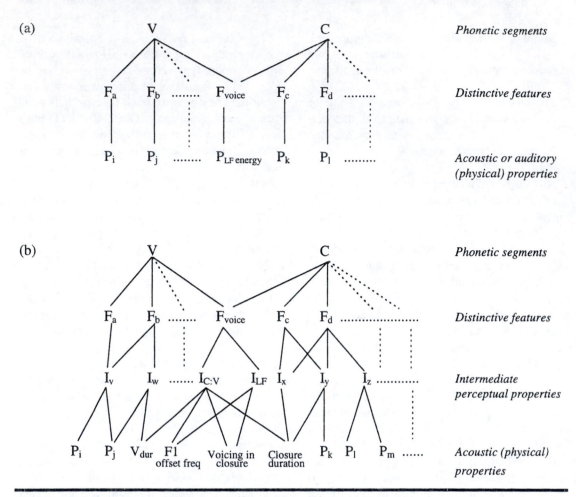

FIGURE 15-1. Schematic relation of some physical properties to higher-order properties in a VC sequence in (a) a traditional distinctive feature system such as that of Stevens and Blumstein (1981), and (b) auditory enhancement theory. Details are given only for the feature *voice*. In (a), the acoustic property $P_{LFenergy}$ is the only correlate of the distinctive feature *voice*, F_{voice}, as in Stevens (1989). In (b), $I_{C:V}$ is the intermediate perceptual property (IPP) C:V duration ratio, and I_{LF} is the IPP low-frequency property. A number of acoustic properties contribute to each of these IPPs, and both IPPs contribute to F_{voice}. (After Nearey, 1995, and Lindau & Ladefoged, 1986)

independently controlled in production, just as the lengths of a vowel and of the stop closure that follows it are believed to be independently controlled. Diehl's position contradicts that taken by the Motor Theorists for many (but not all) properties that enter into trading relations with VOT, for example. Most of the evidence Diehl's group offers comes from data reported in the literature by other researchers.

Another part of their work on trading relations seeks to show that acoustic properties may enter into trading relations with one another because each contributes to, or enhances, a single auditory effect. This position directly contradicts the claim made by gesturalists (Motor Theorists and direct realists) that when two acoustic properties enter into trading relations because they are both the result of a particular gesture, they nevertheless have independent auditory effects. Consider the voicing distinction for stops. Gesturalists suggest that VOT, f0, and F1 cutback are auditorily distinct, but that they all influence the perception of stop voicing in speech because they all result from a single laryngeal gesture for either long-lag or short-lag VOT in stops. Auditory enhancement theorists argue that this assumed auditory independence of the various properties is wrong. Most of this work on enhancement comes from auditory enhancement theorists' own laboratories. It covers a number of phonological contrasts, including the correlates of the voicing distinction in stops (Diehl & Kingston, 1991; Parker et al., 1986) and fricatives (Balise & Diehl, 1994), correlates of the stop-glide distinction, and properties that enhance auditory differences between vowels (Diehl et al., 1990). Since by far the greatest effort has gone into the voicing distinction in stops, we focus on that work, which is most completely discussed in Kingston and Diehl (1994, 1995).

The experiments have become increasingly complex and sophisticated as they try to establish whether nonspeech analogs of the voicing contrast for intervocalic stops can be manipulated to show that auditory percepts are partly "illusions" formed from particular coincidences of acoustic properties. Notice how like direct realism this is, but with a psychoacoustic basis.

Consider Kingston and Diehl's (1995) two main examples of intermediate perceptual properties, or IPPs, the *C:V duration ratio* and the *low-frequency property*. Both contribute to the distinctive feature *voice*. That is, together they determine whether a consonant is phonologically voiced or voiceless, especially in intervocalic position. The acoustic properties that contribute to each are well known and accepted in the literature (Lisker, 1986). They are summarized in parts (i), (ii), and (iii) of Figure 15-2. The spectrograms of naturally spoken *buckeye* and *bugeye* in part (i) illustrate the five acoustic properties listed in part (ii) that distinguish between these stops. The check marks in part (iii) show the traditional view of which acoustic property contributes to which

higher-order complex property, the *C:V duration ratio* (CV) and the *low-frequency property* (LF). Part (iv) is described below.

Although the acoustic properties in Figure 15-2(ii) have been known about for some time, they have not previously been treated very systematically by auditory theories (cf., Klatt, 1989). Normally, it is accepted that some are more important than others, and that some are dependent on others, such as a greater proportion of voicing in a short closure interval. Auditory enhancement theory is not original in suggesting that they combine to produce the two particular complex properties, nor, of course, in pointing out the interdependence between vowel duration and closure duration in the C:V duration ratio. But it is original in making explicit the concept of the IPP and in attempting to demonstrate experimentally that IPPs are general auditory properties, functions of how the auditory system works, rather than inherently learned and linguistic. It is only when the IPPs are combined into distinctive features that the auditory system is linked into the linguistic system.

The general form of Diehl and co-workers' experiments is to synthesize nonspeech stimuli that mimic properties of a vowel-stop-vowel sequence like /aba/ or /apa/. Figure 15-3 illustrates some typical experimental conditions. Each synthetic stimulus is very simple: a pulsing f0 and a single formant with a silent gap in the middle (the "stop closure"). Diehl and colleagues have varied what F1 and f0 do at the boundaries of the gap: They might stay constant, or rise into the gap and fall out of it, or fall into the gap and rise out of it. In Figure 15-3, as explained in the legend, F1 varies in conditions (a) and (b) and stays constant in (c), (d), and (e), while f0 stays constant in conditions (a), (b), and (e) and varies in conditions (c) and (d). In natural VCV sequences, F1 always falls as a stop closure is made and rises again as it is released. When the stop is voiced, f0 tends to fall at the boundary with the closure and rise again at its release, whereas when the stop is voiceless, f0 is constant or might rise slightly as the closure is made and falls again at the release

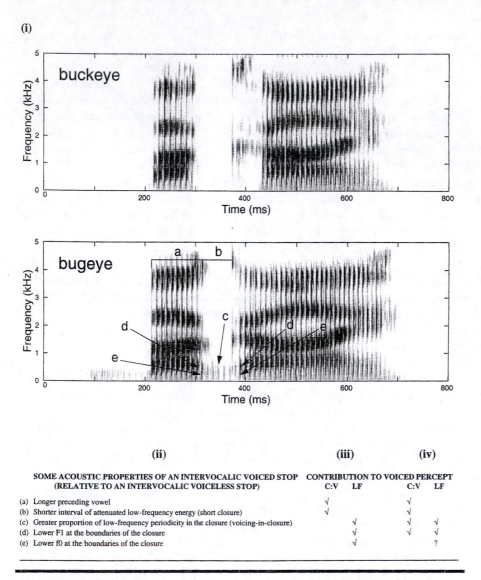

FIGURE 15-2. (i) Spectrograms of naturally spoken *buckeye* (upper) and *bugeye* (lower). The labeled parts correspond to items listed in part (ii). (ii) Acoustic properties that contribute to the perception of a phonologically voiced stop, relative to those for a voiceless stop. (iii) Standard view of how each acoustic property contributes to the perception of voicing: C:V = C:V duration ratio; LF = low-frequency property. Checks indicate a positive contribution; blanks indicate no contribution. (iv) Auditory enhancement theory's view of the respective contributions of each acoustic property: checks and blanks as for part (iii); ? indicates uncertain contribution.

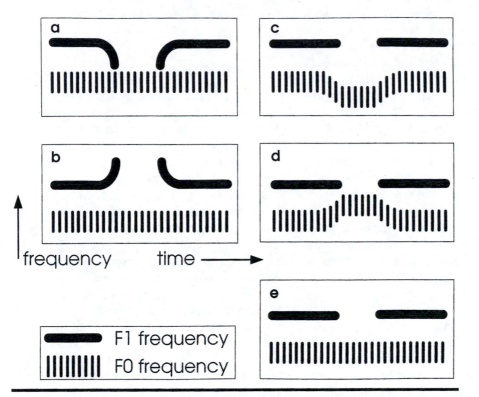

FIGURE 15-3. Schematic spectrograms illustrating some of the conditions used by Diehl and co-workers to test the auditory enhancement model. Here, the frequencies of F1 and f0 are independently varied to test for the Low-Frequency Property in non-speech stimuli that simulate properties of a stop consonant in a VCV sequence. The single formant in each stimulus, F1, is missing in the middle of the stimulus to form a gap that could correspond to the closure interval of a stop consonant. (a) F1 falls as it reaches the gap and rises again when the gap ends; f0 is constant (stays at the same frequency) throughout the stimulus. (b) F1 rises as it reaches the gap and falls again from the end of the gap; f0 is constant throughout. (c) F0 falls as it nears the gap and rises after the gap ends; F1 is constant. (d) F0 rises as it nears the gap and falls after the gap ends; F1 is constant. (e) F1 and f0 frequencies are both constant. Other combinations of F1 and f0 patterns could also be tested. The most speech-like of these patterns is condition (a), with F1 falling into the gap and rising out of it, although in natural speech f0 would normally be lower in the gap, too. Other conditions, not illustrated here, have also been tested.

of closure. More stimuli can be made by varying the duration of the gap in each of the conditions illustrated here: In natural speech, voiced stops tend to have shorter gaps (closure intervals) than voiceless stops. Similarly, f0 might stop during the gap in F1, as for voiceless stops, or it might continue during all or part of the gap, as for voiced stops. These parameters are independently varied. None of these manipulations make the single-formant stimuli sound like speech, but they do mimic acoustic properties of naturally spoken VstopV sequences that have been found to influence the perception of voicing, especially in trading relations experiments.

Listeners are asked to judge whether the gap is long or short, this response being chosen as the nonspeech equivalent of phonologically voiceless and voiced stops respectively. The experimenters look for shifts in the identification curves, in the same way as for trading relations experiments.

Figure 15-2(iv) summarizes auditory enhancement theorists' conclusions about the relevance to real speech of the results of this series of experiments. Consider the C:V duration ratio. We knew already that the duration of the preceding vowel and consonant closure influenced the perception of voicing, but this series of experiments suggests that two other acoustic properties, a low F1 and the presence of voicing in the closure, also contribute to the C:V duration ratio. The theory is that the presence of the low-frequency energy *enhances* the C:V duration ratio. When periodic low-frequency noise fills the gap between the two portions of F1, then the gap is heard as shorter than it really is, and the vowel may be heard as longer than it really is. The contribution of F1 to this auditory illusion is important: When F1 is low at the boundaries of the gap, it is seen as contributing spectral continuity between the filtered pulsing of f0 when F1 is present and the unfiltered pulsing of f0 in the gap. Without this spectral continuity, pulsing in the gap has a much smaller influence on perceived gap duration.

Auditory enhancement theory maintains that the acoustic signal provides all the information that is necessary for the listener to perceive speech. The redundancy of the speech signal is systematic and structured: A number of different acoustic properties combine to enhance perception of particular intermediate properties, and these in turn combine to contribute in varying degrees to the identification of a distinctive feature. This enhancement of perceptual properties is a consequence of the way the auditory system works. There is no reference to motoric gestures, and patterns of production evolved to satisfy the

demands of perception, rather than the other way around.

Evaluation of Auditory Enhancement Theory

Auditory enhancement theory takes a very strong position. It sets itself particularly against the Motor Theory and direct realism, but it is also stronger than many proponents of auditory theories believe is necessary. Nearey describes the emphasis on combining acoustic properties to create illusions of short gaps as follows: "Speakers must be both acrobats and magicians. They must learn to do articulatory cartwheels to produce perceptual illusions" (Nearey, 1995:36). He reasons that although the experimental data are probably reliable, it is not necessary to assume that speakers intentionally produce a lower F1 because it contributes to the low-frequency property and enhances the C:V duration ratio by shortening apparent gap duration. It is known that when the vocal tract narrows towards complete closure, then F1 falls. Listeners can learn this correspondence, and it can be explained by gestural theories as well as by auditory theories. Nearey suggests that a simpler explanation is that each acoustic property is learned by the listener and contributes directly to the identification of a distinctive feature. He further suggests that the listener weights acoustic information according to its importance, which might affect both the nature of phonological categories and allow for variation between languages.

Kingston and Diehl (1994, 1995) argue the case for complex physical properties (IPPs) because their data showing shifts in identification boundaries are for nonspeech stimuli for which it is difficult to believe that listeners have pre-existing categories. The case for IPPs could also be argued from the apparent "auditory illusion" data alone, even if the claim was dropped that articulation is controlled in order to enhance IPPs. Furthermore, it is debatable whether learned category formation is simpler and more straightforward than complex auditory percepts involving some perceptual distortion (illusion) of the physical signal. Both category formation and the types of auditory pattern perception that can be thought of as involving illusions are well documented (cf., Moore, 1997: Chapter 7).

However, Nearey (1995) argues that illusions, like trading relations, normally occur as threshold effects: When one property is relatively weak or ambiguous, it can be enhanced by the presence of a different strong one. He suggests that the entire auditory enhancement model is based on this characteristic of threshold effects. Since a significant proportion of speech sounds do not seem to be close to perceptual thresholds, he asks, to what extent should a theory of speech perception be based on processes that have principally been demonstrated as threshold effects? Nearey's criticism is worth taking seriously, but it is not necessarily damaging to auditory enhancement theory. If a single principle accounts for both clear and threshold cases, then that would normally be taken as a point in its favor. One defense of the theory is that some forms of enhancement are definitely not threshold effects. For example, Diehl (personal communication) points out that lip rounding and tongue backing independently lower the frequency of F2 by amounts that are well above perceptual thresholds, yet they still seem to be used jointly to strengthen the perceptual contrast between front and back vowels. They may be used together because they make the signal robust under a wide range of listening conditions. What is very distinctive in optimal listening conditions may quickly become nondistinctive in noisy or reverberant listening conditions.

Auditory enhancement theory is still in its infancy. Much more work is needed before its worth can be properly assessed. And there has as yet been no attempt to broaden it beyond the identification of selected IPPs and distinctive features. There are no suggestions about how IPPs are combined into distinctive features, and how words are recognized from distinctive features, for example. Even if IPPs prove to be wrong or of restricted

applicability, however, the theory has merits that seem worth pursuing further. Each of these merits is included among the properties we suggest below that a theory of speech perception seems to need.

One merit of auditory enhancement theory is that it explicitly integrates information from across syllables into a single auditory property that maps, exclusively or together with other intermediate properties, onto a linguistically significant feature. In this way, it includes more acoustic-phonetic information than many other theories manage, and, most importantly, accounts for temporally distributed and local information in the same phonological category.

Second, Nearey's objections of articulatory acrobatics notwithstanding, there is no question that speakers know about enhancing sounds. Auditory enhancement theory accounts for this knowledge allowing the same distinctive feature to be signaled by a variety of means according to phonetic (allophonic) and situational circumstances. Consider how you might say *tab* over the phone to distinguish it from *tap*. You would probably increase the vowel length of *tab* and might voice heavily in its final stop closure. The experiments we have summarized suggest that these things contribute both to the C:V duration ratio and to the low-frequency property. If the line were particularly bad, you might even use a lower-than normal f0 for *tab*, and a higher-than-normal one for *tap*, which might further enhance at least the low-frequency property.

A third strength is that this theory of perception is being developed in tandem with ideas about speech production. Since this topic falls outside the scope of this chapter, we shall simply say here that the idea that speakers learn to enhance acoustic properties in their speech, and that enhancement takes different forms in different phonetic contexts and leads naturally to the position that speech production is all tightly controlled, partly so that the speaker can produce the right, language-specific patterns of phonological contrasts. There is no room for "default" articulations. This in turn leads to research on a wider range of languages than is typical for much speech perception research, and our knowledge of what needs to be accounted for increases in consequence. For example, Kingston and Diehl (1994) note that f0 does not vary with stop voicing in Tamil, which leads them to question the assumption that f0 changes are automatic consequences of the state of the vocal folds during long- and short-lag VOTs. Tamil does not "need" the enhancement of the low-frequency property that English does, because in Tamil, voiced stops are short, and voiceless ones are long (geminate), so that phonological voicing is predictable from closure length. Similar proposals for the control of phonological contrasts have been put forward by others, for example, Keating (1985). Notice also that the interpretation of the Tamil data has similarities with Stevens' ideas that "redundant" features can enhance phonological distinctions (Stevens et al., 1986): A feature will be enhanced by another when the auditory distinction would otherwise be unclear. In Tamil, voicing enhances the long-short distinction (or vice versa) and this provides enough contrast. Further enhancement of phonetic voicing is not necessary.

A fourth strength is that the theory, though extreme, has connections with several earlier proposals and with much current thinking by other theorists. We have just noted connections with Stevens and colleagues' (1986) principle of redundant features and with Keating's (1985) ideas on the control of phonetic parameters. The theory could also be relevant to activation models such as TRACE and Massaro's FLMP (see below), although the current position is that IPPs favor the establishment of distinct sound categories, rather like quantal theory. In tying together needs of perception and production, it has similarities with Lindblom's work discussed later in this chapter. Early work from Diehl's group seemed to favor perception determining production patterns, but more recent writing makes it clear that no one aspect drives the others; indeed, IPPs are only one way, and the most complex, of getting to a distinctive feature (Kingston & Diehl, 1994).

Auditory enhancement theory argues that acoustic properties of the signal are integrated first by the auditory system into intermediate perceptual properties (IPPs) that are not specifically linguistic and are only later combined into linguistic distinctive features. This position has two distinctive aspects not shared by all auditory theories. First, it introduces a major theoretical construct, the IPP, to exploit the redundancy and potential variability of the acoustic signal. Second, the particular acoustic properties that contribute to an IPP are said to combine with one another according to lawful psychoacoustic (general auditory) principles to produce a stronger or more coherent effect than each could produce alone. Like trading relations, the principles work by mutual enhancement; but whereas trading relations have classically been restricted to threshold effects, auditory enhancement operates over a wide range of parameter values. The theory does not require the assumption of acoustic or auditory invariance, although it can accommodate invariants with ease.

The theory is very recent, and much more work is needed to establish its worth. At present it goes no further than distinctive features and has not yet explained how IPPs are combined into distinctive features. Nevertheless, it could provide the first stage of a larger auditory theory that allowed words to be identified. It is exciting because it provides at least a partial explanation of the remarkable robustness of natural speech that makes listening and understanding possible even in very difficult listening conditions. A related strength is that the theory explains the perceptual integration of acoustic cues to phonetic distinctions when those cues are distributed across entire syllables and even between syllables; in this, it is unique amongst auditory theories, and offers a challenge to gestural theories.

CATEGORIES OF SOUND?

Although we have suggested that the importance of categorical perception has been exaggerated by early theories of speech perception, we must be careful to distinguish between the premises of the theories themselves and the behavior that they attempt to account for. We might question the ubiquity of categorical perception as an all-or-nothing response, but we do not want to deny that speech, at some point, is structured into categories by the listener, and that one set of those categories corresponds to or is relatable to phonemic or allophonic groupings in the listener's native language. One question is, How do these categories develop as the child begins to speak?; a second is, To what extent are they processed separately from "nonphonetic" acoustic information such as the speaker's gender and personal identity?; and a third is, Do these categories represent phonemes, allophones, features, or some other unit?

The Development of Speech Sound Categories: The Native Language Magnet Model

1. The gross acoustic categories of speech reflect general psychoacoustic boundaries to which babies are innately sensitive, and that are not unique to humans.
2. Experience of a particular language alters perception. Phonetic categories are structured in language-specific ways around prototypes, or best instances, of each category. At least some of these categories are formed by 6 months of age, as demonstrated by the presence of the perceptual magnet effect for vowels in 6-month-olds.
3. The perceptual magnet effect is species-specific and linguistic. It concerns the formation of linguistic categories rather than discrimination of natural boundaries.
4. These structured speech representations are initially auditory, but soon become polymodal as the baby notices connections between speech sounds and movements of speakers it looks at, and between speech movements, resultant feelings and sounds it makes itself. Thus, perception influences production, and production influences perception.

Kuhl's extensive work on the perception of sound categories by human babies and nonhuman animals has been described earlier. She has drawn together her own and others' work into a model of speech perception, the native language magnet (NLM) model. Let us recap part of her work. Kuhl found that the internal structure of categories changes with linguistic experience. She noted that adults can identify best ("prototype") instances and poor ("nonprototype") instances of the vowel /i/ from a number of acceptable /i/s. She conducted experiments that showed that listeners distinguish less well between sounds that are close to a prototype /i/ than between sounds that are close to a "nonprototype" /i/. She named this phenomenon the *perceptual magnet effect*. This demonstration of the internal structure of speech sound categories is distinct from categorical perception. Categorical perception describes enhanced discrimination between closely similar sounds that happen to span a phoneme boundary; discrimination between closely similar sounds that fall within a single phonemic category had been assumed to be uniformly poor. In contrast, the perceptual magnet effect describes variation in discriminability within a single phonemic category, with poorer discrimination close to the most ideal category member. Iverson and Kuhl (1996) offer data to suggest that enhanced discrimination at a category boundary (categorical perception) is a distinct and separate process from reduced discrimination near a phonetic category prototype (perceptual magnet effect).

Iverson and Kuhl (1995) make four points about the perceptual magnet effect. It is present in humans as early as 6 months of age; it is sensitive to early linguistic experience, in that Swedish and American babies show magnet effects for their native vowels, but not for vowels of the other language (this again contrasts with babies' performance on categorical perception tests); monkeys do not show a magnet effect; and the magnet effect is associated with reduced discrimination around a phonetic prototype. They conclude that part of the acquisition of a particular language involves distortion of the perceptual space within a phonetic category: Perceptual distance around a prototype is reduced.

The NLM model describes how an individual baby begins to learn the phonological categories of its native language. A complete description is in Kuhl and Iverson (1995). Following the literature demonstrating that babies can discriminate between most phonemic categories of any language, regardless of whether they have heard the contrast before, Kuhl proposes that the baby is innately endowed with the ability to divide the speech signal into gross categories, the "basic cuts" of the speech sound space. These basic categories are typically more detailed than those used by any single language, because they encompass all gross contrasts that languages could potentially employ. Because animals can also distinguish some of the categories that babies can, Kuhl suggests that the boundaries of these gross categories are natural psychoacoustic boundaries. One of the first tasks the baby is faced with is to work out which of these natural boundaries are used in the language(s) it hears spoken around it. It is helped in doing this by hearing "motherese," the type of babytalk typical of, but not restricted to, mothers of young babies. Motherese has a number of properties thought to help babies focus on speech and the person who is doing the speaking. In many if not all languages, these properties include very long syllables; vowels are especially long. Kuhl suggests that the long vowels of motherese clearly demonstrate the particular vowel qualities of the mother's native language and are especially helpful in establishing the same sound categories for the baby.

From this clear and baby-oriented speech, and within the limits set by the natural psychoacoustic boundaries, the baby learns to reorganize its perceptual space. First, the sound categories appropriate for its native language begin to form, so that by 6 months of age, the baby has learned to recognize good instances, or prototypes, for vowels in its native language but not, of course, for foreign vowels. At this age, then, the baby shows language-specific perceptual magnet effects. Later, the natural boundaries that are not used in the

baby's own language environment cease to be as perceptually important, and this accounts for the loss of discrimination for foreign contrasts at around 10 to 12 months of age that Werker and her colleagues observed. The change from the baby's first representation of the vowel space in terms of natural psychoacoustic boundaries, to one specific to its particular language, is illustrated schematically in Figure 15-4 for English and Spanish.

The NLM model is compatible with observations on what determines whether a foreign sound contrast is hard to hear. We noted earlier that Best (1994, 1995) identified a number of influencing properties of any given foreign contrast, including its inherent acoustic distinctiveness and its relationship to the phonological structure of the listener's native language. For adults, the difficulty of learning a foreign contrast should depend at least partly on the proximity of the contrast to a single magnet of the native language: The closer to the magnet, the harder it will be to perceive the difference. These predictions have not yet been tested.

Consistent with the facts about (re)learning foreign contrasts, Kuhl suggests that the natural psychoacoustic boundaries do not disappear, but only "recede" after language-specific magnet effects develop. This means that the baby's basic sensory abilities are not changed. Instead, the change occurs at a higher level, involving memory or attention. Perceptual space for speech-relevant distinctions is warped, shrinking the perceived difference between good instances of the same phonetic category and stretching the perceived difference between poorer exemplars that are closer to the phonetic category boundary. At the time of writing, experiments are in progress to test these ideas for American English /l/ and /r/ ([ɹ]) with Japanese and American babies. These are data to look out for in the literature.

From her own and others' work, Kuhl proposes that babies' early speech representations are entirely auditory, but that they very soon involve visual, kinesthetic, and motoric elements, too, as the baby makes links between the sight

A.   The natural auditory boundaries
an infant perceives

Dimension related to F2 frequency,
and corresponding to front-back
on the vowel quadrilateral

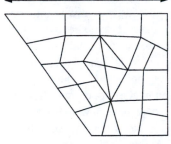

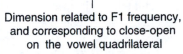

Dimension related to F1 frequency,
and corresponding to close-open
on the vowel quadrilateral

B.   English perceptual magnets

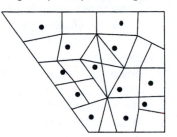

Spanish perceptual magnets

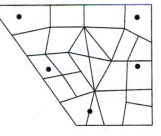

C.   English vowel space   Spanish vowel space

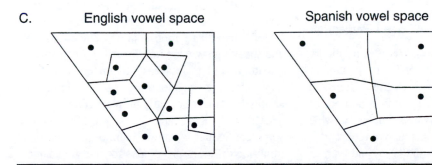

FIGURE 15-4. The development of the vowel space according to NLM theory. (A) At birth babies can perceive all the natural boundaries that underlie differences in vowel quality, but the area within each boundary is unstructured, so there are no perceptual magnet effects for "good" instances of a vowel. (B) Language-specific perceptual magnets have developed by about 6 months of age, but the baby is still sensitive to many natural boundaries that are not used in the language he or she hears. (C) Later, the baby is no longer sensitive to boundaries that are not used in its native language.

and sound of humans talking and between its own vocal-tract behavior and the sounds it makes. Thus, speech perception is polymodal and influenced by experience. Moreover, as the perception of speech is reorganized through the development of language-specific structures, perception in turn begins to influence production.

The NLM model describes the interaction of innate, general auditory abilities with species-specific and language-specific learning about phonetic categories to produce changes in speech representations in a baby's brain that affect both its perception and production of speech and last into adulthood. During the first six months of life, babies begin to form language-specific sound categories from their experience of the language they hear. Natural psychoacoustic boundaries set limits on these categories. Perceptual space is reorganized within the categories so that good and poor exemplars of a sound category are responded to differently, as demonstrated by the perceptual magnet effect. Category boundaries that are not used in the child's native language cease to be responded to in speech-relevant tasks. The perceptual restructuring, though initially auditory, soon becomes polymodal, and the polymodal perceptual structures influence the individual's speech production.

Evaluation: NLM Model of Speech Perception

The NLM model is a new and interesting theory that needs a lot of work before its generality and validity can be properly assessed. Kuhl and Iverson (1995) themselves identify a number of questions as needing answers. One is at what level of representation the perceptual reorganization occurs. Kuhl and Iverson (1995) and Iverson and Kuhl (1996) envisage it as being at quite a late stage of perception, but Kuhl and Iverson (1995) also note evidence that it might happen quite low down in the auditory pathway. Although this is an important question, we shall not pursue it here.

Another question concerns the nature of the phonetic prototypes. Kuhl uses the term prototype

in a relatively neutral way, avoiding committing herself to whether the mental representation is in terms of a set of instances or a single abstract template-like prototype formed from statistical evidence (see the discussion of Rosch's prototype theory in Chapter 13). She also notes that there is no obvious reason why the brain should not hold an abstract average as well as sets of actual instances from which the average is computed. This is an attractive proposition because it allows perception (and production) to change over time, even in adulthood, thus allowing for an individual to adapt to a new regional accent in perception and in his or her own speech.

A third and more pressing question is how context affects prototypes. This question is important because it could determine the level of abstraction at which the perceptual magnet effect is thought to work, but it has barely begun to be addressed. As the preceding chapters have shown, the acoustic properties of vowels are very different when they are spoken in isolation compared with when they are spoken in context. The segmental structure of the syllable, its prosodic properties (especially its degree of stress), the overall rate of speech, and the degree of casualness used all affect how a vowel is realized acoustically, and hence how far it resembles the isolated vowel. Consonants are also affected by these contextual influences and by their position in the syllable. When these modifications due to context and speaking style are missing, the speech sounds unnatural and is less easy to understand. Phonemes may be misidentified, or the signal may simply become essentially unintelligible.

Although Kuhl and Iverson (1995) expect some contextual variation, mentioning that there might be different prototypes for the same sound spoken by people of different genders, they do not discuss variation due to phonetic context, and their own successful experiments have been restricted to isolated high front vowels in American English and Swedish, and to /la/ versus /ra/ in American English (Iverson & Kuhl, 1996). It has proved harder to demonstrate perceptual magnet effects for /ga/ versus /ka/ (see Kuhl & Iverson, 1995). Most of their work has concerned only the vowel /i/ in isolation. However, empirical work by others shows that perceptual magnet effects, and by implication prototypical units of perception, arise for allophones of phonemes. This evidence comes (indirectly) from changes in rate of speech on the perception of VOT, and (directly) from different allophones of /u/ determined by phonemic context.

Miller (1994) discusses evidence on rate of speech. In one experiment, Volaitis and Miller (1992) used two VOT series, ranging from /b/ to /p/ and from /g/ to /k/, to assess the influence of rate of speech and place of articulation on the categorization of stops as voiced or voiceless. The VOT at the boundary between voiced and voiceless stops was shorter for bilabial than for velar stops, and it was shorter for syllables spoken at faster rather than slower rates of speech. Both of these shifts in VOT were expected: Other things equal, VOT is shorter for bilabials than for velars in natural speech, and it is also shorter at fast speaking rates. As well as identifying the sound they heard, listeners rated how good each sound was as an exemplar of its phonemic category. Crucially, the goodness ratings also shifted with shifts in the VOT boundary. So, for example, at fast speech rates, the stimuli that listeners judged to be the "best /p/s" had shorter VOTs than those judged to be best at slower rates of speech. Volaitis and Miller inferred that changes in the pattern of goodness ratings reflect changes in the internal structure of the perceptual category, but did not test for magnet effects directly in a discrimination test.

Direct evidence for perceptual magnet effects for different allophones of the vowel /u/ comes from doctoral work by Barrett (1996). In Southern British and many other accents of English, /u/ varies greatly with segmental phonetic context, especially in the frequency of F2. In the syllables /u/, /lu/, and /ju/, for example, F2 is lowest in /u/ and highest in /ju/. Barrett found that Southern British listeners chose acoustically very different "best exemplars" of /u/ in these syllables, /u/, /lu/, and /ju/, following the patterns found in their

speech. In discrimination experiments, Barrett found three quite separate magnet effects, one for each syllabic context. That is, comparing /u/s with /u/s, /lu/s with /lu/s, and /ju/s with /ju/s, syllables close to the best exemplar of each were harder to discriminate between than were syllables close to a poor exemplar. She also found that the prototype F2 frequency used in one syllable does not induce a magnet effect when it is used in one of the other two syllables. In other words, synthetic /u/, /lu/, and /ju/ must have different F2 frequencies if they are to sound natural; the best exemplars of each of these syllables each produces a magnet effect that is specific to that syllable, and the same vowel F2 frequency in one of the other two contexts does not produce a magnet effect, but acts instead like a nonprototype.

This demonstration of contextually sensitive magnet effects has some intriguing implications. If a perceptual magnet effect implies existence of a phonetic prototype, and if these prototypes play a significant role in speech perception, there must either be an infinite number of contextually sensitive prototypes or else a smaller number of prototypes for larger units than the phoneme, such as syllables. Consider the first possibility. If each phoneme were represented in an unlimited number of contexts, then there would be an unlimited number of prototypes and an unlimited number of magnet effects for different contexts. Presumably there would be a great deal of perceptual overlap, and the organizational advantage of prototypes and associated magnet effects would be lost or significantly weakened. Nevertheless, it has been suggested before that the brain might store a large set of context-sensitive allophones (cf., Wickelgren, 1969). Under the second possibility, where the prototypes were not for phones, but for larger units such as syllables, there could be fewer contexts, and hence less possibility of overlap, though the number of prototypes would still be huge.

Although Kuhl's claim is for *phonetic* categories, and she rarely generalizes beyond isolated vowels or the particular consonants of a given experiment, most of the theoretical discussion is couched in terms of phonemes. In particular, the importance of systematic variability does not seem to have been considered. For example, Iverson and Kuhl briefly discuss the problem that "the best exemplars of phonetic categories tend to have more extreme acoustic values than do average productions" (1996: 1136) but do not mention the systematicity in the variation that causes the average to be different from the most extreme. They suggest that listeners prefer instances that maximize distinctions between phonemic categories, and that they will "undershoot" these extreme targets in natural speech but can attain them when they want to speak especially clearly. The implication of this brief suggestion seems to be that they favor the prototypes as an ideal. It is hard to reconcile this view with one in which there is a perceptual magnet effect for individual syllables.

In summary, if any sort of contextual change produces a shift in the internal structure of the category, either the category must be very fluid, of a sort barely understood at present and not hinted at in the current version of the NLM model, or there must be a potentially infinite number of such categories. The latter possibility is not especially appealing, because the beauty of the NLM model is in the way it relates the sensory signal to phonological categories. An infinite number of categories, including nonphonological information like the sex of the speaker, loses linguistic power. It might be a reasonable description of the development of speech perception, because babies and young children do not have fully organized phonologies, so conflicts between contextual variants and ideal cases either do not arise, or exist in the child's system anyway. But this is not a welcome solution.

Another possibility might be that the organization of each syllable is internally coherent so that each subelement knits perfectly into the whole. In this case, the magnet effects would reflect acoustic coherence arising from vocal-tract dynamics as well as phonological structure. This is an interesting possibility that has yet to be explored,

although it has parallels in the theory of direct realism.

A fourth question is to what extent the development of linguistic structure involves elimination of boundaries, as illustrated in Figure 15-4, compared with the construction of boundaries. In other words, does the baby arrive in the world with *all* speech sound categories as basic cuts in its perceptual space, or does it have to discover some? Data from infants' perception of acoustically similar phonetic contrasts, such as dental versus alveolar stops, is needed here.

The final problem for the NLM model that we discuss here concerns the interpretation of the data from which it has been concluded that the perceptual magnet effect is specific to humans. The NLM model proposes that the ability to discriminate gross category boundaries is a general auditory ability that is not special to speech, nor even to humans. In contrast, reorganization of the perceptual space and the development of the perceptual magnet effect is species-specific in that only humans do it and also language-specific in its details. This represents an appealing and welcomely moderate position in the special-mechanisms debate. However, more work is needed to assess its validity. There are a number of problems. First, to date there is only one published investigation of the perceptual magnet effect in nonhumans, Kuhl's (1991) experiment with monkeys (Chapter 13), which failed to find a magnet effect for American English /i/. Second, if the effect is truly language-specific, then it seems unreasonable to expect monkeys to show magnet effects for a communication system not native to them. A more stringent test would be to look for magnet effects in categories of sound that the monkeys themselves use in communication, and, preferably, to test for them in dialects across monkeys of the same species, if such dialect variations can be found. Another more relevant test for captive monkeys might be to look for magnet effects in syllables of words that are important to them and often used around them, perhaps in the word *applesauce*. Experiments of these types are difficult, so no rapid answers can be expected. There are also other problems in interpreting the existing data from monkeys, but they involve detailed analysis and argument that would take us beyond the scope of this book.

Despite all these potential problems, the NLM model is appealing in a number of ways. It is almost unique in being a potentially general theory whose origin is in child development. The importance of development to theories of both speech production and perception has only begun to be appreciated relatively recently. Another attractive aspect is the emphasis on polymodal information, both from other sensory channels such as vision and internally to the individual. This approach seems rational: The auditory channel is initially primary, for speech is not perceived normally and efficiently in the absence of normal hearing, but perception is subject to other influences. The emphasis on natural categories has connections with quantal theory, offering a useful extension in the proposal that special feature-sensitive auditory mechanisms, and regions of articulatory-acoustic stability, are not necessary to produce percepts of distinct categories: Simply experience of hearing a particular language will distort the perceptual space in ways that predispose the listener to hear distinct categories where none exist physically. The underlying implication is that phonetic categories are formed from statistical distributions of what is heard. This view is the opposite of auditory enhancement theory, in which distinct categories are formed by speakers enhancing particular types of acoustic property, and by the additional auditory distortions that these properties can produce due to general psychoacoustic processes. In the NLM model, perceptual distortions occur as a result of linguistic experience. Though quite different from one another, the NLM and auditory enhancement models are not incompatible, however: Perceptual space may be modified by more than one cause.

The NLM model is intended to describe one aspect of how an individual's phonological structure develops and does not attempt to address the details necessary for a complete model of speech perception. But it is compatible with a number of other approaches. For example, because magnet effects distort perceptual space, they arguably provide a mechanism that would produce language-specific auditory invariance. The model could also be incorporated into activation models based on neural networks, as described below. There are a number of methodological and interpretational problems in the current data, and the model urgently needs, and is receiving, extension to a wider range of speech sound categories. Clarifying to what sound category the magnet effect applies—allophonic, phonemic, and/or syllabic—is especially important. Even if current interpretations of the perceptual magnet effect do not stand the test of time, the model will have stimulated valuable new ideas about the development of speech perception from infancy to adulthood, about relationships between phonetic perception and linguistic structure, and about the nature of linguistic categories themselves.

Decoding a Linguistic-Phonetic Message Independently of Other Acoustic Information?

The theories discussed so far are all based on the implicit or explicit assumption that speech perception must separate information from the signal and classify it into abstract linguistic categories. These categories are usually either relatively clearly defined distinctive features, or so-called "phonetic segments" that are normally treated as equivalent to phonemes. In most cases, these categories are predefined by the linguistic theory and have not themselves been very critically evaluated by the speech scientists who have adopted them. Gestural theories linked with articulatory phonology are less open to this criticism, because articulatory phonology has taken units of speech production, gestures, into phonology, rather than taking phonological constructs into a theory of speech production. However, although the focus is on gestures that make vocal tract constrictions, these constrictions are treated in speech perception theories very like the most criterial distinctive feature(s) of a particular phonemic minimal contrast.

There are two potential problems in uncritically adopting linguistic constructs for speech perception theories. One is that most current linguistic theory deals with the system of language independently of the speaker; the analytical categories appropriate for linguistics may not be the most appropriate for accounts of how human brains work. The second problem is that linguistic categories are themselves the products of a particular way of analyzing language. There are alternative ways of looking at the structure of language, and these lead to different constructs. The theoretical constructs that shape the terminology of a theory also shape the solutions it offers. In our case, we have inherited phonetic units that are rearrangeable into different sequences, namely the phonemes (or feature bundles) that differentiate units of meaning. In this and the next section, we discuss some ideas that suggest that theories of speech perception might profitably take a more critical approach to linguistic constructs.

The assumption that the listener's task is to find abstract linguistic units from the speech signal has encouraged the view that the signal contains linguistically relevant and linguistically irrelevant information. The relevant information includes what we would put in standard systematic narrow and phonemic (phonological) transcriptions (cf., Ladefoged, 1993; Laver, 1994). It helps us get to the words, and so to the meaning, in a fairly nonredundant way. It may include prosodic information, but this is often seen as secondary to "segmental" information, though of course it is not. Some of the irrelevant information tells us personal characteristics of the speaker such as gender, approximate age, aspects of his or her health and emotional state, and so on. Other information is apparently irrelevant to both the linguistic and the social message, and generally remains unanalyzed and unaccounted for. Categorizing the signal in terms of its supposed relevance to linear linguistic-phonetic units has

encouraged the search for invariance and discreteness in the physical signal.

Some research suggests that this view may be mistaken. We have already seen that auditory enhancement theory, though based on early identification of discrete properties (first general perceptual IPPs and then linguistic distinctive features), does not assume discreteness in the signal. Information for any given IPP may come from a number of acoustic properties distributed across at least a whole syllable. Although the NLM model suggests that listeners' perceptual space may be restructured to conform with the sound categories of his or her particular language, loss of discrimination of "irrelevant" attributes only operates in relatively small regions around prototypical values of sound categories, and the restructuring is not seen as permanent, but will change if the language environment changes significantly.

The most systematic body of research on the relevance of "linguistically irrelevant" information to speech perception comes from Pisoni's laboratory. Some has already been described in Chapter 13 (section entitled "Developmental Loss, or Selective Attention? The Effect of Retraining"). There we noted that Pisoni and his co-workers (e.g., Pisoni et al., 1994) demonstrated that robust sound categories can only be relearned when listeners hear a wide range of different instances of the sound; training on single cases of natural speech—or worse still, on synthetic speech with its very reduced and stylized information—tends to be an ineffective way of teaching adults to discriminate foreign sound contrasts. An experiment by Goldinger, Palmeri, and Pisoni (1992) suggests that the variation that listeners find useful is not just "relevant" variation that helps define abstract linguistic-phonetic categories; rather, it is all the physical properties of the speech.

Goldinger and co-workers (1992) report two experiments in which subjects listened to lists of words spoken in isolation. In one experiment, the task was to say whether each word was new or old (had appeared in the list before). The experimenters varied the number of intervening words (between 1 and 64, which introduced lags of up to 3 or 4 minutes), what voice a repeated word was spoken by (the same speaker as the original, a different voice of the same gender, or a different voice and gender), and the number of speakers in the data set (between 1 and 20). Memory for repeated words spoken by the same voice was always better than for repetitions in either of the different-voice conditions, which did not differ from each other. There were of course strong effects of the number of intervening words, and the number of speakers in the data set, but these only affected the overall accuracy of the data; they did not interact with the effects due to whether the repeated words were spoken by the same person.

In the second experiment, Goldinger and colleagues (1992) asked whether these differences would be found when the memory load was higher, and when it was less clear to listeners that the task involved memory. The stimuli were the same as for the first experiment, but this time there were two tests, both demanding more memory because the delays were longer (5 minutes, 1 day, and 1 week). In one test, the *explicit* memory test, the task was the same as in the first experiment: Say whether you've heard the word before. The results for this test were also the same as for experiment 1 (better identification of same-voice repetitions in the second test), although the difference was no longer significant after one week. For the *implicit* test, listeners heard the words in noise, and their task was to identify the word in each of two sessions. Here, the measure of interest was the difference between accuracy of identification in the second session compared with the first. Because the task was to identify the word, subjects' memories were tested only indirectly. Unlike the explicit test, length of delay did not affect the results of the implicit test, although listening was more accurate when there were only two voices. Most crucially from our point of view, even when a whole week separated the two sessions, identification of repeated words was better when the same voice was used, and worse when the word was repeated in a different voice.

These experiments suggest that specific instances of words affect lexical storage and retrieval. Details about specific instances may affect word recognition even when the details are no longer consciously available to the listener, because the implicit test showed advantages for same-voice repeated words after a week, whereas the explicit test did not. In other words, the data suggest that a word's representation in the brain includes, or can include, information about the speaker, and that this information makes it easier to identify the word. Since, at least for short-term memory (less than five minutes) the memory trace is not affected by the number of speakers or their gender, it further suggests that the encoding of detailed voice information is automatic: It is not something that listeners choose to do in order to perform better at a particular task. This "episodic memory" (memory of particular instances) is quite different from the abstract representation commonly assumed by theories of speech perception. Research on cognitive processes suggests that episodic memory contributes importantly to how humans form categories in nonlinguistic systems (Pisoni et al., 1994).

Pisoni (1992) points out that many properties of speech make it particularly suitable for episodic, as opposed to abstractionist, approaches to categorization. These properties include multi-dimensional categories (such as phonemes) that are hard to define, complex relations between the properties of the signal and the categories abstracted from them, high variability in the stimuli, and high redundancy in the signal together with each cue only partially identifying the category of which it is a member.

There are important implications to these conclusions that we remember very detailed episodic information about what we have heard. If episodic memory includes information about the speaker's voice, by implication it can include any sort of information about the stimulus. This suggests that abstract segmental-phonetic information is not separated from "nonlinguistic" information when words are identified. It also suggests that the lexical representation of a word may be continuously updated as more instances are heard. Continuous updating of course allows for learning. Together with Best's (1994, 1995) observations on the inherent acoustic distinctiveness of the foreign contrast and its relationship to the listener's native sound categories, and with Kuhl's perceptual magnets, continuous lexical updating could play a crucial role in (re)learning foreign contrasts. For example, novice learners often understand a foreign language better when the speaker is familiar. Continuous lexical updating of detailed, speaker-specific information could underlie how children acquire the accent and voice quality of their local speech community as they learn its phonology and has also been proposed for gradual adaptation to new accents (cf., Hawkins & Warren, 1994).

There are connecting threads between this work on episodic memory in speech perception and at least two of the theories discussed above. First, like Fowler's application of direct realism to speech, Pisoni and his colleagues are bringing into speech perception concepts that were developed in nonlinguistic psychological research, in this case categorization of nonspeech stimuli. And second, introducing episodic memory as part of lexical knowledge is compatible with Kuhl's suggestion that abstract prototypes and memory for specific instances could co-exist and help define perceptual categories, as well as with their work on the development of perceptual magnets. In both cases, the development of cognitive categories is seen as a dual process whereby a category's criterial attributes become perceptually more distinctive, and noncriterial aspects become less distinctive, so that some differences in the physical stimuli are exaggerated by the perceiver, and other differences are condensed. This approach is worth pursuing because it encourages a more critical look at the assumptions underlying our theories of speech perception, emphasizes more clearly the role of experience and of interaction between the environment and the listener, and places speech perception within a broader framework of human behavior. In short, this type of approach has the merit of trying to make the theory fit the data, instead of forcing the data to fit the theory.

Are Phonemes Necessary for Speech Perception?

If people use very detailed, context-dependent information about particular instances of words they have heard when they identify words from the speech stream, do they also identify the discrete units of standard linguistics, and if so, which units, how abstract are they, and how and when are they abstracted? Questions like these are increasingly being asked in speech perception research (cf., Remez, Fellowes, & Rubin, in press). Like the arguments about the modality of speech perception, the topic is complicated and unlikely to be resolved in the next few years. To give a flavor of the arguments, consider some reasons why the phoneme may not be a basic unit in speech perception, defined as the identification of words. To keep the argument simple and within mainstream thought, we will assume that some linguistically relevant categories are normally identified quite early in the perceptual process, and, because they are familiar, we will call these categories distinctive features, although the argument would be much the same if they were called gestures instead.

Thus, our question becomes, is a phonemic segmental stage necessary? Why not map features directly onto words? One argument against a phonemic stage is that, if phonemes must be identified before a word can be identified, then the phoneme stage must be intermediate between the incoming acoustic signal and the identification of a word. The advantage of an intermediate classification is that it allows you to reduce processing load by throwing away detailed information and keeping only the distinctive parts. So to be worthwhile, the intermediate classification must be reasonably error-free, because it is not safe to throw away the detailed information unless the classification into intermediate categories is correct. If the first classification turns out to be wrong, the detailed information will be needed to make a second classification.

There are at least two sources of evidence that these two conditions are not met: detailed acoustic information is not thrown away, and errors are made and are corrected. The work on episodic memory discussed in the previous section suggests that, far from being thrown away, detailed acoustic information is used when words are identified. Even if you don't accept Pisoni's interpretation of these data, you may be willing to accept that listeners can correct perceptual errors quite a long time after the misperception, reconstructing an entire phrase. If you observe your own misperceptions, you will probably notice that you can back-track to reinterpret acoustic information quite a long time after a misperception; you reconstruct the whole phrase and seem to "hear" that the reconstruction is more satisfactory than the original interpretation (see also Hawkins & Warren, 1994). This too suggests that detailed acoustic-phonetic information is still available after a phonemic string could be assigned.

The second source of evidence in this argument is that the listener sometimes can't be sure that a phonemic classification is error-free until after the acoustic offset of some candidate words. For example, in the sentence *I saw the plum on the tree,* listeners are not sure that the word is "plum" rather than "plumber" until towards the end of the word *on* (Grosjean & Gee, 1987). The listener is presumably able to keep both lexical options available (cf., Cutler, 1986; Swinney, 1979). Logically, therefore, there seems little to be gained by throwing away the detailed sensory information before word strings are identified.

A less commonly made argument against phonemes comes from language acquisition. There is fairly clear evidence that children learn to talk by imitating the general sound pattern of what they hear, having carried out little or no phonological analysis (cf., Eimas, Miller, & Jusczyk, 1987; Ferguson, Menn, & Stoel-Gammon, 1992; Jusczyk et al., 1995). If that is the case, then presumably they operate without a fully systematic phonemic inventory, and if children start by doing that, it is difficult to see that they should be obliged to change as they get older, though they may develop awareness of phonemes.

Klatt (1979, 1989) argued against all intermediate stages of classification, largely on the grounds of the complex and overlapping relationships between acoustic properties and successively higher-order phonetic units like allophones and phonemes—the many-to-one and one-to-many problem that pervades discussion of acoustic phonetics. As we have seen, acoustic properties cannot always be straightforwardly combined into phonetic features; features cannot always be straightforwardly combined into phonemes. Klatt suggested instead that words are represented in the brain as spectral patterns (templates); the acoustic signal, analyzed as a series of short-time spectra, is directly compared with these lexical spectral templates, and the word identified is the one whose stored template best matches the signal. This is known as the LAFS (Lexical Access from Spectra) model of speech perception. Other recent work, such as that of the auditory enhancement theorists, suggests that such a radical approach might not be necessary. However, the emphasis in LAFS on preserving acoustic detail is interestingly similar to the multidimensional, episodic approach of Pisoni and his colleagues.

In summary, it seems reasonable to suggest that words can be identified before their constituent phonemes, and that phonemic identification does not normally precede word identification. This does not mean that phonemes are not accessible to the listener, but only that they do not have to be identified en route to identifying a word. Put another way, it is possible but not obligatory to interpret the signal in terms of phonemes before lexical access. Normally, the phonemic interpretation will come after lexical access, perhaps to the extent that the person is literate in an alphabetic writing system (or perhaps phonetically trained!). Some experimental evidence suggests that only people who have learned to read an alphabetic writing system can reliably identify phonemes (cf., Liberman, Shankweiler, Liberman, Fowler, & Fisher 1977; Morais, Bertelson, Cary, & Alegria, 1986; Morais, Cary, Alegria, &

Bertelson, 1979; Morais & Kolinsky, 1994; Read, Zhang, Nie, & Ding, 1986). Of course, listeners might use phonemes unconsciously to decode speech even when they have no conscious awareness of phonemes (cf., Huang & Hanley, 1995). But evidence that phonemic awareness depends on being literate in an alphabetic system is compatible with a model of perception in which a phonemic stage is not obligatory.

Modeling phonemes as only an optional route resolves the conundrum in which allophonic information is crucial to feature identity and word segmentation but must be ignored in order to assign phoneme status. In a model in which phonemes are not central, we preserve the perceptual cueing value of variation due to phonetic context (including syllabic position) and connected speech processes by relating the input directly to phonological structure. Thus, we preserve the information about syllable-dependent variation in the spectral and temporal properties of phones that is crucial to lexical access. For example, other things equal, /s/ is longer at the beginning of a syllable than the end. The duration of the /s/ therefore signals which syllable it belongs to. If this information is not available to the listener because both syllable-initial and final [s]s are coded simply as the phoneme /s/ before words are identified, then there is a good chance that words will be misidentified because they will be wrongly segmented: *The cat saw dogs* could be interpreted as *the cats or dogs* (in an accent that does not have postvocalic /r/). Similarly, in British English the phoneme string /ðəgɹeɪtɹeɪn/ could be *the gray train* or *the great rain*, and /ʌpəteɪtəklpk/ could be either *up at eight o'clock* or *a potato clock*. You can think up other examples of your own.

The claim that we preserve syllable-dependent allophonic information can have interesting phonological implications. Take the position- and/or style-dependent distinction between clear versus dark or vocalized /l/ found in several varieties of English. Thus *lull* is [lʌɫ] in standard Southern British English, but a "vocalized" pronunciation, [lʌʊ], is rapidly gaining ground as a stylistic

option for some speakers and is the only option for others. In standard phonological theory, all these accents are said to have a phoneme /l/ that can fall either before or after a syllabic nucleus. But are these "l"s the same for speakers who have only the vocalized version syllable-finally? For such speakers, the vocalized version is subject to linking phenomena that cannot occur in the dark /l/ version: consider *legal fees,* [liɡʊfiz], but *legal aid,* [liɡʊweɪd], in the vocalized accent. The dark /l/ accent would say [liɡəɫeɪd], and never [liɡʊweɪd]. This suggests that, in these contexts, vocalized and word-initial /l/ are phonologically distinct. An important consequence of distinguishing syllable position of phones or features is that syllabic constituency is not only signaled, but preserved throughout the interpretation. Correct assignment of syllabic constituency seems basic to correct word segmentation, but this information is lost in a phonemic string unless phonotactic constraints are violated.

In summary, we conclude with Pisoni and Luce that "units like phonemes which are identified within linguistic theory are probably not good candidates for processing units in the real-time analysis of speech. However, units like phones, allophones or context-sensitive diphones may be more appropriate to capture important generalizations about speech and to serve as perceptual units during the earliest stages of speech perception" (1987:26). To this list we could add some type of distinctive features. Consistent with the points made in this section, the remainder of this chapter considers theories of speech perception that are less tightly tied to linguistic constructs and/or that take a more widely functional approach to speech perception than those discussed in earlier sections.

TOWARD A MORE COMPREHENSIVE THEORY OF SPEECH PERCEPTION

What Do We Want to Account For?

None of the theories we have looked at so far can account for everything we know about speech perception. In particular, with the exceptions of

LAFS and LAFF, none directly addresses the goal of speech perception, which is to identify words and meanings. All are still grappling with the problem of how listeners identify phonetic units. In this section, we consider what can be done to place these theories in the broader context of word identification and meaning. This means that we must consider more than careful speaking styles and short, simple phonemic sequences. We want a theory that holds good for all the varieties of speech that speakers standardly produce and understand, and that is able to include all the linguistic and nonlinguistic knowledge that listeners use when they understand what another person is saying. The theory must take account of knowledge from a wide range of sources that contribute to understanding the message.

Let us assume that there is some truth in each theory we have considered. What then should we take from them into a more comprehensive theory? Quantal theory and its developments tell us that certain short stretches of the speech signal provide unambiguous information about a particular place or manner of articulation: These information-rich sections signal the presence of a particular value of a distinctive feature, typically as a short-term event at an acoustic-phonetic boundary. Auditory enhancement theory suggests that some information about distinctive features may be built up from different types of acoustic information that is distributed across a syllable or sequence of syllables. The Motor Theory and direct realism also tell us that information about a single phoneme is distributed in time over the signal. Although their focus is on how listeners use speech gestures to understand the signal, one of their more theory-neutral contributions is to stress that movements of the vocal tract provide the signal with acoustic-perceptual coherence. That is, unless the signal sounds as if it comes from a single vocal tract, listeners will not hear it as a single person's speech. Quantal theory also stresses relationships between vocal tract movements and acoustic and perceptual consequences. Direct realism shows that the listener's own experience and expectations affect how the sensory input is organized and

understood. All theories suggest that we should be seeking to identify phonetic categories of sound, though it is not clear whether those categories include all or only some of the standard linguistic categories such as distinctive features, allophones, phonemes, and syllables. Finally, since experiments show that speaker-specific attributes of the signal can affect some aspects of speech perception, a good theory of speech perception should potentially allow the strictly linguistic part of the message to be linked with its more general properties.

Additionally, if a theory is to account for normal communication, it must allow us to identify words from the stream of speech without ambiguity. This means, at least, that the listener must keep track of allophonic information so that the structure of syllables is clear. We discussed this point when we considered whether phonemes are a necessary stage in the speech perception process, using pairs in which only allophonic information distinguishes the right words, as in *the cats or dogs* and *the cat saw dogs,* or *gray train* and *great rain.*

To summarize, we want a theory that allows linguistically relevant categories of sound to be developed from the speech signal without assuming that immediate perceptual responses are necessarily categorical and that does not require the signal to be equally clear at all times. While some sounds, in some circumstances, are likely to be systematic enough to be considered invariant, others are not, so our theory must be able to accommodate both invariant and variable, or partial, information. The theory must assume that the perceptual system keeps track of both short-term and long-term events and that the sensory signal is understood in the context of the listener's existing linguistic and nonlinguistic knowledge.

The Role of Knowledge and Variability: The H&H Theory and Perception

1. The task of speech perception is to understand meaning.
2. The speaker and the listener cooperate in communicating: The speaker produces as much

coarticulation as the listener can tolerate. The amount the listener can tolerate varies with the purpose and the content of the message.

3. The listener uses all his or her knowledge to interpret the sensory signal: The signal just fills in the missing information.

Lindblom has suggested that variability in the signal is not an unfortunate side effect of the co-articulatory activity of the vocal tract, but a crucially informative part of the linguistic message (Lindblom, 1990, 1996; Lindblom, Brownlee, Davis, & Moon, 1992). Listeners use it, and theorists should therefore make sense of it. He believes that speech organization is based on communication, defined as lexical access and understanding. The patterns of speech (and language in general) that a talker uses will vary systematically with the purpose of the communication. The person doing the talking adapts all aspects of his or her language to the needs of the hearer. We are all aware of choosing our words and grammar to suit the type of message and who we are talking with. This is very obvious when we speak to an adult right after speaking to a child, or to a close friend or family member compared with a stranger, but it affects every spoken communication, not just these extreme cases, and it affects the phonetics of our speech, not just the words and grammar.

Following Roman Jakobson, Lindblom suggests that when the main purpose of talking is to convey information, then speech will be clear because it is important that it is intelligible. When the main purpose is social, then the speaker will use phonetic reductions that make the speech easy to understand only if one is a member of the speaker's social group. When the main purpose is to express emotional closeness, babytalk and similar distinctive patterns will be used. So speech can be used to define oneself as a member of a group in order to preserve either social distance or social cohesion. H&H theory takes its name from this premise that speech varies along a continuum from very clear "hyperarticulated" to very unclear or reduced, "hypoarticulated."

The speaker and the listener cooperate in this act of communication, balancing the talker's need to use as little articulatory effort as possible against the listener's need to be given a clear message. When the subject matter is obvious, the talker can speak less carefully than when the subject matter is less predictable. In short, the speaker produces as much coarticulation as the listener can tolerate. The listener, in turn, understands the spoken message in the context of the entire communicative situation. His or her knowledge and expectations about what is likely to be said are just as important as the spoken message itself. The spoken words, Lindblom suggests, provide only the information that is missing from the act of communication, interacting with the listener's understanding of the general subject matter and the talker's emotional attitude. Lindblom calls this a "signal-plus-knowledge" approach.

A consequence of these arguments is that Lindblom abandons the search for a single primary unit of perception, arguing that no level of organization is privileged enough to be indispensable. In particular, neither articulation nor the acoustic/auditory signal is seen as especially privileged, although he does suggest that the auditory channel probably has some precedence, because it carries the most crucial sensory information.

Another claim of Lindblom's model is that there are probably no absolute invariants in the signal itself. The invariance in a message is in the string of words, or in their meaning. The systematic variability throughout the whole range of speech styles means that it makes no sense to talk of invariants, because they can only apply to a particular type of speech, and no one type of speech is more correct, or more important, than any other.

Evaluation of H&H Theory. Like quantal theory, H&H theory is broadly based and is relevant to speech production as much if not more than to perception. The reasoning behind it is based on data from a wide program of research carried out by Lindblom and his colleagues over more than thirty years, as well as inquiry into evolution and various biological systems. We will evaluate only those aspects of the theory that apply to speech perception.

The H&H theory proper offers a general approach to perception, rather than being a theory in its own right, because it says little about the processes by which speech is perceived. It mainly provides a framework for making sense of the variability found in speech production. But because it stresses the meaning and social function of speech rather than its formal structure, the theory highlights the importance of the listeners' knowledge interacting with the incoming sensory signal and provides a broader context from which a more complete model of perception could be developed. Lindblom (1996) suggests some directions, which we discuss in the next section.

In its current form, the theory is too powerful in at least two ways. It must be constrained to give more appropriate emphasis to information available from the sensory signal and from its systematic variability. First, it takes an extreme position on how the speech signal varies, giving great emphasis to the information that systematic variability conveys while largely ignoring the fact that not all variability is systematic. There can be big differences between different repetitions of the same word in the same context by the same speaker. We need to know a lot more about how much variation is systematic rather than random and how much the systematicity influences perception. Although we have known for a long time that these influences exist (Lieberman, 1963), their widespread study is relatively recent and there is much left to learn (e.g., Engstrand, 1992; Fowler & Housum, 1987; Hawkins & Warren 1994; Hunnicutt, 1987; Nooteboom & Kruyt 1987).

Second, the theory almost certainly underestimates the importance of the sensory signal compared with the speaker's knowledge. A clear sensory signal will override any expectations, as is obvious if a person suddenly starts saying nonsense words or talking in a foreign language, or suddenly changes the subject in the middle of a sentence. It is obviously true that the acoustic signal supplies missing information, but that information is crucial. It almost always defines the message, and it can define expectations. So to stress that the acoustic signal supplies only missing information risks trivializing the role of sensory input. However, it does force us to reevaluate what our perceptual theories should look like and will probably be modified soon. Lindblom (personal communication) has said he will probably give greater emphasis to the auditory channel in future forms of the theory, because his observations of how young children learn to understand and speak suggest that he may have underestimated its importance.

Notice how H&H theory seems to take even further the direct realists' claim that the acoustic signal is meaningless in itself: that the sounds are only the product of speech gestures and have no significance unless they can be related to such gestures. Direct realists maintain that vocal-tract gestures are meaningful because they are the units of phonology, and the goal of speech perception is to derive a phonological interpretation of the spoken signal. It is therefore gestures that listeners recover as the first stage of understanding speech. But in H&H theory, phonological units are meaningless, too, because the goal of speech perception is to identify words or their meanings, not to identify phonological units or any other stage between the signal and its meaning. Lindblom uses the analogy of a hungry rat being forced to run through a maze to find food. It can use any form of locomotion, and it can use the same form each time, or different forms. No one suggests there should be invariants in the rat's movements—the end goal is the only invariant. Applying the analogy to speech perception, it doesn't matter how listeners do it, as long as they reach the goal of understanding the meaning or at least identifying the words. Thus, in H&H theory, phonology, like the physical signal, is only a medium for carrying the message; it is not the message itself.

This viewpoint is not as extreme as those on the roles of variability and the sensory signal, but it does risk being overinterpreted. Just as a rat *can* use any form of locomotion to get through the maze but normally will use much the same movements in the same circumstances, so can listeners use a wide range of information to understand a talker, but, as we know from babies' and foreign listeners' behavior, they will normally be strongly influenced by phonological and grammatical patterns. Despite this risk, this aspect of H&H theory has the merit of breaking away from the sequential phonemic mold that is the hallmark of many phonetic theories of speech perception. In doing so, it opens up possibilities for more flexible models of perception that fit in with the richness, redundancy, and variety of human speech communication and allow perception to involve the combined influences of the sensory signal and the listener's existing knowledge.

Lindblom's theory is also like direct realism in its emphasis on how speech understanding takes place only through the interaction between the listener's experience, or knowledge, and the sensory signal. This appealing aspect of these theories reflects the influence of general biological and psychological theories of perception. The difference between H&H and direct realism is that in Lindblom's thinking the physical signal is what is perceived; as explained above and by Lindblom (1996), the theory does not require that gestures are perceived.

Lindblom (1996) gives examples of how the signal-plus-knowledge approach can help us take a fresh look at old data. In one example, he showed that when acoustic measurements from CV syllables starting with /b/, /d/, or /g/ are plotted in three dimensions rather than the two of standard spectrograms, then the resulting distributions form "clouds" that are fairly distinct for each place of stop articulation, as shown in Figure 15-5. Lindblom reasoned from these data that it should be possible to build up a concept of what each place of articulation looks like in this three-dimensional acoustic space: a sort of statistically based category or cloud. The listener need not

have heard every possible /b/-vowel combination to be able to identify the right place of articulation from patterns he or she has heard before. As long as the vowels that have already been heard with /b/ are spread fairly well across the vowel quadrilateral, they will define a distinctive pattern within whose boundaries most new /b/-vowel syllables will fall.

Lindblom applied this reasoning to data from an experiment by Kluender and colleagues (1987) in which Japanese quail learned to peck when they heard CV syllables that began with /d/, and not to peck when the syllable began with /g/ or /b/. The interesting point about this experiment was that the quail were trained on CV syllables with only four vowels, /ɪ, u, æ, ɑ/, yet they also pecked correctly to /d/ and not to /g/ or /b/ tested with a wide range of other vowels, /ɪ, ɛ, ʊ, ʌ, eɪ, oʊ, ɔɪ, ɚ:/. Vowels in these test syllables lie between the training vowel points, and therefore within the clouds whose boundaries were defined by the training. The trained quail had learned the acoustic properties of the /d/-cloud and used this knowledge to respond correctly to the new stimuli in the test condition.

Notice how the quail can be seen as knowing about human phonetic categories without any predisposition to learn human phonology or other aspects of language. The auditory input allows the knowledge to be systematized into phonetically relevant categories, and this knowledge is then used to respond to new stimuli. The new stimuli themselves further define the properties of the place-specific clouds in acoustic space.

Notice also how these ideas fit in with aspects of a number of other theories. Lindblom's clouds are compatible with Steven's ideas of acoustic or auditory invariants, where different phonetic classes are defined by particular patterns, or relationships, between certain acoustic properties. But Lindblom would stress that these exact cloud shapes may only apply to the particular style of speech used (in this case, prevocalic stops in nonsense syllables spoken in a laboratory) and would certainly be missing in some speech styles. When they were missing, the listener's knowledge would

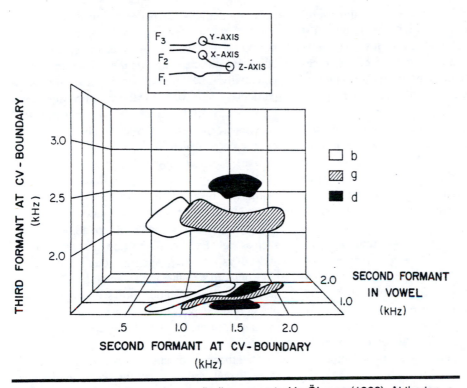

FIGURE 15-5.   A summary of some findings reported in Öhman (1966). At the top, a stylized spectrogram to define the measurements (taken from Öhman's Table IV). They include the onset of the F2 transition at the CV$_2$ boundary (plotted along the x axis), the F3 transition onset at the CV$_2$ boundary (y axis), and the F2 value at the V$_2$ steady state (z axis).

(Reprinted with permission from Björn Lindblom, Role of articulation in speech perception: Clues from production. *Journal of the Acoustical Society of America, 99*(3) 1683–1692. Copyright 1996 Acoustical Society of America)

be more important than the acoustic signal. Lindblom's interpretation of how the quails learn acoustic-phonetic categories from the statistical distribution of the input is similar to direct realism's notion of attunement discussed above: The difference is that direct realists maintain that the motoric gesture must be perceived, whereas Lindblom suggests that the same result can be achieved from systematicities in the acoustic-auditory input alone, without recourse to articulation.

H&H theory proposes that systematic variability transforms speech patterns in principled ways that perform specific linguistic and/or social

functions. One of the speaker's tasks is to work out what style of speech to use to efficiently supply the listener with information that is missing in their communication. Often, the spoken message only supplies partial information, as there are no reliable acoustic or auditory invariants transcending all speech contexts and styles: The invariant is in the word form or meaning. The listener copes with this partial information by interpreting the speech signal in interaction with his or her existing knowledge, using the signals' systematic variability in the process. Some aspects of this theory are almost certainly stated too strongly, so it needs to be constrained. In particular, only some of the variability in speech contains useful information for the listener, and we are only just beginning to find out how much. However, H&H theory is valuable in stressing the communicative function rather than the formal structure of speech, and the flexibility of speech perception within this context.

In H&H theory, then, we have an interesting point of view. Speech perception is seen as a complex, variable process in which no one linguistic unit must be identified in order for the message to be understood. Instead, meaning can be derived from a signal that is only partially informative, in interaction with the listener's linguistic and contextual knowledge. As we all know from our own experience, the listener's knowledge may also be incomplete, if only with respect to his or her understanding of the speaker's expectations and presuppositions. Small wonder, then, that so many communications are only partially successful! In the next section we consider how perception might take place under these conditions of uncertainty.

Continuous-Information Theories of Speech Perception

One question we have given no attention to so far is what the process of identifying a word, or making a phonetic decision, looks like. How is a decision made? Most of the theories we have considered so far implicitly or explicitly hold that phonetic decisions are made more or less instantaneously and without ambiguity. Motor theories (the Motor Theory and direct realism) and the quantal theory are especially good examples of this class: Theories that assume invariance in the signal or in the auditory or phonetic response to the signal generally assume that responses are categorial (either one sound/feature or another). A theoretical focus on invariance has tended to lead to questions about the modality of the invariance and to downplay detailed questions about how decisions are made.

The question of how (rather than in what modality) phonetic decisions are made comes into sharper focus when a theory does not assume

acoustic, auditory, or phonetic invariance. Theories that do not assume invariance give a major perceptual role to variability in the signal. They build on a basic assumption that all information is potentially salient and allow information about a particular feature or phone to vary in clarity. These assumptions lead naturally to the position that speech perception can at times involve a good deal of inference, which we might think of as estimation, or of weighing up the evidence for a particular linguistic unit: a feature, phone, syllable, or word. And this position in turn leads to consideration of how listeners use information from more than one source. The sources might all be sensory, such as sight and sound, or some might be sensory and others cognitive, such as sound and knowledge of word structure in the language. These considerations lead to models of speech perception that continuously evaluate information in order to estimate in some way how likely it is that a particular sound or sounds were spoken.

The theories discussed in the first part of this chapter are compatible with continuous-information models, but although some of those theorists are beginning to consider how such models can be used (cf., Fowler, 1996b), their emphasis has typically been elsewhere. In this section, we consider two theories of speech perception that give primary focus to how decisions are made rather than to the nature of the input. They are Massaro's Fuzzy Logic Model of Perception and Elman and McClelland's TRACE model.

FLMP: The Fuzzy-Logic Model of Perception

1. Each syllable is represented in memory as a prototype, a category made up of features with ideal values.
2. All sources of information are continuously and independently monitored for the information they provide about the message.
3. Perception involves estimating how closely features in the actual message correspond with the expected value of features for each different syllable, and mathematically combining

these estimations into a score for each syllable prototype. The syllable that is perceived is the one whose prototype matches the signal best.

The Model   The Fuzzy Logic Model of Perception (FLMP) was proposed in detail by Oden and Massaro (1978) and has been described in several later publications (e.g., Massaro, 1987a, 1987b, 1994). The model assumes that speech perception follows general principles of matching learned patterns. The patterns that are learned are those that occur repeatedly. They are learned mainly in infancy and childhood and are represented in the brain as prototypes. The prototypes are the perceptual units, or categories, of the particular language. The patterns from which prototypes are learned can be in any modality. For speech, auditory and visual patterns are normally most important, but other modalities such as haptic patterns (from touch) can also be learned.

Each prototype is made up of a number of properties called features. The features represent ideal values of various properties; for example, the attributes that a sound must ideally have in order to be classed as a member of a particular category or prototype. In FLMP, the prototype categories are normally taken to be syllables (although other units could be used), and the features are descriptions of phonetic properties. For example, for the syllable /ba/, one visual feature would be the closed lips and their rapid opening, and a corresponding auditory feature would be a rapid rise in the frequency of all formants. For /da/, corresponding visual features would include lips open, and possibly some view of the tip and blade of the tongue raised against the alveolar ridge and then moving away, while the auditory features would include the second and third formants falling.

Perception comprises a three-stage process of evaluation, integration, and classification decision, as schematized in Figure 15-6. The processes of evaluation and integration apply to the features, and this model is sometimes described

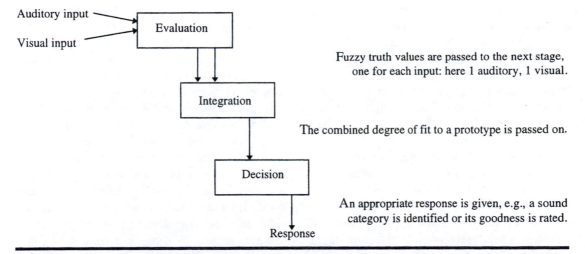

Fuzzy truth values are passed to the next stage, one for each input: here 1 auditory, 1 visual.

The combined degree of fit to a prototype is passed on.

An appropriate response is given, e.g., a sound category is identified or its goodness is rated.

FIGURE 15-6.   Schematic representation of the three stages of perception in the FLMP. Auditory and visual inputs are evaluated separately in terms of how well they fit ideal prototypical values. The resultant fuzzy truth values, one for each feature evaluated, are passed to the second stage, where they are combined into a single value that reflects how well the combined information supports a given prototype. In the decision stage, an appropriate response is made, such as the identification of the linguistic category, for example, /da/ and not /ba/. The boxes representing the three stages overlap to represent how their processes must take place successively, but overlap in time, which is implicit in the left-to-right axis.

as an example of a feature-integration model. During the evaluation stage, each property, or feature, detected in the signal is independently evaluated in terms of the degree to which it matches its expected (ideal) values for each prototype. That is, for each prototype, each feature in the signal is given a score or value. The value can be anything between 0 [absent] and 1 [present in the expected amount]. A value of 0.5 indicates that the signal is completely ambiguous with respect to that feature; a value of 0.8 indicates that the feature is represented quite strongly but there is still some ambiguity, and a value of 0.2 indicates that the signal contains little evidence for that feature. These scores are the fuzzy logic, or fuzzy truth, values. They are called fuzzy because they are continuous, rather than having only two states, 0 or 1, absolutely true or absolutely false, as in a binary model. Each value represents the degree of truth of a statement, rather than the probability of its being true, and it can be thought of as representing how closely a feature detected in the signal matches a feature in a given prototype, or the goodness-of-match between signal and prototype features. Truth values behave in many respects like probability values, but they are not quite the same. Massaro uses the analogy of deciding whether a whale is a fish. If a whale matches the category fish with a fuzzy truth value of 0.2, that means it has some fish-like properties, such as living in water, but it is a long way from being a fish. If a whale's probability of being a fish was 0.2, that would mean that 1 in 20 whales was actually a fish. The end result between matches based on probability and on truth values may not be very different, but the implications are rather different.

At the end of a single evaluation, then, the signal has been analyzed so that, for each prototype, a value has been assigned to each feature. In the integration phase, the independent contributions (values) of each feature are mathematically combined to reach a final value for the whole prototype. The clearest features have more influence on the result than the ambiguous features. The outcome is an estimate of how well each prototype in memory fits the syllable.

In the third phase, the classification decision is made, by evaluating how well each prototype fits the signal compared with other relevant prototypes. This is another mathematical calculation. Technically, the conjoined feature values for a given prototype are divided by the sum of the conjoined values for each other prototype, giving relative goodness-of-match between each prototype and the signal. Thus, the final estimate is of the best match *relative* to all the estimates for the relevant set of prototypes, with clear information having a much bigger effect than ambiguous information.

In this model, the signal is continuously evaluated, and the output from the integration phase is also continuous. Many sources of information are monitored and can contribute to perception. The sources can be both top-down (from knowledge) and bottom-up (from the signal), although the contribution of bottom-up information has received most attention. Their contributions are independent of each other right through the evaluation stage.

Empirical Evidence for the FLMP   Massaro and his colleagues argue that the FLMP accounts for the standard "problems" of speech perception without the need for posing special processes or mechanisms. He uses the FLMP to model data on categorical perception, trading relations, vocal-tract normalization, and duplex perception. Categorical perception, for example, is seen as a pseudo-phenomenon. It is not inherent in the signal or in the immediate percept, but is essentially an artifact of the experimental designs that have been used and the fact that our linguistic labels are categorial. Both identification and discrimination functions are essentially categorization tasks and can be modeled as well by continuous truth-value functions as by models that assume binary responses (see especially Massaro 1987c, 1994). Massaro is not alone in this view—see Chapter Fourteen of this book, Harnad (1987), Studdert-Kennedy (ms).

One of the most interesting and most researched aspects of the FLMP is its ability to model the fusing of different sources of information, because the ability to fuse information from different sources into a *single* percept may hold the key to how we are so good at understanding speech, with its sometimes redundant and sometimes partial auditory information. Typical experiments use the McGurk effect to investigate how sight influences our perception of sound, even to the point of producing auditory-phonetic illusions. For example, when a spoken syllable /ba/ is dubbed onto a videotape of a person saying /ga/, subjects typically report hearing /da/; when spoken /ba/ is dubbed onto a video of someone saying /da/, subjects often report hearing /ða/. The mismatched sounds must be quite similar and, as we shall see, the effects are not symmetrical.

In the original experiment (McGurk & MacDonald, 1976), the syllables *baba* and *gaga* were cross-matched, as summarized in Table 15-1 for adults only (children responded slightly differently).

When subjects heard *baba* and simultaneously saw *gaga*, as in condition (a) of Table 15-1, almost all of them (98%) reported hearing *dada*, which was neither the visual nor the auditory stimulus. On the other hand, when the stimuli were presented in the opposite way, so that subjects heard *gaga* and saw *baba* (condition (b)), there was a wider variety of responses. About a third of subjects (31%) reported hearing *baba*, suggesting that they paid most attention to the visual stimulus, and 11% reported *gaga*. But over half of them reported what McGurk and MacDonald called "combination responses," in which both /g/ and /b/ were heard, sometimes in complicated combinations like *gabga*.

TABLE 15-1. Stimulus conditions and corresponding responses for adults

	STIMULUS		RESPONSE
	Hear	See	Adults
(a)	baba	gaga	98% dada
(b)	gaga	baba	54% gabga/gaba, etc; 31% baba; 11% gaga

From McGurk and MacDonald (1976)

It is important to realize that these percepts seem very real. Although the percepts can sound ambiguous as sounds of English, depending on what visual and auditory syllables are paired, and even the particular speakers and rates or styles of speech involved (cf., Munhall, Gribble, Sacco, & Ward, 1996), subjects do not consciously know that they are getting conflicting information. So although the sound they "hear" may be easy or difficult to describe depending on the precise stimulus conditions, the percept itself is unified, immediate, and compelling. There is no question of consciously weighing up the evidence and deciding which of two conflicting sources of information must be right. When subjects look away from the video screen, they are invariably surprised to hear a different syllable.

The McGurk effect excited a great deal of attention, particularly among theorists who interpreted it as supporting the Motor Theory. But it supports the Motor Theory no more than that it shows that visual information about a speakers' movements can have a profound influence on perception. Neither does it support any theory that assumes that sensory information is processed automatically, without reference to knowledge. What it really shows is that listeners seem to use sensory information intelligently, attending to apparently good quality information, and giving less weight to apparently less reliable information. This argument fits in with one of the major principles of the FLMP (that the least ambiguous information has the greatest influence on classification decisions), and it is also compatible with knowledge-based models of perception such as Lindblom's, discussed above. The argument can be supported on logical grounds from McGurk and MacDonald's (1976) original data, and it has been further developed and tested in other experiments done in the context of FLMP (cf., Massaro, 1994) and lip-reading (cf., Summerfield, 1987).

The asymmetry of the data in Table 15-1 holds the key to explanation of the McGurk effect. The visual stimulus has a profound and consistent influence when the auditory stops are bilabial, but when the auditory stops are velar, the visual influence of lip position is smaller and less consistent, even though the lips are clearly seen. The explanation rests in what the listener knows about the relative quality of each sensory channel: It is normally obvious if the visual channel is unreliable, whereas degradation of an acoustic signal can be less obvious. In other words, it is normally easy to see that a picture is blurred or has irrelevant information superimposed on it, whereas it can be hard to know whether what you hear is due to sloppy articulation or poor listening conditions such as a reverberant room. Bearing this in mind, consider what we know about the acoustic properties of bilabial and velar stops: Acoustically, velar stops are fairly distinctive, whereas bilabials are not. Clearly spoken velars have a high-amplitude burst spectrum with a compact mid-frequency spectral prominence, and for /ga/ this prominence is also seen in the vowel transitions. Bilabials have a flat or falling low-amplitude burst distinguished mainly by its nondistinctiveness; under the right conditions, heard bilabials might easily be misinterpreted as poor pronunciations of other articulations, or as misheard due to environmental interference like room reverberation.

Listeners presumably attach more weight to a clear visual stimulus that conflicts with the auditory input when the auditory information is ambiguous. (This makes sense intuitively, and it is a prediction of the FLMP.) So when it is clear that the lips have not closed, an auditory /baba/ will be interpreted as poorly pronounced, or too quiet to hear, and so on. The combined visual and auditory information matches /dada/ best, because the lips are clearly open so the stop must be /d/ or /g/, lip readers often misread velars as alveolars, and, possibly, outside interference is more likely to mask the high frequencies of an alveolar stop burst than the distinctive mid-frequency peaks of a velar stop's burst and transitions. When the auditory signal is distinctive, as it is with /gaga/, either conflicting (though unambiguous) visual information of closed lips carries less relative weight and produces combination g-b responses, or else one source of information is ignored, and the subject "hears" either /baba/ or /gaga/.

Research in the context of the FLMP on how visual and auditory speech cues are integrated has typically taken two forms. One (e.g., Oden & Massaro, 1978) uses as auditory stimuli a series of synthetic syllables ranging between two clear end points, like /ba/ and /da/, such as might be used in a standard categorical perception experiment. Each auditory stimulus is paired with one of two visual stimuli, a face saying /ba/, or a face saying /da/, or is heard alone. Subjects write down what they hear, but unlike most identification experiments, they can respond freely rather than just with /ba/ or /da/. More recent experiments have paired naturally spoken syllables such as /ba/, /va/, /ða/, and /da/ with a face saying one of the same syllables, so that sometimes subjects see and hear appropriately matched stimuli, and at other times they do not (e.g., Massaro & Cohen, 1995). Some of these experiments have involved children, and languages other than English including Japanese and Spanish. Most are summarized in Massaro (1987d, 1994). The data from all these experiments can be predicted by the FLMP and are consistent with the view that perception involves the integration of information from different sources, in ways that reflect how much weight the subject places on each source, which is in turn influenced by what he or she knows about heard and visible speech.

In summary, auditory information dominates when it is clear, but clear visual information can also have a strong influence. When the visual information is especially informative—that is, when the articulation is bilabial or labiodental—it has a very strong influence, especially if the auditory signal is itself ambiguous. The details of the patterns of influence can be quite complicated, reflecting differences in patterns of mutual confusability among visible speech cues on the one hand and auditory cues on the other, as discussed by Summerfield (1987). We started by suggesting that the McGurk effect led to auditory illusions. In the context of the FLMP, the percept is not an illusion: It is the natural consequence of integrating conflicting visual and auditory signals, with due weight being given to the quality of information that each carries.

Evaluation and summary of the FLMP will be done after the other continuous-information model, TRACE, has been described.

TRACE: A Connectionist, Interactive-Activation Model of Speech Perception

1. A model of spoken-word recognition in which auditory input every 5 ms excites a 3-layer network of units: features, position-sensitive phonemes, and words.
2. All connections between units are bidirectional, so that top-down information flows as readily as bottom-up information, and excitation from one unit directly changes the activation level of units in other layers.
3. Connections between each layer are excitatory; those within a layer are inhibitory. So activation of a unit increases if there is also evidence for that unit in a higher or lower layer, and decreases as a unit in the same layer becomes more active.
4. The word finally perceived is the one with the greatest activation.

The TRACE model of speech perception is the best-known connectionist model of spoken word recognition and is described by Elman and McClelland (1986) and McClelland and Elman (1986). It contrasts with the FLMP because it is highly interactive, emphasizing the role of top-down processing. That is, whereas the FLMP evaluates each feature from each source of information independently of others, only later integrating this information into linguistic categories, TRACE forces units of information to mutually influence one another. TRACE is a model based on probability, and when the probability rises that the signal contains a particular word, the probability levels of each phoneme and phonological feature that comprise that word also rise.

Connectionist models are computer programs that are particularly adept at deriving categories from a lot of data. They have received intensive effort from the speech research community because they can be used as the first stage of speech recognition by machines (see Chapter Sevenn-

teen), and because the way that they work could mirror ways in which brains learn (cf., Hebb, 1949). For this reason, connectionist models are often called neural networks, or neural nets. They are basically sophisticated ways of estimating the probability of a particular category being in the signal. All connectionist models are made up of a large number of simple processing units arranged in different layers or levels. What distinguishes different models is how many units and layers there are, whether the units are predefined in the system or whether the system "learns" what they are from the data, and how the units are connected. A good summary of how connectionist models work can be found in the Appendix to Harley (1995: 397–402); Stemberger (1992) offers a clear description applied to child phonology.

TRACE has a relatively simple architecture, schematized in Figure 15-7. It is strictly hierarchical, with units in three layers of processing corresponding to the standard linguistic units of phonological features, phonemes, and words. Each unit is connected to every other unit in its own layer and the layers adjacent to it. There is some initial processing to make the speech rather like an auditory spectrogram, and then successive 5 ms "time-slices" of the signal are fed to the input units of TRACE. These input units are sensitive to acoustic features. When properties of the acoustic signal activate particular feature-sensitive units in the first layer, excitation from these activated units spreads through the net in a pattern determined by numerical weights placed on the connections. The final result is that a single word is identified because only one output unit (word) remains activated.

Connections between units are excitatory or else inhibitory. Excitation increases the activation levels (probability values) of units, and inhibition reduces them. All connections between *different* layers are excitatory, so they increase the activation levels of units; and all are bidirectional, meaning that excitation flows between layers in both directions. In consequence, excitation from a higher layer feeds back down to increase the sensitivity of relevant units on lower layers, and their

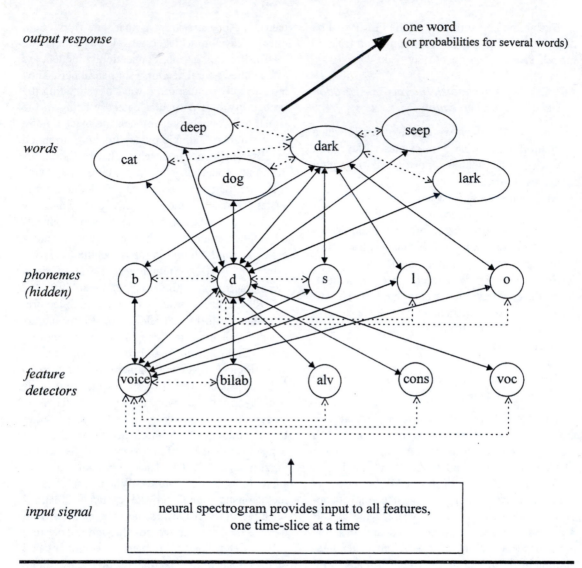

FIGURE 15-7. Schematic structure of part of TRACE. Circles/ellipses are units in each layer. Solid lines with filled arrowheads represent excitatory connections between layers. Dashed lines with open arrowheads represent inhibitory connections within a layer. Weights on connections and activation levels of units are not shown. Full sets of excitatory (between-layer) and inhibitory (within-layer) connections are shown only for the feature unit *voice*, the phoneme unit *d*, and the word unit *dark*. Connections between other units follow the same principles but are not shown, for visual clarity. Feature names are not those used in TRACE, but more familiar phonetic labels that describe the same things. See text for further explanation.

increased excitation feeds back up again. The result is a strongly interactive, top-down model in which lexical excitation directly raises the activation level of its constituent phonemes, and phonemic excitation increases the activation lev-

els of features. In contrast, all connections between units on the *same* layer are inhibitory. So when a given feature unit is excited it reduces activation of competing features that are currently less excited. Similarly, phonemes inhibit competing phonemes and words inhibit competing words. This aspect of the model emphasizes competition between linguistic units of the same type. Thus, excitation of a particular unit tends to create more excitation because it mutually excites compatible units on other layers and simultaneously inhibits competing excitation of other units on the same layer.

For example, if in the first time slice the features corresponding to voice, alveolar, and stop are excited, they will excite /d/ in the phoneme layer, and words beginning with /d/ in the word layer, such as *dog, dark,* and *deep.* Excitation of *dog* will further excite the lower layers that contribute to it. At the same time, inhibitory connections within each layer will reduce the activation level of units that are incompatible with /d/: Features corresponding to voiceless, bilabial, velar, vocalic, and so on will become less active, as will phonemes other than /d/, and words like *cat, lark,* and *seep* that do not begin with /d/. Information in later time slices changes the levels of excitation along the same principles, so that activation (or traces) for different units waxes and wanes over time until eventually one word is identified.

It can be hard to understand how this type of reciprocal excitation produces sensible results, so it is worth going into a little more detail. Each connection is associated with a number, called a weight. The value of the weight on the connection between two units governs how much excitation or inhibition passes between them: A weight of 0.7 is excitatory, and of −0.7 is inhibitory, and a weight of 0.7 passes information faster than a weight of 0.2. There are also limits on the overall ranges of excitation allowed. So although each unit in the network is connected to every other unit in its own layer and the adjacent layers, the connections do not all have the same degree of effect. For example, in Figure 15-7, the connections between the phoneme unit *b* and each word unit shown are positive (excitatory), but their weights will be very small because none of these words contains a *b*: That is, *b* will excite these words very little. In contrast, the connections between the phoneme unit *d* and the word units *deep, dark* and *dog* will be strong because these

words begin with *d,* while connections will be much weaker between *d* and the words *cat, lark,* and *seep.* Top-down excitation will reciprocally excite *d* but not *b,* and any excitation for *b* will gradually decay because there is no top-down excitation, while there is inhibitory excitation from the *d* phoneme on the same layer.

Like the FLMP, TRACE is designed to account for a number of properties of phonetic perception, including categorical perception, trading relations, lexical effects like the Ganong effect (see Chapter Fourteen), and phonetic context effects including the influence of coarticulatory patterns on speech perception. These are discussed in detail in McClelland and Elman (1986). For example, categorical perception arises in this model because there are inhibitory connections within each layer but not between layers, and the Ganong effect arises when top-down excitation from a real word increases the activation level of its constituent phonemes at the expense of competing phonemes that are not part of that word.

Evaluation of Continuous-Information Models

Comparison of the FLMP and TRACE   These two models have many similarities and some important differences. They are similar in that they produce a single response from a number of choices, they operate with relatively continuous interpretation of information, they attempt to account for a wide range of the phenomena of laboratory speech perception but have been tested little or not at all on natural connected speech, and they are explicit and therefore in principle testable.

They differ in domain, or the type of material that they use. TRACE uses relatively constrained information to identify phonemes and words, whereas the FLMP can deal with a lot of sensory information, normally identifies syllables, and has not been tested on word identification, although in principle it could be. Similarly, TRACE could in principle use nonacoustic sensory input. TRACE can process real speech, turning it first into a neural spectrogram (roughly, a spectrogram-like representation in which the frequency parameter mirrors the ear's sensitivity in different frequency bands), and then analyzing it in the network proper. The FLMP models listeners' responses to particular stimuli—data that have already been collected—although ideally it would be connected to a real-speech processor first.

There are two much more important differences between TRACE and the FLMP than the domain they operate on, however. First, TRACE is mainly concerned with the time-course of lexical access, while the FLMP is more concerned with the classification and integration of information. And second, they differ in how they model the actual perceptual processes. TRACE assumes that units are activated or excited, and top-down information directly changes the activation levels of the feature units that pick up sensory information. In other words, top-down information interacts with bottom-up information so that their effects are not independent. In contrast, sources of information in the FLMP are independent. Thus, the FLMP assumes that top-down information supplements information from the sensory system, but does not directly change it. In the FLMP, top-down information is just one more source of information like any other; like all information, it is evaluated independently of other sources and makes its greatest contribution to a decision when information from other sources is ambiguous.

This difference between interactive and independent perceptual processing leads the models to predict different patterns of results for experiments in which information from different sources influences phonetic or lexical decisions. A series of studies presently suggest that, at the time of writing, the FLMP approximates human responses as well as or rather better than TRACE does. In each case, the arguments are detailed and rest on how well predictions from the models fit experimental results from human listeners when sounds are ambiguous between different phonemes, as with phonetic contrast effects due to coarticulatory patterns (cf., Mann & Repp, 1981) and lexical effects such as the Ganong effect. These conclusions are based on work by and Elman and McClelland (1988), Massaro (1989),

McClelland (1991), and Massaro and Cohen (1991), and the series of experiments is summarized in Massaro (1994).

The necessity for TRACE's assumption of interactive activation from top-down processes has also been questioned by Norris (1992), who has shown that a more sophisticated connectionist model can produce Elman and McClelland's (1988) results without interactive activation—that is, from bottom-up processes alone. Norris' (1992) model does use top-down processes (interactive activation) during a training phase so that the net can "learn" about lexical patterns. Errors are corrected by a process of "back-propagation," which changes the weights on connections between units until the desired output is produced. (Harley, 1995, gives a relatively nontechnical explanation of back-propagation.) Top-down effects, therefore, do influence learning in the training phase, but once training is finished, all the excitation travels in one direction only. There is a "memory" built in that takes care of phonetic contrast effects. This is like the long time-window that we have said is needed to track coarticulatory effects; it is not the same as memory that is needed to store information that contributes to phonetic prototypes or other linguistic units.

In summary, experimental tests of the FLMP and TRACE using ambiguous stimuli and different types of information suggest that TRACE overemphasizes the influence of top-down processing in speech perception. Connectionist models that make weaker assumptions about top-down activation can do as well as TRACE, as can the FLMP.

Norris' (1992) model has some interesting properties from our point of view. One is that it is based on a modification of the system that Fowler (1996b) has proposed for speech production Jordan, 1986). Like most connectionist models that work well for speech, it uses long time-windows as well as short ones. That is, as well as analyzing the signal in short chunks of a few milliseconds, it looks at relatively long durations of the signal at a time in order to take care of coarticulatory effects. The FLMP also focuses on relatively long stretches of speech because its main units are syllables, but it would benefit from a still longer window and, indeed, a shorter one.

Another interesting property of Norris' model is that it works well without an explicit phoneme layer. In defense of TRACE, it identifies allophones rather than phonemes, because each phoneme unit is sensitive to the position in the word. But the information for each allophone is still concentrated into a single unit. Unlike TRACE, the intermediate units in the Norris' (1992) net are not predefined, which means that there are no units that must correspond to phonemes. Instead, the net builds up its own system of information as it "learns." The experimenter has no control over how it organizes this information in the net. So any given intermediate unit could, in principle, correspond to a particular phoneme, but in practice phonemic information is typically distributed rather widely across a number of intermediate units. Not only is this view consistent with other experimental data (e.g., Marslen-Wilson & Warren, 1994) and with our earlier argument that it may not be necessary to identify phonemes in order to understand speech, but it also allows for individual differences in how speech is organized in the brain. The speech and language that a child hears affects the details of his or her early linguistic structures, and these details in turn affect how later speech input is organized, so that eventually, although there is much in common between different people, there is room for considerable differences between them too, as every experimenter knows. Research on bilingualism supports this argument, because many bilinguals use slightly different sets of acoustic cues to understand speech from most monolingual speakers of either language, and bilingual children hear a very different type of input from monolingual children.

Another way to assess the relative merits of FLMP and TRACE, or of TRACE and other connectionist models, is to see which can do most with fewest assumptions. On the whole, it seems that TRACE may include an unnecessary variety of processes and be too rigidly specified. For example, TRACE's connections between units in the same layer are inhibitory in order to produce categorical perception. As we have argued above in the context of the FLMP and elsewhere, categorical responses do not require categorical perception. If categorical perception is removed from the list of primary perceptual phenomena that must be accounted for, then one of TRACE's strong assumptions could prove unnecessary. Norris' (1992) arguments in favor of a bottom-up net that includes learning and memory processes point to the same conclusion.

What are we left with? Though TRACE may be incorrect in some of its assumptions, it has served and continues to serve a useful purpose. It is one of a large group of "activation" theories, so called because the signal input activates word representations in proportion to how well the representation matches the signal; the word whose representation best matches the signal has the most activation and is the one that the listener perceives. These theories were developed largely within psycholinguistics to explain lexical access. In the past, most psycholinguistic models paid little attention to phonetic problems in speech perception, tending to assume that phoneme identification was relatively straightforward. This gulf between theories of how we perceive phonetic contrasts and theories of how we perceive words is growing smaller, as evidenced by a number of phonetically sophisticated theories of lexical access such as Luce's neighborhood activation model and Marslen-Wilson's modified cohort theory. These and other models are reviewed by Lively, Pisoni, and Goldinger (1994).

General Evaluation of Continuous-Information Models   For the most part, where TRACE and the FLMP lead to different predictions, we have suggested that the FLMP is probably more satisfactory, or that another connectionist model could be preferable. The two models also share some problems. First, neither has been much tested with connected speech. The FLMP, for example, is unlikely to be able to deal well with perceptual cues from coarticulatory effects that originate in another syllable, because each syllable prototype is defined in ideal terms, so it includes little information about changes due to phonetic context, stress, or style of speech. Thus, although the FLMP is in principle capable of dealing with connected speech, in practice it would need significant modification in order to do so.

Neither model is designed to reproduce the human's ability to correct perceptual errors when later evidence comes in, for example, after the acoustic end of a word or when the sentence does not make sense. This capability could be built in and might be more straightforward to do in TRACE, but it would require considerable broadening of the current models.

However, these and other problems are common to all phonetic theories of speech perception. Despite their limitations, these continuous-information theories are valuable because each provides a working, testable, model and can describe and predict human behavior without resorting to special mechanisms that make speech quite distinct from other processes. Earlier, we argued that one does not want to invoke special mechanisms for speech unless forced to, so we tended to prefer more general theories. But we must strike a balance. While some processes of speech perception are almost certainly general to all auditory processing, there seem to be speech-specific aspects, too. Remez and his colleagues (Remez, 1994; Remez & Rubin, in press; Remez, Rubin, Berns, Pardo, & Lang, 1994) remark perceptively on just where some of the speech-specific processes lie, based mainly on experiments using sine-wave speech. They suggest that principles of general auditory perception such as Gestalt processes and auditory scene analysis (e.g., Bregman, 1990) do not explain how sine-wave speech is understood. This conclusion is independently confirmed for vowel perception by Assmann (1996). They suggest that people can understand sine-wave speech because it reflects the way the vocal tract changes shape over time, so it "makes phonetic sense." These slowly varying properties of speech provide the perceptual glue that makes a significant contribution to the perceptual coherence of the signal, partly through

innate predispositions and partly through learning. Without this glue, speech will not sound like speech and will not be processed like speech. Remez's ideas are compatible with continuous-interpretation models and could be especially valuable in developing more sophisticated ways of dealing with time in theories of speech perception. They are also compatible with the idea that linguistic categories are not found in the signal itself, but are built up as superordinate structures derived from, and then imposed on, the signal.

Another strength of continuous-interpretation models is that they actually use multiple sources of information rather than acknowledging them as important but in practice ignoring them. An attractive consequence of continuous-information models' integration of information from several sources is that there is less necessity to assume a rigid sequence of identification and classification. Evidence increasingly converges to suggest that there is no advantage in postulating a single primary unit of perception. Information is used in ways that get to the probable message fastest. Words can be identified, and meanings understood, without a full specification at each linguistic "layer."

The models all estimate in some way the best fit of the data to some predetermined ideal, which may be an ideal feature specification or a pattern built up from statistical distributions in the input signal. All make decisions in terms of relative merit—the best candidate wins. This means that a signal does not have to be very clear to produce a very clear response: It just has to be clear enough and consistent enough that it outweighs evidence for all other candidates. So quite casual speech can be very easy to understand as long as it obeys rules that the listener knows. These models, then, are compatible with Lindblom's ideas about the significance for perception of variability in speech production.

As we said above, an important aspect of connectionist models is their use of adaptive mechanisms to enable them to "learn": they are "trained" on one set of data, and, if the training data are sufficiently representative, the model can then classify entirely new data very accurately from what it has "learned" about the training data. To learn, connectionist models must have a set of hidden units and a process called back-propagation that changes the weights on and between units. Many connectionist models continue to learn with every new piece of data. The relevance for speech research is obvious. For example, it provides continuity between how children and adults process speech, and it allows people to gradually adapt to a new accent until they no longer notice it as strange.

Connectionist models, then, learn by organizing information in layers of increasingly complex hidden units. The organization is influenced by properties of the net at the outset—how many hidden units it has, in how many layers—but the way it finally looks and behaves depends on how this initial structure interacts with and is reorganized by the stimulus input. So at any given time, the structure depends partly on how it began, and partly on what the stimulus input is like. This is compatible with the development of superordinate categories described by direct realists.

Although it does not currently learn, the FLMP too is seen as part of a larger system that does. Consider the FLMP's features. They are like unconnected descriptions: /b/ has the feature "lips closed"; /d/ has the feature "lips open." To the extent that there is any connection between these two features, it is built up through learning as a superordinate category that has no bearing on primary perception. Details of the prototypes are also built up through learning, so that speakers of different languages respond differently to the same audiovisual stimuli in ways that are predictable from their language backgrounds. Language-specificity is, of course, a property of Kuhl's phonetic prototypes.

TRACE, of necessity, is more explicit than many theories about the role of time. However, a lot more could be done. The FLMP does not deal with time explicitly because it only classifies information (such as identification responses) once it has been gathered. However, to work on real speech, both models would have to make a clear distinction between the slow variation and the fast events that characterize speech and that underlie our earlier assertion that a theory needs both long and short time windows to track them. These modifications are possible and may come. Remez' work provides one source of information that could be incorporated. Its potential is especially obvious for prosodic variation that is crucial to understanding connected speech. Coarticulatory information that spreads over a whole syllable can also be important. Massaro (personal communication) and Hawkins (Hawkins, 1995; Hawkins & Warren, 1994) envisage that the perceiver knows not only about the ideal feature values for each prototype but also about the range of values and their likelihood of occurrence. Notice the parallel with direct perception, in which listeners are said to disentangle the effects of coarticulation, attributing each influence to its correct gesture. These principles are indirectly incorporated in many of the more successful systems for automatic speech recognition by machine developed by engineers. Rather than looking directly for linguistically relevant units, these typically (though not always) use either connectionist or hidden Markov models (see Chapter Seventeen) to look for patterns that have been learned from the statistical distributions of the acoustic speech signal. Those that are currently most successful look at a whole sentence at a time. This solution is not as phonetically insensitive as it is sometimes made out to be: By looking at a whole sentence, the system has a greater chance of decoding assimilations and other connected-speech processes by filling in information from long-term coarticulatory patterns and other, nonassimilated parts of words, and perhaps most importantly, it picks up the patterns due to prosodic effects.

Their compatibility with engineering solutions and psycholinguistic models of spoken-word recognition (lexical access) also makes these models valuable as bridges between disciplines. If we can make compatible theories in phonetics, word recognition, and sentence understanding, then we can begin to hope for broader models of language understanding in general.

However, although neural nets and comparable models are currently a popular and successful way of modeling speech processes, and are said by some to reflect the way the brain works, they bring with them two problems. One is that their performance reflects what the experimenter builds into them (cf., Norris, 1992). This gives them the advantage of being theory-neutral rather than having to depend on particular theoretical constructs such as gestures or a specific set of distinctive features. But it also allows so much flexibility that it can be hard to disprove them. The other problem is that nets reflect the current state of the art in computer science. Behavioral models of how the brain works have always tended to be couched in terms of contemporary models in engineering and, most recently, computer science. We can assume, then, that when neural nets are replaced by another model in computer science, there will soon be changes in models of how the brain works.

In summary, there is as yet no single continuous-information model that incorporates all the features that a theory of speech ideally needs. But these models offer great potential for developing such a theory. The FLMP and TRACE are both testable and flexible, and TRACE deals with overall temporal patterning better than most other phonetic theories. They are thus ideally suited to becoming vehicles for implementing, testing, and developing ideas from other theories.

In the FLMP, perceptual units, normally syllables, are represented as prototypes held in memory. A prototype is a category made up of features with ideal values. All sources of information can contribute to a prototype, and each makes its contribution independently of any of the others. The incoming information goes through a three-stage process: evaluation of features from each separate source, integration of different sources to reach a final score for each prototype, and classification, the final percept being the prototype with the highest value or score. In principle, the signal is continuously monitored and these three processes operate continuously. TRACE is a simple, hierarchical connectionist model with a highly interac-

tive structure. It recognizes phonemes and words. There is evidence that other connectionist models may perform as well or better than either TRACE or the FLMP, and in particular that some of the strong assumptions of TRACE are unnecessary. As examples of a type of theory, these models are valuable for their ability to integrate disparate sources of information and to arrive at linguistically relevant categories without previous segmentation of the signal. Both are compatible with principles from a number of other important theories and, if broadened, could form the basis of a general theory of speech perception. They are also valuable for providing connections between phonetics and other research and applications in understanding speech and language.

Conclusions

The theories discussed in this chapter have many things in common, and where they differ or are incomplete, aspects of each can be combined into a coherent picture. In this section, we suggest what a model developed in this way could look like, although this view would not be shared by all theorists.

The structure of our model is uncontroversial and is in principle like those outlined in the continuous-information theories: From the input signal, the model identifies properties that are linguistically relevant, combines them into higher-order categories, and identifies their linguistic status in a matching process. This process repeats as long as the signal continues. Controversy arises over the details of the process. Here, we outline one viewpoint based loosely on the preceding discussion.

The viewpoint taken here is a simple "best match" model. Words are represented in memory as sets of features with appropriate probability or truth values, together with knowledge of how those values can change with different styles of speech or phonetic contexts. The input signal is also represented as a complete set of features whose values could be represented either as probabilities or truth values. Truth values are appealing because they imply a measure of dissimilarity or similarity, as explained above, but we will use probabilities because they are more familiar. In this discussion, the difference between the two is unimportant. The signal is continuously monitored for information on each unit and continuously interpreted, giving rise to continuous modulation of probability levels of input features. Simultaneously, these probability patterns are matched against the feature patterns for different words in memory, and the best match is chosen. The model allows for the system to track time functions and hence vocal-tract dynamics and their acoustic consequences.

Let us look in more detail at how words could be represented. Words are stored in memory as features organized into hierarchical structures. These features differ in three important ways from standard phonological distinctive features. They are expressed in terms of probability, so that they take continuous values (from 0 to 1) rather than being binary. They are distributed across time rather than bundled into phonemes, so that their probability changes within a single word. And they are integrated into higher-order structures that indicate their syllable structure, the relative stress of each syllable, and its organization into rhythmic feet. In other words, the structure of each word can be conceptualized rather like the waxing and waning probability traces for each feature of TRACE, with the traces being grouped into a hierarchy that reflects syllabic and prosodic structure, much like standard linguistic trees.

This type of structure is illustrated for the word *tasty* in Figure 15-8. The dark gray patches at the bottom of the figure show probability (or truth) values for some of the features of *tasty* heard in isolation, while the light gray patches show additional feature patterns that would be perceived when the word was heard in the sentence. So, for example, when *tasty* is heard in isolation, the feature *consonantal* only takes on a high value at the release burst of the first /t/. In contrast, when the listener hears *What a tasty . . .* , then the value of *consonantal* begins to rise during the schwa and is high throughout the silence due to the closure

period of the first /t/. The tree in the top of Figure 15-8 shows the prosodic structure for *What a tasty tomato*. Words in bold type show "strong" elements: the more strong elements that are above a particular syllable, then the more prominent that syllable is in the utterance. So in this sentence, the first syllable of *tasty* takes the nuclear accent because it has the most strong elements above it: It is the only one whose syllable, foot, and accent group are all strong. If the nuclear accent were to be on *tomato*, then the third foot would be strong, and the second would not. If *tasty* were spoken in isolation, it would have the prosodic structure of just the first two syllables of the middle foot. The strength of the prosodic structure above a word affects how it is spoken, and hence it affects the pattern of featural values, but for simplicity this is not shown in Figure 15-8, and indeed the details are not yet well understood.

Connected with these primary word structures, or "prosodic trees," is knowledge of what changes each word can undergo as the style of speech and/or its phonetic context change. This will particularly affect unstressed syllables and the ends of words and will involve knowledge of permissable ranges of coarticulatory effects like those mentioned in the evaluation of continuous-information models. For simplicity, this type of knowledge is not shown in Figure 15-8, except for the very minimal effects of putting the word in context, as shown by the light gray areas of featural values.

These prosodic trees that represent words can potentially link into structures of grammar and meaning. Some of these other structures may also be hierarchical, while others may be much more like networks of more or less similar items. Grammar would be a good candidate for hierarchy, while associative meanings (*dog-cat-mouse*) and rhymes (*pat-cat*) might be less structured networks. Each of these linked structures is directly connected with other aspects of knowledge and cognitive processing. In this way, words can be seen on the one hand as unique structures, and on the other hand as like, and connected with, non-phonetic and ultimately nonlinguistic structures.

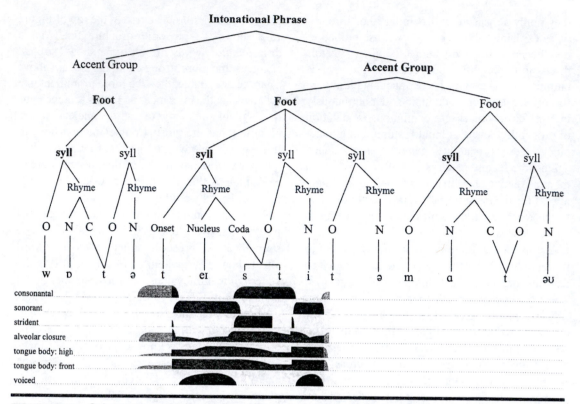

FIGURE 15-8. Schematic partial illustration of the lexical representation of the word *tasty*, together with its representation in the sentence *What a tasty tomato.* The upper part represents the utterance's prosodic structure. Syll = syllable; the syllabic constituents O, N, and C represent onset, nucleus, and coda, respectively. Relatively strong elements in the prosodic structure have bold type; relatively weak elements have normal type. The stronger an element, the more prominent it is—the more it is stressed or accented. The bottom of the figure shows the probability or truth values of some selected features in the word *tasty*. The feature names are chosen to be easily understood and intentionally make no commitment to any existing theory. Dark gray patches indicate values for features when *tasty* is heard in isolation, and light gray patches show additional information available when the word is heard in the whole sentence. The listener uses the spoken signal to build up a picture similar to that of the stored lexical representation and can identify elements at any and all levels of the structure simultaneously. For example, the presence of a stressed syllable could be identified before the place of articulation of its initial consonant, or vice versa. See text for further explanation.

The process of primary perception involves analyzing a sensory signal, together with linguistic knowledge and expectations, into potential words, and matching them with possible word meaning-structures in memory until the best match is found. This process is continuous and allows correction of errors, as described below.

All information, whether sensory from the input signal or from the listener's knowledge, is used to understand the meaning of the communication. Each type of information is weighted according to its apparent value, which will depend on what the listener knows about the source of the information. The information is first resolved into properties or features. These features may correspond directly to lexical (word) features, or they may be subcomponents of lexical features. Properties of the signal that give very clear evidence for a lexical feature include some of those that have been suggested as invariant phonological features by Stevens and his coworkers. Other properties might normally be combined to provide robust evidence for a particular feature that stretches over quite a long part of a syllable; these include the intermediate perceptual properties of auditory enhancement theory and also other features, for example, visual information about the vocal tract and prosodic information. (A truly comprehensive theory would include information about the rest of the speaker's face and body, since it is often very important for the meaning of the message, but this falls outside the scope of this model.) Whether a lexical feature is activated by a single property of the signal or by a combination of several is immaterial: Evidence for each level of the hierarchical lexical structure is always combined and classified using the same basic processes. For simplicity, we suggest that these processes comprise estimating and then matching probabilities, possibly with each source of information being evaluated independently before integration with others.

The input signal is continuously monitored in this way for information about each linguistically relevant feature. Interpretation (or evaluation) of the input is also continuous. The monitoring involves a short time-window to look for short events like stop bursts, and at least one longer window to track intonation, stress, and consistency of other long-term coarticulatory and stylistic effects. Knowledge about the speaking style, for example, allows connected speech processes to be correctly interpreted. Because both fast and slower events are tracked, early decisions affect later decisions. Equally, when an earlier decision is incompatible with later decisions, the earlier decisions can be changed by reference to a more or less complete reanalysis of the signal held in memory.

A word is identified when the best match is found between the input and stored probabilities for features. Unambiguous stimulus input is given great weight and can be in any modality, with precedence given to clear acoustic information, and to sensory information more than to knowledge. Because the system is based on choosing the most likely answer, a signal can produce a clearcut response even if acoustic cues are relatively poor, as long as they are consistent for long enough and there is no strong contradictory information—that is, as long as everything else stays relatively ambiguous.

Since the entire signal is potentially represented in episodic memory, the model system is "holistic": It is not divided strictly into discrete segments, nor into segmental-phonetic and prosodic strands. Such distinctions can be made, but they need not be, and they are not normally made. Normally each phonetic segment is identified as part of its particular syllabic and prosodic context, and each prosodic unit is defined partly in terms of its particular syllables and their particular vowels and consonants. These ideas are not new (cf., Firthian phonology and also Wickelgren, 1969). In traditional terms, allophonic information and coarticulation are represented as central properties of the system, rather than as secondary or intermediate stages relative to phonemic information. Additionally, phoneme strings need not be identified before lexical access, although there is nothing to stop them being so identified, assuming they are represented in the lexical structures. It may be that phonemes are learned about and added into the system only after a person has learned an alphabetic writing system.

Notice that the model preserves the relational, hierarchical structure of contrasts from input through to the highest levels of linguistic interpretation. No one unit is of prime importance, nor can it be functionally separated from the others in the structure of which it is part. For example, a syllable is not just a syllable; it is a strong or a weak syllable, with a complex or a simple onset, and so on. Of course, each type of unit can be analyzed independently, as they are in theoretical linguistics and practical phonetics classes. But in reality, no unit is independent of the units above and below it in the linguistic structure. In other words, because each unit is part of other units, acoustic information feeds several units simultaneously, and each unit uses several types of acoustic information.

Linguistic structures of this type are built up gradually through experience of patterns in the language(s) the child hears. The process may be started by innate or very early sensitivities to relationships between vocal-tract behavior and acoustics, and to a wide variety of sound contrasts. The development—or construction—of linguistic categories might be like the direct realists concept of attunement, or like learning in a connectionist model. The trigger for linguistic-phonetic processing into categories (by adults as well as children) could be time-varying changes in the auditory signal that are characteristic of human vocal-tract output, as suggested by Remez and his colleagues (Remez et al., in press, and the references cited above). Among the first language-specific developments might be sensitivities to the prosodic patterns of the child's native language, as discussed by Juszcyk (1994), and phonetic prototypes of the sort proposed by Kuhl and Iverson (1995). More complicated and complete linguistic structures continue to be built, very fast in early childhood, and continuing more slowly at least into adolescence. Thus, the child builds his or her own linguistic structures, not from the bottom up, phonetics to phonology to morphology and so on, but from the middle (the prosodic and syllabic structure) outwards, both up and down.

When a structure is rich and redundant as in this proposal, there is flexibility in the units used and how the signal is segmented. This provides one source of individual differences in speech production and perception. In speech production, the route the child first learns for a particular articulatory maneuver stands a good chance of being perfected. It will be changed only if subsequent learned patterns conflict with it. Likewise for perception: Some people pay more attention to one set of cues, others to another. Thus, there is room in the model for experience of the individual child to underlie individual differences in adulthood.

Individual differences in experience may mean that people do not have maximally systematic representations of language in their brains. Informal evidence suggests that some people operate throughout life without a complete phonological and syntactic system as a linguist would recognize them. Take /aid əv laɪkt tə gəʊ/, frequently expanded even by adults as *I would of* rather than *I would have*. Similarly, if phonemes are added only as a consequence of learning to read, many people may generate incomplete systems or nonstandard phonemic classes.

Notice also that a relatively direct mapping from signal to lexicon is consistent with the general approach of the more successful systems for automatic speech recognition, whose impressive recent success has depended on the use of all information over long time domains, using fairly minimal linguistic information, as described above. The general pattern-matching approach of statistical solutions to speech recognition is almost certainly relevant to human speech perception. Linguistic structures such as phonetic prototypes could be built up from statistical evidence of recurrent patterns.

SUMMARY

The classical theories of speech perception are distinguished more by details of the mechanisms, or processes, that they propose underlie the perception of speech than by the empirical findings and general processes they try to account for. For example, each tries to account for categorical perception and each postulates an invariant property or referent in, or derivable from, the speech signal. Similarly, each assumes processes that "simplify" the signal by making it as abstract as possible (like a phonemic transcription) as soon as possible, with information that is irrelevant to the linguistic message being stripped off en route.

None of these assumptions is necessary, and some more recent theories have moved away from them.

In particular, some more recent developments in speech perception are moving away from this assumption of early abstract representation and instead are assuming that we *retain* the richness of acoustic information at least until words have been identified. These approaches tend to be those that also emphasize the information-value of the systematic variability mentioned above. The assumptions underlying these newer approaches lead to very different questions that can be asked, and of course to very different theories. The theories we have looked at in this chapter have in common that they try to explain speech perception in terms of more general perceptual processes, and that the listener's experience actively structures speech perception. Although none yet answers all our questions, and it can be difficult or impossible to choose between some competing models, we have suggested that the most promising theories at present are those that continuously evaluate and integrate all sources of information to find the most probable (or most satisfactory) sequence of words.

Some of the most important questions theorists have asked are outlined below, together with more specific questions that have developed from them, and answers suggested by the research we have discussed in the last two chapters.

What does the immediate task of speech perception entail? Or, what is the modality of speech perception? Do we track vocal tract movements or reconstruct the linguistic-motoric plans for those movements, or do we detect linguistically relevant units such as features or phonemes directly from the acoustic signal alone, without reference to articulation? Alternatively, is our interpretation amodal (not modality-specific) or are we perhaps able to use a number of different routes to get to the meaning of an utterance? The answer is clearer than it was, but still not complete. It can be divided into two parts. First, it seems that we do unconsciously keep track of the modality the information comes in, because the McGurk effect suggests we evaluate how reliable the information is, which requires knowing its modality, and because we seem to remember information about the particular speaker's voice for quite a long time. But it may be that modality-specific information is only part of the linguistic information, and that as the message is processed into increasingly abstract linguistic structures, its particular modality becomes less important. Second, the answer depends partly on what the primary goal of speech perception is seen to be. If a phonological analysis is the goal, then the units are normally couched in terms of phonological units: vocal-tract gestures for direct realists, auditory features for auditory theorists, and so on. If the primary goal is to reach the meaning, then the route taken may be seen as less important. Remez argues that speech perception is amodal because all the interpretation is linguistic, occurring entirely inside the listener's head. If we take a moderate position, we could conclude that these questions are worth asking because they can tell us more about what is important in the speech signal and how it is processed, but we may never get to the answer, and in some sense there may be no answer because the modality may depend on the level of abstraction.

What "units" of perception are used? Is there a single primary unit, or more than one? There is no single unit of primary perception in the model of speech perception we suggested in the previous section. Perceptual information can activate any linguistic unit, and activation of one unit automatically begins to specify other units, because each unit is defined partly in terms of others.

Is the acoustic signal automatically decoded by brain cells that are sensitive to specific properties in it, or does the listener treat it as raw material that needs a lot of active interpretation? The second option is clearly right, but that does not rule out the possibility that brain cells are sensitive to specific properties of the speech signal. No individual cells sensitive to properties of speech sounds have been found so far, and if there are any, they only contribute a

TABLE 15-2. Comparative summary of theories of speech perception discussed in Chapters Fourteen and Fifteen.

	THE MOTOR THEORY	DIRECT REALISM	QUANTAL THEORY AND LAFF	AUDITORY ENHANCEMENT THEORY	NATIVE LANGUAGE MAGNET MODEL	CONTINUOUS-INFORMATION MODELS
Main modality	Motor	Motor	Auditory	Auditory	Neutral; auditory bias	Neutral/multi-modal
Philosophy	Perception by reference to speech production	Direct experience of the physical object causing sensation (in any modality)	Auditory neural (psychoacoustic) responses grouped into linguistic categories	Auditory neural (psychoacoustic) responses grouped into linguistic categories	Input compared with prototypes in memory, developed through experience	Knowledge-based information processing
Perceptual primitives	Speaker's intended phonetic gestures (motor commands)	Speaker's actual articulatory gestures	Acoustic or auditory correlates of linguistic distinctive features	General auditory (nonlinguistic) properties	Neutral, but strong bias toward auditory properties	Flexible, but usually a set of phonological features
Output units	Phonemes	Phonological gestures most like phonemes or allophones	Distinctive features mapped onto words	Distinctive features	Language-specific phonetic categories (phonemes?)	Flexible, but usually words (TRACE) or syllables (FLMP)
Mechanism of perception	Specialized phonetic module maps signal onto production	Integrated general perceptual systems & learning from activity	Auditory system and cognitive processes	Auditory system and cognitive processes	Auditory system and cognitive processes: prototypes	Sensory system(s) and cognitive processes
Specificity to speech	Human speech only	All modalities of perception in humans and other species	General auditory basis in humans and other species	General auditory basis in humans and other species	General auditory basis in humans and other species	Neutral

Invariants?	Speaker's intended gestures; none in the signal	Can be in proximal or distal stimuli; higher-order invariances are learned (attunement)	In acoustic signal or auditory response	None proposed, but compatible with a limited number (acoustic or auditory)	Not addressed, but would be cognitive more than acoustic	Not addressed
Role of variability:						
(a) Coarticulation	Enables perceptual access to invariant phonetic gestures	Coproduced gestures are perceived independently	Invariant acoustic properties transcend variation due to coarticulation	Mainly not addressed, but IPPs* account for much variation	Not addressed	Part of "knowledge" (after training)
(b) Speech style	Not addressed	Not addressed	Lexical items include partial knowledge of variation	Not addressed: IPPs* account for some	Possibly different prototypes	Models can be trained with new styles
Acquisition:						
(a) Information babies initially perceive	Linguistic	Nonlinguistic (gestural)	Nonlinguistic (auditory)	Nonlinguistic (auditory)	Nonlinguistic (auditory)	Not addressed
(b) Effect of hearing a language	Parameters in speech module are "tuned"	Native gestural invariants perceived more efficiently (attunement)	Not addressed	Not addressed	Perceptual prototypes and magnet effect develop	Rarely addressed, but can account for learning

---

*Intermediate Perceptual Properties

Other theories mentioned in Chapters Fourteen and Fifteen:

H&H (Lindblom): Functional-linguistic approach emphasizing signal variability, language-specific systemic influences on variability, language-specific knowledge, and common understanding between speaker and hearer; assumes initial auditory rather than motoric perceptual primitives, but as yet no details about the processes involved.

Episodic memory (Pisoni): Acoustic/auditory rather than motoric perceptual primitives, acoustic invariants are probably rare, heavy emphasis on memory and rich acoustic detail, possibly without phonemes.

Remez and Rubin: Linguistic-phonetic perceptual primitives that are abstract and modality-neutral.

small (though possibly crucial) part to the speech perception process.

Are there invariants in the signal or in the percept?   Opinions differ. Almost as many forms of invariance have been proposed as there are theories, and scientists' theoretical positions often determine how they interpret evidence for invariants. The question is not especially important for continuous-information theories and any theory that integrates information from multiple sources and matches it against a stored category. Taking a moderate position, it seems fair to say that patterns of relative invariance do occur, especially within a single style of speech, but they are not so consistently found that a comprehensive theory of speech perception can be based exclusively on them. It might be better to regard them as regions of extremely high reliability in a probability-based system. Looking ahead, some future theory might deny the existence of invariants in the percept too, though none do at present. Connectionist models that distribute information about linguistic categories over a large number of hidden units have moved part way to this position, and if we begin to recognize significant individual differences in perception and linguistic organization instead of focusing on what is common, then it is conceivable that the notion of invariance will be completely redefined.

How are linguistic-phonetic categories formed?   Young babies can discriminate many speech sounds, but they probably do not organize them into linguistic-phonetic categories. Linguistic categories seem to be built up due to experience with speech and language throughout childhood and possibly on into adulthood. They presumably reflect continuing interaction between genetic endowment and the environment: That is, the nature of the categories reflects how the human brain organizes the sensory input. The input changes the brain's organization, which in turn affects the way the input is perceived, until each one's contribution to the mature system cannot be distinguished from the other's.

How are linguistic-phonetic categories identified during perception?   We cannot yet answer this question. Speech perception demands attention to both slow and rapid acoustic changes, but we have no definite answer to how these changes allow us to identify phonetic categories. There may be something like prototypes, defined in ideal or statistical terms, with or without details about variability, but we know little about them as yet. The signal may be evaluated and then matched against such a prototype, but again there are many ways this could happen. These are some of the more recent ideas. They are attractive partly because they can be implemented as computer models and tested. But they are only models. We cannot assume that current neural net technology reflects the way the brain works.

What role does memory play in speech perception?   Memory is very important. Phonetic categories are at least partly, if not wholly, language- and accent-specific, so they must be learned and therefore stored in long-term memory. These categories held in memory may be linked to more general memory processes, given that details of speakers' voices can help in word retrieval. The memory for these categories must be changeable, because listeners adapt to unfamiliar accents. There will be shorter-term phonetic memory processes too, such as those that keep track of prosody and coarticulation. In this chapter, we have described this type of memory as long time-windows. Long phonetic windows must involve memory because spoken sentences take time to arrive at the ear. This is one way in which recognizing spoken and written words differs. How close speech perception is to general memory processes is not yet well understood.

Is speech perception different from other forms of perception?   Opinions differ, but theorists increasingly look towards other forms of perception and cognition to describe speech perception as part of a biological system. Although there are strong links with other types of perception, speech is a relatively self-contained system that links directly with human language; to the extent that it is linguistic, speech perception is special. The answer to this question, then, is "yes and no." The next question is: Are the principles of speech perception different from those of perception of any other self-contained, hierarchical and redundant system? We do not know.

How is nonacoustic information used in understanding speech?   Listeners can get valuable phonetic information from other sensory modalities, such as seeing the talker's mouth, and they use information from their own brains that comes from knowledge and experience. Is nonacoustic sensory input used in the same way as knowledge? Do we interpret the acoustic signal as fully as possible before using other sensory information and knowledge, or do we decode the signal by using all information simultaneously? If information is used simultaneously, are different sources of information independently evaluated and added into a final cognitive-linguistic decision as in the FLMP, or do they interact with and mutually influence one another as in TRACE? Answers to these questions are not yet in, but current evidence suggests that all information can be processed (1) using the same principles, (2)

simultaneously, and (3) independently at first and then combined with other information when linguistic classes are identified. However, the fact that a model produces similar patterns to human responses does not have to mean that it works like a human brain. Interactive models can produce similar results with quite different processes.

Is acoustic information always primary in normally hearing listeners?   If the analysis is integrative, is acoustic information always primary in that it will dominate the response whenever there is a conflict between two sensory signals, or between the acoustic signal and top-down information? The answer is probably yes as long as the acoustic information is clear, but otherwise no: when acoustic information is ambiguous, the clearest information will be primary, regardless of its modality.

How are errors dealt with?   Are decisions about the sensory input always final, or can we "go back" over the signal to correct a first interpretation that turns out to be wrong? What would

TABLE 15-3.   Some issues in speech perception and theories that explicitly address them.

ISSUES	THEORIES
Working model (e.g., implemented as a computer program)	FLMP; TRACE and other activation models; LAFF
Phonemes not obligatory or their status explicitly questioned	LAFF; LAFS; Episodic memory
Attempt to explain children's acquisition and learning	Direct realism; NLM; TRACE; Episodic memory
Variability in speaking style	H&H; NLM: (Episodic memory?)
Identifying and/or understanding words	LAFF; LAFS; TRACE; (Remez; FLMP; H&H)
Strong claim of acoustic invariance	Quantal theory; acoustic invariance theory; LAFF
Strong claim against acoustic invariance	The Motor Theory
Links with nonhuman species	Direct realism; NLM; Auditory enhancement; (Quantal theory/LAFF)
Explicit re role of memory and higher-order cognitive processes	Direct realism; Episodic; TRACE; NLM; H&H; (Remez)

be the implication of these two alternatives? If we can backtrack, how is information re-evaluated once an error of interpretation is noticed? Answers to these questions largely fall outside the scope of this book or are as yet unanswered. However, a system that continuously monitors the signal, uses principles of probability or best match, and has a significant memory component is compatible with relatively easy correction of perceptual mistakes by reevaluating the signal.

These questions have driven and guided theorists in the second half of the twentieth century. Their answers provide an end to our discussion of theories of speech perception and a beginning to decisions about where to go next. Table 15-2 provides a summary of the theories of speech perception discussed in Chapters Fourteen and Fifteen, and research issues are described in Table 15-3.

CHAPTER 16

HEARING LOSS AND THE AUDIBILITY OF PHONEME CUES

SALLY G. REVOILE

Deficits in speech perception are often concomitant with hearing impairment. The nature of these deficits can be partly revealed through description of their phonemic composition and by examining the acoustic-cue structure of the misperceived phonemes. Other important information for explaining speech perception deficits is knowledge of the audibility of phoneme acoustic cues for the hard of hearing listener. This last type of information contributes to understanding of how reduced hearing sensitivity may deter access to phoneme acoustic cues.

The effect of hearing loss on the audibility of speech acoustic cues, and the consequent phoneme perception, is the primary focus of this chapter. The chapter considers why consonant and vowel misperceptions occur, in terms of the audibility of speech acoustic cues. Audibility of cues is described for hypothetical listeners with different degrees of hearing loss: namely, profound, severe, and moderate.[1] The listeners are assumed to receive the speech in a clinical audiometric situation where a word recognition test[2] is presented at comfortable levels via earphone. Descriptions of the listeners' acoustic-cue use are based mainly on graphic displays representing words from the test that have been processed to simulate the portions of the speech signals that are audible for the hypothetical listener from each hearing loss category. The availability of cues to a variety of consonant distinctions will be discussed in relation to findings of perception studies in the literature.

Among qualifications to note regarding this approach[3] for examining hearing loss versus acoustic-cue audibility, the reader should be

---

[1]The hypothetical hearing losses considered in this chapter represent mean data from a sample of Gallaudet University students classified in profound, severe, or moderate loss categories for the purposes of an experiment (Revoile, Kozma-Spytek, Nelson, & Holden-Pitt, 1995b). The hearing level definitions of the categories were chosen for experimental reasons and may not correspond to those used commonly for clinical purposes. Also, according to clinical practice, degree of hearing impairment need not be labeled for a single category of loss; double labels, such as moderate/severe, are often used to characterize losses that cross categories among audiometric frequencies.

[2]In clinical audiometry, word recognition tests are used to assess persons' speech perception capacity.

[3]The speech audibility simulations and related graphic displays used in this chapter probably underestimate the total effects of hearing loss on speech reception, especially for persons with more than moderate losses (see Van Tasell, 1993). Other auditory dysfunctions that can accompany reduced hearing sensitivity, such as deficit frequency and/or temporal resolution and abnormal loudness growth (e.g., sound tolerance problems) were not considered in deriving the simulations. Further, no contributions were included from auditory distortions that may result from the high signal levels used by some hard of hearing persons. Also, the audibility simulations are for words presented in quiet, without the interference of background noise that often occurs in everyday communication. Hearing aids that amplify speech frequency regions encompassing reduced audibility cues can facilitate phoneme perception for hard of hearing listeners. However, hearing aids are not conducive to good speech reception in noisy situations. Many hard of hearing persons seem to experience substantial disruption to speech perception from noise.

cautioned especially against generalizations to specific hard of hearing persons based on the hypothetical losses described in this chapter. People with similar losses of hearing sensitivity can show substantial differences in speech perception, both in error patterns and performance level. Thus, it is important to avoid blanket assumptions about speech perception abilities of a particular hard of hearing listener from the hypothetical listeners considered here. However, knowledge of some of the likely missing cues for a listener whose loss falls within one of the three degrees of loss analyzed here may guide the clinician in hearing aid fitting and counseling of the client in what cues to listen for.

CONSONANT ACOUSTIC-CUE USE BY A HYPOTHETICAL PROFOUNDLY HARD OF HEARING PERSON

The extent of hearing loss that characterizes profoundly hard of hearing persons (generally, 90 – 115 dB Hearing Level [HL][4] at 0.5, 1.0, 2.0 kHz [PTA][5]) greatly restricts their use of acoustic information in speech. Without amplification of the speech signal by conventional hearing aids, speech analyzing hearing aids (Faulkner, 1994), or other assistive listening devices,[6] profoundly hard of hearing people are incapable of receiving audible information from speech. Even with amplification, this population of the hard of hear-

ing is quite limited in the amount of acoustic information that can be accessed from the speech signal. Such listeners often have significant difficulty distinguishing most phonemes in the absence of visual speech cues and typically find amplified speech beneficial only as an aid to lipreading (e.g., Boothroyd, 1984; DeFillipo & Clark, 1993; Faulkner, Ball, & Rosen, 1992).

Some of the constraints imposed on speech reception from profound hearing loss are suggested by considering the audibility differences for speech between normal-hearing persons listening to conversational speech versus profoundly hard of hearing persons listening to amplified speech. Figure 16-1 presents pure tone hearing thresholds (dashed line) expressed in dB sound pressure level (SPL) in the free field (MAF)[7] for the better hearing ear of a hypothetical profoundly hard of hearing listener.[8] Also shown for this listener are some estimates of better-ear loudness discomfort levels[9] (dotted line) expressed in dB SPL re MAF. Other data displayed include an average long-term spectrum of speech (Byrne, Dillon, Tran, Arlinger, Bamford, et al., 1994) at an overall level of about 65 dB SPL (shaded area), which is similar to the

---

[4]Thresholds above 115 db HL may represent tactile rather than auditory perception (Plant, 1982). Persons with such thresholds can be considered deaf. However, cultural factors rather than specific hearing threshold levels may also be used to define deafness. Some people with average losses of 80 to 90 dB HL consider themselves as being deaf, although audiologically, they could be classified as severely or severe/profoundly hard of hearing.

[5]For categorizing hearing loss, the average of detection thresholds across the pure tones of 0.5, 1.0, and 2.0 kHz (pure tone average or PTA) is often used as a summary. Thresholds at these frequencies are used partly because of the preponderance of energy in speech throughout these frequencies.

[6]Assistive listening devices that may be used for speech amplification include induction loop, infrared, and frequency modulation systems (Compton, 1991).

[7]Free field measurements of hearing are those made in an acoustic environment free of sound reflecting surfaces, and presentation of the test signal to a listener is typically via loudspeaker; these thresholds are referred to as minimum audible field (MAF). Most hearing threshold measurements are made by test signal presentation through an earphone of a headset (referred to as minimum audible pressure [MAP]). In Figure 16-1, the hearing thresholds are expressed re dB SPL in a free field for comparison with the average speech spectrum (Byrne et al., 1994), which represents talkers recorded in acoustic environments somewhat resembling a free field. ANSI (1989) standard reference threshold values for TDH-39 phones were used to convert the profound hearing thresholds to dB SPL. The profound thresholds and loudness discomfort levels were transformed to MAF using Bentler and Pavlovic's (1989) monaural MAF data.

[8]The elevated pure tone thresholds in Figure 16-1 are mean data from 15 profoundly hard of hearing (mean PTA 94 dB HL) Gallaudet University students who were subjects in a speech perception experiment (Revoile et al., 1995b).

[9]The loudness discomfort levels were derived from those displayed for profoundly hard of hearing listeners tested by Faulkner et al. (1992).

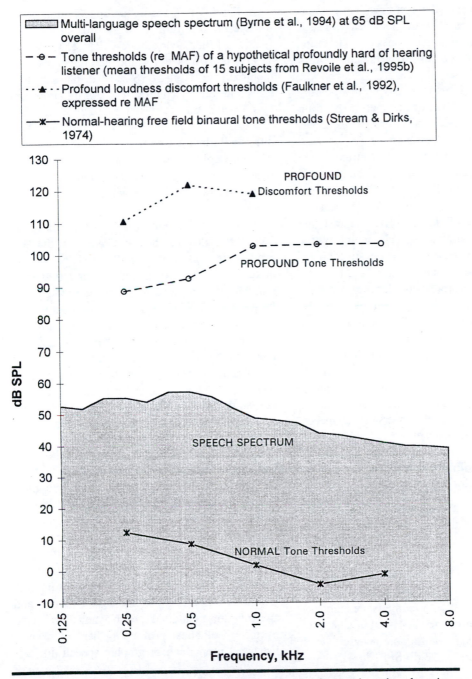

FIGURE 16-1. Acoustic conditions of hearing thresholds of normal- and profound-hearing listener in relation to the overall speech spectrum, without amplification. Notice that the speech spectrum levels are at least 45 dB below the tolerable listening thresholds of the profound-loss listener. See text for further discussion.

level of speech in everyday conversations. For normal-hearing persons, mean free field binaural thresholds are shown for pure tones (solid line) and speech (triangle at vertical axis) (Stream & Dirks, 1974).

The differences between the normal-hearing thresholds and the level of the speech spectrum at the audiometric frequencies provide estimates of the audibility of conversational speech at various frequency regions of the spectrum for a normal-hearing listener. Among the audiometric frequencies, the audibility of the speech signal ranges from about 45 dB at the 0.5 kHz spectrum peak to about 37 dB at 4.0 kHz. Contrast this extent of conversational speech audibility for normal-hearing listeners to the negative differences between the speech spectrum and the tone thresholds of the profound-loss listener. Substantial amplification would be required for the speech to exceed the thresholds of this hard of hearing listener. Also, the listener's loudness discomfort levels (LDLs) impose limitations on the amount of amplification that can be tolerated. Consequently, the attainable audibility of amplified speech for the profound-loss listener is far less than the audibility of conversational speech for a normal-hearing listener.

Acoustic Cue Audibility re a Word Recognition Test for a Hypothetical Profound Loss

To examine further the effects of profound hearing loss on speech reception, presentation of a speech audiometric test to the hypothetical listener is assumed. A word recognition test, the Northwestern University Auditory Test 6 (NU6) (Tillman & Carhart, 1966) is administered monaurally through an earphone (TDH-39) of a headset at the listener's most comfortable listening level (MCL)—equivalent to 123 dB SPL.[10]

In Figure 16-2, the lighter shaded area shows the speech spectrum for the words of the NU6 (Auditec [Sherbecoe, Studebacker, & Crawford, 1993]) transformed for the earphone response (approximate[11]). Figure 16-2 also displays the tone thresholds and discomfort levels of the profound-loss listener transformed for the response of a standard earphone (ANSI, 1989; Table 6, TDH-39). Similarly, for a normal-hearing listener, pure tone thresholds (solid line) and the NU6 speech spectrum (darker shading) are shown; the spectrum is at a 60 dB overall level, a standard conversational level.

The minimal extent of shaded area above the tone thresholds (dashed line) reveals that the available energy in the amplified NU6 words is quite limited both in magnitude and frequency range for the profound-loss listener. In the higher frequencies, 2.0 kHz and above, no components of the signal are audible. At 0.25 kHz and below, the average signal energy is nearly inaudible. The most audible portion of the signal is in the 0.5 kHz frequency region, at the spectral peak of the NU6 words. Here the signal is about 23 dB higher than the listener's threshold. Thus, only a narrow frequency region of the amplified NU6 words is accessible, and at low audibility.

When speech is restricted in audibility and frequency range, what are the consequences for speech reception? Which kinds of acoustic information for correct perception remain accessible in the speech signal? Are there acoustic cues in reduced-level, low-frequency speech energy that can contribute to phoneme perception for profoundly hard of hearing listeners?

We will consider these questions by examining frequency-amplitude patterns in waveforms and spectrograms of audible speech estimates received by the hypothetical profoundly hard of hearing listener. Comparison of graphic speech displays

---

[10]The 123 dB SPL NU6 presentation level of the hypothetical profoundly hard of hearing listener is based on the mean MCLs (self-chosen) of the 15 research subjects (Revoile et al., 1995b) whose mean threshold contour was designated as that of this hypothetical listener (Figures 16-1 and 16-2).

[11]For the transformation of the NU6 spectrum re the earphone response (Figure 16-2), the data of Bentler and Pavlovic (1989; Table 1, Col N) for mean TDH-39/49 standard reference thresholds (ANSI, 1989) were used because they include interoctave and low-frequency reference values.

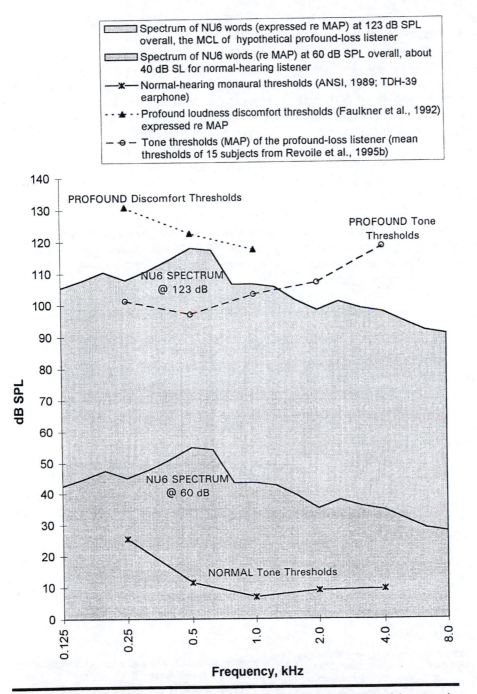

FIGURE 16-2. Acoustic conditions for a standard clinical amplification of the speech spectrum by 63 dB for the profound-loss listener at a comfortable level. The amplification brings speech spectrum information available at relatively low levels of audibility above thresholds from the low frequencies, up to about 1.3 kHz. Implications of this situation for the profound listener's hearing of phoneme cues is discussed in the text.

(prepared via signal processing software [Bunnell, 1998]) before and after adjustment for the profound hearing-loss effects suggests the acoustic information that may be conveyed. The speech graphics showing the profound-loss effects were obtained via processing some NU6 words through a digital filter (Tucker-Davis Technologies) generated to represent the differences in speech audibility between the profound-loss listener and a normal-hearing listener. In brief, the speech audibility differences were based on the relative levels above tone thresholds of the NU6 words presented at a comfortable level per listener.[12]

Note that the derived filter yields merely an approximation of the audibility constraints re the NU6 words for one hypothetical profound hearing loss. The speech graphics are not universally representative of the total effects of profound hearing loss on speech reception. Because auditory dysfunctions other than sensitivity loss were excluded for the filter design, the speech graphic displays probably underestimate the speech reception problems concomitant with profound hearing loss.[13] The graphics are merely intended to suggest the limitations on available speech acoustic information when a signal is confined to a narrow frequency range and is low in audibility, as when received by the profound-loss listener.

NU6 Waveforms Representing Hypothetical Profound and Normal Audibility. Figure 16-3 shows two waveforms of the NU6 test word *jar*, along with the preceding carrier phrase *Say the word*. The word *jar* was chosen because of the lower frequency and greater amplitude of the /ʤ/ affricative noise than seen for other consonants among the NU6 stimuli. Given these acoustic characteristics, some low-frequency energy of the /ʤ/ noise might be retained subsequent to simulation of the profound loss by filtering.

In Figure 16-3A (normal audibility), the waveform represents the phrase as processed through a digital filter simulating monaural presentation via earphone (TDH-39) to a normal-hearing listener. The overall level of the NU6 words is about 60 dB SPL according to the use of a 40 dB sensation level (SL)[14] re the speech standard threshold reference of 12.5 dB above the threshold reference at 1.0 kHz (7.0 dB SPL, TDH-39 phone [ANSI, 1989]) for the normal-hearing listener. In Figure 16-3B (profound audibility), the waveform is of the phrase after filtering to approximate the limited frequency region and audibility of the profound-loss listener. Recall that the NU6 words are administered to the profound-loss listener at an overall level of 123 dB SPL. The estimated SL of the words is about 7 dB, assuming a speech threshold of approximately 116 dB SPL, or 12.5 dB above the listener's 1.0 kHz threshold of 103.9 dB SPL (ANSI, 1989). However, this approach for estimating a speech SL may be overly conservative. Among persons with profound losses similar to the listener here, a mean SL of 27 dB was found based on differences between their thresholds versus self-selected MCLs for the vowels of speech test syllables[15] (Revoile et al., 1995b).

---

[12]The procedure of simulating speech audibility by computing relative differences between audiometric thresholds versus speech at comfortable listening levels and the use of associated speech waveforms and spectrograms are acknowledged to yield only estimates of phoneme audibility. This is because various assumptions were involved in deriving the speech audibility, and also because graphic displays of speech signals may not reveal exact relations among certain signal characteristics, particularly frequency characteristics.

[13]Profoundly hard of hearing listeners typically score quite poorly on word recognition tests, particularly those that use open-response formats (i.e., responses are not restricted to given choices; any word may be used as a response) such as the NU6. For example, nine listeners with PTAs from 90 to 107 dB HL tested by Clark and Snell (1993) obtained mean correct word recognition of less than 10% on the open set subtest of the Speech Pattern Contrast Test (Boothroyd, 1986).

---

[14]A sensation level (SL) of a sound is the relative level of that sound above a listener's threshold.

[15]The 15 listeners whose average tone and speech data were used to represent the hypothetical profoundly hearing impaired listener had a mean threshold of 96 dB SPL and mean MCL of 123 dB SPL for a representative /æ/ of /æCæ/ syllables tested in a study by Revoile et al. (1995b).

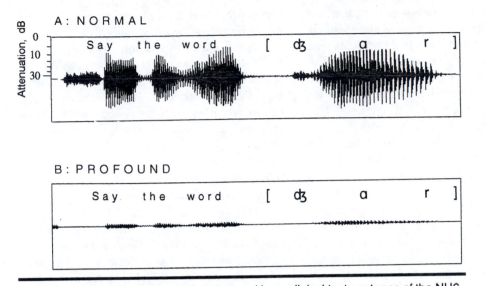

FIGURE 16-3. (A) Waveform of *Say the word jar,* a clinical test sentence of the NU6 audiometric test, as presented to a normal listener. (B) Waveform of the same sentence as heard above the profound-loss listener's threshold after 63 dB of amplification to that listener's tolerable comfort level. The amplitude scale of attenuation on the A waveform shows the amount of attenuation for both waveforms relative to the peak amplitudes received by the normal listener taken as the reference 0 dB. The amount of attenuation between A and B is the level of the peaks of the B wave, read against the scale, subtracted from the level of the peaks of the A wave. It appears that the B peaks are attenuated by as much as 30 dB. See text for more discussion.

The excursions up or down from the midline of each waveform represent the amplitude, or magnitude, of sound energy throughout the phrase. The perimeter of the excursions shows the outline or envelope of the amplitude changes during the phrase. The vertical alignment of Figure 16-3A and B facilitates examination of waveform sections representing the same speech segments between the phrase filtered for normal versus profound audibility. Relative audibility can be compared between analogous sections of Figure 16-3A and B according to the height of waveform excursions at given time locations (horizontal axis). To estimate the waveforms' audibility differences in dB, an attenuation scale of 30 dB range is provided. Zero attenuation represents full-scale waveform excursions in the NU6 test stimuli.

Relative to the normal-audibility waveform, all segments of the profound-audibility waveform are substantially reduced in amplitude. The diminished amplitude is associated with both the limited audibility and the reduced frequency range for hearing of the profound-loss listener. Where smaller excursions occur for the profound than the normal audibility waveform, such as the vowel segment of *jar,* the effect is due mostly to the limited audibility of the profound-loss listener in the 0.5 kHz region—the peak frequency of the NU6 spectrum. However, where the amplitude excursions are absent or nearly so in the profound waveform, that is, the [s] frication segment in *say* and the [dʒ] affricate noise in *jar,* the effect is associated with the listener's extensive hearing loss in the high-frequencies.

NU6 Spectrograms: Hypothetical Profound and Normal Audibility. A more detailed view of the effect on speech transmission of the profound loss in the high frequencies is provided by spectrograms (Figure 16-4) of *Say the word jar*, filtered for normal and profound audibility. Across the normal-audibility spectrogram (Figure 16-4A), shading representing various magnitudes of speech energy can be seen throughout most of the 0 – 5.0 kHz frequency range (vertical axis). This indicates broad frequency representation in the phrase when it is filtered to simulate presentation via headphone to a normal-hearing listener. Visible segments representing acoustic cues to [ʤ] in *jar* are the aperiodic striations of the affricate noise from about 1.5 kHz upward and, at the vowel onset, the transitions in the first through the third formants (F1 transition 0.2 to 0.5 kHz, F2 transition 1.7 to 1.2 kHz, F3 transition 2.0 to 2.5 kHz).

In contrast, the profound audibility spectrogram (Figure 16-4B) shows shading representing speech energy only in the F1 region, around 0.5 kHz. Formants at higher frequencies are not apparent, nor is the segment representing the [ʤ] affricate noise or the [s] of *say*. At the onset of

[ʤ] in [ʤɑr] and at the vowel [ɚ] onset in *word*, the rising incline of the striations indicate some semblance of an F1 transition. Transitions of the first two or three formants in vowels can provide substantial cues to the perception of adjacent voiced consonants. However, it is unlikely that this nascent F1 transition would be usable by the profound-loss listener. Different samples of profoundly hard of hearing young adults at Gallaudet have shown no use of formant transitions for perception of spoken consonants (e.g., Revoile et al., 1995a, 1995b; 1991a, 1991b). On the other hand, for synthetic single-formant (F1) stimuli, some profoundly hard of hearing children demonstrated use of the F1 transition in the vowel onset to distinguish voiced versus voiceless initial stops (Hazan & Fourcin, 1985). Yet, other profoundly hard of hearing children tested with spoken stimuli generally were unable to use vowel onsets containing transitions for initial stop voicing distinctions (Holden-Pitt, Hazan, Revoile, Edward, & Droge, 1995).

The restriction of energy to the narrow frequency region seen in the spectrogram reveals that the profound-loss listener is deprived of the broad

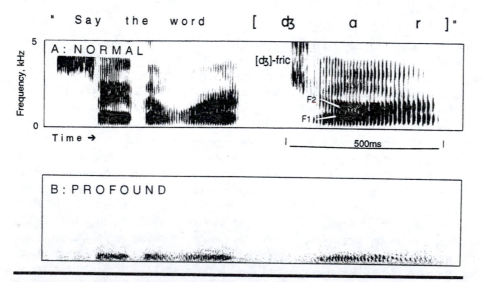

FIGURE 16-4. Spectrograms of the NU6 test sentence of the previous figure. (A) As heard by the normal listener. (B) As heard by the profound listener. See text for discussions of the phoneme spectral cues indicated as available.

range of spectral (i.e., frequency-based) variation in speech. At least with the stimuli and transducer assumed here, we would predict that this listener is generally unable to distinguish the consonants of the NU6 words on the basis of their spectral characteristics. Various studies have reported very poor or no use of spectral cues for consonant distinctions by profoundly hard of hearing listeners (e.g., Boothroyd, 1984, Erber, 1979; Faulkner et al., 1992; Revoile et al., 1995a, 1995b).

Vowel perception based on spectral cues via the NU6 words would also be difficult for the profound-loss listener. As seen in the profound audibility spectrogram (Figure 16-4B), the vowels [eɪ], [ʌ], [ɚ], and [ɑ] show no energy at the F2 frequency region and above. Thus, the listener lacks access to a major cue to vowel identity—the relative patterns of spectral information in the F1 and F2 frequency regions.

Even if speech energy across F1 and F2 frequencies is audible for given profoundly hard of hearing listeners, their vowel perception can be poor due to problems in resolving formants of different frequencies in vowels. Similarly, for consonant spectral cues that are audible, difficulties in resolving the cues can contribute to consonant misperceptions. The basis for such problems is probably the reduced frequency tuning in the cochlea, believed characteristic of many hard of hearing listeners not limited to those with profound losses. With reduced frequency tuning, cochlear auditory nerve (hair) cells do not respond selectively to specific frequencies, as occurs in the normal ear. The reduced frequency tuning is likely exacerbated by the high sound levels profoundly hard of hearing listeners require. An effect of high level sound is to stimulate cochlear nerve cells irrespective of the characteristic frequencies to which they naturally respond. For vowel perception, a consequence of reduced frequency tuning may be inter-formant masking, and/or masking of formants by the fundamental frequency (F0). The spectral complexity of natural vowels may contribute to such masking for profoundly hard of hearing listeners (Deeks & Faulkner, 1994).

To mitigate these masking effects, some investigators have used spectrally simplified vowels in studies of profoundly hard of hearing listeners' vowel perception. Van Son, Bosman, Lamore, and Smoorenburg (1993) reported profoundly hard of hearing listeners' poorer identification of synthetic vowels when F1 and F2 were composed of only one harmonic than when comprising two or three harmonics. In a preliminary experiment, Deeks and Faulkner (1994) have compared identification among different conditions of harmonically simplified vowels and a condition of complex, more naturally structured vowels. For two of four profoundly hard of hearing listeners tested thus far, vowels comprising two formants, each with two harmonics, yielded better identification than their more natural counterparts.

Amplitude Envelope Cues for Phoneme Distinctions by Profoundly Hard of Hearing Listeners

Lacking access to important spectral cues in the NU6 words, the profound-loss listener must rely on changes in the speech amplitude envelope to discern differences among phonemes. The terms "time/intensity patterns" or "time/intensity cues" are used to refer to the amplitude envelope variations in speech that may contribute to some phoneme distinctions by persons with substantial hearing loss. The speech amplitude envelope can provide information about the relative durations (time patterns) among speech segments, as well as the relative magnitude (intensity patterns) of these segments. A hearing level of 96 dB HL PTA or poorer is one criterion that has been applied to characterize profoundly hard of hearing listeners whose speech-cue use is limited to time-intensity patterns (e.g., De Fillipo & Clark, 1993). The PTA of our profound-loss listener is 94 dB HL.

Speech time/intensity patterns can contribute to recognition of voiced versus voiceless consonants and perhaps to certain consonant classes differing for manner of production, that is, fricatives versus stops (sometimes referred to as a continuance contrast). Under controlled test conditions,

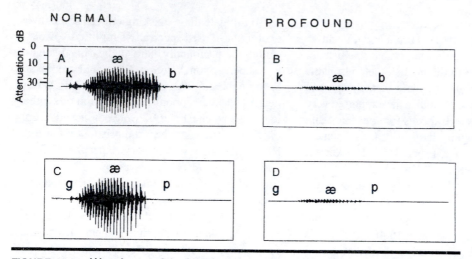

FIGURE 16-5. *Waveforms of the NU6 test words* cab *and* gap *as heard by (A) normal listener, and (B) profound-loss listener. For the profound listener the consonant bursts are inaudible but the vowel is audible at a level about 20 dB lower than for the normal listener.*

certain vowels may also be distinguishable on the basis of time/intensity cues. However, in continuous speech, vowel time/intensity differences are not highly reliable and thus may not be useful as cues in typical speech communication situations.

Temporal Cues in the Amplitude Envelope for Voiced versus Voiceless Consonant Distinctions by Profoundly Hard of Hearing Listeners

Vowel Duration Cues for Word-Final Consonant Voicing Distinctions. The duration of certain speech segments can provide temporal information (i.e., waveform time patterns) of importance for consonant voicing distinctions. For stops and fricatives in word-final position before pauses in speech,[16] duration differences in the preceding vowel may cue whether the consonant is voiced or voiceless. Vowels are roughly 30% longer when preceding voiced consonants than voiceless consonants in pre-pausal positions of continuous speech (Crystal & House, 1982). Such differences

are apparent in Figure 16-5, which shows waveforms of the NU6 words *cab* (Figure 16-5A and B) and *gap* (Figure 16-5C and D) both filtered for normal and profound audibility. The four waveform plots have the same time window (617 ms), providing a constant temporal scale for assessing the durations of speech segments among the waveforms. The waveforms are vertically aligned relative to the onset of the vowel segments to facilitate comparison of the vowel duration differences.

In *cab*, the [æ] is about 78 ms longer than in *gap*, These vowel duration differences obtain regardless of whether the waveform represents profound or normal audibility. Thus, the audibility constraints of the profound-loss listener do not deter use of the vowel duration difference for cueing voicing of final stops and fricatives in prepausal positions in speech.

Experimentally, use of the vowel duration cue for final consonant voicing distinctions was reported for six of twelve profoundly hard of hearing listeners (PTAs 96–110 dB HL, tested by Revoile, Holden-Pitt, Pickett, & Brandt, 1986, Table 3). Also tested was discrimination of stimulus durations. Five of the six listeners with poor use of the

---

[16]The vowel duration cue to word-final consonant voicing also occurs in words spoken in isolation—a context often employed in experiments studying listeners' use of this cue.

vowel duration cue for consonant voicing distinctions also showed the poorest stimulus duration discrimination in the profound loss group. In contrast, nominally normal stimulus duration discrimination (25 ms difference limen [DL] re 200 ms reference) was found for the profoundly hard of hearing listeners who could use the vowel duration cue for consonant voicing distinctions. This finding and the results of Rosen, Faulkner, and Smith (1990) suggest that profoundly hard of hearing listeners who have residual hearing (as opposed to listeners whose reception to acoustic stimuli is limited to tactile perception) are able to discriminate stimulus durations smaller than those associated with temporal cues that are perceptually critical to certain phoneme distinctions.

Stop-Burst Duration Cues for Stop Voicing Distinctions.   For stop consonants in intervocalic or word-initial position, an important characteristic of the speech amplitude envelope that can cue distinctions of voiced versus voiceless stops is the duration of the plosive burst, also referred to as voice onset time (VOT). Examples of some average durations between the onset of the burst transient and the beginning of the following phoneme are about 70 ms for /p, t, k/ in contrast to about 18 ms for /b, d, g/ (Revoile, Pickett, Holden-Pitt, Talkin, & Brandt, 1987). The stop burst durations found in the normal-audibility waveforms of Figure 16-5A and C, respectively, are 59 ms for the [k] of *cab* and the [g] of *gap* (28 ms). However, in the profound-audibility waveforms (Figure 16-5B and D), note that the bursts are not visible. For the profound-loss listener, the VOT cue is unavailable for the initial-stop voicing distinction of *cab* versus *gap*.

Among some profoundly hard of hearing children tested by Boothroyd (1984), the ability to distinguish voicing for word-initial stops and fricatives depended on the degree of loss. Mean perception of consonant voicing was 68% by six listeners with PTAs between 90 and 104 dB HL, while only 40% (chance level) by six listeners with PTAs between 105 and 114 dB HL. That children with as much or more hearing loss than

our profound-loss listener could distinguish initial consonant voicing may be methodologically related. For example, in comparison to the NU6 stimuli considered here, the words presented to the children may have been produced more clearly and with greater articulatory effort. The associated consonant cues could have greater energy, and thus greater audibility than presumed for the velar stops of *cab* and *gap* above.

Intensity Cues in the Amplitude Envelope for Phoneme Distinctions by Profoundly Hard of Hearing Listeners

Silence versus Voicing During Closure as a Cue to Stop Voicing Distinctions.   Stop consonants in word-final or intervocalic position can often be differentiated for voicing by the presence versus absence of periodic low-frequency energy in the closure interval—the brief time (about 50 ms in connected speech [Crystal & House, 1982]) between the offset of the preceding phoneme and the onset of the stop burst release (see Chapter Eight for the articulatory explanation of this effect). Preceding a /p/, /t/, or /k/ burst, the closure interval is typically silent. This silent period is an important cue for the consonant class voiceless stops. For /b/, /d/, or /g/, part or all of the closure interval can contain voicing[17]—cueing the consonant class voiced stops. In Figure 16-5A—the normal audibility waveform for *cab*—the segment preceding the [b] burst shows periodic oscillations representing voicing throughout the closure interval. These oscillations do not appear in the profound audibility waveform (Figure 16-5B). In Figure 16-5C—the normal audibility waveform for *gap*—the closure interval preceding the [p] burst shows minimal perturbations, thus cueing a voiceless stop. However, in Figure 16-5D—the profound audibility waveform for *gap*—note that there is no representation of the

---

[17]Voiced stops in word-initial position *subsequent to a pause* are less likely to manifest closure voicing prior to the burst release to the same extent as found for word-final or intervocalic position.

[p] burst. Thus, the [p] closure is undefined, preventing the listener from assessing whether the closure interval is silent or contains voicing, and consequently, from determining the voicing value (i.e., voiced or voiceless) of the final stop. Research on intentional deletion of stop bursts for final voiceless stops in words tested in isolation has shown reduced identification of voiceless stops for both normal-hearing and hard of hearing listeners (Revoile, Pickett, Holden, & Talkin, 1982). Note that stop consonants in conversational speech may not be released (i.e., a noise burst may not be produced), which can reduce their perceptibility for hard of hearing listeners who rely on the burst presence for stop distinctions.

Some listeners with profound losses greater than that of the listener here have shown distinctions of consonant voicing when perception was tested with audiovisual stimuli and the auditory stimulus was filtered (Faulkner et al., 1992). Eleven profoundly hard of hearing adults (mean PTA of about 110 dB HL) were tested by lipreading alone (visual stimuli) versus by lipreading plus amplified speech (audiovisual stimuli). The group's mean performance for distinction of the consonant classes /b, d, g, v, z/ versus /p, t, k, f, s/ was 57% percent correct[18] for the visual stimuli, while 87% for the audiovisual stimuli. The test stimuli were vowel-consonant-vowel (VCV) nonsense syllables spoken in isolation.[19] The listeners

may have used the presence/absence of voicing during consonant occlusion to distinguish consonant voicing.

In summary, our profound-loss listener seems restricted to use of certain time/intensity patterns of the NU6 words for limited distinctions of consonant classes. Specifically, voiced versus voiceless consonants are discernible on the basis of the vowel duration cue. Voiced versus voiceless stops are distinguishable when stop bursts and/or closure voicing is audible. Lack of audibility of fricative time/intensity patterns prevent voicing distinctions of these consonants, and their distinction from stops. Spectral cues are unavailable for consonant recognition due to the low audibility and restriction of speech energy to a narrow frequency range.

PHONEME ACOUSTIC-CUE USE BY A HYPOTHETICAL SEVERELY HARD OF HEARING PERSON

As our hypothetical model of severe hard of hearing we used the tone threshold data of a group of 40 subjects tested by Revoile and colleagues (1995b). The average threshold contour was rather flat, ranging from 83 to 91 dB, over the audiometric range 0.25 – 4.0 kHz. The severe group's NU6 tolerable spectrum (which was 120 dB overall) was 30 dB above threshold at 0.5 kHz, 15 dB at 1.0 kHz, and 4–6 dB in the 2 to 4.0 kHz region. Thus, it is apparent that this group, at maximum amplification of about 60 dB, would have highly usable hearing for mid-frequency cues, say in the F1 and F2 regions, and possibly some higher frequency information as well, although at very low audibility.

People with severe hearing loss (about 65 to ≤ 90 dB HL PTA) probably vary more as a group in their speech perception abilities than persons in other hearing loss categories. A major factor contributing to this variability is the substantial differences in auditory dynamic range (i.e., the difference in level between the weakest sound detectable versus the loudest sound just beneath discomfort)

---

[18]In computing a listener's performance score for consonant voicing distinctions, each response was scored correctly if the consonant perceived was in the same voicing class (i.e., voiced or voiceless) as the consonant presented. Thus, if a /p/ was the response to presentation of an /s/, the response occurred for an /s/ stimulus the response was considered incorrect for voicing. Responses incorrect for place of articulation (e.g., /k/ for /t/) or for manner (i.e., stop for fricative, or vice versa) were ignored.

[19]For stop consonants, a stimulus context in which the consonant is preceded by another phoneme is important for providing the articulatory conditions that yield voicing or silence during occlusion. A voiced stop consonant occurring after a pause or in a word spoken in isolation usually will not be preceded by voicing. When considering experimental reports of hearing-impaired listeners' use of phoneme cues, the stimulus context should be appraised to assess which acoustic cues may have actually been available.

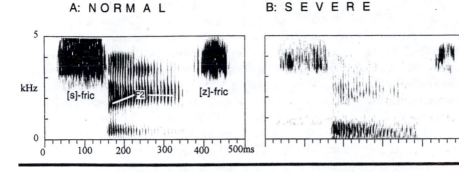

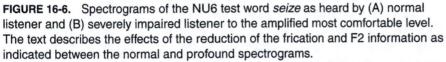

FIGURE 16-6. Spectrograms of the NU6 test word *seize* as heard by (A) normal listener and (B) severely impaired listener to the amplified most comfortable level. The text describes the effects of the reduction of the frication and F2 information as indicated between the normal and profound spectrograms.

that can be found among those with severe hearing loss. Persons in this category with greater hearing loss and/or with low LDLs will have smaller dynamic ranges than those with less hearing loss and higher LDLs. A small dynamic range limits the amount of amplification that a hard of hearing person can tolerate. In such cases, a low speech SL is required, thus constraining speech audibility and access to phoneme acoustic cues. There may be some severely hard of hearing persons whose acoustic cue audibility is as reduced as that seen for the profound-loss listener above. Conversely, significantly greater speech audibility is available to many persons categorized with severe hearing loss who can use higher speech SLs due to broader dynamic ranges. These preliminary comments are to remind the reader that the speech perception abilities discussed for the hypothetical listeners in this chapter are not stereotypical of the listeners' respective hearing loss categories. Also, the descriptions of phoneme acoustic cue use for the hypothetical listeners should be considered only as first approximations, because of the imprecision of specifying phoneme acoustic cue characteristics from waveforms and especially spectrograms, the lack of real-ear speech measurements for more accurate assessment of the

phoneme spectra, and the disregard of listeners' supra threshold auditory abilities.[20]

Acoustic Cues to Fricative Consonants for a Hypothetical Severe Hearing Loss

Spectrograms of *seize* for normal audibility (Figure 16-6A) and severe audibility (Figure 16-6B) indicate the frequency regions containing the energy of the [s] and [z] frications. For normal audibility, the [s] frication encompasses a broad frequency range, extending from about 3.0 kHz upward. Throughout this range, the spectrum is somewhat diffuse, although spectral prominences can be found at about 3.5 and 7.0 kHz. The [z] frication shows a strong spectral prominence between 3.5 and 4.0 kHz. At higher frequencies, energy in the [z] frication noise is quite low compared to the [s] frication.

In the spectrogram of severe audibility *seize*, the light shading across the frication segments

---

[20]Supra threshold auditory abilities is a collective term sometimes used to refer to auditory discrimination performances of frequency, temporal, and/or intensity resolution. The stimuli tested for resolution are presented at levels exceeding a listener's thresholds.

indicates that they contain much less energy than the normal audibility [s] and [z]. Also, the severe audibility [s] and [z] show less spectral diversity; their energy is confined to the 3.5 kHz frequency region. Spectrum measurements showed the peak to be 33 dB lower in amplitude for the severe listener. The apparent weakness of these frications in Figure 16-6B suggests that their audibility is limited for the severely hard of hearing listener.

The continuity of a frication noise over a sufficiently long interval is an important cue for classification of fricative consonants according to continuant versus stop manner of production. In continuous speech, average durations for voiced fricatives of about 51 ms and for voiceless fricatives, about 104 ms have been reported (Crystal & House, 1982). The magnitude of energy can vary across the interval of a frication noise, as suggested by the variation in shading of the severe audibility [s] and [z]. Thus, throughout the frication noise, the audibility of a fricative may not be constant for a hard of hearing listener. Should audibility increase near the terminus of the frication noise, a hard of hearing person might misperceive a fricative as the burst of a stop consonant. Indeed, reduced manner distinctions of voiceless fricatives and stops were found for the thirty hard of hearing listeners tested by Revoile and co-workers (1991a), twenty of whom had severe losses.

Fricative Voicing Cues.   In the *seize* spectrogram for severe audibility (Figure 16-6B), striations for the final two pitch periods of the vowel can be seen below 0.5 kHz. However, representation of the frication noise is not apparent above these two pitch periods, suggesting that the frication occurring at the [i] offset is inaudible. Thus, the severe-loss listener seems unable to use the concurrence of [z] frication and [i] periodicity at the vowel offset as a cue to the voicing status of the [z].

Given the uncertain audibility of frication cues for discerning the voicing value of [z], it may be necessary for the severe-loss listener to rely on the vowel duration cue for word-final fricative voicing distinctions. Recall that in a word spoken

before a pause, a shorter vowel preceding a final stop or fricative typically elicits a voiceless consonant percept, while a longer vowel cues a voiced consonant percept. The [i] of *seize* is 363 ms, a duration exceeding those found in connected speech for vowels preceding voiced consonants in prepausal words (Crystal & House, 1982). This [i] duration could serve as a voicing cue to [z] in *seize*. Revoile and colleagues (1986) found vowel duration to be a useful cue to final fricative voicing distinctions by severely hard of hearing listeners.

An additional cue in the vowel offset that may contribute to voicing distinction of the following fricative is the frequency transition in F1. The F1 frequency at vowel offset is often lower preceding a voiced than a voiceless fricative, assuming a given vowel context and voiced versus voiceless fricatives at the same place of articulation. In laboratory tests of final fricative voicing, normal-hearing listeners correctly distinguished voicing for /dʌC/ syllables in which the final voiced and voiceless fricatives were discarded and the vowels were equalized for duration (Revoile, Holden-Pitt, & Pickett, 1985). The F1 frequency at vowel offset was 25% lower for the vowels preceding the voiced fricatives than the voiceless fricatives. The hard of hearing listeners tested, the majority of whom had severe losses, generally showed poor ability to distinguish fricative voicing on the basis of cues in the vowel offsets. However, performance was nearly perfect for tests of the syllables with natural vowel durations but with frications deleted, indicating the hard of hearing listeners' dependence on the vowel duration cue.

For word-initial voiced fricatives, low-frequency cues in the vowel onset and in the frications seemed equally useful for voicing distinctions by a group of moderately and severely hard of hearing listeners (Holden-Pitt, Revoile, & Pickett, 1991). However, the group's performance via either cue was poorer than normal. About twice as many moderately than severely hard of hearing listeners were tested, which may explain why the group showed some ability to use the vowel onset cues for fricative voicing distinctions, in contrast to the suspected lack of such ability for the severe-loss listener considered here.

Fricative Place Cues.   On the basis of the frication noises, it is practical to limit consideration of place distinctions for the severe-loss listener to alveolar versus palatal fricatives. The frications of these fricatives are relatively strong in comparison to the frication noises of labiodental and linguadental fricatives, which are typically weaker and less likely to be audible for this listener. NU6 *wash* was chosen to examine the possibility of place distinctions for palatal [ʃ] versus alveolar [s] and [z] of *seize* by the severe-loss listener. We found the [ʃ]-noise to average about 10 dB lower in amplitude than the [s] and [z], a condition that should yield lower audibility of [ʃ] than [s] and [z] for the severe-loss listener. Spectrum measurement of [ʃ] showed the spectrum peak to be 22 dB lower for the severe listener than for the normal.

When frications are sufficiently audible, some severely hard of hearing persons may show good

fricative place distinctions. Near-normal perception of synthetic voiceless fricatives was found for the severely hard of hearing listener included among the subjects tested by Zeng and Turner (1990). This result was obtained for frications presented in isolation at levels estimated as yielding 100% audibility. In other research with naturally spoken syllables, the vowel-frication amplitude ratio—and consequently, frication audibility—influenced fricative place perceptibility by hard of hearing listeners (Revoile et al., 1995a). Perception was highest for /aza/ and lowest for /aða/ syllables. Compared to the amplitude of the adjacent vowels, the /ð/ noises were 14 dB lower while the /z/ noises were only about 2 dB lower.

Fricative Place Cues in Vowel Formant Transitions.   In the normal audibility spectrograms, the onset and offset of /i/ in *seize* (Figure 16-6A) and the offset of /a/ in *wash* (Figure 16-7A) show frequency changes in formants that can contribute

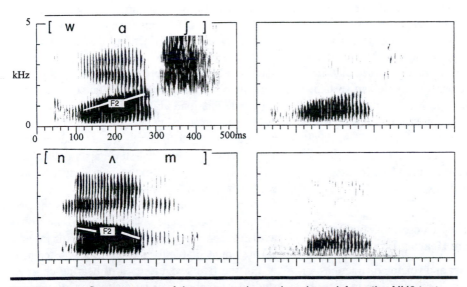

FIGURE 16-7. Spectrograms of the test words *wash* and *numb* from the NU6 test tape, for (A) normal and (B) severe listeners. Note the reduced spectral information for the severe listener, in the F2 region, and virtual absence of the high-frequency frication energy for the fricative [ʃ] of *wash*; the low-frequency spectral information, as in the [w], is available at a reduced level.

to place distinctions of the fricatives. Especially, second formant transitions are important for consonant place distinctions, particularly for voiced consonants. However, various studies have reported poor use of vowel formant transitions for consonant place distinctions by severely hard of hearing listeners (e.g., Revoile et al., 1987, 1995b; Zeng & Turner, 1990). Much of this difficulty may be explained by reduced or no audibility of second formants for these listeners. In addition, poor ability to resolve formant transition frequency changes may also be a factor (Revoile et al., 1995b; Zeng & Turner, 1990). On the other hand, a study with synthetic stimuli suggests that severely hearing- and less-impaired listeners rely more on vowel transitions for certain consonant distinctions than normal-hearing listeners (Nelson, Nittrouer, & Norton, 1995). Because our severe-loss listener has limited audibility for stimuli in second formant frequency regions, the listener's use of F2 transition cues in NU6 words will not be considered.

Reduced distinctions of fricatives according to place of articulation and voicing for the severe-loss listener are probably due predominantly to the high-frequency, relatively low-level frication cues in combination with the listener's poor high frequency thresholds. In comparison, fricative distinctions according to manner of articulation may be easier for this listener, provided that frication noises are sufficiently audible and sustained over an interval characteristic of fricative consonants. Other phonemes with low-level, high frequency cues are stop consonants, especially voiceless stops. The severe-loss listener's distinctions of voicing, manner, and place for stop consonants are examined next.

Acoustic Cues to Stop Consonants for the Hypothetical Severe Hearing Loss

First consider manner and voicing distinctions for the word-final stops. For [g] of *beg* in both the normal- and severe-audibility waveforms (not shown here), excursions were visible for the burst release as well as for the preceding closure voic-

ing. The presence of the [g]-burst contributes to the identity of this consonant as a stop (i.e., manner recognition), and the voicing during closure is important for distinguishing the stop as voiced. The representation of these cues in the severe-audibility waveform indicated their availability for recognition of [g] stop manner and voicing by the severe-loss listener. Spectrum analysis of these final release bursts showed that in the low frequencies they were of the same amplitude, comparing normal with severe listeners; thus a low-frequency burst cue would be available to both.

However, the severe-loss listener was seen to lack access to the [k]-burst. The effect is interference with manner recognition of the [k] as a stop consonant. Also, because the closure interval is undefined due to burst inaudibility, the listener is deterred from using the absence of voicing during closure to classify the stop as voiceless. On the other hand, the severe-loss listener's distinction of final consonant voicing for *beg* and *pick* is facilitated by the vowel duration cue, which appeared to be salient for these words.

For initial stop voicing cues, the burst segments of *beg* and *pick* differed in duration on the normal audibility waveform, indicating that a VOT cue of about 25 ms for the [p] was present for use by the normal hearing listener to distinguish voicing for the [b] versus [p]. On the severe-audibility waveform, however, substantial amplitude was seen for the [b] burst but not the [p] burst. The inaudibility of the [p] burst deters the listener from using cues in the burst for manner and voicing distinctions of the voiceless stop. Thus, between the initial stop bursts of *beg* and *pick*, only [b] voicing and manner cues are audible for the severe-loss listener.

A spectrum analysis of our NU6 words showed that the high-frequency burst cues that contribute to distinctions of place of articulation for [b] and [g] are not available for the severe-loss listener.

For the five severely hard of hearing children studied by Erber (1972), distinction of voicing was similar between voiced and voiceless stop consonants. Stop and nasal consonants were the target phonemes in spoken /æCæ/ syllables. Mean stop voicing of 82% (place errors ignored) was obtained, in comparison to 100% correct stop perception found for the normal-hearing children tested.

Thus, it would appear that perception of some NU6 voiceless stop and fricative consonants for voicing, manner, and place of articulation is difficult for the severe-loss listener because the important high frequency acoustic cues of these phonemes are often inaudible. Voiced stops and fricatives seem distinguishable for voicing and manner since their low frequency cues are generally audible for the listener. Other manner categories of consonants that are characterized by low frequency energy are glides and nasals. Perception of these consonants by the severe-loss listener is considered next.

Glide and Nasal Consonant Acoustic Cues

The occurrence of voicing throughout the production of glide and nasal consonants (and the /l/ and /r/ liquids) yields spectra for these phonemes that show periodic energy predominantly in the low frequencies (see Chapter Six for details about the production and perception of glides and nasals). In utterances of these consonants with vowels, the continuity of strong periodic energy across a phoneme sequence provides a distinguishable contrast to stop or fricative consonants, for which voicing in the speech signal is typically interrupted by continuous or transient noise, respectively. Between glide and nasal consonants, important cues to manner distinctions are in the low-frequency spectral patterns occurring during consonant constriction and in adjacent vowel formant transitions. For glide consonants (and the liquids), it is probable that manner distinctions are also cued by the relatively slow frequency changes in vowel formant transitions associated with these consonants. Cues to consonant place distinctions within the glide or nasal (and liquid) categories occur in the spectral patterns from consonant constriction and typically in the formant transitions of adjacent vowels.

In describing phonetic feature perception by a group of mostly severely hard of hearing persons, Pickett and colleagues (1970) used the label "low-continuant" to refer to the feature of predominant low-frequency energy that characterizes nasal and glide consonants and other semivowel consonants, in contrast to the low-frequency interruption for the obstruent stops and fricatives. Among the 99 listeners examined according to consonant confusions, the feature of low continuant was perceived about as well as voicing, and considerably better than place for consonants in words chosen from a rhyming-words response set. Perception of the low continuant feature improved as degree of loss decreased. Listeners with a mean loss at the maximum in the severe category showed very poor low-continuant perception, while those with the least loss in the severe category perceived the low-continuant feature with few errors. The audibility of the low-frequency energy is probably sufficient for the severe-loss listener to use the uninterrupted periodic energy across the consonant-vowel sequences as a cue to the low-continuant feature of [w], [n], and [m].

Cues to Glide and Nasal Consonant Manner Distinctions. These distinctions appear in the consonants of the NU6 words *wash* and *numb*. Spectrograms for normal and severe listeners are shown in Figure 16-7. In addition to spectrograms, it is helpful to examine spectral slices (or sections) from segments representing the consonant constrictions for determining patterns of some cues that contribute to manner distinctions of glides and nasal consonants. Figure 16-8 shows such spectra for the [w], [n], and [m] constriction segments for normal audibility (panel A) and severe audibility (panel B). These spectra were derived by fast Fourier transformation analysis (FFT, see Chapter Four) of a 51.2 ms window, which encompassed the five highest-amplitude pitch periods of each consonant segment, in the NU6 words *wash* and *numb*. Note that the axes of these spectra are different from those of spectrograms; here the horizontal axis represents frequency and the vertical axis, amplitude.

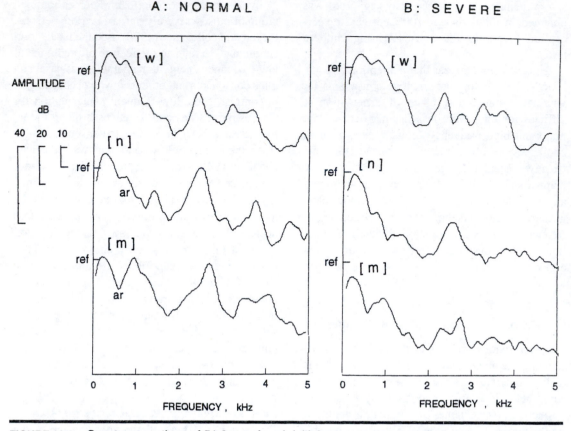

FIGURE 16-8. Spectrum sections of 51.2 ms of each initial consonant murmur in the consonants [w,n,m] in NU6 test words for (A) the normal listener and (B) the severely impaired listener. "ar" designates antiresonant notches in the spectra of the nasal murmurs that are a probable cue for nasal manner versus the oral-only [w]. The depth of the notch is reduced for the severe listener; however, the [w] may be discriminable from the nasals by its wider band of low-frequency energy.

Some characteristics differentiating [w] versus [m] and [n] appear at frequencies below 1.5 kHz in the normal-audibility spectra of these consonants. In the [n] and [m] spectra, a pattern representing an important cue to nasality is the trough, labeled "ar" for antiresonance, subsequent to the first low-frequency peak. An antiresonance (also sometimes referred to as an antiformant or a zero) is a band of reduced energy within a restricted, local frequency region. Antiresonances occurring in nasal consonant spectra are associated with the role of the nasal cavity and the blocked oral cavity in the production of these consonants (see Chapter Seven for details about the production and acoustic properties of nasal consonants).

In the [w] spectrum, the predominant low-frequency band of energy is broad, encompassing an F1 peak at about 0.35 kHz, and F2, at about 0.8 kHz—frequency characteristics similar to those measured in other [w] spectra (Espy-Wilson, 1992). Note that the F1 and F2 peaks are not separated by an amplitude trough as in the antiresonance notch of the nasal spectra.

The severe-audibility spectra of [w], [n], and [m] (Figure 16-8B) represent the same time intervals of the consonant constrictions as those seen for normal audibility. An overall reduction in amplitude of the severe-audibility spectra compared to the normal audibility spectra is related to the lower SL used by the severe-loss listener. For example, the severe audibility spectra lack the high amplitude peaks above about 0.75 kHz seen in the normal audibility spectra. Also, in the low frequencies of the severe audibility spectra, the dominant peak is about 10 dB below the comparable peak in the normal audibility spectra. In the severe audibility nasal spectra, the antiresonance troughs are less apparent, with the [m] antiresonance more distinct than that of the [n]. The [w] severe audibility spectrum exhibits an F2 peak that is at least 15 dB lower than the F1 peak.

These characteristics in the severe-audibility spectra suggest that cues to manner distinctions of the [w] in NU6 *wash* and the [m, n] in *numb* lack salience for the severe-loss listener. However, some new data currently under collection reveal excellent manner distinctions of consonants with the low-continuant feature for some severely and profoundly hard of hearing listeners (Revoile, Barac-Cikoja, Holden-Pitt, & Kozma-Spytek, in preparation). Nasals versus glides versus liquid consonants are distinguishable nearly perfectly by the majority of twenty severely-to-profoundly hard of hearing listeners under test.

Other research has examined distinctions of stops versus consonants with the low-continuant feature. From Erber's (1972) confusion matrices, computations reveal nasal manner distinctions of 92% and stop manner (voicing and place errors ignored) of 95% for five severely hard of hearing children. Five profoundly deaf children performed at or near chance level. Revoile and co-workers (1995b) reported a wide range of ability among severely hard of hearing listeners for distinctions of /n/, /l/, and /d/ in /æCæ/. Factors associated with performance differences were syllable SL and frequency discrimination ability of the listeners. The lowest SLs were used by listeners with

the poorest consonant identification. Between listeners with near normal versus fair consonant identification, the former showed better discrimination of vowel pitch periods identical except for frequency differences. In another study, Revoile and colleagues (Revoile, Holden-Pitt, Edward, Bunnell, & Pickett, 1985) found fairly good distinctions of glide from stop consonants by severely hard of hearing listeners.

Place distinctions of consonants within glide and nasal manner categories by severely hard of hearing listeners have not been reported extensively. For nasal consonants, Erber's (1972) confusion matrices indicate the [n] was identified at chance level, although identification of [m] may have been above chance by five severely hard of hearing children. In the severe audibility glide and nasal spectra (Figure 16-8B) recall the considerable reduction of high-frequency energy and the diminution of low-frequency spectral patterns relative to normal audibility. These characteristics suggest that the severe-loss listener would have difficulty in distinguishing the glide and nasal consonants of NU6 *wash* and *numb*.

In summary, the hypothetical severe-loss listener seems able to distinguish manner of articulation for various consonants in certain NU6 words. Waveforms and spectrograms representing words processed for the severe loss suggest sufficient audibility of low-frequency cues to enable the listener's distinctions between some glides and nasals and distinctions between these low-continuant consonants versus stops and fricatives. The listener can determine the voicing status of voiced stops that show audible voicing during closure. The frequency change in F1 transition of the adjacent vowel may also be a useful cue for stop voicing distinctions by the listener. Cues to manner distinctions of fricatives versus stops appeared audible when the constriction noises of these consonants contained high-amplitude noise in the mid-frequencies. Within manner categories, distinctions of consonants according to place of articulation seem difficult for the severe-loss listener due to the inaudibility of cues at F2 frequency regions and higher.

PHONEME ACOUSTIC-CUE USE BY A HYPOTHETICAL MODERATELY HARD OF HEARING PERSON

For people with moderate hearing loss (about 40 to 65 dB HL PTA), speech perception abilities may be influenced by audiometic threshold configuration[21] more than for persons with greater hearing loss. Severely and especially profoundly hard of hearing listeners often have dynamic range constraints that limit the extent of amplification they can use, regardless of audiometric contour. In turn, this limits the audibility of speech acoustic cues for severe and profound losses, particularly cues in the high frequencies where the speech signal is inherently weaker than in the low frequencies. In comparison, moderate losses are characterized by greater dynamic range, especially if no sound tolerance problems accompany the hearing loss. In such cases, amplified speech may be received at SLs approaching normal, depending upon the audiometric configuration. With a flat configuration, a moderately hard of hearing person can experience relatively normal amplitude ratios among inherently weak versus strong frequencies in speech, assuming linear speech amplification. However, for a moderate degree of loss with a gradually sloping audiometric contour using linear amplification, high frequencies would be received at unnaturally reduced levels relative to low frequencies. When the audiometric contour is steeply sloping above the mid frequencies, high frequency cues may be inaudible for a moderately hard of hearing person, even though low-frequency cues are at or near normal SLs.

Various studies have reported greater reduction in speech perception abilities by hard of hearing persons with sloping audiometric contour than flat (e.g., Dubno, Dirks, & Schaeffer, 1987; Owens, Benedict & Schubert, 1972).

The preceding indicates that inter-listener differences in audiometric threshold contour, in addition to sound tolerance and auditory resolution abilities, are a further reason to avoid generalization about speech perception abilities among persons in a given category of hearing loss. As expressed above relative to severe and profound losses, the acoustic-cue audibility described for the moderately hard of hearing listener here may not be representative of other persons in this hearing loss category.

Consonant acoustic cue audibility is considered below for a hypothetical moderately hard of hearing listener with a PTA of 58 dB HL and a gradually sloping loss, that is, tone thresholds increasing from about 50 to 70 dB HL between 0.25 and 4.0 kHz. Acoustic cues of consonants in words of the NU6 auditory test are examined for the listener's audibility relative to normal audibility. Presentation of the words via headphone (TDH-39) for clinical audiometric purposes is assumed.

The listener's tone thresholds[22] in dB SPL (better hearing ear) are shown in Figure 16-9 (dashed line), as well as tone thresholds for a normal hearing listener (solid line) (ANSI, 1989; TDH-39 reference thresholds). Also displayed is the spectrum of the NU6 words (Auditec [Sherbecoe et al., 1993]) positioned vertically for either listener according to the level[23] at which the NU6 test

---

[21]On an audiogram, the pattern of pure tone thresholds of a hard of hearing person can be labeled according to the plotted change in hearing sensitivity across frequency. A very flat audiometric configuration is one for which hearing thresholds remain within about 15 to 20 dB range across the audiometric frequencies. A sloping configuration shows greater hearing loss as frequency increases. A sloping loss can be gradual, e.g., a 5 to 10 dB threshold decline per octave (Carhart, 1945); steep, e.g., a threshold decline of ≥40 dB; or precipitous, e.g., >30 can also present both flat and sloping components in the audiometric configuration.

---

[22]The elevated pure tone thresholds in Figure 16-9 are mean data from 13 moderately hard of hearing (PTAs from 46–65 dB HL) Gallaudet University students who were subjects in a speech perception experiment (Revoile et al., 1995b).

[23]The 109 dB SPL NU6 presentation level is based on the mean, self-chosen MCLs of the 13 research subjects (Revoile et al., 1995b) whose mean threshold contour was designated as that of the hypothetical moderately hard of hearing listener (Figure 16-9).

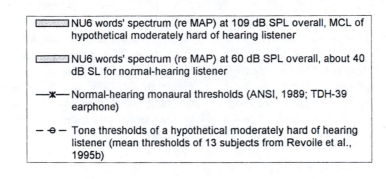

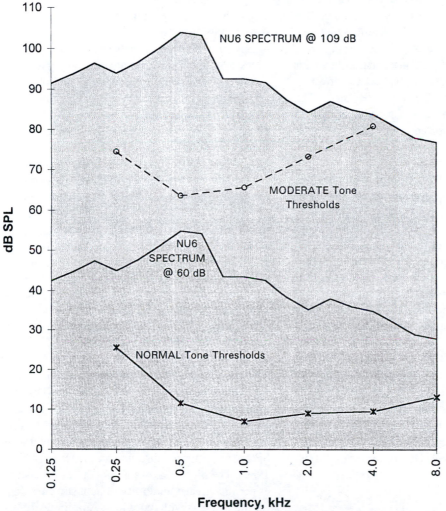

FIGURE 16-9. Acoustic conditions for a standard clinical amplification of the speech spectrum by 40 dB for the moderate-loss listener at a comfortable level. The amplification brings speech spectrum information available to levels 20 to 40 dB above thresholds and encompassing a wide range of speech frequencies up to 4 kHz. Further description and discussion of implications are given in the text.

might be presented clinically. That is, at an over-all level of 109 dB SPL[24] for the moderate-loss listener (lighter shading), and 60 dB SPL for the normal hearing listener (darker shading). The SL associated with these presentation levels is about 40 dB for normal hearing and 30 dB for the moderate loss, based on the speech standard reference SPL relative to either listener's threshold at 1.0 kHz (ANSI, 1989).

Comparison of the NU6 absolute presentation levels used for the two listeners reveals the need for amplification by the moderate-loss listener. From the section above on severe hearing loss, recall that the 60 dB NU6 presentation level for the normal hearing listener approaches conversational speech levels, about 65 dB SPL. The moderate-loss listener would require around 45 dB of amplification for conversational speech to reach the 109 dB SPL assumed here for presentation of the NU6 words.

The differential effects from flat versus sloping moderate hearing loss on the audibility of acoustic cues in different frequency regions may be examined in Figure 16-9. Note the threshold versus NU6 spectrum differences of the moderate-loss listener relative to the normal hearing listener, whose threshold contour approximates that of a flat hearing loss (assuming the thresholds are expressed in dB HL rather than dB SPL). Below 1.0 kHz, the differences between the listeners' thresholds versus the NU6 spectrum are similar, for example, about 40 dB at 0.5 kHz and 19 dB at 0.25 kHz, indicating that cues in the low frequencies are at comparable audibility for normal hearing and the moderate hearing loss. Above about 0.75 kHz, however, the listeners' threshold versus NU6 spectrum differences begin to diverge; for example, at 1.0 kHz, the difference is about

35 dB for normal hearing, while only about 25 dB for moderate hearing loss, and at 4.0 kHz, 25 dB versus 3 dB, respectively. Thus, as frequency increases above 0.5 kHz, the high frequencies decline in audibility for the sloping moderate loss relative to normal. On the other hand, assume that the moderate loss is flat, that is, with a threshold configuration similar to the normal contour. The flat moderate loss would have audibility of acoustic cues more similar to normal across the frequency range, given sufficient linear speech amplification.

Speech waveforms, spectrograms, and spectral slices (via signal processing software [Bunnell, 1998]) are examined to assess the audibility of acoustic cues in some NU6 test words filtered to simulate reception by the moderate-loss listener. First, however, we will consider differences in speech audibility according to moderate, severe, and profound categories of hearing loss. Figure 16-10 shows waveforms of NU6 *Say the word get* for normal audibility (panel A) and moderate audibility (panel B), which can be compared to waveforms of NU6 phrases for severe and profound audibility, respectively, in Figures 16-7 and 16-3. The normal audibility waveforms across the three figures, are quite similar in magnitude of excursions for *Say the word*, providing a reference against which to judge the audibility differences among the phrases according to hearing loss category. The amplitude excursions of the moderate audibility waveform are noticeably greater than those of the severe and profound audibility waveforms. This reflects the different NU6 SLs used among the three hard of hearing listeners: about 30 dB, moderate; 20 dB, severe; and 7 dB, profound, based on the speech standard reference SPL re the listeners' thresholds at 1.0 kHz (ANSI, 1989). The higher SL of the moderate-loss listener permits greater audibility of acoustic cues than for the listeners with more loss. Amplitude differences across the waveforms representing different categories of hearing loss can be estimated by comparison with the 5 dB amplitude steps of Figure 16-4.

---

[24]The 109 dB SPL NU6 presentation level is based on the mean MCLs (self-chosen) of the 13 research subjects (Revoile et al., 1995b) whose mean threshold contour was designated as that of the hypothetical moderately hard of hearing listener (Figure 16-9).

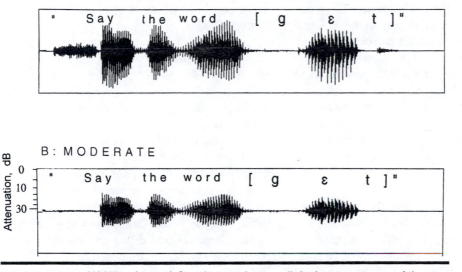

FIGURE 16-10. (A) Waveform of *Say the word get*, a clinical test sentence of the NU6 audiometric test, as presented to a normal listener. (B) Waveform of the same sentence as heard above the moderate-loss listener's threshold after 40 dB of amplification to that listener's most comfortable listening level. The amplitude scale of attenuation on the B waveform (at top right) allows an estimate of the amount of attenuation going from the normal listener to the moderate listener. It appears that the B peaks are attenuated only about 10 dB for the vowels but the frication of [s] in *say* is inaudible above threshold. See text discussion of other differences.

Audibility of Some Acoustic Cues to Consonant Place of Articulation for Moderate Hearing Loss

Cues to consonant place of articulation will be the main focus in our examination of speech audibility for moderate hearing loss. Although reduced use of cues to consonant manner of articulation and/or voicing may occur among moderately hard of hearing persons, consonant place cues are likely to be more problematic (e.g., Dubno, Dirks, & Langhofer, 1982). For the severe and profound losses, we were concerned primarily with consonant manner and voicing cues. Some speech segments containing manner and voicing cues were largely inaudible to the hypothetical severe- and profound-loss listeners. Relative to speech segments with audible cues, severely/profoundly hard of hearing listeners seem able to use constituent temporal acoustic cues to distinguish consonant

voicing and manner (Revoile et al., 1986; Rosen, Faulkner, & Smith, 1990). For moderate-loss listeners, normal use of temporal cues to consonant voicing and manner perception has been found for VCVs altered to eliminate spectral cues (Turner, Souza, & Forget, 1995). While reduced temporal resolution (measured by gap detection) has been found among moderately hard of hearing listeners (e.g., Fitzgibbons & Wightman, 1982), such deficits may involve auditory temporal processing that is not critical to the use of temporal cues for phoneme perception.

Consonant place of articulation is cued primarily by spectral (i.e., frequency-based) characteristics in the speech signal. Important spectral cues to consonant place perception occur in segments resulting from the constriction and/or release of consonants, and also in segments of vowels (i.e., transitions) contiguous with consonant segments (see summary of Chapter Nine for acoustic cues to place of articulation). The critical frequency regions of place cues are usually in the mid, and especially, higher speech frequencies for many consonants. Among stop consonants, for example, important cues to place distinctions are found in the mid to high frequencies (see also the place templates of quantal theory in Chapter Fourteen). For the moderate-loss listener, we will first examine the audibility of place cues to stop consonants, a much-studied class of consonants relative to hearing loss.

Cues to Place of Articulation for Stop Consonants. Spectral cues to stop consonant place reside in the noise burst generated upon release of a stop and in the formant transitions of adjacent vowels. The initial 10 ms or so of the noise burst usually carries the most critical spectral information regarding place of articulation for both voiced and voiceless stops bursts. Zue (1976) measured spoken stop releases and reported broader-band spectra and higher frequencies of spectral peaks for /t/ than /k/ bursts. (Spectra for labial stops were not described due to their variable and indistinct burst frequencies and weak amplitudes.) Depending on the subsequent vowel, mean peak frequencies of /t/ occurred between 3.0 to 4.0 kHz, while for /k/, peaks occurred from about 1.25 to 2.7 kHz. The voiced cognate bursts showed peak frequencies similar to those of the voiceless bursts, although somewhat lower for the /d/ than the /t/. Thus, at a given place of articulation, voiced and voiceless bursts are typically similar for the frequency region in which critical spectral cues reside.

In vowel formant transitions adjacent to a voiced stop consonant, an important cue to place of articulation for the stop is the frequency trajectory of F2 transitions. For word-initial voiced stops, F2 in the adjacent vowel rises in frequency following a [b] and falls in frequency following a [g]. The trajectory of F2 transitions associated with [d] is more dependent upon vowel context, falling in frequency for front vowels and rising or flat for back vowels. For word-initial voiceless stops, vowel formant transitions are generally absent because the articulator movements produc-

ing these consonants have largely occurred prior to the onset of the subsequent vowel (Stevens & Klatt, 1974).

Place Cues in Stop Consonant Noise Bursts Available for the Moderate-Loss Listener. Voiced and voiceless stop consonants for bilabial, alveolar, and linguapalatal place of articulation are present among NU6 *get, book,* and *deep.* Waveforms of these words, respectively, are displayed in Figure 16-11 for normal audibility (A panels) and for moderate audibility (B panels). In the normal-audibility waveforms, the representations of the alveolar noise bursts show greater energy than those of the palatal and, especially, bilabial bursts. These differences are consistent with the burst peak amplitudes measured by Zue (1976). For either the voiced or voiceless stops, the bilabial bursts are somewhat briefer than the alveolar and velar bursts. The diminished intensity and duration of the bilabial bursts suggests they may be the least audible for the moderate-loss listener.

In the moderate-audibility waveforms (Figure 16-11, B panels), the voiceless stop noise bursts are poorly defined, showing weak excursions dispersed irregularly throughout the burst segment. For the [p] burst, no excursions are apparent, revealing its probable inaudiblity for the moderate-loss listener. Among the voiced stops, excursions representing the bursts are seen for each place of articulation, although at much diminished magnitude relative to the bursts in the normal-audibility waveforms. The bursts' reduced amplitude in the moderate-audibility waveforms indicates they are at low audibility, and perhaps their energy is limited to a particular frequency region for the moderate-loss listener.

The frequency regions of stop burst energy available to the listeners in *get, deep,* and *book* can be seen in spectrograms of the words in Figure 16-12 for normal (A panels) and moderate (B panels) audibility.[25] For normal audibility, the

---

[25]The spectrograms of *get, book,* and *deep* for normal and moderate audibility were obtained without high-frequency emphasis to facilitate display of energy in the low frequencies of the moderate audibility stimuli.

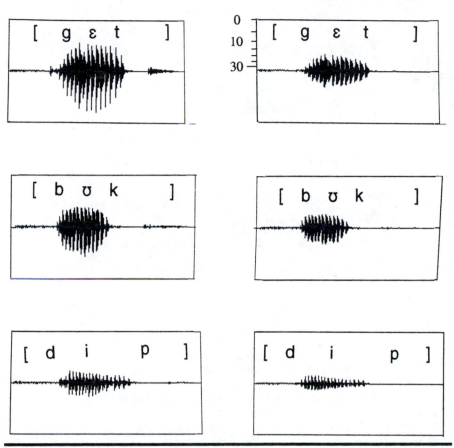

FIGURE 16-11.   Waveforms of NU6 test words *get, book,* and *deep* as received by the normal and moderate-loss listener.

bilabial voiced and voiceless bursts show energy mostly below 1.5 kHz. Both the voiced and voiceless alveolar bursts comprise fairly concentrated energy between 3.0 and 4.5 kHz. Energy of the velar bursts is primarily in the low to mid frequencies, and is somewhat more diffuse for the voiced than the voiceless stop.

The moderate-audibility spectrograms show representations of the stop bursts that are much fainter and considerably less concentrated than found for normal audibility. Energy is apparent mostly in the low frequencies of the noise bursts, regardless of stop place of articulation. Exceptions are the [d]-burst of *deep*, for which some

very faint shading can be seen at about 3.5 kHz; and the [p]-burst, for which no energy appears on the *deep* spectrogram. The apparent low (or no) audibility of the noise bursts and lack of differential energy across frequency regions, reveals that the moderate-loss listener would have difficulty using spectral cues in the bursts to distinguish place of articulation for the stops in *get, deep,* and *book*.

While the full repertoire of burst spectral cues may be unavailable to moderately hard of hearing listeners, some research indicates that such listeners may depend more on the bursts than adjacent vowel transitions for distinctions of stop place.

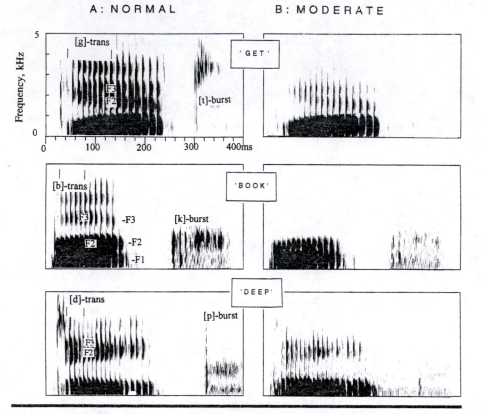

FIGURE 16-12. Spectrograms of the NU6 words of the previous figure, annotated to mark the formant transitions in the vowels that are the cues related to the distinctions among the phonemes /g, b, d/, and the release bursts of /t, k, p/. See text under the heading Cues to Place of Articulation for Stop Consonants, Moderate-Loss Listener.

Hedrick, Schulte, and Jesteadt (1995) found that burst/vowel relative amplitude seemed important for distinctions of synthetic /pa-ta/ by mild-to-moderately hard of hearing listeners. In contrast, the normal hearing listeners tested identified the stops more on the basis of vowel transitions, irrespective of the burst/vowel amplitudes. Greater than normal dependence on release bursts for stop distinctions was also reported by Revoile and colleagues (1995b) for several moderately hard of hearing listeners. When the bursts were intentionally deleted from spoken /Caek/ (C = /b, d, g, w, j/), performances were degraded more for these hard of hearing than for normal hearing listeners. Experimental tests of hard of hearing listeners

using words with intentionally deleted stop bursts may be analogous to their experiences in conversational speech where stops can be unreleased or the released bursts are too weak to be audible.

Explanations offered for poorer-than-normal stop distinctions by mild to moderately hard of hearing listeners include partial audibility of burst spectral cues, as well as other psychoacoustic[26] factors (Turner & Robb, 1987), for

---

[26]The label "psychoacoustic" is putatively associated with auditory tasks requiring discrimination of two or more auditory stimuli presented in succession. Usually, the stimuli are much less complex than a spoken utterance; they may differ in only one acoustic variable, such as frequency or duration.

example, suprathreshold deficits such as impaired frequency selectivity (Raz & Noffsinger, 1985). Findings of recent studies suggest poorer-than-normal frequency selectivity in mild to moderately hard of hearing listeners (e.g., Dubno & Schaefer, 1992). However, these listeners showed consonant recognition comparable to that of normal hearing listeners when both groups were tested under equivalent conditions of speech spectrum audibility.

Place Cues in Vowel Formant Transitions for Stop Consonant Perception by the Moderate-Loss Listener.   Wideband spectrograms of *get*, *deep*, and *book* appear in Figure 16-12 for normal audibility (panel A) and moderate audibility (panel B). These spectrograms were generated with a reduced frequency scale and expanded time scale to display frequency changes[27] of the transitions in more detail.

In the normal-audibility spectrograms, the F2 formants at vowel onset show the expected changes in frequency according to place of articulation for initial voiced stop consonants. Following the burst releases of the alveolar and bilabial stops, F2 rises in frequency, while for the velar stop, F2, falls in frequency. The F2 frequency rise occurs over the initial six to seven pitch periods, increasing approximately from 0.9 kHz to 1.1 kHz in [ʊ], and 1.8 to 2.3 kHz in [i]. In [E], F2 appears to fall in frequency throughout the vowel. However, the transition associated with [g] probably occurs only over the initial six or seven pitch periods. At the vowel offset in *deep* and *book*, notice that changes in F2 frequency are minimal prior to the voiceless stops. Perceptually, vowel offsets tend to provide less information for place distinctions of voiceless stops than voiced (Nelson & Revoile, in review).

In the moderate-audibility spectrograms (Figure 17-12B), the visibility of the formants and associated transitions generally decreases as a function of frequency. Thus, relative to F1, F2 and higher formants are at lower audibility for the moderate-loss listener than for the normal-hearing listener. Although weaker than normal, however, the presence of the initial F2 transitions in *get*, *book*, and *deep* indicate that they are available for use as cues to the moderate-loss listener's perception of voiced stop place.

The extent to which low-audibility transitions are usable for consonant place distinctions by moderately hard of hearing listeners is not known. Some preliminary data show that hard of hearing listeners whose SLs were 20 dB or less for the [ɑ] of stop-[ɑ] syllables were among those whose identification was poorest when the syllables were presented with deleted stop bursts (Nelson & Revoile, 1996). This suggests that the use of transitions for stop distinctions by hard of hearing listeners requires SLs of greater than 20 dB for the adjacent vowel. Other factors that may affect such listeners' use of transitions involve deficient auditory resolution, for example, reduced resolution of vowel transition frequency changes. Resolution may be especially difficult for the frequency changes in vowel formant transitions adjacent to stop consonants, in comparison to those adjacent to say, glide consonants or other semivowels. Frequency changes in vowel formant transitions are typically more rapid for stops than for semivowels. This is because the vocal tract is completely blocked in the production of a stop, causing the articulators to and from the stop constriction move more quickly than in production of a glide, for which the vocal tract is only partially blocked during constriction.

Difficulty in the use of cues in rapid formant transitions may be inferred by the poorer-than-normal identification of burstless /ba-da/ synthetic syllables by nearly all of the listeners tested by Godfrey and Millay (1980). In contrast, these listeners (most of whom had moderate losses) showed normal identification for synthetic /wa-ba/—suggesting that they could use cues in slow-

---

[27]No high-frequency emphasis was used in generating the spectrograms of *get*, *deep*, and *book* in order to obtain better representation of energy below 1.0 kHz for the moderate-audibility versions. Trial spectrograms produced with high-frequency emphasis for moderate audibility yielded much poorer visibility of low-frequency energy, while energy above 1.0 kHz was no more visible than seen in Figure 16-12.

er versus faster transitions. Some other mild-moderately hard of hearing listeners studied by Godfrey and Millay (1978) seemed unable to use either rapid or slower transitions for consonant identification. They showed aberrant labeling of synthetic /be-we/, which differed only for transition duration. For some listeners with moderate losses, Revoile and colleagues (in preparation) found poorer-than-normal place perception of initial stop consonants in /CVk/'s when the stop release bursts were deleted. Thus, the listeners had difficulty using the CV transitions for stop place distinctions. Other moderately hard of hearing listeners tested by Revoile and colleagues (1995b) varied in their identification of /d/ in /aCa/ (C = /d, n, l/) syllables partly depending on their ability to discriminate pitch periods that had been extracted from the onset of the /da/ transitions.

Research with stimuli less complex than speech reveals that both normal hearing and hard of hearing listeners discriminate slower better than more rapid frequency changes in tone glides (Summers & Leek, 1995) or synthetic formant transitions (Revoile, Wilson, & Pickett, 1977). Among hard of hearing listeners per se, however, degree of loss may affect whether frequency change discrimination is poorer than normal. Listeners with mild to moderate losses have shown normal discrimination of rapid and slower tone glides, except when the extent of frequency change was limited (Summers & Leek, 1995). On the other hand, moderately to severely hard of hearing listeners discriminated both rapid and slower synthetic formant transitions more poorly than normal, irrespective of the extent of frequency change (Revoile et al., 1977).

Temporal resolution has received little investigation as a factor in the use of vowel transitions for consonant distinctions. However, in a study with tone glides, discrimination of swept versus stepped frequency changes were deemed to be measuring temporal resolution (Madden & Feth, 1992). Steps of longer intervals were required by mild-to-moderately hard of hearing than normal-hearing listeners to differentiate the stepped frequency changes from the glides. Perhaps this

outcome is analogous to degraded use of rapid transitions for stop place distinctions found for some hard of hearing listeners.

Another factor in the reduced use of transitions by hard of hearing listeners may be within-speech masking, that is, simultaneous and/or temporal masking of high frequency by low frequency components in speech. Danaher and Pickett (1975) reported reduced discrimination of F2 transition frequency extent when F1 was present in the synthetic vowels tested for moderately to severely hard of hearing listeners. Delaying the onset of F1 relative to F2 yielded improved discrimination by the listeners. In an earlier study, hard of hearing listeners showed normal discrimination of frequency extent for synthetic F2 transitions presented in isolation (Danaher, Osberger, & Pickett, 1973). When F1 was added, a decline in F2 transition discrimination occurred, but this was reversed when the F1 energy was reduced. A few of the moderately hard of hearing listeners studied by Van de Grift Turek, Dorman, and Franks (1980) showed improved identification of burstless synthetic /ba, da, ga/ when F1 versus F2/F3 were presented dichotically. For the listeners who received no benefit from the dichotic stimulus presentation, difficulty in resolving the stimulus spectral differences was one explanation offered for the lack of effect.

Glides and voiced stop consonants at the same place of articulation (e.g., /b/ versus /w/ or /g/ versus /j/) usually show similar changes in frequency trajectory of formant transitions in adjacent vowels. Because transitions associated with glides are generally slower than those with stops, place of articulation may be more easily discerned for glides than stops by hard of hearing persons deficient in the use of cues in rapid transitions. Cues to distinctions among glide consonants and other semivowels will be examined next for moderate hearing loss.

Place Cues to Semivowel Distinctions for the Moderate-Loss Listener. An acoustic analysis of semivowels has revealed various spectral differences in F1, F2, and F3 during consonant constriction and in the transitions of contiguous vowels that may contribute to semivowel distinctions (Espy-Wilson, 1992). Here, we will focus on F2 frequency differences of semivowels because the moderate-loss listener's audibility is more marginal for signals in the F2 frequency region; F3 frequencies are largely inaudible while F1 frequencies have near-normal audibility for the listener. Some important F2 characteristics of semivowels appear in the normal-audibility spectrograms of NU6 *wife*, *yes*, and *love* in Figure 16-13 (A panels). In the moderate-audibility spectrograms (Figure 16-13, B panels), these F2 characteristics of the semivowels are also apparent, but not as saliently as in the normal spectro-

grams. The consonant/vowel segments marked on the spectrograms were based on comparisons of the spectrograms versus waveform amplitude changes (Figure 16-14) at points assumed to represent the semivowel constriction boundaries. Although semivowel constrictions may appear on spectrograms as steady state segments (relatively constant formant frequencies), perceptually, it is difficult to identify precise boundaries between semivowels and adjacent vowels because of coarticulatory effects.

In *wife* and *yes*, the glides, [w] and [j], show substantial differences in F2 frequency during the consonant constriction and vowel transition segments. In the frequency nadir at the start of the

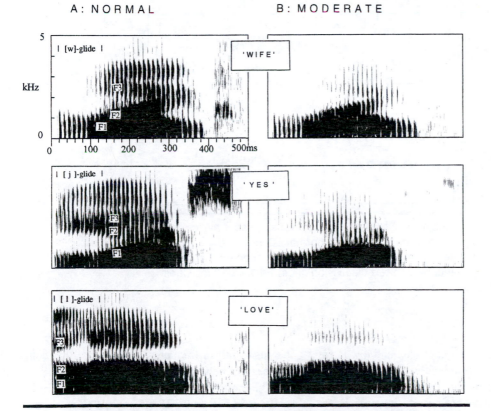

FIGURE 16-13. Spectrograms of the NU6 words *wife, yes,* and *love* for examination of the spectral cues for glide consonant perception. (A) Normal listener, (B) moderate-loss listener. The consonant-glides and formants are labeled for comparison of cues that may be used by the listeners. See text.

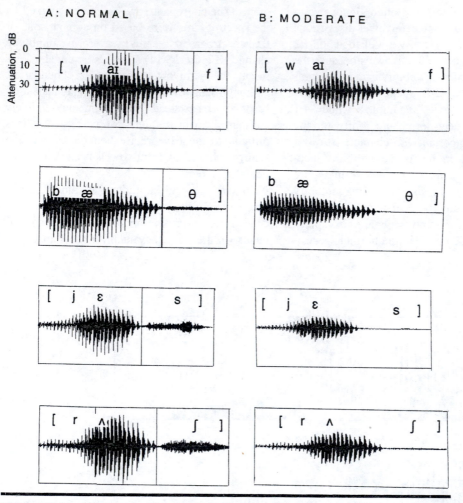

FIGURE 16-14. Waveforms of the NU6 test words *wife*, *bath*, *yes*, *rush* for assessing audibility of fricative place cues as heard by (A) normal listener, and (B) moderate-loss listener. For the moderate-loss listener it appears that the fricatives are largely inaudible. See text discussion under Fricative Place Cues for the Moderate-Loss Listener.

[w] constriction, F2 is quite weak and low in frequency; it appears to merge with F1. Before the end of the constriction, F2 begins rising from about 0.5 kHz and continues to increase in frequency throughout and beyond the transition. Comparatively, F2 of [j] is nearly steady state at about 2.0 kHz during most of the constriction. Toward the end of the constriction, the [j] F2

begins to fall in frequency, a trajectory that continues into the vowel transition.

The moderate-audibility spectrograms of *wife* and *yes* in Figure 16-13 (B panels) show the F2 characteristics of [w] more distinctly than those of [j]. This effect is related to the moderate-loss listener's poorer audibility for high frequencies than low. Thus, in terms of cue audibility, the listener would probably identify the [w] of *wife* more easily than the [j] of *yes*.

For the lateral [l] of *love*, the respective frequency regions of F1 and F2 during constriction are at about 0.4 and 1.2 kHz and remain rather steady state (Figure 16-13, A and B panels, respectively, normal and moderate audibility). Note also during the constriction, that the intensity of F2 appears to approach that of F1, at least in the normal-audibility spectrogram. In comparison, the moderate-audibility spectrogram shows substantially lower F2 amplitude than F1. An effect for the moderate-loss listener could be reduced salience of the F2 cue for /l/, perhaps resulting in a weak or indistinct /l/ percept, confusable with /w/, for example.

Moderately hard of hearing listeners have received limited study for their perception of semivowel distinctions. However, such listeners have been included in some recent experiments with voiced consonants, which included semivowels. Revoile and colleagues (in preparation) reported a significant decline in identification of /l/, /w/, and/or /j/ for the majority of nine moderately hard of hearing listeners when the semivowel constriction segments were deleted from spoken /ɑCɑ/. The deletion did not reduce normal hearing listeners' distinctions of the semivowels. Deficient use of cues in the adjacent vowel transitions may explain the performance decline for the hard of hearing listeners. In another study (Revoile et al., 1995b), moderately to profoundly hard of hearing listeners' identification of /l/ in /ɑCɑ/ syllables (C = /d, n, l/) was associated with their ability to discriminate pitch periods taken from the onset and offset of the /lɑ/ transitions. An earlier experiment revealed poorer identification of /w/ than /j/ in /Cæk/ by twenty-one listeners with moderate to severe losses (Revoile, Holden-Pitt, Edward, et al., 1985b). Performance for /jaek/ was moderately related to discrimination of synthetic /j/-like F2 transitions, suggesting that some listeners' perception of /j/ was associated with their ability to discern frequency changes in the /jæ/ transitions. However, discrimination of /w/-like F2 transitions showed a low relation to identification of /wæk/. The hard of hearing listeners' mean discrimination of both the /j/- and /w/-like transitions was poorer than found for a group of normal-hearing listeners whose identification of /w/ and /j/ was nearly perfect.

The NU6 words chosen for examination of semivowel place distinctions were selected as well to contain final fricatives that vary for place of articulation. The moderate-loss listener's access to place acoustic cues for final voiceless fricatives will be considered next.

Fricative Place Cues for the Moderate-Loss Listener. Among voiced and voiceless fricatives, the major cues to place distinctions are the spectral differences in the frication noises. For example, /f/ and /θ/ frications have rather diffuse energy across 1.8 to 8.5 kHz, compared to /s/ and /ʃ/, which contain spectral peaks at about 3.5 to 5.0 and 2.5 to 3.5 kHz, respectively (Behrens & Blumstein, 1988). Voiced fricatives typically show frication spectra similar to their voiceless place cognates. However, voiced and voiceless fricatives may differ for the frequency extent of transitions in adjacent vowels. Transitions of greater frequency extent have been found for voiced alveolar fricatives than voiceless, at least in F1 (Stevens, Blumstein, et al., 1992). The contributions of vowel formant transitions to place distinctions of adjacent fricatives has received minimal attention in acoustic and perceptual studies. For a given place of articulation, we can infer that vowel transitions should contribute to fricative identification to the same extent as found for stop consonants.

NU6 *yes*, *rush*, *bath*, and *wife*, respectively, enable examination of some cues to fricative distinctions at labiodental, alveolar, palatal, and linguadental place of articulation. In Figure 16-14, the waveforms of these words for normal audibility (A panels) indicate the weak frication energy of the labiodental and linguadental fricatives versus the alveolar and palatal fricatives, which is a difference typically found among these consonants.

In comparison to the normal-audibility waveforms, the moderate audibility waveforms (Figure

16-14, B panels) reveal substantially diminished frication noises. Furthermore, in the moderate-loss waveforms, most of the frications are not sustained, showing substantial amplitude briefly at the frication onset, as in *bath*, or dispersed intermittently throughout the frication noise, as in *wife* and *yes*. The exception is [ʃ], for which the frication noise is continuous and similar in duration to that in normal-audibility *rush*. The comparative weakness and intermittency of these frications, as represented for the moderate-loss listener is due to the declining audibility across mid to high frequencies. Thus, for the situation of moderate loss, we may expect problems in fricative place distinctions and perhaps some manner confusions of voiceless stops for fricatives could occur.

To look for distinctive cues, spectral section graphs were generated of the most intense portion of each frication noise to examine the spectral differences of these noise segments. In the normal-audibility sections (Figure 16-15, A panel), the [f] and [θ] present rather similar spectra—relatively flat across frequency overall, but with two minor peaks below 2.0 kHz. In comparison, the [s] and [ʃ] spectra show greater energy in the high frequencies. In the /s/ noise, a strong peak appears at about 4.2 kHz; it is at least 20 dB greater than the maximum peaks below 1.0 kHz. The [ʃ] displays a broad peak between about 2.5 to 3.5 kHz, which is more than 10 dB higher than the peaks below 1.0 kHz. These spectral differences are critical for distinctions of /s/ versus /sh/. On the other hand, the spectral similarity of the [f] and [θ] is consistent with analyses of these consonants in acoustic studies (e.g., Behrens & Blumstein, 1988), and can yield normal-hearing confusions of these fricatives in perceptual experiments (e.g., Revoile et al., 1991a).

Spectral sections representing the moderate-audibility frication noises (Figure 16-15, B panel) show spectral prominences at frequencies similar to those seen for normal audibility. In comparison, however, the moderate audibility spectra are suppressed in amplitude at 1.0 kHz and above. For example, the high frequency peak in [ʃ] is no greater than peaks below 1.0 kHz. This lack of spectral differentiation would to contribute the moderate-loss listener's difficulty in distinguishing these fricatives for place of articulation.

Although hard of hearing listeners typically show reduced fricative recognition in studies of overall consonant perception (e.g., Bilger & Wang, 1976), few investigations have examined fricative perception specifically. The mild-to-moderately hard of hearing listeners tested by Zeng and Turner (1990) showed fairly good distinctions of voiceless fricatives in synthetic /Ci/ syllables when the frication noises were estimated to be 20% to 100% audible. For syllables with deleted frications and vowel transitions present, comparable performance was obtained but only when the transitions' estimated audibility was about 100%. The stimulus audibility estimates were based on comparisons of listeners' tone thresholds versus computed audibility spectra derived for the frication and transition segments. From a recently completed study, preliminary analyses show that moderately hard of hearing listeners' identification of /v/ depended on the frication noise more than for /z/ in spoken /ɑCɑ/ (Revoile et al., in preparation). For either consonant, these listeners were much less able than normal-hearing listeners to use cues in the adjacent vowels for /v-z/ distinctions. In another study by Revoile and colleagues (in preparation), vowel offset transitions were found more useful for place distinctions (alveolar and labiodental) of final voiced than voiceless fricatives by moderately hard of hearing and normal-hearing listeners.

Nasal Consonant Place Cues for the Moderate-Loss Listener. In the section on severe hearing loss, we found that an important cue to manner distinctions of nasals versus other low-continuant consonants was the presence of an antiresonance in the consonant constriction segment. Antiresonances are also important for distinctions of nasals according to place of articulation. Among /m, n, ŋ/, antiresonance frequencies differ, for example, an antiresonance below 1.0 kHz Hz is more representative of /m/, while an antiresonance in the range of 1.5 to 2.0 kHz is more typical of

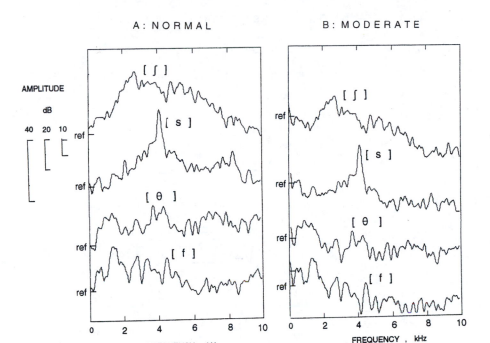

FIGURE 16-15. Spectrum sections of consonant frications in the consonants [ʃ, s, θ, f] in the NU6 test words of the previous figure, for (A) the normal listener, and (B) the moderate-loss listener. The references marks, "ref," are placed at the same amplitude level for each consonant spectrum, enabling exact comparison of the levels of all spectral features between normal and moderate-loss listeners. Each frication was sampled for 51.2 ms of the most intense part.

/n/, and above 3.0 kHz is associated more with /ŋ/. However, according to acoustical analyses, frequencies of antiresonances and formants can vary substantially among utterances of a given nasal consonant, as well as throughout the nasal constriction segment from an individual utterance (Fujimura, 1962). Additional cues to nasal place distinctions can occur in adjacent vowels when nasalization is produced preceding and following the consonant constriction (see Chapter Seven for more details of nasalization). Finally, spectral characteristics of transitions in the adjacent vowels may also contribute important information for nasal place differentiation (e.g., Harrington, 1994).

Figure 16-16 shows spectra for the first five pitch periods (pp) of the [m] and [n] in NU6 *moon*

for normal audibility (panel A). The nasal antiresonances "ar" are visible in the [m] and [n] constriction segments. The antiresonance of [m] falls in frequency from about 0.7 to 0.4 kHz throughout the constriction. In comparison, the antiresonance in the [n] constriction is deeper, more steady state, and at about 1.8 kHz throughout the constriction.

In the moderate-audibility spectra (Figure 16-16, panel B), the antiresonances in both the [m] and [n] constriction segments have less definition than in the normal spectrogram. Especially, the [n] antiresonance lacks salience. Recall that NU6 audibility for the moderate-loss listener was seen to decline from normal above 0.5 kHz. The higher-frequency antiresonance of the [n] relative

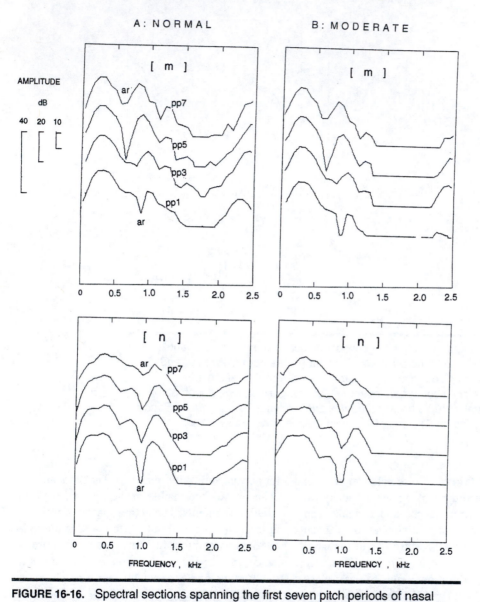

FIGURE 16-16.   Spectral sections spanning the first seven pitch periods of nasal murmurs of [m] and [n] for (A) normal and (B) moderate-loss listeners. Compared to the fricatives in Figure 16-14, there is not much reduction in amplitude level going from normal to moderate, due to the moderate's good hearing for low frequencies. The frequency location of the antiresonances, "ar," falls from .9 to .7 kHz, with time for the [m] but is steady at 1 kHz for the [n]. The text discussion is under heading Nasal Consonant Place Cues for the Moderate-Loss Listener.

to the [m] could yield poorer perception of [n] than [m] by the moderate-loss listener. The lower-frequency antiresonance of the [m] than the [n] could result in the hard of hearing listener perceiving the /m/ more easily than the /n/.

There is little documentation on distinctions of nasal consonants by hard of hearing listeners. Preliminary analysis of recent findings for nine moderately hard of hearing listeners indicated near-normal distinctions of /m-n/ in spoken /ɑCɑ/ syllables (Revoile et al., in preparation). When the nasal constriction segments were deleted, a substantial performance decline for the these listeners suggested deficiencies in their use of cues in the vowels for /m-n/ distinctions. The nasal segment deletion did not reduce performance by normal hearing listeners. In another study, identification of /n/ in /æCæ/ (as well as /d/ and /l/) was investigated for listeners with moderate to profound losses (Revoile et al., 1995b). Most of the listeners relied greatly on the presence of the consonant constriction segment for identification of /ænæ/; that is, cues in the adjacent vowels did not support /n/ perception. Further, the listeners' identification of /n/ in /æCæ/ was well predicted by their ability to discriminate pitch periods that had been extracted from the onset and offset of the /næ/ transitions. However, normal-hearing listeners showed relatively good identification of the /n/ on the basis of nasality cues in the vowels, that is, when the syllables were presented with the vowels unaltered and the nasal consonant segment deleted.

In summary, the sloping hearing configuration of our moderate-loss listener effected reduced audibility in NU6 words of energy above 0.5 kHz, decreasing from about 20 dB at 1.0 kHz to 3 dB at 4.0 kHz. Cues to place of articulation among consonants were affected differently, depending on the extent to which they resided in the frequency regions of reduced audibility. Waveforms and spectrograms of the words filtered to simulate the audibility reduction showed speech energy associated with stop and fricative consonant constrictions that appeared inaudible or greatly reduced in audibility relative to normal. These segments would be unavailable or spectrally indistinguishable for use by the moderate-loss listener to differentiate place of articulation for stops and fricatives. In comparison, the filtered constriction segments of nasal and semivowel consonants appeared to retain sufficient spectral identity to enable place distinctions by the listener. The formant transitions in vowels adjacent to the consonants were partially or fully visible in the speech graphics, indicating that they would be available to some extent for use in consonant place distinctions by the moderate-loss listener.

CHAPTER 17

SPEECH TECHNOLOGY

SPEECH MACHINES

J. M. PICKETT AND JUERGEN SCHROETER

Can we build machines that speak? This query expresses a surprisingly old, basic curiosity about human communication. It eventually led to the development of today's speech technology.

To build a speaking machine, obviously we need to devise some type of articulating mechanism. The machine should be a physical, working model of the speech organs that articulate speech. This was the approach of one of the earliest experimenters. Wolfgang von Kempelen, in experiments from 1769–1791, built a speaking machine that was a hand-controlled model of vocal mechanisms; it used a bellows for lungs to drive air through a buzzing vibrator, feeding the buzz-sound into a deformable horn that served as the vocal-tract resonator (Dudley & Tarnoczy, 1950). Another approach was simply acoustic, to make speech-like sounds by blowing shaped organ pipes, as did Kratzenstein in simulating Russian vowels in 1781.

In our electronic era both routes, articulatory and acoustic, have been intensively investigated, beginning in the 1930s, particularly at AT&T's Bell Telephone Laboratories (Flanagan, 1972), where they built speaking electronic models consisting of electronic voice sources that activated electronic vocal-tract shapes. Other speech scientists readily embraced developments in electronic simulation of speech sounds and used it in their research to understand how speech works, both in production and perception. Then electronic developers used the scientists' findings to improve the performance of their machines. If we know all the relations between speaking maneuvers and the resulting sounds, then we should be able to build a speaking machine that would be an articulatory model (also see Mattingly, 1974).

How can we synthesize speech that would sound completely natural? Ideally, in principle, we could generate the most natural sounding speech by true articulatory synthesis; however, currently not enough is known to do this (see the section below on Articulatory Synthesis). At present, state-of-the art speech synthesis by computers uses one of two methods: (1) formant synthesis by rule or (2) concatenative synthesis by computer-assembly of speech from pieces of natural speech. Formant synthesis uses a set of rules for controlling a source-filter/formant model, an articulatory model that is sufficient, but only partially true. These two methods produce more or less natural-sounding synthetic speech; they will both be described in the following section on Speech Synthesis.

On the way to developing formant-based speech synthesis, it was apparent to researchers that knowing an electronic code that would correctly produce essential speech characteristics might enable us to reverse the process, namely to correctly recognize speech sounds via a decoding machine. The recognition machine would be a

Acknowledgments

The preparation of the section on Automatic Speech Recognition by Kewley-Port was supported by SBIR grants from the National Institutes of Health for Deafness and Other Communication Disorders to Communication Disorders Technology, Inc., Bloomington, IN.

specialized acoustic analyzer capable of deriving the essential characteristics and putting them together to get the phonemes in words that had been spoken. This process is called *automatic speech recognition.*

The current field of computer processing of speech is made up of many subfields in both technology and science. The whole is called *speech processing.* Speech scientists and phoneticians use speech processing for research on speech production and perception, linguists use it in experimental phonology. Technologists use it to enhance speech in noise and for aiding people with hearing impairment, for example. Applications of speech processing are called *speech technology,* which includes programs and devices for speech recognition, speech coding, speech synthesis, and talker identification/recognition and verification. Simple speech recognizers are used every day in the telephone directory service and in business for tasks where it is inconvenient or inefficient to write or type information. Examples of tasks are: recording inspection data on the production line, taking product inventory, and computer control by voice. Technology developers work to improve and expand the use of recognizers to type out anything that anyone might say, correct to the last phoneme or word. They have developed some impressive voice dictation systems for use by individuals on their personal computers. But universal recognition is still far in the future, as we will describe in the section entitled Speech Recognition by Computer.

Some recognition tasks are feasible for all speakers, if the task is well constrained, as it is for using the telephone directory and for recording product data, or if meaningful tasks can be accomplished even with imperfect recognizers (e.g., word recognition rates below 50%), as long as the intent (meaning) of what the speaker is saying is recognized reliably (e.g., the user wants information on flights from Chicago to Detroit; see Gorin, 1995). In addition, a useful constraint is a fixed, limited vocabulary of words. An example of such a constrained but meaningful task is making travel reservations by speaking to a computer that is equipped with programs and information to carry out the reservation process. The computer would speak to the traveler using a speech synthesis program and listen to the traveler using a speech recognition program. Synthesizer programs often employ the same production principles and relations between formant frequencies and the consonants and vowels that we have already studied in Chapters Four through Nine. Recognition programs encounter the more complex problems, acting like speech perceivers, that we studied in Chapters Eleven through Fifteen.

SPEECH SYNTHESIS

CORINE BICKLEY, ANN SYRDAL, AND JUERGEN SCHROETER

In a spoken language system (see the section entitled Speech Recognition by Machine below) for making travel reservations by voice (e.g., over the telephone) the synthesizer program would first ask the traveler to speak the city where she or he wished to go. The recognizer would identify the city name and the synthesizer would then speak back the city. If the traveler confirms the computer's recognition, then it would speak a list of choices of flights and the reservation process could continue back and forth between the traveler and the computer.

The task of the synthesizer is to go from written text (stored in or generated by a computer) to an intelligible acoustic version of the utterance. The text input to the synthesizer can be in ordinary words that are then converted to phonetic symbols and amended by prosodic information (fundamental frequency F0 and duration information). Then the converted and amended text of the utterance is fed into the synthesizer backend that generates as its output an acoustic waveform for the utterance. This general process is called *text-to-speech,* or "TTS" for short.

The optimal method used for synthesizing speech from text depends on the requirements of the intended application. For some applications, for example, for proofing the flow of this writing by listening to speech synthesized from a high-lighted paragraph or section, the speech from a synthesizer doesn't need to sound completely natural; it needs only to be highly intelligible and have a reasonably pleasant and smooth quality. Today, there are two types of speech synthesis techniques in common use: formant techniques and waveform techniques. Formant synthesis strings together formant patterns corresponding to the phoneme string to be synthesized; wave synthesis strings together segments consisting of consonant-vowel pairs taken from the waveform of a natural utterance of that phoneme string.

For formant synthesis we know how to program the course of formant tracks for all the vowels and consonants, and this speech knowledge can be "coded" into rules interpreted by the text-to-speech program when it converts running text into synthetic speech. Waveform techniques for concatenative synthesis are used in applications where a higher degree of intelligibility and naturalness is desired. In concatenative synthesis, snippets of speech are cut from several recorded utterances and are recombined on the fly during synthesis of a target utterance. Further below we will compare formant synthesis and concatenative synthesis. After learning about these two methods we will describe articulatory synthesizers used for basic speech research.

Synthesis for Text-to-Speech

The general process of converting text into speech is shown in Figure 17-1. The first operation is to convert the text from words and punctuation marks into a string of phonemes and prosodic marks. This step is called *letter-to-sound* conversion. For several languages, including American and British English, Swedish, French, German, and others, rules are known for the correspondence between spelling and sounds, or quite extensive dictionaries may be used where pronunciations are looked up. In any case, some details of the conversion process must be specified explicitly as exceptions to general rules. For some

aspects of the conversion, there are several possibilities that are acceptable, particularly to allow variations in the prosody of the spoken utterance. Current research efforts are aimed at understanding the possible variations and the constraints on pronunciations and prosody. The final step in the process is the synthesis of the speech waveform from the phonetic and prosodic specifications. Today's systems commonly employ two techniques for the final synthesis stage: formant techniques and concatenative waveform techniques. Formant synthesis strings together formant patterns corresponding to the input phoneme string; concatenative synthesis strings together waveform segments taken from a natural utterance containing the required segments. We will now describe and compare formant synthesis and concatenative synthesis in more detail.

Formant Synthesis for Text-to-Speech. The last block in Figure 17-1, the block for synthesis of the speech waveform, may be implemented with a formant synthesizer. High-quality commercial text-to-speech systems that use formant synthesis include DecTalk (based primarily on the research of Dennis Klatt of the Massachusetts Institute of Technology) and Multi-Talk (developed at the Royal Institute of Technology in Stockholm). Synthesizers of this type employ the source-filter theory of speech production. They utilize formant tracks, "basic" formant patterns for each phoneme, and tracks of F0 that specify source variations and other aspects of articulation (Carlson, Granstrom, & Hunnicutt, 1988; Klatt & Klatt, 1990). The source excitation can be either voice pulses or noise. For example, for the word *saw* the /s/-phoneme pattern might specify noise excitation of a filter that passes mostly the higher frequencies with a formant at about 5000 Hz followed by the /aw/-pattern of voice excitation of three formant filters with peak frequencies at 600, 1300, and 2500 Hz representing formants F1, F2, and F3.

Because spoken phonemes are articulated in a context of adjacent phonemes and various stress

TEXT-TO-SPEECH SYNTHESIS

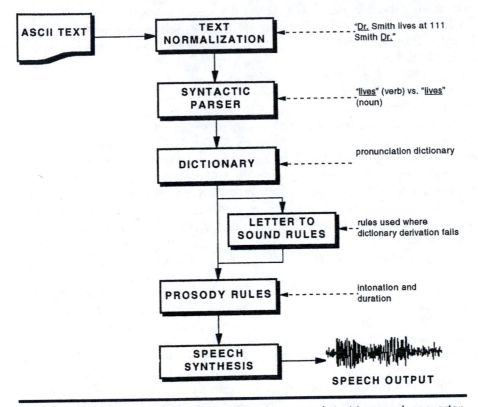

FIGURE 17-1.   Diagram of computer functions for a generic text-to-speech converter. The blocks represent processes necessary for the computer to carry out to convert the input text to a spoken output. The text input in the example, *Dr. Smith lives at 111 Smith Dr.*, first goes to a normalizer that must convert the abbreviation *Dr.* as *Doctor* only if it begins the sentence, but otherwise as *Drive*. This expanded text then goes to a parser that can determine from the context that *lives* should be interpreted as a verb rather than a noun. The dictionary stage then looks up the pronunciation sequence of phonemes for each word, sometimes using letter-to-phoneme rules. The prosody rules are consulted to decide on the intonation and duration to be used, say on each syllable. Finally, the phonemes, prosodically marked, are fed to the speech synthesizer to be converted to sound output.

patterns, there needs to be rules for modifying the basic phoneme formant patterns to create natural connections between them in the synthesized speech. This need to connect together parameter tracks (these are the control signals that set formant frequencies F1, F2, and F3, fundamental frequency F0, and source changes) between adjacent speech sounds is one of the crucial problems for good synthesis. For example, if the text is *saw me*, then the basic /aw/-pattern would need to be modified just prior to the /m/-murmur by lowering the offgoing frequencies of F1 and F2 to mimic the anticipatory coarticulation of the /m/ in *me*, but if that text is *saw Dee*, the coarticulation adjustment at the end of /aw/ would be to raise F2 and lower F1, in anticipation of the /d/ in *Dee*.

General rules for formant-based synthesis of individual segments are well known. Short utterances that are completely intelligible (series of consonants and vowels, words, and sentences of a few words) have been synthesized by many researchers for a variety of purposes. When the control parameters of a formant synthesizer are hand-tuned for a given utterance by repeatedly adjusting the source spectrum and individual formants to those of the speaker, the result is so realistic that it can be very difficult to distinguish the synthetic from the original natural speech. However, it is hard to match the quality of hand-tuned synthetic speech using an automatic system to acquire the necessary synthesis control parameters.

A difficulty in using formant synthesizers results from the precise coordination needed among the many parameters. Although high-quality speech can be synthesized when careful attention is paid to parameter specification, unnatural sounds can result from some combinations of parameter values. It can be determined, though, which combinations of parameter values are sensible, based on understanding sound generation in the vocal tract. Stevens (1998) has documented many of these constraints in what the vocal apparatus can do. A commercial system based on this research, HLsyn (high-level synthesis), has been developed. From just a few HL parameters, all of the detailed acoustic parameters for a formant-based synthesizer are derived by rule in the program. The HL parameters include both acoustic ones such as resonances and articulatory ones such as vocal tract configuration.

Another general problem is the assignment of the correct prosody for the text utterance. This is attempted by the MITalk system, a text-to-speech system that was developed at MIT by a team of researchers led by Jonathan Allen including Sheri Hunnicutt and Dennis Klatt (1987). The system accepts unrestricted English text and converts it to synthesized speech. MITalk decomposes words into morphemes and assigns syntactic structure. It then applies letter-to-sound rules and prosodic analysis to create a representation that is used to control the speech synthesizer. The morphemic analysis provides information needed to distinguish pronunciations of "un" in the word *unit* and *uninitialize*. A parser that processes words sequentially starting from the beginning of a sentence assigns syntactic structure. Some words in English are pronounced differently depending on their part of speech; the word *project* receives stress on the first syllable if it is used as a noun, and on the second if it is used as a verb. The parser builds the longest possible phrase based on the parts of speech of each word. In this way, only one parse is found for any sentence, even sentences that are syntactically ambiguous such as *She gave her dog food*. Letter-to-sound rules specify the pronunciation of sound sequences depending on context and syntactical structure. For instance, "ea" is pronounced differently in the words *reach, react, create, breath*, and others. Also, *down* is pronounced somewhat differently each time in *Down Fido! Put down the down pillow.* and *It was a big letdown to go down the ramp with no trophy*. In addition, realistic production of segmental acoustics as well as timing and intonation are all important for natural-sounding speech. In all these areas, MITalk has contributed important first steps toward good-quality text-to-speech.

Uses of formant synthesizers. Many uses of formant synthesizers have been developed over the past forty or so years. As with all TTS systems, the goal of more natural-sounding synthesized speech for text-to-speech applications continues to drive refinement of formant synthesizers. They are very efficient because they do not require a large storage capacity for an inventory and the computational demands are relatively simple. This makes formant synthesis attractive for use in text-to-speech systems.

Formant synthesizers are frequently used to create stimuli for experiments that explore the perception of speech and speech-like sounds. The independent manipulation of acoustic parameters needed for perceptual experiments can be achieved easily with formant synthesizers, but is more difficult with synthesizers based on concatenation of pieces of natural speech. Most textbooks of acoustic phonetics treat formants as the primary vehicle of speech information. Therefore, it is relatively easy to apply this knowledge directly when employing a formant synthesizer.

Formant synthesizers allow researchers to control very precisely the acoustic differences between two sounds. Formant synthesis was used in most of the studies we described in Chapters Eleven and Twelve. One way to study the perception of sounds by human listeners is to synthesize sounds that differ from each other in small steps along an acoustic continuum, and then to present these stimuli in random order to listeners. In one kind of experiment, listeners are asked to judge "same" or "different" for pairs of sounds, some of which are the same stimulus and same pairs of which are composed of two different stimuli. In this way, researchers try to understand how much of an acoustic difference is needed to cause listeners to decide "different." In another kind of experiment, the synthesized sounds are created to be similar to or different from naturally produced sounds in certain characteristics, and listeners are asked which phoneme each stimulus sounds most like. Researchers then try to infer which variations in acoustic characteristics are most important for phoneme identity. Understanding these aspects of human speech perception has been useful in diverse areas such as hearing aid design, speech training, and speech recognition, as well as in further refining the synthesis of speech.

The relationship between speech acoustics and speech perception has been studied using synthesized stimuli in many languages, including American English, several European languages, some Asian languages, and others. Most of these experiments have used listeners with normal hearing and stimuli based on normal articulation. Much work remains to be done in both the acoustics and the perception of other languages of the world and of disordered speech. Synthesized stimuli will also be useful in studying speech and hearing across the life span.

Both spectral and temporal characteristics of speech have been studied using synthesized stimuli. In early work, continua of vowel sounds differing only in the frequency of one formant were used to investigate the relationship between formant frequency and the perception of vowel features such as height and backing. The perceptual effect of temporal changes such as differences in voice onset time or vowel duration have also been studied extensively.

Another very important use of formant synthesizers is in reading machines for the blind. Visually challenged people use their screen readers (software or hardware that allows a blind person to obtain synthetic speech for any information displayed on a computer screen) or reading devices (optical character recognition, OCR, combined with a TTS-system) for many hours every day. They prefer a rather high speaking rate of up to about 600 words per minute. Since formant synthesizers can easily accommodate such a high speaking rate, they have an advantage over concatenative synthesizers where a speed-up factor of 10 or more would be needed that, at present, is likely to produce very disturbing distortions in the resulting synthetic speech. (For more information on screen readers, see the section on Comparison of Formant versus Concatenative Synthesis below.)

Coded Voice and Concatenative Speech Synthesis

Concatenative synthesis methods result in highly intelligible and potentially very natural-sounding speech. Such methods consist of storing, selecting, and smoothly concatenating snippets of speech (see below) in and from their specific acoustic inventory. Imagine that one would record, in all desired voices, all existing words spoken in all sensible intonations: Such a system would be a truly smart speech playback system that would sound absolutely natural. The caveat of such a system, of course, would be the prohibitive cost of the required storage and the cost for the fast computer to find and retrieve the desired recording of an utterance given just the text of the utterance. In addition, it would be highly impractical (if not impossible) to ask any voice talent to speak such a large inventory of words. The task would take years, and one would run the risk that the talent's voice could change during the course of the recordings. Therefore, compromises have to be made in terms of what kind of "atomic" units to store in the acoustic inventory. In addition, since we want the acoustic inventory to occupy as little space as possible, voice coding techniques may be used to compress the inventory while keeping the number of units in the inventory constant.

For voice coding, the process begins with a recording of a natural version of a desired utterance (or acoustic inventory unit; see below). Then the recorded signal is coded efficiently, in as few bits as possible for the desired quality, and stored with name tags for retrieval. The stored data are then used to resynthesize a version of the original element of the acoustic inventory of the TTS system. In other words, the basic goal for voice coding is to lower the speech coding rate (the number of kilobits per second of speech that need to be stored) while maintaining a high quality of the synthesized speech.

Various coding techniques are used to represent the acoustic inventory units used for concatenative synthesis. LPC methods were widely used ten to twenty years ago; more recently, a waveform coding technique called *pitch-synchronous overlap add* (PSOLA; Moulines & Charpentier, 1990) has been popular. Most recently, however, sinusoidal speech coding techniques that decompose the periodic portions of the signal into its harmonics, have become commonplace (see, e.g., Stylianou, Dutoit, & Schroeter, 1997). For more information on the latter two methods, see, for example, Dutoit (1997). Independent of what kind of speech coding is used, speech coding of acoustic inventory units for concatenative synthesis must allow a unit to expand or compress in duration, must provide for smooth concatenation of units, and must tolerate changes in the original

fundamental frequency of the unit while still retaining its natural speech quality.

Voice Coding Techniques. The efficiency of a speech coding method can be expressed in terms of the perceptual quality of the decoded speech versus the required amount of information storage and transmission capacity to move it (the bandwidth). Rate of information is measured in bits per second or kilobits per second, kb/s. Consider the information rates of the two basic types of speech coding: *waveform coding* and *voice coding*, or *vocoding*. Waveform coders aim to capture and reproduce the original time-domain audio waveform as faithfully as possible to preserve the perceptual quality, naturalness, and intelligibility of the original speech. Waveform coding is widely used in digital telecommunications in the form of standard 64 kb/s pulse code modulation (PCM) and 32 kb/s adaptive differential PCM (ADPCM). More recently, researchers have succeeded in compressing audio waveforms transparently (i.e., no distortions are detectable) at rates down to 16 kb/s by taking advantage of perceptual (auditory hearing) models. Distortions produced by (bad) waveform coders are generally perceived as containing more background noise in the resynthesized version than was present in the original. Still lower bit rates can be achieved by more complex vocoding techniques. These techniques assume a speech production model, usually separating the speech signal into estimated vocal tract shape (derived from the spectral envelope) and its excitation (periodic pulses for voiced portions or aperiodic noise for unvoiced portions). Vocoders attempt to recreate equivalent perceptual quality rather than waveform accuracy with respect to the original speech. Vocoding techniques are widely used commercially for stored voice applications such as voice messaging, for which a bit rate of 8 kb/s is common. Even the "classical" 2.4 kb/s vocoders can yield intelligible speech, though it may sound unnatural (with distortions that can be described as gurgles, whistles, buzziness, harshness, or a muffled quality). Some newer voice coding techniques (such as multipulse-excited LPC or code-excited linear prediction [CELP]) combine aspects of waveform coding (for the excitation) and vocoding (for the spectral envelope) to enhance speech quality at low bit rates. For an overview of the current state of the art in speech coding, see, for example, Kleijn and Paliwal (1995).

Concatenated Stored Speech. Stored voice response systems rely on coding, storing, and reconstructing speech. For applications that involve voice responses or messages with variable numeric amounts or digit strings—for example, telephone numbers, account numbers, order numbers, dates, times, and account balances—it is clearly impossible to record all possible messages in advance. In these cases, messages are typically constructed by concatenating smaller words and phrases. For example, to report a checking account balance of $146.95, the following sequence might be concatenated from a series of recorded segments: "Your" "checking" "account balance is" "one" "hundred" "forty" "six" "dollars" "and" "ninety" "five" "cents." Often, variants of a word with different intonations are stored in order to approximate better natural prosody. However, without sufficient skill and understanding of speech, the quality of concatenated stored voice announcements can be disfluent, choppy, unnatural, and hard to understand or remember. Other disadvantages of stored speech include the lack of dynamic control, the need for time consuming rerecording, editing, and application redesign whenever updated or expanded information must be conveyed, and practical limitations on how many words and phrases can be stored.

Concatenative Synthesis. Concatenative synthesis uses an inventory of pieces of natural recorded speech as building blocks from which any arbitrary utterance may be constructed. The size of the inventory units is limited by various constraints. Whole word units are impractical because there are too many words to store and access readily, and lack of coarticulation and phonetic recoding at word boundaries would result in unnatural connected speech. The syllable is also

impractical for much the same reasons. Although there are only a relatively small number of phonemes in a language, the phoneme is unsatisfactory as an inventory unit because of the large coarticulatory effects between adjacent phonemes. There are two types of inventory units, smaller than syllables that have been used for concatenative synthesis, the diphone and the demi-syllable.

A diphone is the acoustic piece of speech from the middle of one phoneme to the middle of the next phoneme. (Note that the average length of a diphone is identical to that of a phoneme!) The middle of a phoneme tends to be its acoustically most stable region, and diphones thus represent acoustic transitions from one phoneme to the next. A minimum inventory of about 1000 diphones is required to synthesize unrestricted English text (Olive, 1977; Peterson, Wang, & Sivertsen, 1958). Because concatenative synthesis preserves the acoustic detail of natural speech, diphone synthesis is generally highly intelligible. A disadvantage of diphone synthesis is that coarticulation is only provided with the immediately preceding and following phonemes, whereas in some cases, such as in /r/ contexts, coarticulation can occur over several phonemes. Another problem is that the transitions between diphones may not be sufficiently smooth, and perceptually disruptive discontinuities can be introduced in the middle of a phoneme when diphones are concatenated. Recently, some diphone-based concatenative speech synthesizers have been extended to include multi-phone units of varying length to better represent highly coarticulated or commonly occurring sequences. Because of recent advances in automating many of the processes involved in creating a diphone inventory, there are numerous diphone concatenative synthesis systems available commercially for a variety of languages, including English.

The demi-syllable is an alternative unit for concatenative synthesis (Fujimura & Lovins, 1978). A demi-syllable is half a syllable; that is, either the syllable-initial portion up to the first half of the syllable nucleus, or the syllable-final portion starting from the second half of the syllable nucleus. The number of demi-syllables in English is roughly comparable to the number of diphones. Although demi-syllable units allow for more coarticulation than diphones, they can have problems with discontinuities at syllable nuclei and particularly with transitions between syllables. Although less common than diphone systems, demi-syllable concatenative synthesis systems are also commercially available.

Very recently, a new approach, called *automatic unit selection*, has been introduced by Sagisaka and Iwahashi (1995), Hunt and Black (1996), and Campbell and Black (1995). In automatic unit selection, an algorithm selects the longest snippet of speech in the inventory, thus avoiding many concatenation problems by drastically reducing the number of concatenation joints. In addition, if multiple versions of an acoustic unit exist in the inventory, the one which best matches specified quality, for example, prosodic targets, is chosen. Clearly, automatic unit selection has great promise for producing the most natural-sounding synthesis to date, but many hurdles, such as guaranteeing a minimum quality, have still to be overcome. However, this is a very promising new technique, which, at present, has a good chance for dominating the marketplace a few years from now.

Uses of Concatenative Synthesis.   Concatenative text-to-speech synthesis shares many applications in common with formant synthesis: Terminal-based applications include talking terminals and training devices, proofreading, warning and alarm systems, talking aids for the hearing-impaired and vocally handicapped, and reading aids for the blind (for moderate speaking rates). Telephone network-based services allow users to retrieve information from public or private databases using the telephone. The information may include names and addresses from a telephone directory, financial accounts, stock quotations, weather reports, reservations, sales orders and inventory information, or locations of commercial dealers. Text-to-speech systems are most appropriate for accessing a large and frequently changing database, since storage needs are greatly reduced from many thousands

of bits per second for stored speech to only a few dozens of bits for the equivalent text. Database maintenance is also simplified, since only the textual data needs updating. For case studies of various applications of speech synthesis, as well as of other speech technologies, see Syrdal, Bennett, and Greenspan (1994).

Comparison of Formant Concatenative Synthesis

Formant synthesis has the advantages of extreme flexibility, the ability to generate smooth transitions between segments, and relatively small storage requirements. A disadvantage is the difficulty of specifying detailed rules to synthesize acoustically robust, natural sounding segments, and particularly consonants. This constraint leads to another disadvantage, that of long development time for a formant synthesis system and the need for researchers who are very knowledgeable in speech acoustics and perception to develop the system. Concatenative synthesis is generally highly intelligible because much of the acoustic detail of recorded natural speech is preserved in the acoustic inventory elements. However, since the prosody of concatenative synthesis is generated by rule, the prosody imposed on the concatenated units is often just as limited in naturalness as that of formant synthesis. The storage required for an extensive inventory of acoustic units is a disadvantage for concatenative synthesis, but with the costs of computer storage decreasing rapidly, and with the development of rapid database access techniques, this disadvantage is not as serious as it once was. Because concatenative synthesis is not so intensively knowledge-based as formant synthesis, but rather more data driven, it has the advantage of more rapid development, in particular, when modern techniques of speech recognition discussed below are used to label and segment automatically the large corpora of speech required.

For both techniques, intense research is currently underway to discover how to control voice quality, such as female voices or children's voices, including how to generate different female and different child voices. Research is also aimed at understanding the ways in which speech conveys emotions, such as happiness or anger.

Special Applications of Speech Synthesis

Clinical Uses of Synthesized Speech. To a clinician, synthesized speech has several uses. One of the most obvious is for speech output of augmentative communication devices—devices used by persons who are either unintelligible or whose speech is difficult to understand in situations such as speaking over a telephone or in a classroom (e.g., the famous physicist Stephen Hawking). Few persons have disabilities that affect only their speech. Usually the cause of the speech disability, such as head trauma or neurological disease, also affects motor control of a person's arms, hands, and feet, and may affect cognitive processing of language, such as word sequencing or vocabulary retrieval or recognition of letters or words. Whether the user controls a device with scanning or symbol selection or text entry, the augmentative communication device then translates the input into a phonetic representation and string of prosodic markers, which together are translated by the synthesizer into speech. The synthesized speech generated by high-quality devices is very intelligible.

A report entitled "Voice Output Communication Aids" (Galyas, Fant, & Hunnicutt, 1992) chronicles part of the testimony of Rick Creech (the testimony originally appeared in *Conversations with Disabled Persons,* published by the Canadian Rehabilitation Council for the Disabled):

> Communication is the key that releases the soul of man. All of us are continuously sending messages. However, for some of us, messages become confused, distorted, and garbled before reaching their destination. Imagine forever being on the transmitting end of a bad connection. This is how it is for people with a communication problem. Sometimes they feel like completely breaking the connection—

some do by committing suicide—but most cling to whatever connection they have to the world, praying that someone will finally understand. Communication is not a luxury; it is a necessity. Speech is not a privilege; it is an inalienable right.

In addition to being an integral part of voice output aids, synthetic speech is important to clinicians because it is part of a variety of tests, treatment plans, and devices. Several of these uses are speech training, hearing screening, reading training, and talking toys.

Whatever the clinical application of synthetic speech for persons with speech disabilities, the issues of intelligibility, naturalness, individuality, and communication rate are critical.

Text-to-Speech Systems for the Blind. Computer users who are blind rely on so-called "screen readers" to translate the textual information on their screens into speech. With the transition to graphical user interfaces (GUIs), the problem of how to render the information on the screen acoustically is becoming very important. One issue we already discussed when we listed the advantages of formant synthesizers is the desire for higher-than-normal-speaking rates. The average user of screen readers prefers a rate of 300 to 500 words per minute; some users adjust their readers to speak at a rate as high as 600 words per minute. In addition, efficient and easy-to-use browsing capabilities, as well as several modes of auditory presentation, following a sensible hierarchical structure, are very important. Contrary to the case of a visual page/screen layout, it is nontrivial to render optimally—by acoustic means alone—different parts of a page or screen with multiple overlaying windows, designed mainly with a seeing person in mind (titles, paragraphs, figure captions, etc., in the case of printed information; title bars, button text, icon text, control information, textual content, etc., in the case of a graphic display on a computer screen). Once the different elements are identified, naturally, it is relatively easy to use different voices, different pitch ranges, or different speaking styles. However, the difficult problem is how to identify these elements. One solution to this problem is the use of specific tags, much like in the Hypertext-Markup Language (HTML) used in your favorite web browser. Therefore, it is not surprising that some commercial solutions (e.g., the "WebSpeak" project), and the use of "auditory style sheets" favored by the World Wide Web Consortium (W3C; http://www.w3.org), exist already for "acoustic web browsers" that work quite well as long as some care is taken by webmasters when designing their pages, for example, by providing alternate text tags for images. However, for general computer applications, much more work needs to be done to provide specific tags within application programs and operating systems to be spoken correctly by the screen reading software. For further information, see, for example, Raman (1997a, 1997b).

Articulatory Synthesis for Research in Speech Production.

Articulatory synthesis is accomplished by computing the desired speech sounds directly from the physical structure and movements of the vocal tract, in response to an input of text that represents the phoneme-sequence of the utterance to be produced. An all-out, "pure" phoneme-to-articulation-to-utterance machine would need to assemble the correct combination and timing of many speech muscle groups, corresponding to the different articulators (e.g., tongue, lips, and glottal muscles); this information would need to generate and control the acoustic output of a three-dimensional dynamic model of the vocal tract. This truly articulatory synthesizer could be developed, if no limits were placed on time and expense. And researchers indeed pursue various avenues toward this goal (for a nonexhaustive list, see Sondhi & Schroeter, 1997). The pure text-articulator would embody everything anyone would need to know about the biomechanics of speech production. It could act as a test-bed for (possibly) conflicting theories of speech production and contribute to our knowledge in this field. However, it is unlikely to ever lead to practical, low-complexity implementa-

tions that would be part of any typical text-to-speech system (see below).

Some of the research in articulatory synthesis explores how the shape of the vocal tract is controlled by the action of the many muscles acting to move and shape the tongue and lips, and to move the jaw. Here, we need to develop complicated dynamic (moving) models for these articulators. Good models demand complete and accurate measurements of vocal tract changes. These measurements are obtained by nuclear magnetic resonance (Baer, Gore, Gracco, & Nye, 1991), ultrasound pictures of the tongue shapes (Stone, 1990), combined with computational tongue modeling from muscle actions to tongue-shape changes (Wilhelms-Tricarico, 1995). Beyond vocal tract shapes, Honda (1996) describes the transformation of nerve signals to muscle action for some of the articulators. A group lead by Titze (see, e.g., Titze, 1994) investigates the mechanics and gestures of the vocal folds.

In order to have a practical synthesizer capable of running on a reasonably priced computer at tolerable speed, we have to make "engineering" approximations to our speech production models. One approximation that most researchers working in the area of articulatory synthesis make is to rely on two-dimensional data from x-ray pictures and even x-ray movies. Most of this type of data originated in the 1950s and 1960s and is documented in the works of Fant (1960) and others. Since it is nontrivial to "guess" the width data not shown in sagittal (side) views of the vocal cavity, techniques have been devised to fill in this information, for example, by demanding that certain acoustic properties measured from the simultaneously recorded speech should be matched (see, e.g., Maeda, 1990). So-called "articulatory models" (static models, e.g., Mermelstein, 1973; Coker, 1967; or dynamic models, such as the task-dynamic model of Saltzman & Munhall, 1989) then convert positional coordinates of the articulators to the two-dimensional area functions of the vocal tract that can be used to compute the vocal-tract acoustics.

Now, in principle, a "no compromises" articulatory synthesizer should produce good-quality speech, provided that the multiple layers of models (nerve-to-muscle, muscle-to-articulator-position, articulator-to-tract-shape, and tract-shape-to-source/cavity-acoustics) perform correctly. In fact, given good input data, many articulatory synthesizers fulfill the dream of reproducing some portions of speech very well; vowels and all-voiced sentences are the "easiest." To our knowledge, however, there is not one articulatory synthesizer in existence right now that, as far as the quality of the synthesized speech is concerned, comes close to the quality of other "competing" techniques. Why is this?

Obviously, given the facts stated above, the answer to why articulatory synthesis is losing ground relative to other techniques is multifaceted. First, there still might be missing knowledge of speech production to push the accuracy of our models to the necessary level. This notion, naturally, is driving further research in how speech is produced. Second, we have to solve the problem of how to obtain input/control data for our synthesizer. Third, given that any of the cascaded models in our synthesizer might be slightly less than perfect, and even assuming the ideal case of having available all the control data—such as measured nerve action potentials, muscle forces, articulator positions, and vocal-tract area functions—to resynthesize a full sentence, there is no guarantee that our synthesizer produces high-quality speech. These three caveats lead to the following observation: In practice, we always obtain the best quality synthetic speech when we are able to "close the loop" around one or more of the cascaded models, that is, when we start from a recorded "original" of an utterance, guess the "trial" input data at a given level of the cascaded models, synthesize, compare the synthetic speech to the desired original, modify the input data, and iterate (Parthasarathy & Coker, 1992; Schroeter & Sondhi, 1991). This approach, although practical, suffers from the additional hard problem of having to "invert" the speech production process,

that is to perform synthesis by analysis, in order to estimate the necessary control data. This inversion is not always possible due to fundamental ambiguities of the acoustic-to-articulatory mapping. For a detailed look at practical approaches to solving the inverse problem, see, for example, Schroeter and Sondhi (1994). For some introductory insights about quality of synthetic speech and how research in speech production/articulatory synthesis could contribute to improve it, see Schroeter (1997).

SPEECH RECOGNITION BY MACHINE

DIANE KEWLEY-PORT

Students in speech acoustics appreciate the difficulty of providing exact acoustic descriptions for phonemes, especially phonemes in words and sentences. Theories of speech perception invoke complex cognitive processes to derive meaning from acoustic input. How then can a computer be programmed to recognize speech? The effort to develop automatic speech recognition (ASR) algorithms is almost as old as the computer itself, although even today only partial progress has been made. The original motivation to develop ASR techniques was that communication with computers was highly constrained and unnatural and the idea that speech could be used as input was very appealing. As it became evident that the general goal of recognizing spontaneous speech input would be difficult to achieve, ASR technology pursued less ambitious goals. For example, the first commercial ASR success was to recognize just the ten digits, 0 to 9, over the phone (White & Neely, 1976). However, since speech is the natural mode for communication by humans, rather more ambitious goals are currently the targets for ASR development such as airline reservation systems and translators between languages (Cole, Hirschman, Atlas, Beckman, Bierman, et al., 1995).

Given the huge domain of communication problems that ASR could benefit, it is helpful to understand how scientists and engineers have approached the problem. It is generally understood that the first useful step is for recognizers to covert speech to symbols, either phonemes or words, without deriving the "meaning" of those symbols. Algorithms to map acoustics to symbols are generally referred to as speech recognition systems, while speech understanding systems extract meaning from the symbols, and the most advanced systems, spoken language systems, interact with humans completely with spoken language using speech synthesis (rather than printed text) for computer output. Thus, it is not surprising that advancements in recognition systems require broad expertise from many disciplines, including engineering, artificial intelligence, linguistics, and speech and hearing sciences. It is also not surprising that cooperation from such a diverse team is hard to achieve and, therefore, that solutions to ASR problems have often been biased towards one discipline with suboptimal contributions from other areas. This has resulted in ASR systems that are so different that integrating the benefits from one system into another has been difficult. Nonetheless, currently there are many successful applications of rather limited speech recognition systems for commercial and military use. More importantly, speech recognizers are now widely available on personal computers, and applications for education or to improve the lives of disabled citizens are numerous. The purpose of this chapter is describe the basic issues that apply to speech recognition technology. These include many problems in speech acoustics familiar to readers of this book. In addition, future approaches to spoken language systems will be described. Finally, a specific application of ASR to speech training for disordered speech will be discussed.

Speech Recognition Problems

Consider the standard ASR task of playing one recorded sentence as input and printing out the corresponding words. The first big problem is how the speech can be segmented into smaller units, whether words, syllables or phonemes. As anyone who has tried to read a spectrogram knows, this is a difficult problem. In the case of ASR, the choice of a specific unit is the fundamental decision for the entire system. (A more detailed discussion of this problem is provided in the section on Automatic Segmentation.) The unit selected for segmenting the sentence affects how knowledge is stored in a "dictionary" that is accessed by the recognizer. That is, recognizers must store both reference models of these units and rules for combining the models into a printed sentence. If the models are words, then the output rules are simple and basically string the words together. If the models are phonemes, then complex rules that reflect English phonology, such as vowel reduction ("buy you" pronounced as "buy ya"), must be included in order to access words in an English dictionary and then produce the printed sentence.

The second big problem is how to handle variability in the speech signal. All the classic problems in speech acoustics occur here: acoustic differences due to coarticulation, talkers, speaking rate, dialect, sentence prosody, and so on. While these problems are very challenging in their own right, in ASR another set of challenges related to the acoustic environment in the real world exist as well (Acero, 1993; Cole et al., 1995). These are referred to as the problem of robust speech recognition and include degrading of the speech signal due to background noise or talkers (the cocktail-party effect), reverberation, characteristics of the microphone, and quality of the recordings (for example, speech recorded over phone lines). Many people consider these as strictly engineering problems. However, we must keep in mind that humans are amazingly good at ignoring nearby noises and conversations and they talk over telephones quite successfully. That is, understanding of how humans perceive speech, including selective attention and the frequency properties of the auditory system, bear directly on the these "engineering" problems. Thus, the solutions to both speech variability and robust speech recognition problems will come from understanding human sensory and cognitive processes as well as improving acoustic analysis and engineering techniques.

Speech Recognition Systems

The basic components of most speech recognition systems are shown in Figure 17-2. The first component is a device called an analog-to-digital converter (A-to-D). This involves a complicated process that measures voltages in the signal, and then filters, samples, and converts the voltages into digital numbers (see Rosen & Howell, 1991). Presently, the standard representation for digital signals is the one used on compact digital disks and it is also widely available for personal computers in the Sound Blaster PC cards.

For speech signals, less information must be stored about sound than is required for high fidelity music since the important frequency range for speech is smaller (8000 Hz compared to 20000 Hz). Because digital waveforms take up large (expensive) amounts of computer storage as high fidelity signals, engineers have developed efficient and specialized methods of speech coding (see the Speech Coding section in Atal, Miller, & Kent, 1991). Thus, the second component in a speech recognizer is an acoustic processor that codes the digital waveform. All processing techniques take advantage of the redundancy in the acoustic waveform since information about phonemes overlaps in time due to coarticulation. After processing, temporal information is reduced to 10 to 50 coded samples for each second of speech (Makhoul, Roucos & Gish, 1985). Some processors even attempt to model the physiological properties of the auditory nerve cells, and these are termed "auditory front ends" (Ghitza, 1994). Whatever the acoustic processing that is applied, the output is a small set of coded samples for each second of speech that are ordered in time. Information about time, energy and frequency in the coded samples is greatly reduced from the original digital signals.

Depending on the overall approach of the recognition system, the next component is that of feature extraction. This process generates a set of

Speech Recognition

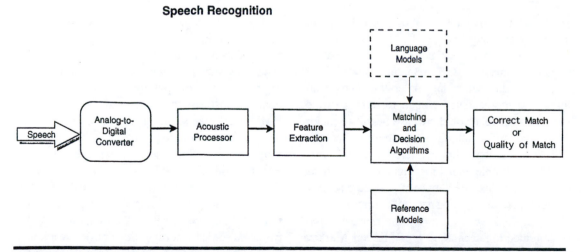

FIGURE 17-2.   Diagram of computer functions for a generic model for automatic speech recognition. The speech input, the acoustic signal from a microphone, is first digitized by analog-to-digital conversion. This digital acoustic data is analyzed, for example, into a series of spectral patterns. Then the features to be used for syllable, word, or phrase recognition are extracted. Finally, the feature information is recognized by deciding which of the stored reference patterns most closely match the features derived from that input.

features that represent the units of speech stored as the reference models. Two extreme examples illustrate the relation between the acoustic processor and the final matching algorithms. One approach (closely related to speech science) uses the phoneme for the recognition unit. The coded words from the acoustic processor are analyzed to extract phoneme-like features based on principles of acoustic phonetics. These acoustic features are combined to represent the phonemes stored as the reference models for the final matching process (Cole, Phillips, Brennan, & Chigier, 1986; Deng & Sun, 1994). In contrast, many engineering approaches frequently have no separate feature extraction module. Algorithms in the acoustic processor are refined such that the coded samples are presented directly to the final matching component, which selects the recognition units. Frequency coding has always taken advantage of the fact that frequency resolution in the ear that is better at low frequencies than at high frequencies. For example, these processes often incorporate specific algorithms to account for both frequency and masking properties of the auditory system (Schroeder & Atal, 1985; Schroeder, Atal, & Hall, 1979).

The last component in a speech recognition system is the one that actually "recognizes" the speech input. Logically there are two parts, matching the feature set to the reference models, and then rules that select and order the recognized units into the sentence output. Referring to the examples above, again there have been two major procedures for matching. Those that use acoustically based features in the reference models usually have simple matching algorithms such as calculating a distance between the feature set and the reference models that account for normal variability word length. Currently, the most successful engineering technique uses Hidden Markov Models (HMMs) (Rabiner, 1989; Rabiner & Juang, 1993). HMMs represent the units of speech as small networks (a set of connected states). These networks become the reference models after they are trained with a large set of carefully constructed sentences. During training, the probabili-

ties for every sequence of units that can occur are statistically calculated. During recognition, coded words are compared against these probabilities to determine which was the most likely sequence of units.

In both of the above cases, matching produces an ordered sequence of the speech units. The decision algorithms that examine the sequences and produce the final written sentence may be more or less elaborate. In the simple case of word units, the word sequence is the output sentence. In the case of phoneme units, the phoneme sequence may be analyzed by phonological rules to map the observed phonemes into corresponding English words. This latter process incorporates some linguistic knowledge about the constraints of the English language. In some recognition systems, additional linguistic knowledge is incorporated in the decision process, say a simple grammar of the order of words. In such cases, the recognizer may be thought of having a language model as an additional component to the system. While many simple recognizers with small vocabularies have no language component, a language component is obviously essential for speech understanding systems.

The previous paragraphs have described the flow of information shown in Figure 17-2 from the speech input to the recognized sentence as series of processes. However, the important step of how the reference patterns are stored in the recognizer must also be addressed. In the case of HMM recognizers, the units and the models are defined in the training process in terms of the probabilities within and between the networks. For most other recognizers, the units are predefined, and the training of the associated reference patterns is independent of the recognition process. For example, acoustically based features may be extracted for several repetitions of one word, and then a simple average of that information provides the reference model (Kewley-Port, Watson, Elbert, Maki, & Reed, 1987).

This overview of speech recognition has referred to some of the many different ways to design an ASR system. The complexity of the ultimate goal to recognize spontaneous, conversational speech has forced ASR designers to subdivide the problems into manageable pieces. Below we consider the particular subdivisions of speech recognition problems used in research and development. Unfortunately, descriptions of commercial systems often obscure the particular speech recognition problem a device is designed to solve.

Continuous, connected, and isolated (or discrete) are terms that refer to how the problem of word segmentation has been resolved. Isolated word recognition requires that a half-second (500 ms) or greater pause be inserted between spoken words. Connected word recognition only requires that a very short pause be inserted between rather carefully spoken words. The popular series of Dragon systems are examples of connected-word recognizers (Baker, 1989). Continuous speech recognizers require no pauses between words and accept fluent speech pronunciation. Restrictions on the size and nature of the vocabulary of words differentiate speech recognition devices. Vocabulary size is usually divided into small, large, and very large, with corresponding size limitations of roughly 200, 1000, and greater than 20,000 words. For example, two quite different sizes of vocabularies are required for recognition of digits or alarm messages, and, on the other hand, the operation of voice typewriters. While the size of the vocabulary poses obvious restrictions on speech recognition, the nature of the vocabulary should also be considered. One primary consideration of vocabulary size is the extent to which users may specify their own vocabularies. Fixed vocabularies are usually found for devices that are tailored to specific tasks, and that need to be extremely reliable across talkers. Very large fixed vocabulary systems (greater than 30,000 words) are now commercially marketed for dictation purposes with human editing correcting the 4 to 10% errors produced by the recognizer.

Another major subdivision of recognizers specifies whether they recognize speech from many talkers (speaker independent), or only from one speaker at a time (speaker dependent). Clearly, users of speech recognizers would prefer speaker independent systems, but these algorithms are far more difficult to construct at acceptable levels of accuracy (Rabiner & Wilpon, 1987). Recognizers that claim speaker independence are usually not, in fact, totally independent of such things as a talker's dialect and individual voice characteristics. Typically these speaker independent systems require a short training period called enrollment to adjust to each talker.

As an example of speech recognizers that students may encounter, many personal computers come equipped with a feature called a "voice navigator" that is intended to recognize basic computer commands such as "change directory." The speech recognizer that identifies these commands is usually a small, fixed-vocabulary, speaker-independent, isolated-word recognizer. There are already plans to equip computers with more powerful recognizers in the future. However, it is important to match the specific features of a recognizer carefully to the application of the user. As discussed in the section on speech training below, a less powerful recognizer may match the specific needs better than a more powerful one with different, but less appropriate features.

Spoken Language Systems

The main focus of this chapter is speech recognition systems. Although many problems need to be resolved before such systems can transcribe spontaneous speech into written English, current research has the much more ambitious goal of spoken language systems. Two recent articles provide overviews of the key problems that need to be solved to achieve this goal (Cole et al., 1995; Gorin, 1995). The scope of these systems is to combine speech recognition with the capability to assign meaning to sentences (generally called natural language processing) and also to provide spoken output. Systems that produce the spoken output include many components as well: databases that store knowledge about the world, algorithms to interpret the input in order to retrieve a response from the databases, generation of meaningful sentence output; and finally, intelligible speech synthesis.

There are several reasons for aspiring to spoken language systems as the next generation of ASR technology. First, the potential applications and benefits to society are very high. These applications go beyond benefits to improve human-computer interaction. As examples, they can enable people with a variety of disabilities to significantly improve their lives, or they can bridge language barriers with multilingual translation systems. Second, the scientific infrastructure needed to develop spoken language systems are both enormous and multidisciplinary. Given the diversity of the training required for the scientists and the cost of the physical resources, it makes sense to establish an infrastructure that addresses as many aspects of spoken language systems as possible. The collaboration needed both across disciplines and between academics, governments, and industry has fostered new consortiums. For example, speech databases are being shared through the Linguistic Data Consortium located at the University of Pennsylvania. Overall, research on spoken language systems will result in advancements in speech recognition including robust performance, input of spontaneous speech, and general solutions to the speaker variability problem.

Speech Training Application

The use of computers as interactive, multimedia systems for training speech and language is an obvious application for speech recognition. There are many potential areas, such as acquisition of reading skills, speech production and speech perception training for impaired populations, foreign accent reduction, and second language acquisition. Collectively these applications will be called computer-based speech trainers (CBST). A group of researchers in Bloomington, Indiana has been working on various aspects of CBST systems since 1985. This section reflects the collaborative thinking of that group (Anderson & Kewley-Port, 1995; Watson, Reed, Kewley-Port, & Maki, 1989).

The core of CBST systems is the feedback that will be given the student during speech training. Although CBST systems might derive feedback from a number of different signals, such as articulatory movement, the only systems to be discussed here use acoustic signals processed from a speech recognizer. We caution that some commercial systems sold as speech trainers in fact do not provide any feedback but only play speech as examples and never actually record speech from the student. More information about feedback can be found in Watson and Kewley-Port (1989), who provided a theoretically motivated description of the nature of feedback in speech training.

Speech recognizers can provide several kinds of feedback in speech drill as shown in Figure 17-3. The first is a response that identifies whether a particular word spoken was correct or incorrect. This might be used in learning to read words. To improve intelligibility, a different kind of feedback should be used clinically: Feedback that evaluates the quality of the utterance (for example, "That's terrific," or "You can do better.") As discussed in Watson and colleagues (1989) and Anderson and Kewley-Port (1995), evaluative feedback derived from a speech recognizer can substitute for human ratings of speech quality. That is, humans can reliably rate speech quality on a scale of 1 (normal production) to 7 (unintelligible) for many types of disordered speech. Thus, the research question is whether a metric calculated from the output of speech recognizers can substitute for these human ratings in speech training. Results of several studies demonstrated that metrics from acoustically based recognizers generally correlated well with human ratings, while metrics from HMM recognizers did not. On the other hand, Anderson and Kewley-Port (1995) found that a HMM recognizer was the best at identifying correct from incorrect speech spoken by children with speech disorders. The conclusion of this line of research is that while several different types of information might serve as feedback in speech training, it is essential to demonstrate that particular feedback is a valid substitute for human judgments.

What kind of ASR technology is likely to be most useful for speech training applications? Powerful spoken language systems (not yet commercially available) would be useful in second language trainers. These very large vocabulary, speaker-independent, continuous speech systems could recognize words and sentences from many different talkers and determine whether the utterance was meaningful or not. Contrast this to a limited, but widely available, low-cost system, one that is a small vocabulary, speaker-dependent, isolated-word recognizer. It has been argued by Kewley-Port and Watson (1995) that in fact such recognizers have important properties for training disordered speech. Training in speech therapy concentrates largely on a limited vocabulary tailored for each student (i.e., small-vocabulary recognition). Moreover, if the student is quite unintelligible (for example, a deaf speaker), it is important to train reference models for just that individual (e.g., speaker-dependent recognition), since the student's speech is very different from normal standards that are found in speaker-independent recognizers. And finally, standard clinical practice in speech-language pathology initiates training on isolated syllables and words, so isolated-word recognition is useful at the beginning of training.

Since limited speech recognition capabilities are appropriate for speech trainers, it is not surprising that several have been commercially developed. Of course, feedback in commercial systems can be presented in video game format to motivate students to practice their speech drills. To illustrate the potential uses of speech recognizers, feedback displays from a few speech trainers will be described (see Figure 17-3). *SpeechViewer* from IBM (Pratt, Heintzelman, & Deming, 1993) implements both identification and evaluative feedback in speech drills. One drill identifies which of several vowels was spoken in order to allow a penguin to climb an iceberg. Another drill prompts the user to produce a single vowel and, using an evaluative metric from the recognizer, a penguin climbs higher up a mountain upon better pronunciation. *ISTRA* from Communication Dis-

orders Technology (Kewley-Port & Watson, 1995) implements evaluative feedback in a set of drills incorporated into a full training curriculum. For example, the rating of speech quality is represented in a bull's-eye target game and a baseball game where higher scores result in singles, doubles, and home runs (Figure 17-3).

While the obvious benefits of CBST systems to motivate students and to free teachers to attend to other, more challenging tasks stimulates the market for these trainers, consumers should demand some evaluation of their performance. It has already been mentioned that validation of

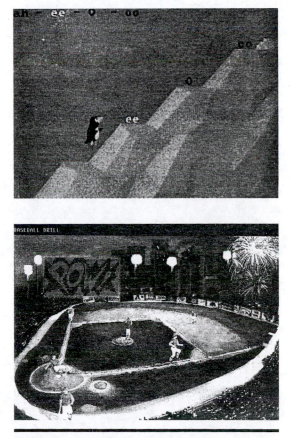

FIGURE 17-3. Computer screen displays for two speech trainers. Top: Penguin climbs the vowel mountain on IBM's Screen Viewer II. Bottom: Baseball game, home run display on the Indiana Speech Trainer ISTRA.

the feedback, usually in a direct comparison with human listeners, is the first step. Such evaluations are expensive, and one of the few published is for ISTRA (Watson et al., 1989). Equally important is verification that the disordered speech of an individual improves with training (Gierut, Morrisette, Hughes, & Rowland, 1995). Such clinical effectiveness studies are also costly, and again, not many have been published (for ISTRA, Kewley-Port & Watson 1995; for SpeechViewer, Pratt et al., 1993). As speech recognition becomes more widely available in second language trainers, the concern of performance evaluation should be kept in mind by all potential purchasers and users.

Conclusions

Speech recognition systems with powerful capabilities are available commercially in dictation systems, and in laboratories as prototype speech understanding systems. The ultimate goal of communication with computers entirely through speech will be achieved in the future and prototypes exist for very limited tasks, such as the airline reservation vocabulary (ATIS, Price, 1990; Cole et al., 1995). In general, the complexities of speech recognition have forced researchers to subdivide the problem into areas that have limited, but potentially useful applications. In fact, several successful speech trainers for disordered speech have been designed for very limited, low-cost recognizers. Knowledge to improve the recognition technology of today will be contributed from a variety of disciplines. While obviously the first stages of the recognition process rely on knowledge of sound and speech acoustics, the structure of language and cognitive processes used to derive meaning also interact with lower levels of processing. As multidisciplinary teams integrate all this knowledge into spoken language systems, more natural communication between humans and computers will provide many educational and social benefits in the twenty-first century.

APPENDIX A

EXPERIMENTING WITH SPEECH

TO LEARN ACOUSTIC PHONETICS: EXPERIMENT!!

This book by itself will not teach you acoustic phonetics because it lacks sounds that you hear. It describes speech sounds, using text and diagrams, with explanations you can use if your career involves the language sciences. To really know what you may be writing and talking about you must experiment with speech sounds: by listening, by feeling your articulation, and by activities with a sound laboratory.

Listening Around

Listen for speech sound details when you don't need to listen for meaning, for example, during redundant conversations, TV and radio commercials, and speeches that are boring, predictable, or perfunctory. It is really surprising how differently people talk, even those of the same sex and dialect. A lot of phonetics can be done by ear; for example, when Winston Churchill heard an àctor's imitation of him, he noticed, "Why, he even has my teeth!"

Articulating Silently to Feel Speech

J. C. Catford, in the British linguistic tradition for teaching phonetics, found that you can easily feel the shapes and movements of your own articulations, especially if you speak silently. Try it: First speak a word or phrase, then repeat it with closed glottis, making no sound at all; you'll find that, silently, you can very clearly feel the shapes of your tongue and its movements to contacts, but not so clearly when speaking. Thus, Catford published a remarkable set of 124 exercises with

which you can experiment systematically using your own articulation and ear. In the book above I adapt some of his maneuvers for self-illustration of the major phonetic differences in English that we will study. Apprentice linguistic and phonetic practitioners should have all of Catford's "experiments" on hand, together with his remarks on their uses for learning the many other sounds encountered in a variety of world languages (Catford, 1988).

From Experiment to Expertise

A complete CD-ROM course in acoustic phonetics can be purchased from Sensimetrics Corporation; the title is "Speech Production and Perception I"; inquire for an illustrated brochure from products@sens.com (Berkovitz & Pickett, 1992). The course is systematically arranged in units with more than 40 interactive experiments that use speech analysis and synthesis to reinforce the principles taught in each unit. The course is designed to teach efficiently independently of a student's verbal or reading facility. Our book may be used as a more academic back-up to primary instruction via the computer course.

Acoustic Analysis of Speech in the Laboratory

It is now easy to do acoustic experiments on speech using any one of several computer programs. We present below a set of Laboratory Exercises, keyed to our chapters on acoustic differences, that we have used in teaching. We believe the experiments can be performed with any of the speech programs on the market. Some computer programs available are also listed below.

Speech Synthesis for Learning

The Sensimetrics CD-ROM course incorporates some speech synthesis exercises. Our readers should use that synthesizer or a similar one to learn by listening to the sound patterns used as examples here in our book. You can also use a synthesizer to study the acoustic cues in perception by synthesizing speech sounds based on an analysis of natural speech and then changing some elements in the synthetic version and making a re-comparison.

LABORATORY EXERCISES

To thoroughly learn acoustic phonetics students should analyze the sounds of speech themselves; they should measure the spectral and temporal features corresponding to the important phonetic features. The laboratory exercises that follow are designed for this purpose. They can be used in conjunction with the text; each exercise is related to a text chapter.

The exercises are not completely self-explanatory. Successful use requires supervised interpretation by an instructor who has experience in speech analysis and who has tried each exercise and modified it if necessary.

The major equipment needed is a desktop computer system with simple basic facilities for speech analysis. There are several good software and sound-board packages available for PCs. We made our 3D Perspectrograms with the Sensimetrics SpeechStation, a modestly priced package with a very wide range of functions that are easy to use. It runs in Windows 95 with any standard sound card. SpeechStation will also derive, display, and print standard spectrograms like those in our figures, incorporating graphic read-outs of frequency values and time points. Sensimetrics Corporation (48 Grove St., Somerville, MA 02144-2500; e-mail: products@sens.com) also

developed the computer-based instruction course titled Speech Acoustics and Perception I.

The Computer Speech Research Environment, developed at the Department of Communicative Disorders, University of Western Ontario, is available from Avazz Innovations, London, Ontario; for Macintosh computers the Signalyze system, developed at the Swiss Technical University is offered by InfoSignal, Inc., C.P. 73, CH1015, Lausanne (Americas Representative: Network Technology Corp., 91 Baldwin St., Charlestown, MA 02129); both of these systems offer cone kernel analysis in addition to the more standard Fourier analyses and standard spectrograms. Tiger Electronics (Fax: 206-367-2672) offers a suite of programs for clinical and research use called Dr. Speech. The SPEECHLAB, a multimedia CD-ROM, is available from Media Enterprise-Ingolf Franke, Gottbillstrasse 34A, 564294 Trier, Germany.

University laboratories also offer packages, such as the SPECTO system of the BoysTown National Research Hospital, Omaha, Nebraska 68131; Bunnell's Edwav developed at the Center for Auditory and Speech Sciences, Gallaudet University, Washington, DC, and the A. I. Dupont Research Institute is available free from Tim Bunnell on the University of Delaware computer (302-831-6150), at castle.asel.udel.edu; also check out the DSPS Realtime Signal Lab from DSPS Inc., P.O. Box 5348, Station F, Ottawa, Canada K2C 3J1; and Unix-based instruction sequences were under development in 1992 at the Linguistics Department, University of Edinburgh, Scotland (turk@ling.ed.ac.uk).

For Macintosh computers, linguistics and phonetics laboratory-type demonstrations are available at extremely modest cost from the Phonetics Laboratory, Linguistics Department, University of California, Los Angeles.

Workstations for acoustic analysis are available as advertised in the Acoustical Society of America's Meeting Programs by Kay Elemetrics Corp. and GW Instruments. The capabilities of various packages have been reviewed in a series of articles in the *Journal of Speech and Hearing*

Research; for example, see Read, Buder, and Kent (1992).

Good tutorials are available on how speech waves are represented digitally in computers, and the necessary wave analog-to-digital settings and compromises. The student may be interested and the instructor *must* be familiar with speech-digital principles found in texts such as Denes and Pinson (1995), Ladefoged (1996), Kent and Read (1992).

Lab 1. Introduction to the Sound Spectrograph (Text Chapter Two)

The purposes of this lab are to learn how to make spectrograms and to get a general idea of what a speech spectrogram presents. As a background, before lab, the student should briefly review Chapter Two to be familiar with how speech waves are represented by spectrum values and plotted in a spectrogram.

Making a Spectrogram. The instructor will demonstrate how to set and change the parameters of the acoustic analysis program, to first record speech and then reproduce the analysis in a spectrogram. Use the 4 kHz frequency range (sample rate of 8 kHz) and broadband analysis (analysis window 10 ms or less). Record the utterance *The spectrum of speech in time*, spoken very distinctly by a male talker.

Each student should then go through the same procedures as demonstrated. If the spectrogram is not fairly clear, the analysis parameters should be readjusted and another spectrogram made.

Try to locate the center point in time of each vowel in the speech spectrogram. Then calculate the syllable rate. There is always one vowel per syllable, so the time between syllables is indicated by the time between vowel centers.

What, approximately, is the average time in ms between vowel centers? Based on this, what is the average syllable rate?

Syllable rate = 1 / Average time in ms between vowel centers

Notice the gross changes between higher and lower frequency sounds. For example, the [s] and [ʃ] sounds do not have strong energy in the same frequency ranges as the vowels. What are these frequency ranges, approximately, as indicated in your spectrogram?

Lab 2. Length Rule for Tube Resonances (Text Chapter Three)

The purpose of this experiment is to demonstrate by measurement the dependence of the frequency of the main resonance of a tube on its length. The main tube resonance is due to repeated reflections of the sound disturbances between the ends of the tube. In speech it is the reflections of the vocal pulses between the ends of the pharyngeal-oral tube that produces the main voice resonance (the first formant).

If we use a tube that is very long, the reflections are far enough apart in time to be seen on a spectrogram as separate pulses. Thus, in this experiment we first use long tubes so we can measure the time between reflections and calculate from this the main resonant frequency. We then turn to short, vocal-tract size tubes and measure their resonant frequencies on the spectrograph frequency scale.

The main resonance of a tube in response to an air pulse is caused by the reflection of the pulse at the ends of the tube and the consequent reversal of the travel of the pulse wave. The frequency of the resonance is determined by two factors: (1) the length of the tube and (2) the types of reflection at the ends. The longer the tube, the longer the time for the pulse to travel between the ends, and thus the lower the frequency of appearance of pulses at the open end. The vocal tract is a tube that is closed at the glottis end and open at the lip end. The reflection from the open end is the inverse in orientation of the original pulse arriving from the closed end; this "inverse pulse" then travels back down the tube, is reflected at the closed end, travels back out, is reinverted at the open end, makes another round trip of the tube, and reappears at the open end with the same orientation as the original pulse. Thus, two round trips are required for a complete cycle of repetition of the appearance of the original pulse orientation. Therefore, the main resonant frequency of a tube that is closed at one end and open at the other is dependent on the necessity of four traverses of the tube per cycle, and the frequency is equal to 1 second divided by four times the traverse time.

Measure the time between reflections of a sound pulse in long tubes. Pulse the large tubes at one end by hitting the open end with the palm of the hand. After the hand hits, keep it against the end to close off that end while leaving the other end open near the microphone of the spectrograph. A good resonance of the pulsed tube is fairly loud and long, lasting about 1 second; it sounds like a brief low organ tone or a "boing. " If only a short, dead thud is heard, the hit was not solid enough. Record and make a spectrogram of two solid hits.

What is the time between reflections of a sound pulse in the following tubes, closed at one end?

1. A 20-foot tube
2. A 10-foot tube

(Two 10-foot sections of 2 inches in diameter Amoco Underground Electrical Duct Type 11 can be used with a matching sleeve for connecting the two 10-foot sections to make the 20-foot tube.)

Sound propagates at 344.4 meters per second or 1130 feet per second, taking approximately 0.9 ms to travel 1 foot. Are the pulse reflections on the spectrograms the correct distance apart in time, according to the two different lengths of tube and the time required to travel 1 foot? Remember that, after the pulse first reaches the open end, where the microphone is located, it must travel down the tube and back again before another pulse arrives at the open end.

Also, there are two intervals between pulses for each four traverses of the tube length. What are the resonant frequencies corresponding to four traverses of each tube?

Measure the main resonant frequencies of model vocal tract tubes. Two short plastic tubes are provided, which are model vocal tract tubes:

1. An 18 cm tube; model of adult male vocal tract
2. A 9 cm tube; model of an infant length vocal tract

Using the model vocal tract tubes, record and measure the sound resulting from pulsing the tubes. Pulse the tube by making a "Bronx cheer" between pursed lips held tightly pressed to one end of the tube, as you would in playing a trumpet, trombone, or bass horn. Record the sound from the open end of the tube and make spectrograms.

Assume that the 18 cm tube is 7 inches long. What would be the time between appearances of reflections at the open end? (This cannot be measured on the spectrogram because the pulses are too close together on the spectrogram.)

Every other reflection is inverted. What is the time period between the inverted reflections and what is the corresponding frequency? How is this frequency represented in the spectrogram?

Notes to Instructor. The tricky thing in this exercise is that the inverted polarity pulses and the noninverted pulses appear in the spectrogram in the same upward-pointing orientation. On close examination it will be seen that the "original orientation," noninverted pulses are marked differently from the inverted. The first pulse recorded is the "original" (only its reflection is inverted, not the pulse radiated from the open end to the microphone). The interval between any two pulses is the time for one round trip down the tube toward the closed end and back out to the microphone.

The 18 cm and 9 cm tubes should be rigid, about 1 inch inside diameter, and smooth walled. The author has found Lucite tubes of about 1/8-inch thickness to be satisfactory.

Lab 3. Tube Constriction/Formant Rules (Text Chapter Three)

This exercise can be done in two different ways: (1) with the computer-based course: Speech Acoustics and Speech Perception I, available from Sensimetrics Corporation or (2) using lengths of rubber tubing that can be constricted by pinching as described below. The computer course is more accurate and easier to use for measurement. The "real" tubes make a more personal demonstration.

The purpose is to see how different constrictions affect the location of formant frequencies. A flexible tube, 18 cm long and about 1 inch in diameter, is provided. The tube is excited with air pulses by blowing through pursed lips applied to one end, which is held tightly against the lips, as in the previous experiment. Record the sound output on the spectrograph from pulsing the tube under four different conditions of constriction:

1. Varying, for a single spectrogram, the amount of an "alveolar" constriction by squeezing the tube between thumb and forefinger at a point 13 cm from the pulsed (closed) end of the tube. Measure the frequencies of F1, F2, and F3 for several amounts of constriction.
2. Varying amounts of back constriction at 6 cm from the closed end. Repeat the formant measurements.
3. Rounding plus back constriction; repeat (2) with "front" constriction at the open end of the tube. Repeat the formant measurements.
4. Constriction of the "pharynx" area of the tube (constrict the tube over the portion near the closed end over a distance of about 3 cm toward the open end). Measure the frequencies of F1, F2, and F3.

Notes to Instructor.   The tubing used for this exercise should be semi-rigid but not too difficult to squeeze to a narrow constriction. If the tubing is too thin and flexible the tube formants can be damped by the loss of sound energy through the tube walls, and zeros in the tube response can cause the formant frequencies to appear to be shifted. Heavy rubber tubing from a chemistry lab works well if it is about 1/8-inch in wall thickness. The tubes should be marked off in cm from the "closed end."

Lab 4. Voice Pitch (Fundamental Frequency), Harmonics, and Formants (Text Chapter Four)

The purpose is to learn how to measure pitch and to see how it is independent of formants. This can be adapted using the computer course but it is easier to measure harmonics with the "live" talker and spectrograms as here.

Select and record a vowel using a male talker who pronounces it with slow changes in pitch, up and down. The vowel [æ] is especially good for this. Make both broadband and narrowband spectrograms.

Independence of Voice Pitch and Formants. The broadband spectrograms show the frequency positions of the formants, which should be relatively steady frequencies if the vowel shape was held constant by the talker while he changed his pitch. Measure the approximate formant frequencies.

The narrowband spectrogram shows each individual harmonic of the vowel sound. The harmonics are multiples of the fundamental frequency and therefore will be seen to move up or down in frequency as the voice pitch changes up or down. The harmonics are strong or weak depending on their frequency relations to the steady formant frequencies of the vowel. When a harmonic is near a formant frequency, it is strong (darker on the spectrogram), and when it is not near a formant, it is weak or not visible on the spectrogram. Note on the spectrograms that the pitch of the voice, that is, the fundamental frequency, is independent of the formants. As the voice pitch changes, gliding up or down, the formants remain at the same frequencies.

Measurement of Pitch.   The voice pitch (fundamental frequency) can be measured in two different ways: (1) by counting the number of voicing pulses in a given time period on the broadband spectrogram and (2) by measuring the frequency spacing of harmonic intervals on a narrowband spectrogram.

Pitch by Number of Voice Pulses per Unit of Time.   During vowels the broadband spectrogram shows vertical striations that correspond to the individual pulses of airflow from the glottis as they excite the resonances of the vocal tract. The voice pitch or fundamental frequency is equal to the pulse rate of the airflow pulses. You can measure the pitch by finding the number of striations (pulses) per unit of time. A convenient subunit to use is 200 ms; 200 ms is 1/5 second; you can measure the pitch by counting the number of striations in 200 ms and multiplying this number by 5. Measure the pitch at points of high and low pitch in the broadband spectrogram.

You can also measure the pitch by using the principle that the harmonics are multiples of the fundamental frequency and thus are spaced at frequency intervals equal to the fundamental frequency. At any time point on the narrowband spectrogram, the pitch can be determined by measuring the frequency range spanned by a given number of intervals between harmonics and dividing by the number of intervals. This is a more accurate method. Make the measurements at a point midway in the 200 ms time intervals used previously. Some harmonics may be too weak to see but must be counted anyway. Taking the span of 10 successive harmonic intervals is a convenient way to measure the fundamental frequency; the fundamental frequency is then the frequency range spanned by 11 harmonics (10 harmonic intervals) divided by 10.

Note to Instructor.   No more problems after this one.

Lab 5. Spectra of Front Vowels (Text Chapter Four)

The purpose is to study the formant patterns of the front vowels.

1. Record and analyze the isolated vowels [i, ɪ, ɛ], [æ], or [a]. Record and analyze [i] with a slow pitch change of about one octave.
2. Measure the formant frequencies and amplitudes of F1 and F2. Note that the F1 and F2 frequencies follow a certain progression from the more constricted [i] to the least constricted [æ].
3. Make a narrowband spectrogram of the [i] that was recorded with the pitch change. Note that the pitch changes over a large range but the formant frequencies do not change.

Lab 6. Spectra of Back Vowels and Diphthongs (Text Chapter Four)

The purpose of this lab is to study the formant patterns of the back vowels and diphthongs.

1. Make broadband spectrograms of the back vowels [ɑ, ɔ, o, ʊ, u] and the diphthongs [ɪu, ou, aɪ, au].
2. Measure the F1 and F2 frequencies and note how they change with different locations and degrees of tongue constriction.
3. The large contribution of lip-rounding to formant lowering can be studied by recording a spectrogram beginning with [o] and smiling while holding the same tongue position.

Lab 7. Prosodic Features (Text Chapter Five)

The prosodic features of a sentence are embodied in variations in pitch, duration, and spectral balance. The purpose of this lab is to demonstrate all three of these variations. Part 3 should be done with perspectrograms made in SpeechStation as we did in our text for Figure 5-6.

1. Of first concern are the pitch contours that typically differentiate the grammatical function of a statement versus that of a question. Record on the spectrograph the statement "That's a buy" and the question "Is that a buy?" Make a narrowband spectrogram.

We also use the prosodic features to make emphatic statements with the same inverted order of subject and verb employed for questions. For example, we can say "Is that a buy!", a statement expressing enthusiastic emphasis. The emphasis can be put on any word we wish to especially impress on the listener.

Record and study these effects, putting the emphasis on "that" in one statement and on "buy" in another. Make both narrow- and broadband spectrograms of the two statements:

"Is *that* a buy!"
"Is that a *buy!*"

Trace the pitch contours of all the sentences along either the fifth or tenth harmonic of the voiced sounds.

Measure the pitch at the beginning, middle, and end of each vowel. The pitch at any point is easily obtained by measuring the frequency level of a harmonic and then dividing this frequency by the harmonic number. For example, if the fifth harmonic is at 550 Hz, then the pitch is 550/5 = 110 Hz. Make sure you have identified the harmonic number correctly; this can be difficult when the pitch is low and the harmonics are closely packed together in the spectrogram. How can you make the pitch easier to measure?

How do the statements and question differ in overall trend of pitch from beginning to end?

How does the pitch vary with emphasis, between words and within words?

2. Measure the duration of each syllable. How does duration vary with emphasis?

3. See whether there is a change in spectrum balance by comparing intensities of F2, F3, F4, relative to that of F1, depending on emphasis.

Lab 8. Formant Transitions-Diphthongs versus Glide Consonants versus Stop Consonants (Text Chapter Six)

The purpose is to measure the formant transitions, including the rate and amount of transition, for glide consonants versus diphthongs versus stop consonants.

Make broadband spectrograms of the following phrases:

"That's a wow."
"That's a bow [bau]."
"Paint a yacht."
"Paint a dot."

Measure the F1 transitions, comparing durations of transition between diphthongs, glides, and stop consonants; observe transitions in F2.

The rate of change in articulation governs the duration of F1 transition. Change in articulation occurs fastest for stops, slower for glides, and slowest for diphthongs.

In looking at the formation of [w], in "That's a wow," we can see that, as the lips start to round, the formants are all lowered, and in the transition to the vowel following the [w] the formants go up again as the mouth opens.

For [b] in "That's a bow [bau]" there is a period of complete closure followed by a burst and a rapid F1 transition as compared to the glide and diphthong.

In "Paint a yacht" versus "Paint a dot," again we see that the F1 transition for glides is longer than the transition for stop consonants.

The difference between the alveolars [d] and [j] and the labials [b] and [w] is in the F2 transitions. Constriction at an alveolar position causes F2 to rise in frequency whereas constriction or rounding at the lips causes F2 to decrease in frequency.

The F1 patterns are nearly the same for both alveolars and labials. F1 is lowered in frequency during the transition from vowel to consonant and rises in frequency during the transition from consonant to vowel.

Lab 9. Nasals and Glides (Text Chapter Seven)

The purpose is to study the acoustic features of nasals and glides and compare them with other consonant groups.

Record the following phrases on four or five spectrograms: (1) "a nod, anon, a Dodd"; (2) "a mob, a bob, a bomb"; (3) "a bang on, a bag on, a ban on"; (4) "a yacht, a lot, a watt, a rot."

Study the spectrograms for the following characteristics:

a. Similarity of nasals and stops in a given spectrogram (same place of articulation) of the F2 formant transitions.

b. Spectra of the nasal murmurs during constriction.

c. Note effects of any zeros in vowels adjacent to nasals.

d. Differences among glides.

e. Differences between glides and nasals in speed of F1 transition and spectra during the constrictions.

Lab 10. Fricative/Stop Distinction
(Text Chapter Seven)

The purpose is to study the sound patterns of stops and fricatives.

Record the following phrases in four spectrograms: (1) "a top, a sop, a shop"; (2) "a dog, a zog, a jog [ʤɑg]"; (3) "a pop, a fop, a thop [θap]"; (4) "a bog, a vog [vɔg], a shog [ʃɔg]."

Compare the following characteristics: fricative/stop formant transitions, fricative/stop constriction durations, unvoiced fricative spectra among [s, ʃ, f, θ], and male versus female [ʃ].

Answer the following questions, based on the spectrograms: What are the main differences between stops and fricatives? How do the unvoiced fricatives differ among each other in constriction spectrum and in formant transitions? How does voicing affect these differences?

How are male and female size differences reflected in the friction spectrum?

Other questions may be posed by further comparisons.

Lab 11. Voiced/Unvoiced Distinction
(Text Chapter Eight)

The purpose is to study differences between voiced and unvoiced consonants by comparing spectrograms of both.

Make a spectrogram of the phrases "a D" and "a T." For the voiced bilabial stop [b] there is a period of weak sound during the complete occlusion of the lips. This is followed by a release burst of sound before the following vowel begins. Vocal fold pulsing continues for most of the closure period and the burst at the release is short and weak. On the spectrogram this appears as a transient "spike" followed by the immediate resumption of the vocal fold pulsing for the vowel. (Make a very dark spectrogram to see the transient best or make a perspectrogram with SpeechStation.) Why is the voicing during the [b] closure weak or absent in part?

For the unvoiced [t] there is no vocal fold pulsing during the closure and the burst on release is strong and of longer duration. On the spectrogram this appears as a strong transient burst followed by further turbulent sound, called aspiration, before the vowel begins. Describe the spectrum of the aspiration.

Because the release burst is longer for the unvoiced consonant, the resulting voiced phase of the syllable is shorter for the unvoiced consonant than it is for the voiced consonant.

The vowel preceding the voiced stop is longer than the vowel preceding the unvoiced stop, perhaps because the closing movement for voiced stops is a little slower. Is such a difference seen in rate of movement in the formant transitions, especially in F1?

Make a spectrogram of the phrases "a buy" and "a pie." All of the preceding comments about the voiced-unvoiced labial stop distinction also apply here to the labial stops. There is one main difference between the alveolar stops and the labial stops, because the consonant closures are made at different locations in the vocal tract. This difference appears in the frequency transitions of F2. For the labial stops, F2 is lowered in frequency by the labial constriction. For the alveolar stops F2 is raised by the constriction. Often the unvoiced F2 transition occurs only in the release burst. (See Chapter Nine on place effects.)

Make a spectrogram of the Phrases "a V" and "a fee" (be sure to use the high-frequency emphasis). The essential difference between the fricatives and the stops studied previously is that the stops make a complete closure of the oral tract whereas the fricatives are produced with a narrow constriction. The duration of this constriction period is usually longer than the closure period of a stop. During the constriction a high-frequency friction sound is seen, provided there is sufficient playback level when making the spectrogram.

The release of the fricatives is not as sharply defined as it is for the stops because there is no release burst for fricatives.

Voicing pulses are usually seen during the constriction of voiced fricatives like [v], but partial or complete devoicing can occur just as for voiced stops. The glottal pulsing provides the air flowing into the mouth and this causes a corresponding pulsing in the friction sound in the high frequencies. Is there an intensity difference between the voiced and unvoiced friction sound in the high frequencies? Why?

Is the vowel preceding the voiced fricative consonant longer than the one preceding the unvoiced fricative, as it was for stops?

Make a spectrogram of the sentence "He sued the zoo." For the unvoiced [s] we see a more intense high frequency friction sound than for [z]. This is a typical difference between unvoiced and voiced fricatives. For unvoiced consonants, the glottis is held wide open, allowing a high flow into the vocal tract and a high flow through the constriction. For the voiced fricatives, the glottis is continuously closing and opening; it is constricted a great deal of the time, thus reducing the airflow through the upper constriction, causing less turbulence and a lower intensity of high frequency friction.

Lab 12. Coarticulation Effects (Text Chapter Ten)

Make spectrograms to observe and analyze the following coarticulation effects: (1) effect of following vowel on preceding consonant and (2) effect of following vowel on two consonants.

The following words and utterances may be grouped in three spectrograms: (1) seat [sit], sought [sɔt], suit [sut]; (2) sweep [swipl, swap [swap], swoop [swup].

Take care that the words and sounds are spoken rapidly with natural fluency because a very careful, formal, or stilted style reduces normal coarticulatory effects.

How does the spectrum of [s] depend on the following vowel? How is the compound consonant [sw] affected by the following vowel?

SKETCHES OF SOME INTERESTING BOOKS FOR PHONETICIANS

J. M. PICKETT

Most of the references in our book are original research literature. Consult them when you want more detail but often they are too narrowly focused to give you broad or tutorial views of their topics. For larger perspectives I like the following books, some written by the researchers themselves, for the reasons I give for each. Some are for the beginner in speech acoustics and others will take you well beyond the scope of our study here.

GENERAL PHONETICS

The following books are intended for introductory courses in phonetics where the goal is to learn the classical descriptions and notation (International Phonetic Alphabet) of the speech sounds of all languages. Anatomical, physiological, and acoustic descriptions are subordinated to gaining initial appreciations and definitions of linguistic contrasts and how they are discussed by linguists in exploring the many fascinating ways that languages employ speech for communication. These books teach by providing student pronunciation exercises and brief self-quizzes at every desirable point. They provide bibliographies of advanced books where references to original scientific papers may be found.

Ladefoged, P. (1993) *A Course in Phonetics*, 3rd edition. Harcourt Brace Jovanovitch, 6277 Sea Harbor Drive, Orlando, FL 32887. The current edition of this classic, by a distinguished experimental linguist, includes many new examples and exercises. The sections on intonation patterns (Chapters 5 and 10) are excellent introductions for the speech scientist.

Catford, J. C. 1988. *A Practical Introduction to Phonetics*. Clarendon Press, Oxford University Press, Oxford. This book uses participatory, feel-your-own-speech techniques for learning the classic phonetic categories and their symbols in the International Phonetic Alphabet. The method is traditional in British phonetics teaching (Sweet, *A Primer of Phonetics*, 1906, 3rd edition). The student is instructed how to sense the organs, movements, constrictions, and contacts of her or his own pronunciations of examples of phonetic contrasts, and how they are employed in a wide variety of languages. There are 124 such "experiments," many using silent articulation "since the auditory sensations of loud speech tend to mask the motor sensations." Together with Ladefoged's *Course*, which introduces physiological and acoustic analysis, and listening to world language examples from the UCLA database of utterances available on Macintosh Hypercard, this book should provide the beginning student with a real feel for phonetics.

UCLA Phonetics Lab. (Currently available from Linguistics Department, University of California, Los Angeles, CA 90024-1543). Macintosh computer programs in phonetics. A set of computer materials using Hypercard illustrations of speech sound examples from Ladefoged's general *Course* and Maddiesons's phonological *Patterns*, with native speakers. The *Course* exercises may be listened to.

ACOUSTICS

Strong, W. J., and Plitnik, G. R. 1992. *Music Speech Audio.* (Expanded edition of *Music Speech Hi Fidelity,* 1977, 1983), Soundprint, 2250 North 800 East, Provo, UT 84606. This is a unique textbook, combining as it does elementary acoustical physics with the study of speech science, musical acoustics, and audio reproduction. It is the product of two physicists at Brigham Young University. BYU might be called the birthplace of American speech acoustics. From there Harvey Fletcher joined Bell Laboratories in 1916, where he pioneered U.S. research on hearing and speech and founded the Acoustical Society of America. Other prominent BYU people in speech research are OSU's G. Oscar Russell, who made the first movies of the vocal folds, the first author Strong, who was a student of Fletcher, and Iowa's Ingo Titze (see his 1994 book below).

The book is an extensive series of tutorial diagrams and explanations that provide an excellent introduction to acoustics, followed by a major section on each of the three humanistic applications of the title. Everything needed is here, for a beginning study of any combination of hearing, speech, music, and audio technology. The level is undergraduate, assumes only high school mathematics, but the acoustics is presented in thoroughly rigorous physical terms that prepare the way for very clear, scientific treatments of our favorite uses of sound: namely, performing and listening to speech and music. Each of the 46 chapters is supplemented by laboratory exercises, suggested demonstrations, specific further readings, and multimedia available. Appendices review the necessary math, graphical analysis, and acoustical units.

Taylor, C. 1992. *Exploring Music: The Science and Technology of Tones and Tunes.* Institute of Physics Publishing, Bristol (UK). This enchanting and highly tutorial book on the acoustic principles of musical instruments is highly recommended for its interesting demonstrations and crystal clear illustrations of acoustic analysis. Both musicians and speech scientists may find this author's explanations and demonstrations to be a more enticing and lucid introduction to acoustics than our linguistically motivated approach. The book would be an effective complement to our Chapters Two and Three.

Campbell, M., and Greated, C. 1987, 1988. *The Musician's Guide to Acoustics.* Schirmer, New York (1988); Dent, London (1987). This is a complete tutorial treatment, in 600 pages, of music acoustics; it covers principles of acoustics, instrumental sound production, radiation, environmental effects, and the families of instruments (including of course the voice). The first one-third of the book is a remarkable presentation of elementary acoustics, both physical and psychological. It is intended for musicians but any student of an acoustical subject could enjoy it, especially as supplemental reading. The level assumes high school math and then you learn the needed musical terms as you go along.

Sundberg, J., Nord, L., and Carlson, R. 1991. *Music, Language, Speech and Brain.* Macmillan, London. A proceedings book with 40 extended abstracts from the International Symposium at the Wenner-Gren Center in Stockholm, September 1990, covering many different research facets about relations among the title topics. This book provides a fairly complete presentation for advanced students who may be studying or researching methods and experimental work and need a quick overlook of the issues. It provides a green browsing pasture for selecting a dissertation topic in these exciting areas of scientific knowledge. The editors and symposium leaders are investigators at The Royal Institute of Technology's Department of Speech, Music and Hearing, a research center founded by Gunnar Fant 30 years ago (see a fine photo of Fant and encomium on p. xi). There are several tutorial papers and summaries. Halle and Stevens, in the first chapter, provide a nice summary of a current version of distinctive features theory, useful especially to linguistics students.

GENERAL SPEECH SCIENCE AND EXPERIMENTAL PHONETICS

Borden, G. L., Harris, K. S., and Raphael, L. 1994. *Speech Science Primer*, 3rd edition. Williams and Wilkins, Baltimore. This book, presented by prominent researchers, is (deservedly) the most popular text for introductory courses in speech science. The treatment is simple but authoritative and complete, with copious examples and illustrations. The basic acoustics, vocal sound production, speech articulations for vowels and consonants, and speech perception are the four major chapters, making up most of the book. This part includes important explanatory theories, such as the source-filter theory of production and the motor theory of perception. Ancillary chapters present biographies of pioneers of speech science, language and thought, research tools, and speech evolution. The pioneers' biographies contain some hyperboles, but then why not praise the great work of scientists like Helmholtz, Stetson, Sweet, Bell, Dudley, Cooper, Liberman, and Delattre? There is even more history of our field than can be covered here; it has been sixty years since Haskins Labs' Cooper began his development of a device that would convert light patterns to sound as an aid for the blind. For an introductory book, the chapter on research tools is unique in its thorough descriptions of methods, including many examples of data displays. There is an extensive glossary and good index. References are listed separately from each chapter, rather than obtruding them into the text.

Denes, P. B., and Pinson, E. N. 1995. *The Speech Chain. The Physics and Biology of Spoken Language*, 2nd edition. W. H. Freeman, New York. This classic, a primer on speech acoustic communication, the original nearly twenty-five years in paperback, has been completely revised. And there are new chapters that extend the book's elementary, tutorial approach to explanations of analysis, synthesis, and automatic recognition of speech via computers.

Lass, N. (ed.). 1996. *Principles of Experimental Phonetics*. Mosby, St. Louis. An excellent collection of advanced discussions and reviews by distinguished authorities in their fields; covers methods of research, speech production, speech acoustics, and perception. The book has a fine outline of topics heading each chapter. The level as a textbook is what I would call "graduate seminar," somewhat more advanced and less tutorial than my present book. The editor is preparing an undergraduate level book as well for Allyn and Bacon. Thus, a sequence of texts could start with his undergraduate text, proceed with my book for advanced undergraduates, and use Lass's 1996 *Experimental Phonetics* for the graduate seminar.

Miller, J. L., Kent, R. D., and Atal, B. S. (Eds.) 1991. *Papers in Speech Communication*. Speech Production, Acoustical Society of America, Woodbury, NY. This is one of a series of three reprint volumes of seminal journal papers on speech communication, from various sources, selected and edited with some comment on how they fit into the speech research scene of the past fifty years. A gold mine of recent history of theory and experiment on speech production covering topics of respiration, phonation, vocal tract acoustics, and speech synthesis. See also the other series volumes, one on speech processing and one on speech perception.

Lindblom, B., and S. Öhman (Eds.). 1979. *Frontiers of Speech Communication Research*. Academic Press, London. A collection of important research papers of the 1970s, suitable for the advanced student, covering a wide range of acoustic, physiologic, and perceptual topics in speech science.

Malmberg, B. (Ed.). 1970. *Manual of Phonetics*. North-Holland, Amsterdam. Not really a manual for doing phonetic research but contains good chapters by Fant, Fry, and Jakobson/Halle (on distinctive feature theory).

Minifie, F., T. Hixon, and F. Williams. 1973. *Normal Aspects of Speech, Hearing, and Language*. Prentice-Hall, Englewood Cliffs, NJ. A good introductory text to the broad field of the speech and hearing sciences.

Zemlin, W. R. (1988) *Speech and Hearing Science, Anatomy and Physiology*, 3rd edition. Prentice-Hall, Englewood Cliffs, NJ. This monumental text is near-encyclopedic in its illustrations and discussions of speech anatomy, innervation, and circulation to the speech organs. It is highly instructive on mechanisms of hearing.

Zinkin (Zhinkin), N. I. 1968. *Mechanisms of Speech*. Mouton, The Hague. (A translation of the original 1958 Russian treatise of the eminent Moscow phonetician.) This is a remarkable book relating much of its contemporary experimental knowledge of speech to explanations of phonologic, morphologic, pragmatic, and even artistic phenomena. The basic production factors of vocal tract shape and larynx ("pharyngeal") valving, seen in his X-ray studies, are the starting point for building an encyclopedic theory of such classic speech-science issues as variance/invariance of features, coarticulation, cortical/subcortical control of articulation/breathing, and emotional expression. Although this book is not easy to read, and even outdated at many points, any modern theorist might take it as a model of organization.

Flanagan, J. L. 1972. *Speech Analysis Synthesis and Perception*, 2nd edition. Springer-Verlag, New York. This classic is still the most complete technical book that treats all aspects and ramifications of speech communication from the acoustic and engineering points of view.

SPEECH ACOUSTICS

Boothroyd, A. 1986. *Speech Acoustics and Speech Perception*. Allyn and Bacon, Boston. This book replaces our first-edition entry of the classic Fry (1979) as a brief introductory book to speech acoustics. It presents a startlingly clear, yet thoughtful and authoritative treatment of all the basic acoustic principles and issues for beginning students in audiology and speech.

Stevens, K. N. 1998. *Acoustic Phonetics*. MIT Press, Cambridge, MA. Kenneth Stevens is the American leader in acoustic study of speech. His book presents the most thorough, complete account of the acoustic principles of speaking and speech perception that is currently available, particularly focused on the phonological component of languages. Three chapters present the acoustic theory of speech sound production. Two following chapters explain auditory processing and phonology. Then four chapters describe the four basic classes of speech sounds: vowels, stop features, obstruents, and sonorants. The treatment especially develops the Quantal Theory originated by Stevens via his own research. The final chapter is devoted to speech sound variability in relation to phonological constancy for linguistic function. Historically, this book may be considered the culmination of the theory of distinctive features, the acoustic development of which began with the research of Jakobson, Fant, and Halle, 1951.

Kent, R. D., and Read, C. (1992). *The Acoustic Analysis of Speech*. Singular Publishing, San Diego. This little book (eight chapters) efficiently covers all the basics of speech acoustics and related factors in production at an introductory level, without any diversions (or enticements?) into linguistics, phonology, or perception theory.

Fant, G. 1960. *Acoustic Theory of Speech Production*. Mouton, The Hague. This is our classic technical treatise on the acoustic analysis and synthesis of speech production, the first complete derivation and thorough application of the source-filter theory. It covers all major sound classes and features, with considerable emphasis on distinctive feature theory. A very important aspect of Fant's presentation are his graphs (nomograms) showing how the formant frequencies of the model vocal tract are affected by the two major constriction factors: place of constriction and degree of constriction, in combinations. Using these graphs you can find theoretical formant formant frequencies for many types of vocal tract configurations and examine trends of changes with changes in place or amount of constriction. Effects of degree of nasality and liquid and retroflex articulations are also charted and explained via the theory.

Fant, G. 1973. *Speech Sounds and Features.* MIT Press, Cambridge, MA. This book presents further studies and extensions of Fant's analysis of speech sounds, production, and their relation to the theory of distinctive features (for expositions of this theory see Jakobson et al., and Chomsky and Halle, below under Acoustic Linguistics).

Halle, M. 1959. *The Sound Pattern of Russian.* Mouton, The Hague. A distinctive feature analysis of Russian with spectrograms and tables of acoustic characteristics. There is an important chapter on the history of acoustic analysis of speech, unique for the author's earlier European associations with the phonologists who promulgated distinctive features theory from its origins in St. Petersburg and then in Prague.

PROSODICS

Lieberman, P. 1967. *Intonation, Perception, and Language.* MIT Press, Cambridge, MA. An extended experimental study and discussion, presenting the original version of the breath group theory of intonation and stress, and its linguistic implications.

Lehiste, L. 1970. *Suprasegmentals.* MIT Press, Cambridge, MA. A thorough review of research on the acoustics, production, and perception of prosodic features.

Cohen, A., and Nooteboom, S. G. 1975. *Structure and Process in Speech Perception.* Springer-Verlag, New York. Sponsored by the Netherlands government's Institute for Perception Research (I.P.O.), Eindhoven, prominent speech researchers from around the world met to discuss their research and theorizing on suprasegmental (above the phoneme) factors. Here are some interesting beginnings of issues that are still under extensive investigation: the size and nature of perceptual units; interactions of prosody, syntax, and meaning.

Devine, A. M., and Stephens, L. D. 1994. *The Prosody of Greek Speech.* Oxford University Press, New York. These authors reconstruct the spoken rhythms and melody patterns of a dead language, Ancient Greek. They do this by establishing relationships between the musical frequency intervals found in ancient Greek song manuscripts and modern prosodic analysis, confirmed by examples seen in Greek poetry. An amazing performance in any language!

SPEECH PHYSIOLOGY

Lieberman, P., and Blumstein, S. E. 1988. *Speech Physiology, Speech Perception, and Acoustic Phonetics.* Cambridge University Press, Cambridge. This textbook, by two distinguished linguist/phoneticians, offers a concise introduction to basic acoustics, to how all the factors in speech production work for the speech code, and to relationships with language development and evolution of speaking. The approach is rather unique in presenting, within an introductory context, several explanatory models related to current researchers' issues, such as the breath group as an archetypical prosodic pattern, declination theory in phonation, cue invariance, motor perception theory, and speech evolution.

Gauffin, J., and Hammarberg, B. (Eds.). 1991. *Vocal Fold Physiology: Acoustic Perceptual and Physiological Aspects of Voice Mechanisms.* Singular Publishing, San Diego, CA. A collection of 36 research papers on phonation presented at a 1989 conference in the Royal Institute of Technology, Stockholm, the 6th Conference on Vocal Fold Physiology. All aspects mentioned in the title are represented. The reports are rather technical but the broad range of interests covered gives the most recent total picture of phonatory research and its applications in related voice fields.

Hixon, T. J. (and Collaborators). 1987. *Respiratory Function in Speech and Song.* College-Hill Press, Boston. This thoroughly detailed book presents the author's fundamental studies of the mechanisms of breathing that underlie speech production. Particularly the functions of the chest and abdominal musculature and their control of the breath stream and pressures via the movements (kinematics) of the body walls and the resulting lung pressure dynamics are elucidated. Special attention is given to new experimental measuring methods and resulting modifications of conclusions from the preceding "classic" studies. Separate chapters treat abnormalities of speech breathing.

Titze, I. R. (Ed.) 1993. *Vocal Fold Physiology: Frontiers in Basic Science*. Singular Publishing, San Diego, CA. This is the report of technical papers and research discussions at the 7th Conference on Vocal Fold Physiology, held at the Denver Center for the Performing Arts, Denver, CO, in 1991. The focus here examines the structure and phonating mechanisms of the vocal folds per se and presents in one source the latest available anatomical, biomechanical, respiratory, and computer models.

Fujimura, O., and Hirano, M. (Eds.) 1995. *Vocal Fold Physiology: Voice Quality Control*. Singular Publishing, San Diego, CA. This is the report of technical papers and research discussions at the 9th Conference on Vocal Fold Physiology. See description of the 7th Conference report edited by Titze, above.

Titze, I. R. 1994. *Principles of Voice Production*. Prentice-Hall, Englewood Cliffs, NJ.; Allyn and Bacon, Boston. Prof. Titze, a physicist, is our foremost researcher on phonation, voice production by the larynx. His book is unique in its engaging, yet precise presentation of the biomechanics of voice. I like especially his phonation model (see his model diagrams in our Chapter Four) and his explanation of factors for voice efficiency. These principles of efficiency are valuable to voice teachers of singers and politicians. His mechanisms of voice pitch control explain how prosodic melodies in speech are produced.

BIOLOGY OF SPEECH

Lenneberg, E. 1967. *Biological Foundations of Language*. John Wiley & Sons, New York. This book is a classic, pioneering, and highly original discussion of its subject that is still often quoted, criticized, and researched experimentally.

Lieberman, P. 1975. *On the Origins of Language, An Introduction to the Evolution of Human Speech*. Macmillan Publishing Co., New York.

Brings together evidence from the acoustic theory of speech, the brain size and vocal tract shapes of early man from fossil skull measurements, and the development of tool-making behavior, to argue that highly articulate speech was a precondition for the evolution of our present spoken languages and related human culture.

Lieberman, P. 1984. *The Biology and Evolution of Language*. Harvard University Press, Cambridge, MA. This is a masterly presentation of a theory of language evolution that brings to bear an enormous range of anatomical, neural, acoustical, phonetic and linguistic information to explain the workings of human language. All communications students who are curious about the biological background of what they observe should begin with this book.

Lieberman, P. 1991. *Uniquely Human: The Evolution of Speech, Thought, and Selfless Behavior*. Harvard University Press, Cambridge, MA. Lieberman takes his theory of evolution of spoken language to the brink of formal philosophy as he presents evidence of the speech origins of thinking in the human cultural transmission of tool-making methods and the survival advantages of the uniquely human tradition of protecting weaker human beings. Parallels in child language development are presented. He argues that language structure and human thought evolved together on the basis of common biological mechanisms, such as the logical cause-effect and categorizing capacities of the brain.

Lieberman, P. 1999. *The Functional Language System of the Human Brain*. Harvard University Press, Cambridge. Following is excerpted from Prof. Lieberman's abstract for this book:

Data from studies of aphasia, Parkinson's disease, and normal subjects are consistent with the human brain's having a functional language system that evolved to produce and comprehend spoken language; the system regulates speech production, accesses the phonetic addresses of words, and derives the meaning of utterances taking into account morphemic and syntactic information. The system appears to be a distributed network that includes neural structures such as basal ganglia and cerebellum traditionally associated with motor control as well as structures such as prefrontal cortex, often associated with higher "non-linguistic" aspects of cognition. The particular structures that form the system also play a part in other distributed functional systems. Therefore, damage to the brain that disrupts language can also affect manual motor control and/or "non-linguistic" reasoning. These linkages reflect the probable evolutionary history of the system. Basic principles and facts derived from evolutionary biology such as the universal presence of genetic variation and the time depth of hominid evolution argue against a detailed Chomskian "Universal Grammar" that specifies the syntax of all possible human languages.

Leroi-Gourhan, A. 1993. *Gesture and Speech*. MIT Press, Cambridge, MA. (This is a translation by Anna Berger of *Le Geste et La Parole*, Paris, A. Michel, 1964). Contrary to its title, this book doesn't deal directly with motor parallels between manual gesturing and speaking. It is a book on the evolution of representational behavior, ranging from the functional evolution of the human skeleton, particularly the cranium and brain, to contemporary art and future culture (p. 396 on). Along the way it touches many topics of peripheral fascination to the language scientist, although actually there is very little on speech per se. Definitely worth a detour in the library stacks, far removed from any real concerns of the laboratory and consequent loss of a few "manual discoveries" (p. 397).

Barkow, J. H., Cosmides, L., and Tooby, J. (Eds.). 1992. *The Adapted Mind. Evolutionary Psychology and the Generation of Culture*. Oxford University Press, New York. This collection of research reviews carries that curious student further into the broad field of psychobiological research on the origins of language. The acoustic phonetician will be fascinated by the paper on prosodics of "motherese" and its prehuman evolution, by Anne Fernald. The biolinguist will find explorations of many links between language behavior and human evolution, for example, in a speculative chapter linking social evolution to language structure by Steven Pinker and Paul Bloom.

SPEECH PERCEPTION

Miller, J. L., Kent, R. D., and Atal, B. S. (Eds.) 1991. *Papers in Speech Communication: Speech Perception*. Acoustical Society of America, Woodbury, NY. This is one of a series of three reprint volumes of seminal journal papers on speech communication, from various sources, selected and edited with some comment on how they fit into the speech research scene of the past fifty years. A gold mine of recent history of theory and experiment on speech perception covering all relevant topics. See also the other series volumes, one on speech production and one on speech processing.

Liberman, A. M. 1996. *Speech, A Special Code*. MIT Press, Cambridge, MA. A legend among speech scientists, Liberman chronicles his half-century of experiments studying speech perception and production at Haskins Laboratories. He recounts the major twists and turns of hypothesis, strategy, experiments, and outcomes by which he and his colleagues developed the first complete theory of speech perception, the "Motor Theory" of Liberman and Mattingly (1985, 1989). Each major step is described in the introductory chapter, "Some assumptions about speech and how they changed"; then twenty-three subsequent chapters reproduce major journal publications issued from Haskins projects 1951–1992. The topics of investigation, each with its separate commentary relating to the sequences of theorizing presented in the introduction chapter, are "I. On the spectrogram as a visible display of speech; II. Finding the cues; III. Categorical perception; IV. An early attempt (1957) to put it all together; V. A mid-course correction; VI. The revised motor theory; VII. Some properties of the phonetic module; VIII. More about the function and properties of the phonetic module; IX. Auditory vs. phonetic modes; X. Reading/writing are hard just because speaking/listening are easy." In some ways this book is the perception complement of *Producing Speech*, which covers much of the Haskins research on speech production (reviewed below).

Brady, S. A., and Shankweiler, D. P. 1991. *Phonological Processes in Literacy*. Erlbaum Associates, Hillsdale, NJ. This book honors the career of Dr. Isabelle Y. Liberman of Haskins Laboratories and the University of Connecticut School of Education. Her scientific achievements were in the science of reading/phonology relations and its applications to reading and writing disabilities. The book is an advanced presentation of recent research on phonological awareness in children and its relation to their success in learning to read. Its primary interest to speech scientists lies in its extended treatments of the fundamental problem of the highly complex relationship between the phonemic structure of speech and orthographic, alphabetic representation of that structure, and the attendant complexity of the learning processes for successful reading. Motor theories of speech perception explain why speech perception is so easy to learn whereas reading, although based on speech, is so difficult: Speech is motorily coded for direct phonetic perception whereas orthography is an arbitrary cipher for the phonetic units.

Mattingly, I. G., and Studdert-Kennedy, M. 1991. *Modularity and the Motor Theory of Speech Perception*. Proceedings of a Conference to Honor Alvin M. Liberman. Erlbaum Associates, Hillsdale, NJ. This conference of star participants was held in 1988, then the papers, comments, and discussions were revised and finally published here. The result is a highly polished presentation of evidence pro and con the Motor Theory, plus extended critical comments by authors and other participants. For readers already familiar with the theory via our Chapter Fourteen and Liberman's 1996 book, this book would be a valuable source for detailed information on the development of the theory, particularly in relation to biological module theories of perception (more than half the conference). There are several chapters on animal and early child perception.

Ryalls, J. 1996. *A Basic Introduction to Speech Perception*. Singular Publishing, San Diego. This small book presents a remarkably concise course of easy-reading chapters that cover nearly all aspects of speech perception. The approach is highly theoretical, yet clearly tutorial. The core of our knowledge of speech perception, about half the book, is presented in terms of theoretical concepts, represented by Motor Theory, Disctinctive Feature Theory (including infant feature detection) and Quantal (Invariance) Theory.

Perkell, J. S., and Klatt, D. H. 1986. *Invariance and Variability in Speech Processes*. Erlbaum Associates, Hillsdale, NJ. This presents conference papers, comments, and discussion on the title subject, a conference honoring Prof. Kenneth N. Stevens (see his Quantal Theory in our Chapter Fourteen). Highly recommended are the four child language papers; they present well the beginning background of the current enormous interest in child phonological behavior. Ask how, faced with the wide variation of the phonetic pattern for each and every phoneme, we come as adults to use phoneme classes and thus successfully decode everyday variant speech? The answers will be found in children's learning to use phonemic processing that leads to perceiving phonemes as invariant, permutable units of spoken language. Quantal theory says that children are aided in this task by the built-in invariants of hearing and by acoustic speech features that are relatively invariant, that is, not so susceptible to variation by context.

Rosner, B. S., and Pickering, J. B. 1994. *Vowel Perception and Production*. Oxford University Press, Oxford, UK. This book is a remarkably complete and detailed review of research on the psychoacoustic processes of vowel perception, tied to the authors' development of a vowel perception theory. For further study of auditory theoretical issues in our Chapters Thirteen through Fifteeen, this book would be an excellent starting point. It presents an auditory, non-motor theory for explaining how the acoustic input patterns of vowels are transformed by hearing and phonetic classification, to yield correct decisions about vowel identity. In the theory, specific mathematical descriptions of the frequency-integrating and amplitude-to-loudness transforms of hearing are used for analyzing the speech input to a decision model. Factors of speaker style variation, phonetic environment (coarticulation), syllable rate and stress, are reviewed and discussed in relation to the theory; they are deemed to be accountable for correct vowel perception via transforms of the major auditory variables.

Carlson, R., and Granström, B. (Eds.) 1982. *The Representation of Speech in the Peripheral Auditory System*. Elsevier, Amsterdam. These are the papers presented at a conference with the same title, held in Stockholm in 1982 and dedicated to the memory of the late Valerij Kozhevnikov (see Kozhevnikov & Chistovich, 1965). This was a seminal conference that brought together many different approaches to the complex analytic functions of the ear: sensory physiology, automatic speech recognition, phonetic perception, singing, and studies of impaired auditory systems. Despite the early dates of this work, many papers represent good starting points for current review of their respective problems, as these are still concerned with the same complex issues. This book is definitely worth a glance through.

MOTOR AND NEURAL ORGANIZATION OF SPEECH

Fagard, J., and Wolff, P. H. (Eds.) 1991. *The Development of Timing Control and Temporal Organization in Coordinated Action*. North-Holland/Elsevier, Amsterdam. For the advanced student of speech motor activity this volume, collected by investigators of motor development in children, presents detailed experimental studies and theoretical discussions on how human rhythmic expression in movements, such as toddling, walking, speaking, become organized. There are important papers by two speech researchers, Ray Kent and colleagues on the how speech rhythms develop in infancy and childhood, and by Zanone and Scott Kelso on adaptive mechanisms for rhythmic control. For advanced students of the motor

environment for the rhythmic factors in speech prosody, this volume goes far back into early development and deeply into motion dynamics that eventually may be found to relate speech prosodics to findings and theory in basic movement control research.

Bell-Berti, F., and Raphael, L. J. 1995. *Producing Speech: Contemporary Issues*. AIP Press, New York. This is a marvelous collection, on the major issues today about the motor organization of speech, in honor of the Haskins Labs' leader on speech motor research, Katherine S. Harris. Its 34 chapters cover every aspect of theory and experiment by eminent figures in that field. Highly recommended for all advanced students. For a complete review, see Pickett (1996).

Hardcastle, W. J., and Marchal, A. (Eds.) 1990. *Speech Production and Speech Modelling*. (NATO Advanced Science Institutes Series, D: Behavioral and Social Sciences - Vol. 55). Kluwer Academic, Dordrecht. Time was, 1900–1920, when virtually all physiological research on speech was European. Even American pioneers did their doctoral or post-doctoral work in Europe, for example, R. H. Stetson with Rousellot in Paris, and E. W. Scripture with Wundt in Leipzig. In our electronic era of speech modeling, c. 1950 onward, Europeans Roman Jakobson, Gunnar Fant, and Morris Halle spawned the MIT efforts in 1950. Later, Peter Ladefoged, from Edinburgh, began a major branch of physiological research at UCLA in 1962. By the 1989 date of this NATO conference we seem to have caught up: This book is half North American, half European, even though the conference organizers are European. Major international researchers present their theories of speech production, exemplified by computer modeling correlated with the motor structures revealed in speech gestural events. My star-award papers are by Keller on the possible neural mechanisms of the timing coordination of speech gestures and by MacNeilage and Davis on brain-development parallels of infant speech transition from babbling to "phonemic" syllables.

LINGUISTICS

Warning! Students who read Burgess' *Mouthful* and Burling's *Patterns*, listed next, run the risk of life as Linguists.

Burgess, A. 1992. *A Mouthful of Air. Language, Languages . . . Especially English*. William Morrow, New York. This introduction to the history, sounds, and structure of our language is thoroughly enjoyable and still manages to be scholarly.

Burling, R. 1989. *Patterns of Language. Structure, Variation, Change*. Academic, San Diego. A more academic introduction covering linguistics in general, with straightforward, clear explanations of all the major linguistic definitions and phenomena. Especially good on families of the world's languages and sound changes within them.

Pinker, S. 1994. *The Language Instinct*. Morrow, New York. This is an extensive popular introduction to psychobiological linguistics that, on the publisher's cover, is said to explain "How the Mind Creates Language," a cover subtitle that the author did not put on his title page, perhaps because if language is an instinct, why would the mind need to create it? Pinker uses many pop-culture examples to stimulate the reader to understand psycholinguistic principles. The book is an engaging odyssey through the major territories of psychobiological knowledge about language, with titillating excursions such as a smelly demeaning of New Guinea aborigines' method of finding that the white linguists are not Gods. Still it's an enjoyable intellectual romp with a brilliant scientist, through linguistic theory, speculations on speech, evolution, and current psycholinguistic research. As an advanced reader, you may be put off by minor loose ends and misstatements. Despite some discussion of speech acoustic facts, the only illustrations in the book are trees of linguistic units. At one point the author's "torrent of relevant detail" misstates an experimental effect, on p. 264, where the tempo-normalization of formant transitions for perception of [b/w] is stated in reverse. There is an occasional misuse of linguistic terms; on p. 263 it is stated that infants "retrieve phonemes" when only a few weeks old; however, the Glossary properly defines phonemes in terms of meaningful word units that usually would not be in common use until at least a year of age. Perhaps it depends on how you define infancy. For an antidote to this book, see Lieberman (1999) above. Nevertheless, Pinker is an important thinker in socio-evolutionary psychology and his book will attract many students who might not respond to the more conventional enticements of Burgess' and Burling's books above.

Pinker, S. 1996. *Language Learnability and Language Development*. Harvard University Press, Cambridge, MA. This is a reprint, with the author's new commentary and further references, of his very comprehensive exposition, 1986, of a detailed theory of language learning tied closely to the large literature of findings in developmental psycholinguistics. Linguist students of development may use this update to bring together a mass of information bearing on the innate mechanisms supporting language behavior. Another Pinker odyssey, *How the Mind Works* (Norton, 1997), takes us on an exhaustive pop-science tour of his functionalist philosophy of human behavior where speech sounds are only a very minor stop.

PHONOLOGY

Phonology, the study of the sound systems employed by languages, has often been the source of advances in phonetics *per se* when phonological linguists want to explain their findings using principles of auditory perception, articulatory capabilities and constraints, and acoustic speech patterning. In fact, one could argue that phonetic research proper should be motivated and guided by phonological questions. The following books will introduce the curious student of acoustic phonetics to some of the big thinking and demanding experimentation of the major players in a field that one of them, John Ohala, calls "experimental phonology."

Maddieson, I. 1984. *Patterns of Sounds*. Cambridge University Press, Cambridge, UK. A remarkable compilation and original analysis of information on the sounds of the world's languages. Not only does it lay out the magnificent array of sounds produced by vocal maneuvers for speech communication but it analyzes these sound types quantitatively and constructs hypotheses about how various phonemic structures (phonologies) came about.

Kelly, J. and Local, J. 1989. *Doing Phonology.* Manchester University Press, Manchester, UK. This interesting, idiosyncratic book, highly critical of phonological theories and "received," "standard" feature systems, will serve the avid reader of the enticing general linguistics books above as a damper to giving over one's life to the fascinations of language science. The elaborate phonetic marking system, deemed necessary to record data for discovery of all of the hidden systematicities of phonetic segments in fluent communication, by itself indicts the sometimes simplistic insights of modern feature theories and serves notice of the complexities of discovering effective systems for explaining just the wonders of segmental detail, especially in natural speaking situations.

Ohala, J. J., and Jaeger, J. J. (Eds.) 1986. *Experimental Phonology.* Academic Press, New York. This is the first book collection of experimental studies of phonological phenomena. It deals with things like the acoustics of phonemic nasalization, quantitative relations among phonemic contrasts, perceptual salience, modeling of optimum contrastive systems, cognitive tests in linguistic research, and contemporary age-generations' perceptual parallel of a small sound-change in their language.

Papers in Laboratory Phonology, I (1990), II (1992), III (1993), IV (1994). Cambridge University Press, Cambridge, UK. A kind of sequel series to *Experimental Phonology* above, these are research collections of studies covering the expanding field of linguistically motivated investigations of speech production and perception.

Diehl, R. L. (Ed.) 1992. Articulatory Phonology. Special Issue of *Phonetica,* 49 (3–4). This discussion consists of a "target" article presenting a phonological system that employs speech gestures as the basic units of utterances, followed by extended commentaries on the system. Articulatory phonology is intended to base phonemic

lexical contrasts on contrasts of vocal-tract configuration changes in response to speech gestural constellations. Phonological phenomena discussed are allophonic variation, fluent speech changes, coarticulation, speech errors, and phonological development in children.

ACOUSTIC LINGUISTICS

This section highlights books that are primarily linguistic but with more emphasis on speech acoustic patterns than other linguistics books.

Hammerich, L. L., Jakobson, R., and Zwirner, E. (eds.). 1971. *Form and Substance.* Akademisk Forlag, Copenhagen. Research and theoretical papers on phonology, speech acoustics, and phonetic perception.

Chomsky, N., and Halle, M. 1968. *The Sound Pattern of English.* Harper & Row Publishers, New York. For the advanced student, a complete exposition of distinctive feature theory applied to English.

Delattre, P. 1965. *Comparing the Phonetic Features of English, French, German, and Spanish.* Chilton Books, Philadelphia. A detailed description of the acoustic pattern differences of four major languages.

Kavanagh, J., and Cutting, J. 1975. *The Role of Speech in Language.* MIT Press, Cambridge, MA. This book is hard to classify because it contains interdisciplinary research and discussions of why such a complex coding in phonology and grammar is necessary to go from meaning to speech sound. Discussions of sign language codes are also included, to compare with the speech code.

Fromkin, V. A. (Ed.) 1985. *Phonetic Linguistics.* Academic Press, New York. This is a collection of papers honoring Prof. Peter Ladefoged, the distinguished linguist/phonetician who may be credited with creating the current blend of linguistic and acoustic research that is now common in the best laboratories of acoustic phonetics. There is a complete biography and an interview. The papers range as widely as the title suggests, reporting research and theory of very high quality, commensurate with that of Ladefoged himself.

SPOKEN LANGUAGE DEVELOPMENT

Jusczyk, P. W. 1997. *The Discovery of Spoken Language.* MIT Press, Cambridge, MA. For advanced students and language scientists looking for a complete summary of acoustical, psycholinguistic research on how infants and children start to be accomplished users of their language, this book may be the answer. It is a detailed description and interpretation of the findings of many scientists, including the author and his co-workers, on the development from birth of the perceptual processing of heard speech to the level of early word-learning and storage, which is thought to begin at about 7 1/2 months of age. "The focus is on the sound structure of the native language and how the infant's perceptual capacities are developed and optimized for perceiving fluent speech." A chapter is devoted to research studies on relations between early speech-sound discrimination capacities and speech production of first words in age-ranges up to 47 months. The final chapter is on theoretical models of phonetic storage of words in the child's lexicon; the author presents and discusses his WRAPSA model (Word Recognition and Phonetic Structure Acquisition). There is a 17-page appendix on the behavioral methods used in testing infant perception of speech sounds.

Werner, L. A., and Rubel, E. W. (Eds.) 1992. *Developmental Psychoacoustics.* American Psychological Association, Washington, DC. The Association held a conference of distinguished workers in the field of infant and child auditory function. The resulting papers collected here are an excellent summary of current knowledge and theory on the basic hearing functions and mechanisms that support speech perception. Interesting chapters specific to speech: Kuhl's chapter, related to our Chapter Thirteen, gives us a brief historical sketch of how psychologists researching infant speech perception have tried to resolve the problem of categorical effects in discrimination: Are they innate or learned? And Carney's chapter brings the material into relation with pediatric problems.

Ferguson, C. A., Menn, L., and Stoel-Gammon, C. (Eds.) 1992. *Phonological Development, Mod-* *els, Research, Implications.* York Press, Timonium, MD. This is a book of basic research papers and commentary, one of an ongoing series of chronicles of language development conferences sponsored by NIH's National Institute of Child Health and Human Development. This International Conference on Phonological Development was held in 1989 by the Stanford (University) Child Phonology Project. This group instigated and carried out the first wide-scale collection of phonological observations on developing infants and children. The resulting book is a very extensive, far-reaching volume for scientists who are investigating how phoneme perception and phonological access to the adult-level lexicon develop in infants and children, including even relationships to disorders and animal models of communication development. Theories and findings are presented by all the major scientists in this field: linguists, psychologists, phoneticians, and developmental researchers. Among the many star papers, two of special interest to motor and acoustic phoneticians are the biological model of development of Ray Kent and the gesture-oriented model of babbling of Marilyn Vihman who directed the Stanford Project in its final half, 1980–1988.

Bloom, L. 1993. *The Transition from Infancy to Language: Acquiring the Power of Expression.* Cambridge University Press, Cambridge. Lois Bloom pioneered the scientific study of early word acquisition from the point of view of psychological function, beginning with a study of her infant daughter in 1973. Before that, acquisition of linguistic structure had been the primary focus of developmental researchers. Effects of the infant's concurrent conceptual, cognitive, and emotional development, language function factors, had been largely ignored. This book presents the theories and results of the author's subsequent study of a diverse large group of infants, from early infancy through the word-acquisition stage, following the coordinated psychosocial and language development of word-use by each child. An integrative theory of the interdependence of early language and social development is constructed from controlled observations of infants' word-communication.

Bloom, L. 1991. *Language Development from Two to Three*. Cambridge University Press, New York. Somewhat more distant from the interests of phoneticians than the previous citation of Bloom's work on word acquisition, this book deals with the psychosocial factors in child acquisition of grammar and is noted here for readers in that field.

Locke, J. L. 1993. *The Child's Path to Spoken Language*. Harvard University Press, Cambridge, MA. This book is a candidate for a pioneering classic, in the tradition of Lenneberg's, nearly thirty years ago. It is a unique, encyclopedic study of the astonishingly rich research literature on babies' and infants' speech behavior, including the author's own work and thought. Locke brilliantly lays out all the interactions of social and biological stages of development that lead to the infant's first use of spoken words (at about age 1). The process of "vocal accommodation" is key to Locke's analysis of how babies progress from their visual and vocal imitation behaviors at birth, toward their eventual adult language behavior.

Gopnik, A., and Meltzoff, A. N. 1997. *Words, Thoughts, and Theories*. MIT Press, Cambridge, MA. For the phonetician or psycholinguist who wonders about the basic structure of her or his science, or how we know what we think we know: This book is a fascinating amalgam of theory of knowledge (epistomology) in current philosophy with early child language behavior and cognition. Its overall thesis is that very young children theorize about their world like little scientists and scientists think like "big children." The crux of this claim are in the close analogies, demonstrated here, between children's changing theories, seen in their changing construals of named categories for kinds of objects/events, and scientists' changing theories as they build scientific knowledge.

Yavas, M. (Ed.) 1994. *First and Second Language Phonology*. Singular Publishing, San Diego. Phonology is the classic discipline of linguistics that studies the phonemic patterning of languages, usually as a given language is employed by native mature language users: first language phonology. Recently, a vigorous field of enquiry has developed on how speakers acquire phonological facility with a second language. This book is designed to supplement the first course in general phonology with more information on second language phonology and relate this information to phonological acquisition, both normal and disordered, as well as to phonological theory.

Vihman, M. 1996. *Phonological Development: The Origins of Language in the Child*, Blackwell, Cambridge MA. Clear, thorough, by a recognized phonologist; all that's known on the early course of child speech. Highly recommended for all students and their teachers. Especially strong emphasis on the role of prosody and baby-talk.

Johnson, C. E., and Gilbert, John H. V. 1996. *Children's Language*, Vol. 9. Erlbaum, Hillsdale, NJ. This is the ninth of the series of selections from the proceedings of meetings, titled Children's Language, of the International Association for the Study of Child Language. The first volume was *Baby Talk and Infant Speech*, edited by Raffler-Engler and Lebrun. The present book is a broad sample from the 1993 meeting in Trieste. It emphasizes lexical and syntactic research rather than phonological or prosodics research. There are seventeen chapters. I assume that my readers will be interested mainly in the phonology studies. Although there is not much phonetic data involved, certain chapters have interesting implications. Phonological structuring of normal and retarded language learners receives a thorough theoretical basis in markedness theory in the chapter by Bernhardt and Stoel-Gammon. Other phonological chapters are on the issue of continuity in German and Spanish acquisition, developmental function of filler syllables, and acquisition of object shift in Swedish and noun-classifiers in Zulu. The Swedish study has implications for the interaction of intonation patterns with syntax, an area of phonological research that I and the book's editors believe to be extremely important.

Goodman, J. C., and Nusbaum, H. C. (Eds.) 1994. *The Development of Speech Perception: The Transition from Speech Sounds to Spoken*

Words. MIT Press, Cambridge, MA. An excellent source for the acoustically oriented student of language acquisition, this collection of papers, from a conference of psychologists at the University of Chicago, features startlingly clear presentations by star scientists of issues and evidence that expanded cognitive research on speech, from the psychoacoustic level to broader language functions. The editors' introductory chapter is an excellent review. The major subdomains of enquiry are: Innate Sensory Mechanisms and Constraints on Learning; Perceptual Learning of Phonological Systems; Interactions of Linguistic Levels: Influences of Perceptual Development. The final chapter lays out the major research questions remaining, to arrive at a flexible, functional account of how speech perception develops in full language contexts.

GENERAL PHONETICS

Ladefoged, P. 1993. *A Course in Phonetics*. Harcourt Brace Jovanovich, New York. An excellent introductory text that is linguistically oriented; includes some coverage of acoustics and speech physiology. An authoritative approach by a distinguished experimental linguist.

Singh, S., and Singh, K. S. 1976. *Phonetics: Principles and Practices*. University Park Press, Baltimore. This introductory text is interesting for its still frames from motion pictures of the front facial view of articulations and correlated soundtracks and spectrograms, for numerous vowels and consonants.

PSYCHOLINGUISTICS

Altmann, G. T. M. (Ed.) 1991. *Cognitive Models of Speech Processing*. MIT Press, Cambridge, MA. This book is an excellent place to begin for the student who wishes to advance from the basic phonetics of speech perception presented in our book toward a knowledge of how continuous speech messages are understood, a process only partially introduced in our Chapter Fifteen explanations of phonetics of lexical access. The editor

presents an extensive review of the issues and a number of his own studies in subsequent chapters. There are four thorough discussion chapters that are critical reviews of sections of the book. One of the most interesting chapters to the phonetician is Exploiting Prosodic Probabilities in Speech Recognition by Anne Cutler, which brings English word-stress statistics to bear on listeners' processes for segmenting words for lexical access from the stream of continuous speech.

Levelt, W. J. M. 1989. *Speaking. From Intention to Articulation*. MIT Press, Cambridge, MA. This is a remarkably extensive book on meaningful intercourse by speaking. It is tutorial at a fairly advanced level, primarily for students interested in relating all the linguistic and many of the articulatory/acoustic factors involved in speaking.

Handel, S. 1989. *Listening. An Introduction to the Perception of Auditory Events*. MIT Press, Cambridge, MA. Another fairly advanced book of wide scope, covering the scientific research on all auditory perception, including speech, it is the only textbook on auditory perception in general.

Miller, J. L., and Eimas, P. D. (Eds.) 1995. *Speech, Language, and Communication*. Academic Press, New York. This is a collection of advanced discussions by some of the major researchers in psycholinguistics. Topics range from linguistic structures and cognition, through perception issues such as auditory-motor theory (Direct Realist, Fowler) and developmental psychoacoustics of phonemic communication (Jusczyk), to neuroscience of linguistic perception (Blumstein) and theory of social cooperation between speaker and listener. This book presents some of the best theoretical and critical thinking of its field.

Strange, W. (Ed.) 1995. *Speech Perception and Linguistic Experience: Issues in Cross-Language Research*. Academic Press, New York. This is an extensive presentation of recent research in developmental psycholinguistics by major scientists of the field. It is excellent further reading for our Chapter Thirteen, providing much experimental detail and theoretical interpretation, as well as some applications to problems in learning language.

SPEECH TECHNOLOGY

Miller, J. L., Kent, R. D., and Atal, B. S. (Eds.) 1991. *Papers in Speech Communication: Speech Processing*. Acoustical Society of America, Woodbury, NY. This is one of a series of three reprint volumes of seminal journal papers on speech communication, from various sources, selected and edited with some comment on how they fit into the speech research scene of the past fifty years. A gold mine of recent history of theory and experiment on speech processing covering topics of speech analysis, synthesis, coding and automatic recognition,. See also the other series volumes, one on speech production and one on speech perception.

Cherry, C. 1966. *On Human Communication*, 2nd edition. MIT Press, Cambridge, MA. A classic introduction to the seminal 1960s in communication sciences and technology; the book explains relevant mathematical theories and applies this approach to the nature of languages, speech analysis, information theories, linguistics, perception, and cognition. Primarily for the advanced student of the history of speech technology.

Flanagan, J. L., and L. R. Rabiner. 1973. *Speech Synthesis*. Dowden, Hutchinson, & Ross, Stroudsburg, PA. A reprint collection of forty-six classic researches on speech analysis, perception, and synthesis of speech, that lead up to our current technology of computer speech from printed text.

Syrdal, A., Bennett, R., and Greenspan, S. (Eds.) 1995. *Applied Speech Technology*. CRC Press, Boca Raton. This is a wide-ranging collection of twenty-four chapters written by speech technologists who are working on applied problems and devices in the field. There is particular emphasis on human speech interactions with speech-processing devices, for example, speech trainers for therapy, toys that talk, voice mail strategies, and industrial devices. The book provides critical review and discussion of nearly every speech-processing application, with the exception of processing designed to enhance speech for listening in noise or with hearing impairments.

Roe, D. B., and Wilpon, J. G. (Eds.) 1994. *Voice Communication Between Humans and Machines*. National Academy Press, National Academy of Sciences, Washington. The twenty-six chapters in this book form the proceedings of a 1993 colloquium, Human/Machine Communication by Voice, sponsored by the Academy. Most chapters are comprehensive technical discussions by prominent researchers of the current status of speech technologies, including speech synthesis, speech recognition, and natural language understanding. There are also several chapters on applications, technology deployment, and likely future developments.

Proceedings of the International Conference on Speech and Language Processing, 1996. Alfred I. Dupont Institute, Center for Applied Science and Engineering, Speech Research Program, P.O. Box 269, Wilmington, DE 19899. These proceedings contain extended summaries of all papers presented, covering the widest conceivable range of its relatively new field, human and machine understanding of speech. Available in print and CD-ROM.

HISTORY OF PHONETICS

This list includes both old and modern books of historical interest.

Asher, R. E., and Henderson, E. J. A. 1981. *Towards a History of Phonetics*. Edinburgh University Press, Edinburgh. This history, written by seventeen prominent British phoneticians, presents in satisfyingly expert detail the many phonetic and phonological problems and issues, historical and some current, to which the authors themselves have made fundamental contributions. The major area topics are: History of Ideas in Phonetics: Concepts, Processes, Voice; Greek, Early Chinese, and German Phonetics; Individual Contributions; Writing Systems and Phonetics.

Amman, J. C. 1700. *Dissertatio de Loquela*. J.

Wolters, Amsterdam. English translation, *A Dissertation on Speech,* published by Charles Baker, Headmaster of the Yorkshire School for the Deaf, 1873, Doncaster, Yorkshire; reprinted 1965 by North-Holland, Amsterdam. This tiny, concise book, with introductory commentary by the reprint publisher and the original translator, gives us a highly revealing look into the remarkable sophistication of practical phonetic knowledge of the seventeenth century. Amman was a physician, renowned in his time for success in teaching intelligible speech to deaf children; he mentions that it required intensive hands-on-the-lips guidance for up to a year. His method, described here in a tabular outline, shows a fine appreciation of how vowels and consonants are produced. In particular, he summarizes his classification of the speech sounds in a binary, treelike table that covers many of the articulatory features that we currently accept as well established by articulatory and acoustic science. He claimed that these basic articulatory maneuvers easily generalize in the speech-teaching process. For example, to speak consonants correctly, only the relatively few, basic articulations, such as stop, voiced, and fricative, need to be learned, that can then be combined to form all the many consonants.

Steele, Joshua. 1775. *An Essay Towards Establishing the Melody and Measure of Speech to be Expressed and Perpetuated by Peculiar Symbols.* J. Almon, London. Facsimile reprint, 1969, by Scolar Press, Menston, Yorkshire, England. This remarkable treatise is the first scientific study of English intonation. It is expressly tutorial and didactic, and could still serve any serious student as an introduction to the basics of English prosody. The form of the work is a detailed debate and correspondence with James Burnet, who claimed in his *Of the Origin and Progress of Language* (Edinburgh, 1774), that English syllables had no intonation "except that of louder and softer." One wonders if Lord Burnet may have been almost totally deaf. However, Steele directly gives Burnet an honorable excuse, saying that the extant usage of terms "accent, emphasis, quantity, pause and force" was hopelessly confused "without any

clear and sufficient rules for their use and measurement." This is what Steele sets out to accomplish, including a set of simple marking signs for intonation. His method is, beginning with simple musical notation (musicians were also hopelessly confused in their parlance about melodic expression), to develop a systematic notation system for intonational changes and rhythmic timing. The system is applied in many didactic examples to prove a high sufficiency. Steele also hoped that the study of language ("letters") and music would be more closely joined at Oxford and Cambridge, "those renowned seminaries of the Muses on the banks of the Isis and Cam" (pages xvi-xvii of his Preface). He was successful in persuading Burnet, who apparently was influential in musical circles, to change his mind about the tonal nature of speech accents. I note that, even though Steele could not measure voice pitch, he could and did use musical intervals that have a physical measurement basis, for example, in ratios of string-length; so, in effect he was referring his statements to quantitative pitch data that had a notation system and could be corroborated via personal perceptual and production behavior, in listening to and singing melodies.

CLINICAL PHONETICS

Shriberg, L. D., and Kent, R. D. 1995. *Clinical Phonetics.* 2nd edition. Allyn and Bacon, Boston. This is a very interesting introduction to phonetics for those intending or practicing in the field of speech development and disorders. It is a combined text and practicum-lab program. Linguistic and general articulatory phonetics is first presented via numerous diagrammatic illustrations that are very clear and cover all the major types of speech articulation. A complete articulatory transcription system is presented. Text and diagrams are keyed to audiotapes of examples that are provided for phonetic transcription exercises, listening to the taped examples and then taking taped quizzes. The tapes are actual clinical sessions of interviewers and responding children, designed to illustrate and train the student in recognizing and transcribing different phonetic classes of articulatory problems. In the last part of the study, acoustic phonetics is briefly presented in terms of some clinical problems. This order of presentation of phonetics seems eminently suitable for clinically oriented students. For those interested in acoustic phonetic analysis, there is a discussion of its future clinical use and a vendors listing of personal computer programs and systems. Another feature of the book is its well-chosen and keyed-to-text references to original clinical and research literature.

Fletcher, S. 1992. *Articulation: A Physiological Approach*. Singular Publishing, San Diego, CA. Samuel Fletcher is Dr. Palatograph, maestro of theory, instrumentation, and practice, in recording contact patterns of the tongue to the palate. Every phonetician can profit from a knowledge of the history and current contributions of palatography. The purpose for Fletcher's book is "to pave the way for the clinician to use the palatometer effectively and efficiently." The paving smooths out all the bumps the student might encounter in understanding the importance of tongue-palate events in speech articulation and the principles of recording and analysis of those events. Articulation of vowels, consonants, coarticulation and prosodics are presented. Issues of learning procedures for correct articulation skills are the basis for the second half of the book, on motor skill training in general, then speech articulations.

Baken, R. J. 1987. *Clinical Measurement of Speech and Voice*. Allyn and Bacon, Boston. This interesting textbook grew out of a Columbia University graduate seminar in speech pathology that reviewed the speech science literature for measurement methods, both current and future, that are used for diagnostic and therapeutic procedures. The text and its copious diagrams thoroughly explain all methods, beginning with a chapter on elementary electronic principles and ending with speech movement recording. Two middle chapters, on laryngeal function and on measuring velopharyngeal movements, are especially well worked out. The methods are largely pre-computer-age, but the basics of measurement here remain the same today. Tables of normative data for reference

are included and extended lists of original literature are provided.

Minifie, F. D. (Ed.) 1994. *Introduction to Communication Sciences and Disorders*. Singular Publishing, San Diego. To introduce first-course students to the enormous gamut of clinical and scientific interests that support the field of communication disorders four distinguished teachers and the publisher/speech scientist, Dr. Sadanand Singh, selected eighteen colleagues to write descriptions of their specialties, resulting, at 695 pages, in a volume of seemingly daunting scope. As study guides, each of the sixteen chapters begins with a few questions that the student should be able to answer from his or her study. These ask, for example, Who are speech-language pathologists, what do they do, and where? How do communication specialists take into account the cultural diversity of their clients? How is speech produced acoustically? How do infants and younger children learn to identify the sound patterns of the vowels and consonants? How does full language use develop? How are developmental disorders detected and rehabilitated? Other chapter topics present an environmental interactive systems approach to treating disorders, neural substrate and disordered brain functions, genetic factors, stuttering, hearing and its disorders, and "A Vision of the Future." Each chapter includes a glossary of special terms, references to selected original literature and further text readings.

PHONOLOGY

These books deal with phonology, the linguistics of phonetic patterns. Phonology describes the relationships between the sound-units or acoustic events of speech and the grammatical structures of languages. Grammar, in this broad linguistic sense, means the organizational, structural relations among all speech units: phonemes, syllables, phrases, word formation (morphology), syntax, sentences and paragraphs. Phonology is studied by linguists and by advanced students in communication sciences.

Maddieson, I. (1984). *Patterns of Sounds*.

Cambridge University Press, Cambridge. An omnibus of experimental phonology, except tonology and suprasegmentals, based on the UCLA Phonetics Laboratory's Phonological Segment Inventory Data Base, this remarkable book studies the consonant and vowel systems of 317 diverse languages to explore for universal phonetic tendencies and correlations with experimental data in the literature. For example, any of the languages that employs a given voiced fricative is likely also to employ the voiceless cognate; the tendency is unexceptional for /z, s/ (96 languages) but true for only 40 of the 51 languages here that employ /v/. Intense fricatives ought to be employed by more languages than use weak fricatives; for example /s/, intense as it is, occurs most frequently (in 83% of these languages). Separate chapters explore interesting tendencies for stops, fricatives, nasals, liquids, approximants, laryngealized consonants, vowels and vowel spacing. Chapters 1 and 10, on the design of the study, describe many of the endeavors of experimental linguists. Chapter references and a language data bibliography complete the encyclopedic, scholarly coverage. Appendices classify the languages by genetic relations and again by which languages employ each of the 668 phonemes, in phonetic classes; phonemes are also given in a manner-by-place chart for each language.

Pierrehumbert, J. and Beckman, M. 1988. *Japanese Tone Structure*. (No. 15 in Linguistic Inquiry Monographs). MIT Press, Cambridge, MA. An extended research report on generative theory of tonal phonology, the syllabic variations of voice pitch that are linguistically significant. A complete theory is formulated and investigated, covering the tonal phenomena of word-accent, phrasal accent, and the larger intonational structures of Japanese. English, Hausa, and Swedish tonal phenomena are briefly studied, for comparison with the Japanese findings. A theory of universal, hierarchical levels of tonal variation is proposed. This book is an exemplary research treatise for the advanced linguistics student in its melding of a universal theory with empirical phonetic measurement.

Liberman, M. Y. 1979. *The Intonational Sys-*

tem of English. Garland, NY. This is a discursive but intensive study of a model designed to generate intonational patterns of sentences from unit specifications of stress, emphasis or focus, and speaker's intention. A dissertation from MIT (1975), it presents an original, generative theory to account for voice pitch contours as affected by factors of sentence syntactic stress, speaker's intentions, and informational focus or emphasis. Examples of contours are given to illustrate each theoretical principle. Relations of the theory to other linguistic problems are analyzed. This work was seminal to the most important recent advances in intonation research, and it still provides a fascinating tutorial to introduce investigators to the current advances of linguistic phonetics toward a science of ordinary speech communication.

IMPAIRED SPEECH COMMUNICATION AND AIDS FOR THE HANDICAPPED

Gozy, M. 1992. *Speech Perception*. Forum Phoneticum n. 50, Hector, Frankfurt-am-Main. This extensive study was originally published in Hungarian in 1989, then supplemented and translated for publication in English. The work consists largely of experimental studies of acoustic-phonetic perception of Hungarian, by listeners with hearing impairment and by developing children. Some unusual variables tested are phonotactic structure, interference effects between speech bands for certain listeners and speech melody/stress-pattern perception. A hearing assessment test battery, GMP, employing well-researched synthetic words, some natural sentences, and other tests of speech perception, is developed. Preliminary studies are described to use the tests in prescribing frequency-selective hearing aids and other auditory rehabilitation procedures.

Plant, G., and Spens, K-E. (Eds.) 1995. *Profound Deafness and Speech Communication*. WHURR Publishers, London. In honor of Dr. Arne Risberg, a research engineer and Professor of Hearing Technology at the Royal Institute of Technology in Stockholm, Sweden, this volume summarizes some of the recent progress in processing and presenting speech to profoundly deaf people. The complete story of these developments over the past fifty years is now available with this book together with the 1979 reprint collection of Levitt, Pickett, and Houde, described below. There are twenty-six chapters on five major topics: Tactile Aids, Cochlear Implants, Speech Perception, Speech Production, and Computer-Based Training, written by many of the current prominent figures in speech trechnology for the deaf.

Levitt, H., Pickett, J. M., and Houde, R. (Eds.). 1979. *Sensory Aids for the Hearing-Impaired.* Institute of Electrical and Electronics Engineers, New York. (Order from IEEE Service Center, 445 Hoes Lane, Piscataway, NJ. 08854.) This is a reprint collection of over sixty important research papers and theoretical discussions on speech acoustics related to the following subjects: hearing aids, residual hearing aids and frequency lowering, visual and tactile speech for the deaf, and electrical hearing. The reader is oriented to each major area by extensive critical comments written by the editors. Some historical landmark papers are included. This compendium is a complete summary of the topic up to the burgeoning of the field in the computer age.

Ling, D. 1976. *Speech and the Hearing-Impaired Child: Theory and Practice.* Alexander Graham Bell Association, Washington, DC. A book reviewing the speech production problem of deaf children from a phonetic point of view and prescribing a systematic series of speech training procedures. This is a classic, unique in combining the practice and science of its time.

Winitz, H. (Ed.) 1995. *Human Communication and Its Disorders, A Review, Vol. IV.* York Press, Timonium, MD. This is a collection of extended review articles by prominent scientists in research on communication disorders. The authors and topics of the reviews are as follows: D. K. Oller, Development of Vocalizations in Infancy; M. L. Edwards, Developmental Phonology; N. Cowan and J. S. Saults, Memory for Speech; M. M. Parnell, Characteristics of Language-Disordered Children; J. L. Lauter, Visions of Speech and Language: Noninvasive [brain-] Imaging Techniques

and Their Applications to the Study of Human Communication. Excellent indexes for cited studies and authors are included.

Ohde, R. N., and Sharf, D. J. 1992. *Phonetic Analysis of Normal and Abnormal Speech.* Merrill/Macmillan, New York. This is an acoustic phonetics textbook designed especially for speech and language pathologists. It begins with the rudiments of spectrographic analysis of speech and then follows with a series of chapters covering all the articulatory features of most speech units and their perceptual distinctions for phonological function. Text explanations are copiously illustrated with spectrographic examples of normal and abnormal productions, and followed up for each major distinction with quiz questions, glossaries of the many phonetic terms introduced, and audiotape listening.

READING AND DYSLEXIA

The skill of reading is a phonetic ability to go "in reverse," from printed symbols to the phonetic code in which we mentally store linguistic information, and thus to understand the written-down speech of an author. So the scientific study of reading and its disorders has much to tell us about encoding and decoding in speech. The following books will give the phonetician an appreciation of some of this growing field.

Drake, D. D., and Gray, D. B. (Eds.) 1991. *The Reading Brain.* York Press, Timonium, MD. Neurologically minded pediatricians carry out biologically oriented research on reading. This book presents their research on developmental disorders of reading, relating clinical findings to brain function data, genetic background, phonetic perception research, diagnostic testing, and classification problems. The final chapter by Drake presents a detailed summary of the state of the science in bio-behavioral reading research.

Kavanagh, J. F. (Ed.) 1991. *The Language Continuum, from Infancy to Literacy.* York Press, Parkton, MD. This book collects the papers discussed at a conference on child reading problems in 1991, sponsored by the New York Branch of the Orton Dyslexia Society to present "current information about the acquisition and development of language, the uses to which it is put, and the difficulties some experience with it" . . . for "teachers, therapists, and parents." Learning of language is explained in terms of social interactions between very young children and their parents via special types of facilitation behaviors. Breakdowns in learning and difficulties such as dyslexia are due to insufficient or poorly integrated oral-to-print experiences. Sample normal language development schedules are presented. Phonetic decoding abilities are given primary remedial attention. The book is rich with references to the important scientific literature.

See also Brady and Shankweiler, under Speech Perception.

ENCYCLOPEDIAS

When working in the library, it's always rewarding to take a break with an encyclopedia: You get a respite from what you should be working on but are still learning something new. If the encyclopedia deals with speech, then you don't feel so guilty; you can even gain new perspectives due to the distinguished capabilities of the many authors of articles. For the phonetics student or scientist there are two new encyclopedias to look for:

Koerner, E. F. K., and Asher, R. E. 1994. *Encyclopedia of Language and Linguistics*. Ben-

jamins, London. This compendium emphasizes the classical topics in linguistics, but these are complemented by a wide variety of articles on phonetics and speech technology. There are many useful cross-references within articles.

Bright, W. (Ed.) 1992. *International Encyclopedia of Linguistics*. Oxford University Press, Oxford. See articles with the following titles: Acquisition of Language. Autosegmental Phonology. Generative Phonology. Metrical Phonology. Phonetics. Phonology. Prosodic Phonology. Syllables.

VIDEOS

Searchinger, Gene. Equinox Fifty Ways of Knowing, Inc. "The Human Language Series." This is a series of distinguished linguists filmed as lecturers or demonstrators on three videos: 1. Discovering the Human Language, "Colorless Green Ideas" (Universal Grammar). 2. Acquiring the Human Language. "Playing the Language Game." 3. The Human Language Evolves "With and Without Words." Ecstatic reviews. Shown on PBS in 1995. Some of the famous names who explain their work and theories are: Philip Lieberman, Noam Chomsky, Morris Halle, Alvin Liberman, Peter Ladefoged, Kim Oller, Rebecca Eilers, George Miller, Carol Padden, Steven Pinker, Ursula Bellugi, Russel Baker, Sid Caesar. Missing are many more acoustic scientists like Gunner Fant, Ludmilla Chistovich, John Ohala, Harry Levitt, Kathy Harris, Louis Pols, Janet Baker, Kenneth Stevens, Arthur House, Osamu Fujimura. (Available for rent or purchase from Transit Media, 22 Hollywood Ave., Hohokus, NJ 07423, purchase $200 per video; rent $75).

Abramson, A. S., & Lisker, L. (1967). Discrimination along the voicing continuum: Cross-language tests. *Status Report on Speech Research*, Haskins Laboratories, pp. 17–22.

Acero, A. (1993). *Acoustical and Environmental Robustness in Automatic Speech Recognition.* Boston: Kluwer Academic Publishers.

Acero, A., & Stern, R. M. (1990). Environmental robustness in automatic speech recognition. *Proceedings IEEE-ICASSP,* 849–852.

Allen, J., Klatt, D. H., & Hunnicutt, S. (1987). *From Text to Speech: The MITalk System.* Cambridge, UK: Cambridge University Press.

American National Standards Institute (ANSI). (1989). *Specification for Audiometers (ANSI S3.6-1989).* New York: Acoustical Society of America.

Anderson, S., & Kewley-Port, D. (1995). Evaluation of speech recognizers for speech training applications. *IEEE Speech and Audio Processing, 3,* 229–241.

Assmann, P. F. (1996). The role of formant transitions in the perception of concurrent vowels. *Journal of the Acoustical Society of America, 97,* 575–584.

Assmann, P. F., Nearey, T. M., & Hogan, J. T. (1982). Vowel identification: Orthographic, perceptual, and acoustic aspects. *Journal of the Acoustical Society of America, 71,* 975–989.

Atal, B. S., Miller, J. L., & Kent, R. D. (1991). *Papers in Speech Communication: Speech Processing.* Woodbury, NY: Acoustical Society of America.

Atkinson, J. (1978). Correlation analysis of the physiological factors controlling fundamental voice frequency. *Journal of the Acoustical Society of America, 63(1),* 211–222.

Baer, T. (1975). *Investigation of Phonation Using Excised Larynges.* Doctoral dissertation, Massachusetts Institute of Technology.

Baer, T. (1981). Investigation of the phonatory mechanism. *ASHA Reports, 11,* 38–47.

Baer, T., Gore, J. C., Gracco, L. C., & Nye, P. W. (1991). Analysis of vocal tract shape and dimensions using magnetic resonance imaging: Vowels. *Journal of the Acoustical Society of America, 79,* 799–828.

Bailey, P. J., & Summerfield, Q. (1980). Information in speech: Observations on the perception of [s]-stop clusters. *Journal of Experimental Psychology: Human Perception and Performance, 6,* 536–563.

Baker, J. (1989). DragonDictate—30K: Natural language speech recognition with 30,000 words. *Proceedings of Eurospeech 89,* Vol. II.

Balise, R. R., & Diehl, R. L. (1994). Some distributional facts about fricatives and a perceptual explanation. *Phonetica, 51,* 99–110.

Barrett, S. E. (1996). *The Influence of Phonetic Context on the Internal Structure of Speech Categories.* Department of Linguistics, University of Cambridge, manuscript.

Barry, W. J., Diehl, R. L., & Kohler, K. J. (Eds.). (1993). Prosody and information structure. *Phonetica, 50,* 145–210.

Beckman, M. E., Edwards, J., & Fletcher, J. (1992). Prosodic structure and tempo in a sonority model of articulatory dynamics. In G. Docherty & D. R. Ladd (Eds.), *Papers in Laboratory Phonology II: Segment, Gesture, and Tone.* Cambridge, UK: Cambridge University Press.

Beckman, M. E., Jung, T-P., Lee, S., de Jong, K., Krishnamurthy, A. K., Ahalt, S. C., Cohen, K. B., & Collins, M. J. (1995). Variability in the production of quantal vowels revisited. *Journal of the Acoustical Society of America, 97,* 471–490.

Behrens, S., & Blumstein, S. (1988). Acoustic characteristics of English voiceless fricatives: A descriptive analysis. *Journal of Phonetics, 16,* 295–298.

Benade, A. H. (1960). *Horns, Strings, and Harmony.* New York: Doubleday.

Bentler, R., & Pavlovic, C. (1989). Transfer functions and correction factors used in hearing aid evaluation and research. *Ear and Hearing, 10,* 58–63.

Berkovitz, R. A., & Pickett, J. M. (1992). Developments toward a computer-based course in acoustic phonetics (Abstract). *Journal of the Acoustical Society of America, 92,* 2320. (Full paper available from Sensimetrics Corp.)

Berry, D., & Titze, I. R. (1994). Unpublished data, courtesy Ingo R. Titze, Director, National Center for Voice and Speech, University of Iowa, Iowa City, IA.

Best, C. T. (1994). The emergence of native-language phonological influences in infants: A perceptual assimilation model. In J. C. Goodman & H. S. Nusbaum (Eds.), *The Development of Speech Perception: The Transition from Speech Sounds to Spoken Words* (pp. 167–224). Cambridge, MA: MIT Press.

Best, C. T. (1995). A direct realist view of cross-language speech perception. In W. Strange (Ed.), *Speech Perception and Linguistic Experience: Issues in Cross-Language Speech Research* (pp. 171–206). Baltimore: York Press.

Best, C. T., McRoberts, G. W., & Sithole, N. N. (1988). The phonological basis of perceptual loss for non-native contrasts: Maintenance of discrimination among Zulu clicks by English-speaking adults and children. *Journal of Experimental Psychology: Human Perception and Performance, 14,* 345–360.

Best, C. T., Morrongiello, B., & Robson, R. (1981). Perceptual equivalence of acoustic cues in speech and nonspeech perception. *Perception and Psychophysics, 29,* 191–211.

Bickley, C., & Stevens, K. N. (1986). Effects of a vocal tract constriction on the glottal source: Experimental and modeling studies. *Journal of Phonetics, 14,* 373–382.

Bilger, R., & Wang, M. (1976). Consonant confusions in patients with sensorineural hearing loss. *Journal of Speech and Hearing Research, 19,* 718–748.

Bladon, A., & Fant, G. (1978). A two-formant model and the cardinal vowels. *STL-QPRS, 1,* 18, Royal Institute of Technology, Stockholm, Sweden.

Blumstein, S. E., & Stevens, K. N. (1979). Acoustic invariance in speech production: Evidence from measurements of the spectral characteristics of stop consonants. *Journal of the Acoustical Society of America, 66,* 1001–1017.

Blumstein, S. E., & Stevens, K. N. (1980). Perceptual invariance and onset spectra for stop consonants in different vowel environments. *Journal of the Acoustical Society of America, 67,* 648–662.

Boothroyd, A. (1984). Auditory perception of speech contrasts by subjects with sensorineural hearing loss. *Journal of Speech and Hearing Research, 27,* 134–144.

Boothroyd, A. (1986). *SPAC Version II: A Test of Perception of Speech Pattern Contrasts (Report #RC120).* New York: City University.

Braude, W. G. (1992). *The Book of Legends from the Talmud and Midrash.* New York: Schocken Books. English translation of Bialik, H. N. & Ravnitsky, Y. H., *Sefer-Ha-Aggadah,* Odessa, 1908–1911.

Bregman, A. S. (1987). The meaning of duplex perception, Sounds as transparent objects. In M. E. H. Schouten (Ed.), *The Psychophysics of Speech Perception* (pp. 95–111). Dordrecht: M. Nijhoff.

Bregman, A. S. (1990). *Auditory Scene Analysis: The Perceptual Organization of Sound.* Cambridge, MA: MIT Press.

Browman, C. P., & Goldstein, L. M. (1986). Towards an articulatory phonology. *Phonology Yearbook, 3,* 219–252.

Browman, C. P., & Goldstein, L. M. (1992). Articulatory phonology: An overview. *Phonetica, 49,* 155–180.

Bunnell, H. T. (1998). Edwav: A PC-based program for interactive graphical display, measurement, and editing of speech and other signals. Freeware available from BUNNELL@asel.udel.edu.

Burgess, A. (1992). *A Mouthful of Air; Language, Languages...Especially English.* New York: William Morrow.

Burling, R. (1992). *Patterns of Language.* San Diego: Academic Press.

Byrne, D., Dillon, H., Tran, K., Arlinger, S., Bamford, J., et al. (1994). An international comparison of long-term average speech spectra. *Journal of the Acoustical Society of America, 96,* 2108–2120.

Cahn, J. E. (1990). The generation of affect in synthetic speech. *Journal of the American Voice Input/Output Society, 8,* 1–19.

Campbell, L. (1986). Testing phonology in the field. In J. J. Ohala & J. J. Jaeger (Eds.), *Experimental Phonology* (pp. 163–173). New York: Academic Press.

Campbell, N., & Black, A. W. (1995). Prosody and the selection of source units for concatenative synthesis. In J. P. H. van Santen, R. W. Sproat, J. Olive, & J. Hirschberg (Eds.), *Progress in Speech Synthesis* (pp. 279–292). New York: Springer.

Carhart, R. (1945). An improved method for classifying audiograms. *Laryngoscope, 55,* 640–642.

Carlson, R., Fant, G., & Granstrom, B. (1975). Two-formant models, pitch and vowel perception. In G. S. Fant & M. A. A. Tatham (Eds.), *Auditory Analysis and Perception of Speech* (pp. 55–82). New York: Academic.

Carlson, R., Granstrom, B., & Fant, G. (1970). Some studies concerning perception of isolated vowels.

Speech Transmission Laboratory: Quarterly Progress Report, 3–4, 84–104.

Carlson, R., Granstrom, B., & Hunnicutt, S. (1988). *Rulsys—The Swedish Multilingual Text-to-Speech Approach.* SST-88.

Carterette, E. C., & Jones, M. H. (1974). *Informal Speech.* Berkeley and Los Angeles: University of California Press.

Catford, J. C. (1988). *A Practical Introduction to Phonetics.* Oxford, UK: Clarendon Press.

Chiba, T., & Kajiyama, M. (1941). *The Vowel, Its Nature and Structure.* Tokyo: Tokyo-Kaiseikan.

Chigier, B., & Leung, H. C. (1992). The effects of signal representations, phonetic classification techniques, and the telephone network. *Proceedings ICSLP '92, 1,* 97–100.

Chistovich, L. A. (1985). Central auditory processing of peripheral vowel spectra. *Journal of the Acoustical Society of America, 77,* 789–805.

Chistovich, L. A., Pickett, J. M., & Porter, R. L. Jr. (1998). Speech research at the I. P. Pavlov Institute. *Proceedings of the International Congress of Acoustics and Acoustical Society of America,* June 1998, Seattle, WA.

Chomsky, N., & Halle, M. (1968). *The Sound Pattern of English.* New York: Harper & Row.

Clark, C., & Snell, K. (1993). Performance on speech perception measures by prelingually severely and profoundly hearing impaired young adults. *The Volta Review, 95,* 143–156.

Coker, C. (1967). A model of articulatory dynamics and control. *Proceedings of the IEEE, 64(4),* 452–460.

Cole, R., Hirschman, L., Atlas, L., Beckman, M., Bierman, A., et al. (1995). The challenge of spoken language systems: Research directions for the nineties. *IEEE Transactions on Speech and Audio Processing, 3(1),* 1–21.

Cole, R., Phillips, M., Brennan, R., & Chigier, B. (1986). The C-MU phonetic classification system. *Proceedings IEEE-ICASSP, 86,* 2255–2258.

Collier, R., Lisker, L., Hirose, H., & Ushijima, T. (1979). Voicing in intervocalic stops and fricatives in Dutch. *Journal of Phonetics.* (Collier.eml email requested reprint)

Compton, C. (1991). *Assistive Devices: Doorways to Independence.* Annapolis, MD: VanComp Associates.

Cooper, F. S., Delattre, P. C., Liberman, A. M., Borst, J. M., & Gerstman, L. J. (1952). Some experiments on the perception of speech sounds. *Journal of the Acoustical Society of America, 24,* 597–606. (reprinted as Chapter 3 in Liberman, 1996)

Crothers, J. H., Lorentz, J. P., Sherman, D. A., & Vihman, M. M. (1979). *Handbook of Phonological Data from a Sample of the World's Languages.* Palo Alto, CA: Stanford University.

Crystal, H., & House, A. (1982). Segmental durations in connected speech signals: Preliminary results. *Journal of the Acoustical Society of America, 72,* 705–716.

Cutler, A. (1986). Forbear is a homophone: Lexical prosody does not constrain lexical access. *Language and Speech, 29,* 201–220.

Danaher, E., Osberger, M., & Pickett, J. M. (1973). Discrimination of formant frequency transitions in synthetic vowels. *Journal of Speech and Hearing Research, 16,* 439–451.

Danaher, E., & Pickett, J. M. (1975). Some masking effects produced by low-frequency vowel formants in persons with sensorineural hearing loss. *Journal of Speech and Hearing Research, 18,* 261–271.

Dart, S. N. (1991). Articulatory and acoustic properties of apical and laminal articulations. *Working Papers in Phonetics, No. 79,* Linguistics Department, University of California, Los Angeles.

Darwin, C. J. (1991). The relationship between speech perception and perception of other sounds. In I. G. Mattingly & M. Studdert-Kennedy (Eds.), *Modularity and the Motor Theory of Speech Perception* (pp. 239–259). Hillsdale, NJ: Lawrence Erlbaum Associates.

Davis, B. L., & MacNeilage, P. F. (1995). The articulatory basis of babbling. *Journal of Speech and Hearing Research, 38,* 1199–1211.

Dechovitz, D. (1977). Information conveyed by vowels: A confirmation. *Status Report on Speech Research, SR 51/52,* 213–219 (Haskins Laboratories, New Haven, CT).

Deeks, J., & Faulkner, A. (1994). Residual spectral and temporal processing signaling timbre contrasts in synthetic vowels. *Speech, Hearing and Language, 8,* 141–162.

De Fillipo, C., & Clark, C. (1993). Use of ambiguous visual stimuli to demonstrate the value of acoustic cues in speech perception. *Journal of Communication Disorders, 26,* 29–51.

Delattre, P. (1965). *Comparing the Phonetic Features of English, French, German, and Spanish.* Heidelberg, Germany: Julius Groos Verlag.

Delattre, P. (1969). An acoustic and articulatory study of vowel reduction in four languages. *International Review of Applied Linguistics, 7,* 295–325.

Delattre, P., Liberman, A. M., Cooper, F. S., & Gerstman, L. J. (1952). An experimental study of the acoustic determinants of vowel color; observations on one- and two-formant vowels synthesized from spectrographic patterns. *Word, 8,* 195–210.

Denes, P. B. (1963). On the statistics of spoken English. *Journal of the Acoustical Society of America, 35,* 892–904.

Denes, P. B., & Pinson, E. N. (1995). *The Speech Chain. The Physics and Biology of Spoken Language* (2nd ed.). New York: W. H. Freeman.

Deng, L., & Sun, D. (1994). Phonetic classification and recognition using HMM representation of overlapping articulatory features for all classes of English sounds. *Proceedings IEEE-ICASSP, 94,* 45–48.

DiBenedetto, M-G. (1989a). Frequency and time variations of the first formant: Properties relevant to the perception of vowels' height. *Journal of the Acoustical Society of America, 86,* 67–77.

DiBenedetto, M-G. (1989b). Vowel representation: Some observations on temporal and spectral properties of the first formant frequency. *Journal of the Acoustical Society of America, 86,* 55–66.

Diehl, R. L. (1989). Remarks on Stevens' quantal theory of speech. *Journal of Phonetics, 17,* 71–78.

Diehl, R. L., & Kingston, J. (1991). Phonetic covariation as auditory enhancement: The case of the [+voice]/[-voice] distinction. In O. Engstrand & C. Kylander (Eds.), *Current Phonetic Research Paradigms: Implications for Speech Motor Control* (pp. 139–143). Stockholm: University of Stockholm, PERILUS 14.

Diehl, R. L., & Kluender, K. R. (1989a). On the objects of speech perception. *Ecological Psychology, 1,* 121–144.

Diehl, R. L., & Kluender, K. R. (1989b). Reply to the commentators. *Ecological Psychology, 1,* 195–225.

Diehl, R. L., Kluender, K. R., & Walsh, M. A. (1990). Some auditory bases of speech production and perception. In W. A. Ainsworth (Ed.), *Advances in Speech, Hearing and Language Processing* (pp. 243–268). London: JAI Press.

Dooling, R. J., Okanoya, K., & Brown, S. D. (1989). Speech perception by budgerigars (*Melopsittacus undulatus*): The voiced-voiceless distinction. *Perception and Psychophysics, 46,* 65–71.

Draper, M. H., Ladefoged, P., & Whitteridge, D. (1959). Respiratory muscles in speech. *Journal of Speech and Hearing Research, 2,* 16–27.

Dubno, J., Dirks, D., & Langhofer, L. (1982). Evaluation of hearing-impaired listeners using a nonsense-syllable test. II. Syllable recognition and consonant confusion patterns. *Journal of Speech and Hearing Research, 25,* 141–148.

Dubno, J., Dirks, D., & Schaefer, A. (1987). Effects of hearing loss on utilization of short-duration spectral cues in stop consonant recognition. *Journal of the Acoustical Society of America, 81,* 1940–1947.

Dubno, J., & Schaefer, A. (1992). Comparison of frequency selectivity and consonant recognition among hearing-impaired and masked normal-hearing listeners. *Journal of the Acoustical Society of America, 91,* 2110–2121.

Dubno, J., & Schaefer, A. (1995). Frequency selectivity and consonant recognition for hearing-impaired and normal-hearing listeners with equivalent masked thresholds. *Journal of the Acoustical Society of America, 97,* 1165–1174.

Dudley, H., & Tarnoczy, A. (1950). The speaking machine of Wolfgang von Kempelen. *Journal of the Acoustical Society of America, 22,* 151–166.

Dunn, H. K. (1950). The calculation of vowel resonances in an electrical vocal tract. *Journal of the Acoustical Society of America, 22,* 740–753.

Dutoit, T. (1997). *An Introduction to Text-to-Speech Synthesis.* Dordrecht/Boston/London: Kluwer.

Ehret, G. (1987). Categorical perception of sound signals: Facts and hypotheses from animal studies. In S. Harnad (Ed.), *Categorical Perception: The Groundwork of Perception* (pp. 301–331). Cambridge, UK: Cambridge University Press.

Eilers, R. E. (1980). Infant speech perception: History and mystery. In G. H. Yeni-Komshian, J. F. Kavanagh, & C. A. Ferguson (Eds.), *Child Phonology, Vol. 2 Perception* (pp. 23–39). New York: Academic Press.

Eilers, R. E., Gavin, W., & Oller, D. K. (1982). Cross-linguistic perception in infancy: Early effects of linguistic experience. *Journal of Child Language, 9,* 289–302.

Eimas, P. D., & Corbit, J. D. (1973). Selective adaptation of linguistic feature detectors. *Cognitive Psychology, 4,* 99–109.

Eimas, P. D., & Miller, J. L. (1978). Effects of selective adaptation on the perception of speech and visual patterns: Evidence for feature detectors. In R. D. Walk & H. L. Pick (Eds.), *Perception and Experience* (pp. 307–345). New York: Plenum Press.

Eimas, P. D., Miller, J. L., & Jusczyk, P. W. (1987). On infant speech perception and the acquisition of language. In S. Harnad (Ed.), *Categorical Perception: The Groundwork of Perception* (pp. 161–195).

Eimas, P. D., Siqueland, E. R., Jusczyk, P., & Vigorito, J. (1971). Speech perception in infant. *Science, 171,* 303–306.

Elman, J. L., & McClelland, J. L. (1986). Exploiting lawful variability in the speech waveform. In J. S. Perkell & D. H. Klatt (Eds.), *Invariance and Variability in Speech Processes* (pp. 360–385). Hillsdale, NJ: Erlbaum.

Elman, J. L., & McClelland, J. L. (1988). Cognitive penetration of the mechanisms of perception: Compensation for coarticulation of lexically restored phonemes. *Journal of Memory and Language, 27,* 143–165.

Engstrand, O. (1992). Systematicity of phonetic variation in natural discourse. *Speech Communication, 11,* 337–346.

Erber, N. (1972). Auditory, visual, and auditory-visual recognition of consonants by children with normal and impaired hearing. *Journal of Speech and Hearing Research, 15,* 413–422.

Erber, N. (1979). Speech perception by profoundly hearing impaired children. *Journal of Speech and Hearing Research, 44,* 255–270.

Espy-Wilson, C. (1992). Acoustic measures for linguistic features distinguishing the semivowels /wjrl/ in American English. *Journal of the Acoustical Society of America, 92,* 736–757.

Fant. G. (1959). Acoustic description and classification of phonetic units. Ericsson Technics No. 1 (reprinted in Fant, 1973).

Fant, G. (1960). *Acoustic Theory of Speech Production.* The Hague: Mouton.

Fant, G. (1968). Analysis and synthesis of speech processes. In B. Malmberg (Ed.), *Manual of Phonetics* (pp. 173–277). Amsterdam: North-Holland.

Fant, G. (1973). *Speech Sounds and Features.* Cambridge, MA: MIT Press.

Fant, G., & Kruckenberg, A. (1995). Notes on syllable duration in French and Swedish. *Proceedings of the International Congress of Phonetic Sciences,* pp. 158–161.

Fant, G., & Kruckenberg, A., & Nord, L. (1991). Durational correlates of stress in Swedish, French and English. *Journal of Phonetics, 19,* 351–365.

Fant, G., & Lin, Q. (1991). Comments on glottal flow modelling and analysis. In J. Gauffin & B. Hammarberg (Eds.), *Vocal Fold Physiology* (pp. 47–56). San Diego: Singular.

Farnsworth, D. W. (1940). High-speed motion pictures of the human vocal cords. *Bell Laboratories Record, 18,* 203–208.

Faulkner, A. (on behalf of the STRIDE Consortium). (1994). The stride project. *Speech, Hearing and Language: Work in Progress, 8,* 165–179. Department of Phonetics and Linguistics, University College, London.

Faulkner, A., Ball, V., & Rosen, S. (1992). Speech pattern hearing aids for the profoundly hearing impaired: Speech perception and auditory abilities. *Journal of the Acoustical Society of America, 91,* 2136–2155.

Ferguson, C. A. (1986). Discovering sound units and constructing sound systems: It's child's play. In J. S. Perkell & D. H. Klatt (Eds.), *Invariance and Variability in Speech Processes* (pp. 36–51). Hillsdale, NJ: Erlbaum.

Ferguson, C. A., Menn, L., & Stoel-Gammon, C. (1992). *Phonological Development: Models, Research, Implications.* Timonium, MD: York.

Fernald, A. (1992). Human maternal vocalizations to infants as biologically relevant signals: An evolutionary perspective. In J. H. Barkow, L. Cosmides, & J. Tooby (Eds.), *The Adapted Mind* (pp. 391–428). New York: Oxford University Press.

Finkelhor, B. K., Titze, I. R., & Durham, P. L. (1988). Effect of viscosity changes in the vocal folds on range of oscillation. *Journal of Voice, 1,* 320–325.

Fitch, H. L., Halwes, T., Erickson, D. M., & Liberman, A. M. (1980). Perceptual equivalence of two acoustic cues for stop-consonant manner. *Perception and Psychophysics, 27,* 343–350.

Fitzgibbons, P., & Wightman, F. (1982). Gap detection in normal and hearing-impaired listeners. *Journal of the Acoustic Society of America, 72,* 650–655.

Flanagan, J. L. (1958). Some properties of the glottal sound source. *Journal of Speech and Hearing Research, 1,* 99–116.

Flanagan, J. L. (1972). *Speech Analysis Synthesis and Perception.* New York: Springer.

Flanagan, J. L., & Landgraf, L. (1968). Self-oscillating source for vocal tract synthesizers. *IEEE Transmission, Audio, and Electroacoustics, AU-16(1)*.

Flanagan, J. L., Rabiner, L., Christopher, D., Boch, D., & Shipp, T. (1976). Digital analysis of laryngeal control in speech production. *Journal of the Acoustical Society of America, 60,* 446–455.

Fletcher, N. H. (1992). *Acoustic Systems in Biology.* New York: Oxford University Press.

Fletcher, W. W. (1950). *A Study of Internal Laryngeal Activity in Relation to Vocal Intensity.* PhD thesis, Northwestern University, Evanston, IL.

Fodor, J. (1983). *The Modularity of Mind.* Cambridge, MA: MIT Press.

Fowler, C. A. (1984). Segmentation of coarticulated speech in perception. *Perception and Psychophysics, 36,* 359–368.

Fowler, C. A. (1986). An event approach to the study of speech perception from a direct-realist perspective. *Journal of Phonetics, 14,* 3–28.

Fowler, C. A. (1989). Real objects of speech perception: A commentary on Diehl and Kluender. *Ecological Psychology, 1,* 145–160.

Fowler, C. A. (1994). Speech perception: Direct realist theory. In R. E. Asher (Ed.), *The Encyclopedia of Language and Linguistics* (pp. 4199–4203). Oxford: Pergamon.

Fowler, C. A. (1996a). Listeners do hear sounds, not tongues. *Journal of the Acoustical Society of America, 99,* 1730–1741.

Fowler, C. A. (1996b). Speech production. In J. L. Miller & P. D. Eimas (Eds.), *Speech, Language, and Communication* (pp. 30–61). San Diego: Academic.

Fowler, C. A., Best, C. T., & McRoberts, G. W. (1990). Young infants' perception of liquid coarticulatory influences on following stop consonants. *Perception and Psychophysics, 48,* 559–570.

Fowler, C. A., & Housum, J. (1987). Talkers' signalling of "new" and "old" words in speech and listeners' perception and use of the distinction. *Journal of Memory and Language, 26,* 489–504.

Fowler, C. A., & Rosenblum, L. D. (1991). The perception of phonetic gestures. In I. G. Mattingly & M. Studdert-Kennedy (Eds.), *Modularity and the Motor Theory of Speech Perception: Proceedings of a Conference to Honor Alvin M. Liberman* (pp. 33–59). Hillsdale, NJ: Erlbaum.

Fowler, C. A., & Smith, M. R. (1986). Speech perception as vector analysis: An approach to the prob-lem of invariance and segmentation. In J. S. Perkell & D. H. Klatt (Eds.), *Invariance and Variability in Speech Processes* (pp. 123–136). Hillsdale, NJ: Erlbaum.

Fox, R. A. (1984). Effect of lexical status on phonetic categorization. *Journal of Experimental Psychology: Human Perception and Performance, 10,* 526–540.

Frauenfelder, U. H., & Tyler, L. K. (1987). *Spoken Word Recognition.* Cambridge, MA: MIT Press. (Reprinted from *Cognition: International Journal of Cognitive Science, 25*)

Fromkin, V. (1972).On the reality of linguistic constructs. In A. Rigault & R. Charbonneau (Eds.), *Proceedings of the VIIth International Congress of Phonetic Sciences* (pp. 1107–1110), Montreal. The Hague: Mouton.

Fry, D. B. (1964). The function of the syllable. *Z. Phon. Sprachwiss. Kommunikationsforsch, 17,* 215–221.

Fry, D. B., Abramson, A. S., Eimas, P. D., & Liberman, A. M. (1962). The identification and discrimination of synthetic vowels. *Language and Speech, 1,* 35–58.

Fujimura, O. (1961). Bilabial stop and nasal consonants: A motion picture study and its implications. *Journal of Speech and Hearing Research, 4,* 233–247.

Fujimura, O. (1962). Analysis of nasal consonants. *Journal of the Acoustical Society of America, 34,* 1865–1875.

Fujimura, O. (1972). Acoustics of speech. In J. Gilbert (Ed.), *Speech and Cortical Functioning* (Chapter 3). New York: Academic. (On various voicing features, see especially pp. 131–137.)

Fujimura, O., & Lovins, J. (1978). Syllables as concatenative phonetic elements. In A. Bell & J. B. Hooper (Eds.), *Syllables and Segments* (pp. 107–120). New York: North-Holland.

Fujisaki, H., & Kawashima, T. (1968). The role of pitch and the higher formants in the perception of vowels. *IEEE Transmission, Audio, and Electroacoustics, AU-16,* 73–77.

Galyas, K., Fant, G., & Hunnicutt, S. (1992). *Voice Output Communication Aids.* Stockholm, Sweden: Swedish Handicap Institute.

Ganong, W. F. (1980). Phonetic categorization in auditory word perception. *Journal of Experimental Psychology: Human Perception and Performance, 6,* 110–125.

Gaur, A. (1992). *A History of Writing.* New York: Cross River Press.

Gay, T. (1977). Articulatory movements in VCV sequences. *Status Report on Speech Research, SR-49*, 121–147. Haskins Laboratories, Yale University, New Haven, CT.

Gay, T. (1978). Effect of speaking rate on vowel formant movements. *Journal of the Acoustical Society of America, 63(1)*, 223–230.

Ghitza, O. (1994). Auditory models and human performance in tasks related to speech coding and speech recognition. *IEEE Speech and Audio Processing, 2(1)*, part ii, 115–132.

Gibson, E. J. (1991). *An Odyssey in Learning and Perception.* Cambridge, MA: Bradford Books (MIT Press).

Gibson, J. J. (1966). *The Senses Considered as Perceptual Systems.* Boston: Houghton Mifflin.

Gibson, J. J. (1979). *The Ecological Approach to Visual Perception.* Boston: Houghton Mifflin.

Gierut, J. A., Morrisette, M. L., Hughes, M. T., & Rowland, S. (1995, in press). Phonological treatment efficacy and developmental norms. *Language, Speech and Hearing Services in Schools.*

Godfrey, J., & Millay, K. (1978). Perception of rapid spectral change in speech by listeners with mild and moderate sensorineural hearing loss. *Journal of the American Audiological Society, 3*, 200–206.

Godfrey, J., & Millay, K. (1980). Perception of synthetic speech sounds by hearing-impaired listeners. *Journal of Auditory Research, 20*, 187–203.

Goldinger, S. D., Palmieri, T. J., & Pisoni, D. B. (1992). Words and voices: Perceptual details are preserved in lexical representations. In J. J. Ohala, T. M. Nearey, B. L. Derwing, M. M. Hodge, & G. E. Weibe (Eds.), *Proceedings ICSLP-92 (1992 International Conference on Spoken Language Processing), 1*, 591–594.

Goldsmith, J. A. (1990). *Autosegmental and Metrical Phonology.* Oxford: Blackwell.

Gorin, A. (1995). On automated language acquisition. *Journal of the Acoustical Society of America, 97(6)*, 3441–3461.

Gottfried, T. L., & Strange, W. (1980). Identification of coarticulated vowels. *Journal of the Acoustical Society of America, 68*, 1626–1635.

Gregory, R. L. (1970). *The Intelligent Eye.* London: Weidenfeld and Nicolson.

Grosjean, F., & Gee, J. P. (1987). Prosodic structure and spoken word recognition. in U. H. Frauenfelder & L. K. Tyler (Eds.), *Spoken Word Recognition* (pp. 135–155). Cambridge, MA: MIT Press.

Halle, M. (1992). Phonological features. In W. Bright (Ed.), *International Encyclopedia of Linguistics* (pp. 207–212). Oxford: Oxford University Press.

Halle, M., & Stevens, K. N. (1991). Knowledge of language and sounds of speech. In J. Sundberg, L. Nord, & R. Carlson (Eds.), *Music, Language and Brain* (pp. 1–19). London: Macmillan.

Harley, T. A. (1995). *The Psychology of Language: From Data to Theory.* Hove, UK: Erlbaum (UK: Taylor and Francis).

Harnad, S. (1987). *Categorical Perception.* Cambridge, UK: Cambridge University Press.

Harrington, J. (1994). The contribution of the murmur and vowel to the place of articulation distinction in nasal consonants. *Journal of the Acoustical Society of America, 96*, 19–32.

Harris, K. S. (1974). Physiological aspects of articulatory behavior. In T. A. Sebeok (Ed.), *Current Trends in Linguistics* (12, Part 4, pp. 2281–2302). The Hague: Mouton.

Harris, K. S., & Bell-Berti, F. (1984). On consonants and syllable boundaries. In L. Raphael, G. Raphael, & M. Valvinos (Eds.), *Language and Cognition* (pp. 89–95). New York: Plenum.

Hawkins, S. (1992). An introduction to task dynamics. In G. J. Docherty & D. R. Ladd (Eds.), *Papers in Laboratory Phonology II: Gesture, Segment, Prosody* (pp. 9–25). Cambridge, UK: Cambridge University Press.

Hawkins, S. (1994). Quantal theory of speech. In R. E. Asher (Ed.), *The Encyclopedia of Language and Linguistics* (6, pp. 3417–3420). Oxford: Pergamon.

Hawkins, S. (1995). Arguments for a nonsegmental view of speech perception. In K. Elenius & P. Branderud (Eds.), *Proceedings of the XIIIth Congress of Phonetic Sciences* (3, pp. 18–25). Stockholm, Sweden: KTH and Stockholm University.

Hawkins, S., & Stevens, K. N. (1985). Acoustic and perceptual correlates of the nasal-nonnasal distinction for vowels. *Journal of the Acoustical Society of America, 77*, 1560–1575.

Hawkins, S., & Warren, P. (1994). Implications for lexical access of phonetic influences on the intelligibility of conversational speech. *Journal of Phonetics, 22*, 493–511.

Hazan, V., & Fourcin, A. (1985). Microprocessor-controlled speech pattern audiometry. *Audiology, 24*, 325–335.

Hebb, D. O. (1949). *The Organization of Behavior.* New York: Wiley.

Hedrick, M., Schulte, L., & Jesteadt, W. (1995). Effect of relative and overall amplitude on perception of voiceless stop consonants by listeners with normal and impaired hearing. *Journal of the Acoustical Society of America, 98,* 1292–1303.

Heinz, J. M., & Stevens, K. N. (1961). On the properties of voiceless fricative consonants. *Journal of the Acoustical Society of America, 33,* 589–596.

Henton, C., Ladefoged, P., & Maddieson, I. (1992). Stops in the world's languages. *Phonetica, 49,* 65–101.

Hirano, M., & Kakita, Y. (1985). Cover-body theory of vocal cord vibration. In R. G. Daniloff (Ed.), *Speech Science* (pp. 1–46). San Diego: College-Hill Press (now Singular).

Hirano, M., & Ohala, J. J. (1969). Use of hooked-wire electrodes for electromyography of the intrinsic laryngeal muscles. *Journal of Speech and Hearing Research,* 12, 362–373.

Hirano, M., & Sato, K. (1993). *Histological Color Atlas of the Human Larynx.* San Diego: Singular.

Hirose, H., & Gay, T. (1972). The activity of the intrinsic laryngeal muscles in voicing control: An electromyographic study. *Phonetica, 25,* 140–164.

Hixon, T. J. (and collaborators). (1987). *Respiratory Function in Speech and Song.* Boston: College-Hill Press.

Holden-Pitt, L., Hazan, V., Revoile, S., Edward, D., & Droge, J. (1995). Temporal and spectral cue-use for initial-plosive voicing perception by hearing children and adults and hearing-impaired children. *European Journal of Disorders in Communication, 30,* 417–434.

Holden-Pitt, L., Revoile, S., & Pickett, J. M. (1991). Hearing-impaired and normal-hearing adults' use of low-frequency cues to initial fricative voicing. *Proceedings of the International Congress of Phonetic Sciences,* Aix-en-Provence, France.

Holmberg, E. B., Hillman, R. E., & Perkell, J. S. (1988). Glottal airflow and transglottal air pressure measurements for male and female speakers in soft, normal, and loud voice. *Journal of the Acoustical Society of America, 84,* 511–529.

Holmberg, E. B., Hillman, R. E., & Perkell, J. S. (1989). Glottal airflow and transglottal air pressure measurements for male and female speakers in low, normal, and high pitch. *Journal of Voice, 3,* 294–305.

Honda, K. (1996). Organization of tongue articulation for vowels. *Journal of Phonetics, 24,* 39–52.

Houde, R. A. (1968). *A Study of Tongue Body Motion during Selected Speech Sounds.* SCRL Monograph No. 2. Santa Barbara, CA: Speech Communication Research Laboratory.

House, A. S. (1957). Analog studies of nasal consonants. *Journal of Speech and Hearing Disorders, 22,* 190–204.

House, A. S., & Stevens, K. N. (1956). Analog studies of the nasalization of vowels. *Journal of Speech and Hearing Disorders, 21,* 218–232.

Huang, C. B. (1985). *Perceptual Correlates of the Tense/Lax Distinction in General American English.* Master's thesis, MIT, Cambridge, MA.

Huang, H. S., & Hanley, J. R. (1995). Phonological awareness and visual skills in learning to read Chinese and English. *Cognition, 54,* 73–98.

Hunnicutt, S. (1987). Acoustic correlates of redundancy and intelligibility. *Speech Transmission Laboratory-Quarterly Progress and Status Report, 2–3,* 7–14. Stockholm, Sweden: KTH.

Hunt, A. J., & Black, A. W. (1996). Unit selection in a concatenative speech synthesis system using a large speech database. *Proceedings of IEEE-ICASSP, 96,* 373–376.

Ishizaka, K., & Flanagan, J. (1972). Synthesis of voiced sounds from a two-mass model of the vocal cords, *Bell System Technology Journal, 51,* 1233–1268.

Ishizaka, K., & Matsudaira, M. (1968). What makes the vocal cords vibrate. *Reports of the VIth International Congress of Acoustics,* paper B1-3. Tokyo: Maruzev.

Iverson, P., & Kuhl, P. K. (1995). Mapping the perceptual magnet effect for speech using signal detection theory and multidimensional scaling. *Journal of the Acoustical Society of America, 97,* 553–562.

Iverson, P., & Kuhl, P. K. (1996). Influences of phonetic identification and category goodness on American listeners' perception of /r/ and /l/. *Journal of the Acoustical Society of America, 99,* 1130–1140.

Jakobson, R., Fant, G., & Halle, M. (1951). *Preliminaries to Speech Analysis: The Distinctive Features and Their Correlates.* Technical Report 13, Acoustics Laboratory, MIT, Cambridge, MA. (reprinted 1967 by MIT Press, Cambridge, MA)

Jenkins, J. J., Strange, W., & Edman, T. R. (1983). Identification of vowels in "vowelless" syllables. *Perception and Psychophysics, 34,* 441–450.

Johnson, K. (1990). The role of perceived speaker identity in F0 normalization of vowels. *Journal of the Acoustical Society of America, 88,* 642–654.

Johnson, T. L., & Strange, W. (1982). Perceptual constancy of vowels in rapid speech. *Journal of the Acoustical Society of America, 72,* 1761–1770.

Joos, M. (1948). Acoustic phonetics. *Language, 24 (suppl. 2)* (also published in 1948 as Language Monograph No. 23, Linguistic Society of America, Waverly Press, Baltimore).

Jordan, M. (1986). *Serial Order: A Parallel Distributed Process.* La Jolla/San Diego: University of California, Institute for Cognitive Science, Report 8604.

Jusczyk, P. W. (1986a). Toward a model of the development of speech perception. In J. S. Perkell & D. H. Klatt (Eds.), *Invariance and Variability in Speech Processes* (pp. 1–19). Hillsdale, NJ: Erlbaum.

Jusczyk, P. W. (1986b). Speech perception. In K. R. Boff, L. Kaufman, & J. P. Thomas (Eds.), *Handbook of Perception and Human Performance* (pp. 27–57). New York: Wiley.

Jusczyk, P. W. (1994). Infant speech perception and the development of the mental lexicon. In J. C. Goodman & H. C. Nusbaum (Eds.), *The Development of Speech Perception: The Transition from Speech Sounds to Spoken Words* (pp. 227–270). Cambridge, MA: MIT Press.

Jusczyk, P. W. (1997). *The Discovery of Spoken Language.* Cambridge, MA: MIT Press.

Jusczyk, P. W., Hohne, E. A., & Mandel, D. R. (1995). Picking up regularities in the sound structure of the native language. In W. Strange (Ed.), *Speech Perception and Linguistic Experience: Theoretical and Methodological Issues in Cross-Language Speech Research* (pp. 91–120). Baltimore: York.

Kakita, Y., Hirano, M., & Ohmaru, K. (1981). Physical properties of vocal fold tissue: Measurements on excised larynges. In K. N. Stevens & M. Hirano (Eds.), *Vocal Fold Physiology.* Tokyo: University of Tokyo Press.

Karlsson, I. (1985). Glottal waveforms for normal and female speakers. *Quarterly Progress and Status Report, Speech Transmission Laboratory, 1985/1,* 31–36. Royal Institute of Technology, Stockholm, Sweden.

Keating, P. A. (1985). Universal phonetics and the organization of grammars. In V. Fromkin (Ed.), *Phonetic Linguistics* (pp. 115–132). San Diego: Academic.

Keating, P. A. (1991). Phonetics in the next ten years. *Proceedings of the XIIth International Congress of Phonetic Sciences, 2,* 112–119.

Kelso, J. A. S., & Munhall, K. G. [K&M]. (1988). *R. H. Stetson's Motor Phonetics: A Retrospective Edition.* Boston: College-Hill (Little Brown).

Kelso, J. A. S., Saltzman, E. L., & Tuller, B. (1986). The dynamical perspective on speech production: Data and theory. *Journal of Phonetics, 14,* 29–59.

Kent, R. D., & Moll, K. L. (1969). Vocal tract characteristics of the stop cognates. *Journal of the Acoustical Society of America, 46,* 1549–1555.

Kent, R. D., & Read, C. (1992). *The Acoustical Analysis of Speech.* San Diego: Singular.

Kewley-Port, D. (1982). Measurement of formant transitions in naturally produced stop consonant-vowel syllables. *Journal of the Acoustical Society of America, 72,* 379–389.

Kewley-Port, D. (1983). Time-varying features as correlates of place of articulation in stop consonants. *Journal of the Acoustical Society of America, 73,* 322–335.

Kewley-Port, D., & Watson, C. S. (1995). Computer assisted speech training: Practical considerations. In A. Syrdal, R. Bennett, & S. Greenspan (Eds.), *Applied Speech Technology* (pp. 565–582). Boca Raton, FL: CRC.

Kewley-Port, D., Watson, C. S., Elbert, M., Maki, D., & Reed, D. (1987). Speaker-dependent speech recognition as the basis for a speech training aid. *Proceedings IEEE-ICASSP, 87,* 372–375.

Kingston, J., & Diehl, R. L. (1994). Phonetic knowledge. *Language, 70,* 419–454.

Kingston, J., & Diehl, R. L. (1995). Intermediate properties in the perception of distinctive feature values. In B. Connell & A. Arvaniti (Eds.), *Phonology and Phonetic Evidence: Papers in Laboratory Phonology IV* (pp. 7–27). Cambridge, UK: Cambridge University Press.

Klatt, D. (1973). Interaction between two factors that influence vowel duration. *Journal of the Acoustical Society of America, 54,* 1102–1104.

Klatt, D. (1975). Vowel lengthening is syntactically determined in a connected discourse. *Journal of Phonetics, 3,* 129–140.

Klatt, D. (1976). Linguistic uses of segmental duration in English: Acoustic and perceptual evidence. *Journal of the Acoustical Society of America, 59,* 1208–1221.

Klatt, D. (1979). Speech perception: A model of acoustic-phonetic analysis and lexical access. *Journal of Phonetics, 7,* 279–312.

Klatt, D. (1989). Review of selected models of speech perception. In W. Marslen-Wilson (Ed.), *Lexical Representation and Process* (pp. 169–226). Cambridge, MA: MIT Press.

Klatt, D., & Klatt, L. C. (1990). Analysis, synthesis, and perception of voice quality variations among male and female talkers. *Journal of the Acoustical Society of America, 87,* 820–857.

Kleijn, W. B., & Paliwal, K. K. (Eds.). (1995). *Speech Coding and Synthesis.* Amsterdam: Elsevier.

Kluender, K. R. (1991). Effects of first formant onset properties on voicing judgments result from processes not specific to humans. *Journal of the Acoustical Society of America, 90,* 83–96.

Kluender, K. R., Diehl, R. L., & Killeen, P. R. (1987). Japanese quail can learn phonetic categories. *Science, 237,* 1195–1197.

Kluender, K. R. & Lotto, A. J. (1994). Effects of first formant onset frequency on [-voice] judgments result from auditory processes not specific to humans. *Journal of the Acoustical Society of America, 95,* 1044–1052.

Kozhevnikov, V. A., & Chistovich, L. A. (1965). *Speech: Articulation and Perception* [Rech: Artikulyatsiya i Vospriyatiye, Moscow-Leningrad]. Translated by the Joint Publications Research Service, Clearinghouse for Federal Scientific and Technical Information, U.S. Department of Commerce, Washington, DC 20043 (publication nos. JPRS: 30, 543; TT: 65–31233).

Krakow, R. A., Beddor, P. S., Goldstein, L. M., & Fowler, C. A. (1988). Coarticulatory influences on the perceived height of nasal vowels. *Journal of the Acoustical Society of America, 83,* 1146–1158.

Kuehn, D. P., & Moll, K. L. (1976). A cineradiographic study of VC and CV articulatory velocities. *Journal of Phonetics, 4,* 830–843.

Kuhl, P. K. (1979). Speech perception in early infancy: Perceptual constancy for spectrally dissimilar vowel categories. *Journal of the Acoustical Society of America, 66,* 1668–1679.

Kuhl, P. K. (1980). Perceptual constancy for speech-sound categories in early infancy. In G. H. Yeni-Komshian, J. F. Kavanagh, & C. A. Ferguson (Eds.), *Child Phonology, Vol, 2, Perception* (pp. 41–66). New York: Academic.

Kuhl, P. K. (1983). Perception of auditory equivalence classes for speech in early infancy. *Infant Behavior and Development, 6,* 263–285.

Kuhl, P. K. (1986). Infants' perception of speech: Constraints on characterisation of the initial state. In B. Lindblom & R. Zetterstrom (Eds.), *Precursors of Early Speech* (pp. 219–244). Basingstoke: Macmillan.

Kuhl, P. K. (1987). The special-mechanisms debate in speech research: Categorization tests in animals and infants. In S. Harnad (Ed.), *Categorical Perception* (pp. 355–586). Cambridge, UK: Cambridge University Press.

Kuhl, P. K. (1991). Human adults and human babies show a "perceptual magnet effect" for the prototypes of speech categories, monkeys do not. *Perception and Psychophysics, 50,* 93–107.

Kuhl, P. K., Andruski, J. E., Chistovich, I. A., Chistovich, L. A., & Kozhevnikova, E. A. (1997). Cross-language analysis of phonetic units in language addressed to infants, *Science, 277,* 684–686.

Kuhl, P. K., & Iverson, P. (1995). Linguistic experience and the "perceptual magnet effect." In W. Strange (Ed.), *Speech Perception and Linguistic Experience: Theoretical and Methodological Issues in Cross-Language Speech Research* (pp. 121–154). Baltimore: York.

Kuhl, P. K., & Miller, J. D. (1975). Speech perception by the chinchilla: Voiced-voiceless distinction in alveolar plosive consonants. *Science, 190,* 69–72.

Kuhl, P. K., & Miller, J. D. (1978). Speech perception by the chinchilla: Identification functions for synthetic VOT stimuli. *Journal of the Acoustical Society of America, 63,* 905–917.

Kuhl, P. K., & Padden, D. M. (1983). Enhanced discriminability at the phonetic boundaries for the place feature in macaques. *Journal of the Acoustical Society of America, 73,* 1003–1010.

Kuhl, P. K., Williams, K. A., Lacerda, F., Stevens, K. N., & Lindblom, B. (1992). Linguistic experience alters phonetic perception in infants by 6 months of age. *Science, 255,* 606–608.

Kuhl, P. K., Williams, K. A., & Meltzoff, A. N. (1991). Cross-modal speech perception in adults and infants using nonspeech auditory stimuli. *Journal of Experimental Psychology: Perception and Performance, 17,* 829–840.

Kurowski, K., & Blumstein, S. E. (1987). Acoustic properties for place of articulation in nasal consonants. *Journal of the Acoustical Society of America, 81,* 1917–1927.

Labov, W. (1972). *Sociolinguistic Patterns*. Philadelphia: University of Pennsylvania Press.

Ladefoged, P. (1963). Some physiological parameters in speech. *Language and Speech, 6,* 109–119.

Ladefoged, P. (1967). *Three Areas of Experimental Phonetics*. London: Oxford University Press.

Ladefoged, P. (1971). *Preliminaries to Linguistic Phonetics*. Chicago: University of Chicago Press.

Ladefoged, P. (1993). *A Course in Phonetics* (3rd ed.). Orlando, FL: Harcourt, Brace, Jovanovich.

Ladefoged, P. (1995). The sounds of disappearing languages. *Echoes,* newsletter of the Acoustical Society of America, *5(1).*

Ladefoged, P. (1996). *Elements of Acoustic Phonetics* (2nd ed.). Chicago: University of Chicago Press.

Ladefoged, P., & Bhaskararao, P. (1983). Non-quantal aspects of consonant production: A study of retroflex consonants. *Journal of Phonetics, 11,* 291–302.

Ladefoged, P., & Broadbent, D. E. (1957). Information conveyed by vowels. *Journal of the Acoustical Society of America, 29,* 98–104.

Ladefoged, P., & Maddieson, I. (1988). *Language, Speech and Mind: Studies in Honour of Victoria Fromkin* (pp. 49–61). London: Routledge.

Ladefoged, P., & Maddieson, I. (1995). *Sounds of the World's Languages*. London: Blackwell.

Lahiri, A., Gewirth, L., & Blumstein, S. E. (1984). A reconsideration of acoustic invariance for place of articulation in diffuse stop consonants: Evidence from a cross-language study. *Journal of the Acoustical Society of America, 76,* 391–404.

Lane, H. L. (1965). Motor theory of speech perception: A critical review. *Psychological Review, 72,* 275–309.

Lasky, R. E., Syrdal-Lasky, A., & Klein, R. E. (1975). VOT discrimination by four to six and a half month old infants from Spanish environments. *Journal of Experimental Child Psychology, 20,* 221–225.

Laver, J. (1994). *Principles of Phonetics*. Cambridge, UK: Cambridge University Press.

Lehiste, I. (1970). *Suprasegmentals*. Cambridge, MA: MIT Press.

Lehiste, I. (1977). Isochrony reconsidered. *Journal of Phonetics, 5,* 253–263.

Lehiste, I., & Meltzer, D. (1973). Vowel and speaker identification in natural and synthetic speech. *Language and Speech, 16,* 356–364.

Lehiste, I., & Peterson, G. E. (1961). Transitions, glides and diphthongs. *Journal of the Acoustical Society of America, 33,* 268–277.

Lenneberg, E. (1967). *Biological Foundations of Language*. New York: Wiley.

Liberman, A. M. (1979). Duplex perception and integration of cues: Evidence that speech is different from nonspeech and similar to language. In E. Fischer-Jorgensen, J. Rischel, & N. Thorsen (Eds.), *Proceedings of the IXth International Congress of Phonetic Sciences* (II, pp. 468–473). Copenhagen: University of Copenhagen.

Liberman, A. M. (1996). *Speech: A Special Code*. Cambridge, MA: MIT Press.

Liberman, A. M., Cooper, F. S., Shankweiler, D. P., & Studdert-Kennedy, M. (1967). Perception of the speech code. *Psychological Review, 74,* 431–461.

Liberman, A. M., Harris, K. S., Eimas, P. D., Lisker, L., & Bastian, J. (1961). An effect of learning on speech perception: The discrimination of durations of silence with and without phonemic significance. *Language and Speech, 54,* 175–195.

Liberman, A. M., Harris, K. S., Hoffman, H. S., & Griffith, B. C. (1957). The discrimination of speech sounds within and across phoneme boundaries. *Journal of Experimental Psychology, 54,* 358–368.

Liberman, A. M., & Mattingly, I. G. (1985). The motor theory of speech perception revised. *Cognition, 21,* 1–36.

Liberman, A. M., & Mattingly, I. G. (1989). A specialization for speech perception. *Science, 243,* 489–494.

Liberman, I. Y., Shankweiler, D., Liberman, A. M., Fowler, C. A., & Fisher, W. F. (1977). Phonetic segmentation and recoding in the beginning reader. In A. S. Reber & D. L. Scarborough (Eds.), *Toward a Psychology of Reading* (pp. 207–225). Hillsdale, NJ: Erlbaum.

Lieberman, P. (1963). Some effects of semantic and grammatical context on the production and perception of speech. *Language and Speech, 6,* 172–187.

Lieberman, P. (1967). *Intonation, Perception, and Language*. Cambridge, MA: MIT Press.

Lieberman, P., & Blumstein, S. (1988). *Speech Physiology, Speech Perception, and Acoustic Phonetics*. Cambridge, UK: Cambridge University Press.

Lieberman, P., Sawashima, M., Harris, K., & Gay, T. (1970). The articulatory implementation of the breath-group and prominence: Cricothyroid muscular activity in intonation. *Language, 46,* 312–327.

Lindau, M., & Ladefoged, P. (1986). Variability of feature specifications. In J. S. Perkell & D. H. Klatt (Eds.), *Invariance and Variability in Speech Processes* (pp. 464–478).

Lindblom, B. (1963). Spectrographic study of vowel reduction. *Journal of the Acoustical Society of America, 35,* 1773–1781.

Lindblom, B. (1986). Phonetic universals in vowel systems. In J. J. Ohala & J. J. Jaeger (Eds.), *Experimental Phonology* (pp. 13–44). New York: Academic.

Lindblom, B. (1990). Explaining phonetic variation: A sketch of the H&H theory. In W. Hardcastle & A. Marchal (Eds.), *Speech Production and Speech Modeling* (pp. 403–439). Dordrecht: Kluwer.

Lindblom, B. (1996). Role of articulation in speech perception: Clues from production. *Journal of the Acoustical Society of America, 99,* 1683–1692.

Lindblom, B., Brownlee, S., Davis, B., & Moon, S-J. (1992). Speech tranforms. *Speech Communication, 11,* 357–368.

Lindblom, B., & Engstrand, O. (1989). In what sense is speech quantal? *Journal of Phonetics, 17,* 107–121.

Lindblom, B., Lyberg, B., & Holmgren, K. (1977). *Durational Patterns of Swedish Phonology: Do They Reflect Short-Term Memory Processes?* Stockholm: Department of Phonetics, Institute of Linguistics, Stockholm University.

Lindblom, B. E. F., & Studdert-Kennedy, M. (1967). On the role of formant transitions in vowel recognition. *Journal of the Acoustical Society of America, 30,* 693–703.

Lindblom, B. E. F., & Sundberg, J. E. F. (1971). Acoustical consequences of lip, tongue, jaw, and larynx movement. *Journal of the Acoustical Society of America, 50,* 1166.

Lisker, L. (1978). Rapid vs. rabid: A catalogue of acoustic features that may cue the distinction. *Status Report on Speech Research, SR-54,* 127–132. Haskins Laboratories, Yale University, New Haven, CT.

Lisker, L. (1986). "Voicing" in English: A catalogue of acoustic features signaling /b/ versus /p/ in trochees. *Language and Speech, 29,* 3–11.

Lisker, L., & Abramson, A. (1964). A cross-language study of voicing in initial stops: Acoustical measurements. *Word, 20,* 384–422.

Lisker, L., & Abramson, A. (1967). Some effects of context on voice onset time in English stops. *Language and Speech, 10,* 1–28.

Lively, S. E., Pisoni, D. B., & Goldinger, S. D. (1994). Spoken word recognition: Research and theory. In M. A. Gernsbacher (Ed.), *Handbook of Psycholinguistics* (pp. 265–301). New York: Academic.

Lofqvist, A. (1995). Laryngeal mechanisms and interarticulator timing in voiceless consonant production. In F. Bell-Berti & L. J. Raphael (Eds.), *Producing Speech: Contemporary Issues.* Woodbury, NY: Contemporary Press.

Locke, S., & Kellar, L. (1973). Categorical perception in a nonlinguistic mode. *Cortex, 9,* 355–369.

Macchi, M. J. (1980). Identification of vowels spoken in isolation versus vowels spoken in consonantal manner. *Journal of the Acoustical Society of America, 68,* 1636–1642.

MacNeilage, P. F., & deClerk, J. L. (1969). On the motor control of coarticulation in CVC monosyllables. *Journal of the Acoustical Society of America, 45,* 1217–1233.

MacNeilage, P. F., Rootes, T. P., & Chase, R. A. (1967). Speech production and perception in a patient with severe impairment of somesthetic perception and motor control. *Journal of Speech and Hearing Research, 10,* 449–467.

Madden, J., & Feth, L. (1992). Temporal resolution in normal-hearing and hearing-impaired listeners using frequency-modulated stimuli. *Journal of Speech and Hearing Research, 35,* 436–442.

Maddieson, I. (1984). *Patterns of Sounds.* Cambridge, UK: Cambridge University.

Maeda, S. (1990). Compensatory articulation during speech: Evidence from the analysis and synthesis of vocal-tract shapes using an articulatory model. In W. J. Hardcastle & A. Marchal (Eds.), *Speech Production and Speech Modeling* (pp. 131–149) (NATO Advanced Study Institute Series). Boston: Kluwer.

Makhoul, J., Roucos, S., & Gish, H. (1985). Vector quantization in speech coding. *Proceedings of the IEEE, 73,* 1551–1588.

Malécot, A. (1956). Acoustic cues for nasal consonants, an experimental study involving a tape-splicing technique. *Language, 32,* 274–284.

Malécot, A. (1970). The lenis-fortis opposition: Its physiological parameters. *Journal of the Acoustical Society of America, 47,* 1588–1592.

Mann, V. A. (1980). Influence of preceding liquid in

stop consonant perception. *Perception and Psychophysics, 28,* 407–412.

Mann, V. A., & Liberman, A. M. (1983). Some differences between phonetic and auditory modes of perception. *Cognition, 14,* 211–235.

Mann, V. A., & Repp, B. H. (1980). Influence of vocalic context on perception of the [ʃ]-[s] distinction. *Perception and Psychophysics, 28,* 213–228.

Mann, V. A., & Repp, B. H. (1981). Influence of preceding fricative on stop consonant perception. *Journal of the Acoustical Society of America, 69,* 548–558.

Marslen-Wilson, W. D., & Warren, P. (1994). Levels of perceptual representation and process in lexical access: Words, phonemes, and features. *Psychological Review, 101,* 653–675.

Martin, J. G., & Bunnell, H. T. (1981). Perception of anticipatory coarticulation effects in /stri, stru/ sequences. *Journal of Experimental Psychology: Human Perception and Performance, 8,* 473–488.

Martony, J. (1965). Studies of the voice source. *Speech Transmission Laboratory Quarterly Progress Report, 1,* 4.

Massaro, D. W. (1987a). A fuzzy logical model of speech perception. Tallinn, Estonia: Academy of Sciences of the Estonian SSR. *Proceedings of the XIth International Congress of Phonetic Sciences, 5,* 334–337.

Massaro, D. W. (1987b). Psychophysics versus specialized processes in speech perception: An alternate perspective. In M. Schouten (Ed.), *The Psychophysics of Speech Perception* (pp. 46–65). Dordrecht: Martinus Nijhoff.

Massaro, D. W. (1987c). Categorical partition: A fuzzy-logical model of categorization behavior. In S. Harnad (Ed.), *Categorical Perception: The Groundwork of Cognition* (pp. 254–283). Cambridge, UK: Cambridge University Press.

Massaro, D. W. (1987d). Speech perception by ear and eye. In B. Dodd & R. Campbell (Eds.), *Hearing by Eye: The Psychology of Lip-Reading* (pp. 53–83). Hillsdale, NJ: Erlbaum.

Massaro, D. W. (1989). Testing between the TRACE model and the fuzzy logical model of perception. *Cognitive Psychology, 21,* 398–421.

Massaro, D. W. (1994). Psychological aspects of speech perception. In M. A. Gernsbacher (Ed.), *Handbook of Psycholinguistics* (pp. 9–263). San Diego: Academic.

Massaro, D. W., & Cohen, M. M. (1991). Integration versus interactive activation: The joint influence of stimulus and context in perception. *Cognitive Psychology, 23,* 558–614.

Massaro, D. W., & Cohen, M. M. (1995). Perceiving talking faces. *Current Directions in Psychological Science, 4,* 104–109.

Mattingly, I. G. (1974). Speech synthesis for phonetic and phonological models. In T. A. Sebeok (Ed.), *Current Trends in Linguistics, Vol. 12* (pp. 2451–2487). The Hague: Mouton.

Mattingly, I. G., & Liberman, A. M. (1990). Speech and other auditory modules. In G. M. Edelman, W. E. Gall, & W. M. Cowan (Eds.), *Signal and Sense: Local and Global Order in Perceptual Maps* (pp. 501–520). New York: Wiley-Liss.

Mattingly, I. G., Liberman, A. M., Syrdal, A. K., & Halwes, T. (1971). Discrimination in speech and nonspeech modes. *Cognitive Psychology, 2,* 131–157.

McClelland, J. L. (1991). Stochastic interactive processes and the effect of context on perception. *Cognitive Psychology, 23,* 1–44.

McClelland, J. L., & Elman, J. L. (1986). The TRACE model of speech perception. *Cognitive Psychology, 18,* 1–86.

McGovern, K., & Strange, W. (1977). The perception of /r/ and /l/ in syllable-initial and syllable-final position. *Perception and Psychophysics, 21,* 162–170.

McGurk, H., & MacDonald, J. (1976). Hearing lips and seeing voices. *Nature, 264,* 746–748.

Mermelstein, P. (1973). Articulatory model for the study of speech production. *Journal of the Acoustical Society of America, 53,* 1070–1082.

Miller, J. D. (1989). Auditory-perceptual interpretation of the vowel. *Journal of the Acoustical Society of America, 85,* 2114–2134.

Miller, J. D., Wier, C. C., Pastore, R. E., Kelly, W. J., & Dooling, R. J. (1976). Discrimination and labeling of noise-buzz sequences with varying noise-lead times: An example of categorical perception. *Journal of the Acoustical Society of America, 60,* 411–417.

Miller, J. L. (1981). Effects of speaking rate on segmental distinctions. In P. Eimas & J. L. Miller (Eds.), *Perspectives on the Study of Speech* (pp. 39–74). Hillsdale, NJ: Erlbaum.

Miller, J. L. (1994). On the internal structure of phonetic categories: A progress report. *Cognition, 50,* 271–285.

Miller, J. L., & Grosjean, F. (1981). How the components of speaking rate influence perception of phonetic segments. *Journal of Experimental Psychology: Human Perception and Performance, 7,* 208–215.

Miller, J. L., & Liberman, A. M. (1979). Some effects of later occurring information on the perception of stop consonant and semivowel. *Perception and Psychophysics, 25,* 457–465.

Moon, S. Y., & Lindblom, B. E. F. (1994). Interaction between duration, context, and speaking style in English stressed vowels. *Journal of the Acoustical Society of America, 96,* 40–55.

Moore, B. C. J. (1997). *An Introduction to the Psychology of Hearing* (4th ed.). San Diego: Academic.

Morais, J., Bertelson, P., Cary, L., & Alegria, J. (1986). Literacy training and speech segmentation. *Cognition, 24,* 45–64.

Morais, J., Cary, L., Alegria, J., & Bertelson, P. (1979). Does awareness of speech as a sequence of phones arise spontaneously? *Cognition, 7,* 323–331.

Morais, J., & Kolinsky, R. (1994). Perception and awareness in phonological processing—the case of the phoneme. *Cognition, 50,* 287–297.

Moulines, E., & Charpentier, F. (1990). Pitch-synchronous waveform processing technique for text-to-speech synthesis using diphones. *Speech Communication, 9(5-6),* 453–467.

Munhall, K. G., Gribble, P., Sacco, L., & Ward, M. (1996). Temporal constraints on the McGurk effect. *Perception and Psychophysics, 58,* 351–362.

Nearey, T. M. (1989). Static, dynamic, and relational properties in vowel perception. *Journal of the Acoustical Society of America, 85,* 2088–2113.

Nearey, T. M. (1995). A double-weak view of trading relations: Comments on Kingston and Diehl. In B. Connell & A. Arvaniti (Eds.), *Phonology and Phonetic Evidence: Papers in Laboratory Phonology IV* (pp. 28–39). Cambridge, UK: Cambridge University Press.

Nelson, P., Nittrouer, S., & Norton, S. (1995). "Say-stay" identification and psychoacoustic performance of hearing-impaired persons. *Journal of the Acoustical Society of America, 97,* 1830–1838.

Nelson, P., & Revoile, S. (1996). Predicting recognition of stops and glides by listeners with moderate to severe hearing loss. 19th meeting of the Association for Research in Otolaryngology, *Abstracts,* p. 157. St. Petersburg Beach, FL.

Nelson, P., & Revoile, S. (in review). Carrier phrase contributions to stop consonants recognition, I: Normal-hearing listeners. *Journal of Speech and Hearing Research.*

Netsell, R. (1969). Subglottal and intraoral air pressures during the intervocalic contrast of /t/ and /d/. *Phonetica, 20,* 68–73.

Nittrouer, S., Munhall, K., Kelso, J. A. S., Tuller, B., & Harris, K. S. (1988). Patterns of interarticulator phasing and their relation to linguistic structure. *Journal of the Acoustical Society of America, 84,* 1653–1660.

Nooteboom, S. G., & Kruyt, J. G. (1987). Accents, focus distribution, and the perceived distribution of given and new information: An experiment. *Journal of the Acoustical Society of America, 82,* 1512–1524.

Norris, D. (1992). Connectionism: A new breed of bottom-up model? In N. Sharkey & R. Reiley (Eds.), *Connectionist Approaches to Language Processing* (pp. 351–371). Hove, UK: Erlbaum.

Oden, G. C., & Massaro, D. W. (1978). Integration of featural information in speech perception. *Psychological Review, 85,* 172–191.

Ohala, J. J. (1974). A mathematical model of speech aerodynamics. In G. Fant (Ed.), *Proceedings of Speech Communication Seminar* (II, pp. 65–72). Stockholm, Sweden: Almquist & Wiksell.

Ohala, J. J. (1977). The physiology of stress. In L. M. Hyman (Ed.), *Studies in Stress and Accent* (pp. 145–168). Los Angeles: Southern California Occasional Papers in Linguistics, No. 4.

Ohala, J. J. (1990). The phonetics and phonology of aspects of assimilation. In J. Kingston & M. E. Beckman, *Papers in Laboratory Phonology, I. Between the Grammar and Physics of Speech* (pp. 258–275). Cambridge, UK: Cambridge University Press.

Ohala, J. J. (1992). Alternatives to the sonority hierarchy for explaining segmental sequential constraints. In Chicago Linguistic Society, *Papers from the Parasession on the Syllable* (pp. 319–338). Chicago: Author.

Ohala, J. J. (1996). Speech perception is hearing sounds, not tongues. *Journal of the Acoustical Society of America, 99,* 1718–1725.

Ohala, J. J., & Jaeger, J. J. (Eds.). (1986). *Experimental Phonology.* New York: Academic.

Öhman, S. (1966). Coarticulation in VCV utterances:

Spectrographic references. *Journal of the Acousti-cal Society of America, 39,* 151–168.

Olive, J. P. (1977). Rule synthesis of speech from diadic units. *Proceedings IEEE-ICASSP, 77,* 568–570.

Owens, E., Benedict, M., & Schubert, E. (1972). Consonant phonemic errors associated with pure-tone configurations and certain kinds of hearing impairment. *Journal of Speech and Hearing Research, 15,* 308–322.

Paget, R. A. S. (1924). The nature and artificial production of speech sounds. *Proceedings of the Royal Society, Series A, 106,* 150–174.

Paliwal, K. K., Lindsay, D., & Ainsworth, W. A. (1983). A study of two-formant models for vowel identification. *Speech Communication, 2(4),* 295–303.

Parker, E. M., & Diehl, R. L. (1984). Identifying vowels in CVC syllables: Effects of inserting silence and noise. *Perception and Psychophysics, 36,* 369–380.

Parker, E. M., Diehl, R. L., & Kluender, K. R. (1986). Trading relations in speech and nonspeech. *Perception and Psychophysics, 39,* 129–142.

Parthasarathy, S., & Coker, C. (1992). On automatic estimation of articulatory parameters in a text-to-speech system. *Computer, Speech, and Language, 6,* 37–75.

Perkell, J. S. (1969). *Physiology of Speech Production: Results and Implications of a Quantitative Cineradiographic Study.* Research Monograph No. 53. Cambridge, MA: MIT Press.

Perkell, J. S., & Nelson, W. L. (1985). Variability in the production of the vowels /i/ and /a/. *Journal of the Acoustical Society of America, 77,* 1889–1906.

Perlman, A. L., & Durham, P. L. (1987). In vitro studies of vocal fold mucosa during isometric conditions. In T. Baer, C. Sasaki, & K. S. Harris (Eds.), *Laryngeal Function in Phonation and Respiration* (pp. 291–303). San Diego: College-Hill (now Singular).

Peterson, G. (1961). Parameters of vowel quality. *Journal of Speech and Hearing Research, 4,* 10–29.

Peterson, G., & Barney, H. (1952). Control methods used in a study of vowels. *Journal of the Acoustical Society of America, 24,* 175–184.

Peterson, G., & Lehiste, I. (1960). Duration of syllable nuclei in English. *Journal of the Acoustical Society of America, 32,* 693–703.

Peterson, G., Wang, W., & Sivertsen, E. (1958). Segmentation techniques in speech synthesis. *Journal of the Acoustical Society of America, 30,* 739–742.

Pickett, J. M. (1957). Perception of vowels heard in noises of various spectra. *Journal of the Acoustical Society of America, 29,* 613–620.

Pickett, J. M. (1980). *The Sounds of Speech Communication.* Baltimore: University Park.

Pickett, J. M. (1955). Shadows, echoes, and the auditory analysis of speech. *Speech Communication, 4,* 19–30.

Pickett, J. M. (1996). Review of Bell-Berti and Raphael, "Producing Speech." *Journal of the Acoustical Society of America, 100,* 1931–1934.

Pickett, J. M., Bunnell, H. T., & Revoile, S. (1995). Phonetics of intervocalic consonant perception: Retrospect and prospect. *Phonetica, 52,* 1–40.

Pickett, J. M., Martin, E., Johnson, D., Smith, S., Daniel, Z., Willis, D., & Otis, W. (1970). On patterns of speech feature reception by deaf listeners. In G. Fant (Ed.), *International Symposium on Speech Communication Ability and Profound Deafness, Stockholm, 1970* (pp. 119–134). Washington, DC: A. G. Bell Association.

Pierrehumbert, J., & Beckman, M. (1988). *Japanese Tone Structure.* Linguistic Inquiry Monographs, No. 15. Cambridge, MA: MIT Press.

Pierrehumbert, J., & Hirschberg, J. (1990). The meaning of intonational contours in the interpretation of discourse. In P. R. Cohen, J. Morgan, & M. E. Pollack (Eds.), *Intentions in Communication* (pp. 271–311). Cambridge, MA: MIT Press.

Pisoni, D. B. (1973). Auditory and phonetic memory codes in the discrimination of consonants and vowels. *Perception and Psychophysics, 13,* 253–260.

Pisoni, D. B. (1977). Identification and discrimination of the relative onset time of two component tones: Implications for voicing perception in stops. *Journal of the Acoustical Society of America, 61,* 1352–1361.

Pisoni, D. B. (1980). Variability of vowel formant frequencies and the quantal theory of speech. *Phonetica, 37,* 285–305.

Pisoni, D. B. (1992). Some comments on invariance, variability, and perceptual normalization in speech perception. In J. J. Ohala, T. M. Nearey, B. L. Derwing, M. M. Hodge, & G. E. Wiebe (Eds.), *Proceedings ICSLP-92 (1992 International Conference on Spoken Language Processing), 1,* 587–590.

Pisoni, D. B., Lively, S. E., & Logan, J. S. (1994). Perceptual learning of nonnative speech contrasts: Implications for theories of speech perception. In J. C. Goodman & H. C. Nusbaum (Eds.), *The Development of Speech Perception: The Transition from Speech Sounds to Spoken Words* (pp. 121–166). Cambridge, MA: MIT Press.

Pisoni, D. B., & Luce, P. A. (1987). Acoustic-phonetic representation in word recognition. In U. H. Frauenfelder & L. K. Tyler (Eds.), *Spoken Word Recognition* (pp. 21–52). Cambridge, MA: MIT Press.

Plant, G. (1982). Tactile perception by the profoundly deaf: Speech and environmental sounds. *British Journal of Audiology, 16,* 233–244.

Polka, L., & Strange, W. (1985). Perceptual equivalence of acoustic uses that differentiate /r/ and /l/. *Journal of the Acoustical Society of America, 78,* 1187–1197.

Port, R. F. (1986). Translating linguistic symbols into time. In *Research in Phonetics and Computational Linguistics* (pp. 155–174) (No. 5). Bloomington: Departments of Linguistics and Computer Science, Indiana University.

Pratt, S. R., Heintzelman, A. T., & Deming, S. E. (1993). The efficacy of using the IBM Speech-Viewer Vowel Accuracy Module to treat young children with hearing impairment. *Journal of Speech and Hearing Research, 36,* 1063–1074.

Price, P. J. (1990). Evaluation of spoken language systems: The ATIS domain. *Proceedings of the Third DARPA Workshop on Speech and Natural Language* (pp. 91–95). Washington, DC: Department of Defense.

Price, P. J. (in press). Combining linguistic with statistical methods in automatic speech understanding. In J. Klavans & P. Resnick (Eds.), *Combining Symbolic and Statistical Approaches to Language.* Hillsdale, NJ: Erlbaum.

Rabiner, L. R. (1989). A tutorial on hidden Markov models and selected applications in speech recognition. *Proceedings of the IEEE, 77,* 257–286.

Rabiner, L. R., & Juang, B. (1993). *Fundamentals of Speech Recognition.* Englewood Cliffs, NJ: Prentice Hall.

Rabiner, L. R., & Wilpon, J. G. (1987). Some performance benchmarks for isolated word speech recognition systems. *Computer Speech and Language, 2,* 343–357.

Raman, T. V. (1997a, March). Netsurfing without a monitor. *Scientific American* (special Internet edition).

Raman, T. V. (1997b). *Auditory User Interfaces.* Boston: Kluwer.

Rand, T. C. (1974). Dichotic release from masking for speech. *Journal of the Acoustical Society of America, 55,* 678–680.

Raz, I., & Noffsinger, D. (1985). Identification of synthetic, voiced stop-consonants by hearing-impaired listeners. *Audiology, 24,* 437–448.

Read, C. A., Buder, E. H., & Kent, R. D. (1992). Speech analysis systems: An evaluation. *Journal of Speech and Hearing Research, 35,* 314–332.

Read, C. A., Zhang, Y., Nie, H., & Ding, B. (1986). The ability to manipulate speech sounds depends on knowing alphabetic reading. *Cognition, 24,* 31–44.

Remez, R. E. (1994). A guide to research on the perception of speech. In M. A. Gernsbacher (Ed.), *Handbook of Psycholinguistics* (pp. 145–172). San Diego: Academic.

Remez, R. E., Fellowes, J. M., & Rubin, P. E. (in press). Talker identification based on phonetic information. *Journal of Experimental Psychology: Human Perception and Performance.* Also in Barnard College Speech Perception Laboratory, *Technical Report* (April 1996), 1–19.

Remez, R. E., & Rubin, P. E. (in press). Acoustic shards, perceptual glue. In J. Charles-Luce, P. A. Luce, & J. R. Sawusch (Eds.), *Theories in Spoken Language: Perception, Production, and Development.* Norwood, NJ: Ablex. Also in Haskins Laboratories, *Status Report on Speech Research, SR-111/112,* 1–10.

Remez, R. E., Rubin, P. E., Berns, S. M., Pardo, J. S., & Lang, J. M. (1994). On the perceptual organization of speech. *Psychological Review, 101,* 129–56.

Repp, B. H. (1982). Phonetic trading relations and context effects: New experimental evidence for a speech mode of perception. *Psychological Bulletin, 92,* 81–110.

Repp, B. H. (1984). Categorical perception: Issues, methods, findings. In N.J. Lass (Ed.), *Speech and Language: Advances in Basic Research and Practice, Vol. 10* (pp. 243–335). New York: Academic Press.

Repp, B. H. (1986). Perception of the [m]-[n] distinction in CV syllables. *Journal of the Acoustical Society of America, 79,* 1987–1999.

Repp, B. H. (1991). Around duplex perception. In I. G. Mattingly & M. Studdert-Kennedy (Eds.), *Modularity and the Motor Theory of Speech Perception* (pp. 261–267). Hillsdale, NJ: Erlbaum.

Repp, B. H., Liberman, A. M., Eccardt, T., & Pesetsky, D. (1978). Perceptual integration of acoustic cues for stop, fricative, and affricate manner. *Journal of Experimental Psychology: Human Perception and Performance, 4,* 621–637.

Revoile, S., Barac-Cikoja, D., Holden-Pitt, L., & Kozma-Spytek, L. (in preparation). The use of spectral cues to voiced consonants by hard of hearing listeners.

Revoile, S., Holden-Pitt, L., Edward, D., Bunnell, H., & Pickett, J. M. (1985). Transition discrimination versus use for glide perception by impaired listeners. Presentation at the annual convention of the American Speech-Language-Hearing Association, Washington, DC.

Revoile, S., Holden-Pitt, L., & Pickett, J. M. (1985). Perceptual cues to the voiced-voiceless distinction of final fricatives for listeners with impaired or with normal hearing. *Journal of the Acoustical Society of America, 77,* 1263–1265.

Revoile, S., Holden-Pitt, L., Pickett, J. M., & Brandt, F. (1986). Speech cue enhancement for the hearing impaired. I. Altered vowel durations for perception of final fricative voicing. *Journal of Speech and Hearing Research, 29,* 240–255.

Revoile, S., Kozma-Spytek, L., Holden-Pitt, L., Pickett, J. M., & Droge, J. (1991a). VCVs vs CVCs for stop/fricative distinctions by hearing-impaired and normal-hearing listeners. *Journal of the Acoustical Society of America, 89,* 457–460.

Revoile, S., Pickett, J. M., & Kozma-Spytek, L. (1991b). Spectral cues to perception of /d, n, l/ by normal- and impaired-hearing listeners. *Journal of the Acoustical Society of America, 90,* 787–798

Revoile, S., Kozma-Spytek, L., Holden-Pitt, L., Pickett, J. M., & Droge, J. (1995a). Acoustic-phonetic context considerations for speech recognition testing of hearing-impaired listeners. *Ear and Hearing, 16,* 254–262.

Revoile, S., Kozma-Spytek, L., Nelson, P., & Holden-Pitt, L. (1995b). Some auditory indices related to consonant and vowel-transition use by hard of hearing listeners. Hearing Aid Research and Development Conference; National Institute on Deafness and Other Communication Disorders, and Veterans Administration, Bethesda, MD.

Revoile, S., Pickett, J. M., Holden, L., & Talkin, D. (1982). Acoustic cues to final stop voicing for impaired- and normal-hearing listeners. *Journal of the Acoustical Society of America, 72,* 1145–1154.

Revoile, S., Pickett, J. M., Holden-Pitt, L., Talkin, D., & Brandt, F. (1987). Burst and transition cues to voicing perception for spoken initial stops by impaired- and normal-hearing listeners. *Journal of Speech and Hearing Research, 30,* 3–12.

Revoile, S., Wilson, M., & Pickett, J. M. (1977). Discrimination of formant transition tempo by hearing-impaired listeners. *Journal of the Acoustical Society of America, 62,* S60.

Rosch, E. (1975). Cognitive reference points. *Cognitive Psychology, 7,* 532–547.

Rosch, E. (1977). Human categorization. In N. Warren (Ed.), *Studies in Cross-Cultural Psychology, 1,* 1–49.

Rosen, S., & Howell, P. (1991). *Signals and Systems for Speech and Hearing.* London: Academic.

Rosen, S., Faulkner, A., & Smith, D. (1990). The psychoacoustics of profound hearing impairment. *Acta Otolaryngologica* (Stockholm), *469,* 16–22.

Rothenberg, M. (1973). A new inverse-filtering technique for deriving the glottal air waveform during voicing. *Journal of the Acoustical Society of America, 53,* 1632–1645.

Rothenberg, M. (1981). Acoustic interaction between the glottal source and the vocal tract. In K. N. Stevens & M. Hirano (Eds.), *Vocal Fold Physiology.* Tokyo: University of Tokyo Press.

Ryalls, J. H., & Lieberman, P. (1982). Fundamental frequency and vowel perception. *Journal of the Acoustical Society of America, 72,* 1631–1634.

Sachs, M. B., & Young, E. D. (1980). Effects of nonlinearities on speech encoding in the auditory nerve. *Journal of the Acoustical Society of America, 68,* 858–875.

Sagisaka, Y., & Iwahashi, N. (1995). Objective optimization in algorithms for text-to-speech synthesis. In W. B. Kleijn & K. K. Paliwal (Eds.), *Speech Coding and Synthesis* (pp. 685–706). Amsterdam: Elsevier.

Saltzman, E. L., & Munhall, K. G. (1989). A dynamic approach to gestural patterning in speech production. *Ecological Psychology, 1,* 333–382.

Sandhu, S., & Ghitza, O. (1995). A comparative study

of mel cepstra and EIH for phone classification under adverse conditions. *Proceedings IEEE-ICASSP 95, 1,* 409–412.

Sawashima, M. (1968). Movements of the larynx in the articulation of Japanese consonants. *Annual Bulletin of the Research Institute of Logopedics and Phoniatrics* (University of Tokyo), *2,* 11–20.

Sawashima, M., & Miyazaki, S. (1973). Glottal opening for Japanese voiceless consonants. *Annual Bulletin of the Research Institute of Logopedics and Phoniatrics* (University of Tokyo), *7,* 1–10.

Scherer, R., & Titze, I. R. (1983). Pressure-flow relationships in a model of the laryngeal airway with a diverging glottis. In D. M. Bless & J. H. Abbs (Eds.), *Vocal Fold Physiology: Contemporary Research and Clinical Issues* (pp. 179–183). San Diego: College-Hill.

Scripture, E. W. (1902). *Experimental Phonetics* (p. 450). New York: Charles Scribner's Sons.

Schroeder, M. R., & Atal, B. S. (1985). Code-excited linear prediction (CELP): High-quality speech at very low bit rates. *Proceedings IEEE-ICASSP, 85,* 937–940.

Schroeder, M. R., Atal, B. S., & Hall, J. L. (1979). Optimizing digital speech coders by exploiting masking properties of the human ear. *Journal of the Acoustical Society of America, 66,* 1647–1652.

Schroeter, J. (1997). Bridging the gap between speech science and speech applications. In J. P. H. van Santen, R. W. Sproat, J. P. Olive, & J. Hirschberg (Eds.), *Progress in Speech Synthesis* (pp. 179–184). New York: Springer.

Schroeter, J., & Sondhi, M. M. (1991). Speech coding based on physiological models of speech production. In S. Furui & M. M. Sondhi (Eds.), *Advances in Speech Signal Processing* (pp. 231–268). New York: Marcel Dekker.

Schroeter, J., & Sondhi, M. M. (1994). Techniques for estimating vocal-tract shapes from the speech signal. Special issue on neural networks for speech processing, Part II. *IEEE Transactions on Speech and Audio, 2(1),* 133–150.

Sherbecoe, R., Studebaker, G., & Crawford, M. (1993). Speech spectra for six record monosyllabic word tests. *Ear and Hearing, 14,* 104–111.

Slis, I. H. (1975). Consequences of articulatory effort on articulatory training. In G. Fant & M. Tatham (Eds.), *Auditory Analysis and the Perception of Speech* (pp. 397–411). New York: Academic.

Slis, I. H., & Cohen, A. (1969). On the complex regulating the voiced-voiceless distinction (Parts I and II). *Language and Speech, 12,* 80–102; 137–155.

Soli, S. D. (1982). Structure and duration of vowels together specify fricative voicing. *Journal of the Acoustical Society of America, 72,* 366–378.

Sondhi, M. M., & Schroeter, J. (1997). Speech production models and their digital implementations. In *The Digital Signal Processing Handbook.* New York: CRC and IEEE Press.

Stalhammer, U., Karlsson, I., & Fant, G. (1974). Contextual effects on vowel nuclei. *Quarterly Progress and Status Report, 4/73,* Speech Transmission Laboratory, Royal Institute of Technology, Stockholm.

Steele, J. (1775). *An Essay Towards Establishing the Melody and Measure of Speech to be Expressed and Perpetuated by Peculiar Symbols.* London: J. Almon. (facsimile reprint, 1969, by Scolar Press, Menston, Yorkshire, UK)

Stemberger, J. P. (1992). A connectionist view of child phonology: Phonological processing without phonological processes. In C. A. Ferguson, L. Menn, & C. Stoel-Gammon (Eds.), *Phonological Development: Models, Research, Implications* (pp. 165–189). Timonium, MD: York.

Stetson, R. H. (1928). Motor phonetics. *Arch. Neerl. Phon. Exper. 3,* 1–216.

Stetson, R. H. (1945). *Bases of Phonology.* Oberlin, OH: Oberlin College. (corrected printing, 1954)

Stetson, R. H. (1951). *Motor Phonetics* (2nd ed.). Amsterdam: North-Holland.

Stevens, K. N. (1972). The quantal nature of speech: Evidence from articulatory-acoustic data. In E. E. David & P. B. Denes (Eds.), *Human Communication: A Unified View* (pp. 51–66). New York: McGraw-Hill.

Stevens, K. N. (1977). Physics of laryngeal behavior and larynx models. *Phonetica, 34,* 264–279.

Stevens, K. N. (1980). Acoustic correlates of some phonetic categories. *Journal of the Acoustical Society of America, 68,* 836–842.

Stevens, K. N. (1983). Design features of speech sound systems. In P. F. MacNeilage (Ed.), *The Production of Speech* (pp. 247–261). New York: Springer-Verlag.

Stevens, K. N. (1985). Evidence for the role of acoustic boundaries in the perception of speech sounds. In V. Fromkin (Ed.), *Phonetic Linguistics* (pp. 243–255). New York: Academic.

Stevens, K. N. (1986). Models of phonetic recognition

II: A feature-based model of speech recognition. In P. Mermelstein (Ed.), *Proceedings of the Montreal Satellite Symposium on Speech Recognition* (pp. 67–68). Twelfth International Congress of Acoustics.

Stevens, K. N. (1988). Phonetic features and lexical access. Ministry of Education, Science, and Culture, Japan: *The Second Symposium on Advanced Man-Machine Interface Through Spoken Language* (pp. 10–23).

Stevens, K. N. (1989). On the quantal theory of speech. *Journal of Phonetics, 17,* 3–45.

Stevens, K. N. (1994). Phonetic evidence for hierarchies of features. In P. Keating (Ed.), *Phonological Structure and Phonetic Form* (pp. 242–258). Cambridge, UK: Cambridge University Press.

Stevens, K. N. (1998). *Acoustic Phonetics.* Cambridge, MA: MIT Press.

Stevens, K. N., & Blumstein, S. E. (1978). Invariant cues for place of articulation in stop consonants. *Journal of the Acoustical Society of America, 64,* 1358–1368.

Stevens, K. N., & Blumstein, S. E. (1981). The search for invariant acoustic correlates of phonetic features. In P. D. Eimas & J. L. Miller (Eds.), *Perspectives on the Study of Speech* (pp. 1038). Hillsdale, NJ: Erlbaum.

Stevens, K. N., Blumstein, S. E., Glicksman, L., Burton, M., & Kurowski, K. (1992). Acoustic and perceptual characteristics of voicing in fricatives and fricative clusters. *Journal of the Acoustical Society of America, 91,* 2979–3000.

Stevens, K. N., & House, A. S. (1955). Development of a quantitative description of vowel articulation. *Journal of the Acoustical Society of America, 27,* 484.

Stevens, K. N., & House, A. S. (1961). An acoustical theory of vowel production and some of its implications. *Journal of Speech and Hearing Research, 4,* 303.

Stevens, K. N., & House, A. S. (1963). Perturbation of vowel articulations by consonantal context: An acoustical study. *Journal of Speech and Hearing Research, 6,* 111–128.

Stevens, K. N., Keyser, S. J., & Kawasaki, H. (1986). Toward a phonetic and phonological theory of redundant features. In J. S. Perkell & D. H. Klatt (Eds.), *Invariance and Variability in Speech Processes* (pp. 426–449). Hillsdale, NJ: Erlbaum.

Stevens, K. N., & Klatt, D. H. (1974). The role of formant transitions in the voiced-voiceless distinction for stops. *Journal of the Acoustical Society of America, 55,* 653–659.

Stevens, K. N., Manuel, S. Y., Shattuck-Hufnagel, S., & Liu, S. (1992). Implementation of a model for lexical access based on features. In J. J. Ohala, T. M. Nearey, B. L. Derwing, M. M. Hodge, & G. E. Weibe (Eds.), *Proceedings ICSLP-92 (1992 International Conference on Spoken Language Processing), 1,* 499–502.

Stone, M. (1990). A three-dimensional model of tongue movement based on ultrasound and x-ray beam data. *Journal of the Acoustical Society of America, 85,* 2207–2217.

Strange, W. (1989). Dynamic specification of coarticulated vowels spoken in sentence context. *Journal of the Acoustical Society of America, 85,* 2135–2153.

Strange, W., Edman, T. R., & Jenkins, J. J. (1979). Acoustic and phonological factors in vowel identification. *Journal of Experimental Psychology: Human Perception and Performance, 5,* 643–656.

Strange, W., Jenkins, J. J., & Johnson, T. L. (1983). Dynamic specification of coarticulated vowels. *Journal of the Acoustical Society of America, 74,* 695–705.

Strange, W., Verbrugge, R. R., Shankweiler, D. P., & Edman, T. R. (1976). Consonant environment specifies vowel identity. *Journal of the Acoustical Society of America, 60,* 213–224.

Stream, R., & Dirks, D. (1974). Effect of loudspeaker position on differences between earphone and free-field thresholds (MAP and MAF). *Journal of Speech and Hearing Research, 17,* 549–568.

Studdert-Kennedy, M. (1976). Speech perception, In N. J. Lass (Ed.), *Contemporary Issues in Experimental Phonetics* (pp. 243–293). New York: Academic.

Studdert-Kennedy, M. (1986). Two cheers for direct realism. *Journal of Phonetics, 14,* 99–104.

Studdert-Kennedy, M. (ms). Listening and speaking. Unpublished manuscript (available from The Haskins Laboratories).

Stylianou, Y., Dutoit, T., & Schroeter, J. (1997). Diphone concatenation using a harmonic plus noise model of speech. *Proceedings of Eurospeech '97, 2,* 613–616.

Summerfield, Q. (1981). Articulatory rate and perceptual constancy in phonetic perception. *Journal of Experimental Psychology: Human Perception and Performance, 7,* 1074–1095.

Summerfield, Q. (1987). Some preliminaries to a comprehensive account of audio-visual speech perception. In B. Dodd & R. Campbell (Eds.), *Hearing by Eye: The Psychology of Lip-Reading* (pp. 3–51). Hillsdale, NJ: Erlbaum.

Summerfield, Q., & Haggard, M. P. (1975). Vocal tract normalization as demonstrated by reaction times. In G. Fant & M. Tatham (Eds.), *Auditory Analysis and Perception of Speech* (pp. 115–141). New York: Academic.

Summers, V., & Leek, M. (1995). Frequency glide discrimination in the F2 region by normal-hearing and hearing-impaired listeners. *Journal of the Acoustical Society of America, 97,* 3825–3832.

Sundberg, J. (1973). The source spectrum in professional singing. *Folia Phoniatr., 25,* 71–90.

Sussman, J. E., & Lauckner-Morano, V. J. (1995). Further tests of the perceptual magnet effect in the perception of [i]: Identification and change/no-change discrimination. *Journal of the Acoustical Society of America, 97,* 539–552.

Swinney, D. A. (1979). Lexical access during sentence comprehension: (Re)Consideration of context effects. *Journal of Verbal Learning and Verbal Behavior, 18,* 645–659.

Syrdal, A. K., & Gopal, H. S. (1986). A perceptual model of vowel recognition based on auditory representation of American English vowels. *Journal of the Acoustical Society of America, 79,* 1086–1100.

Syrdal, A. K., Bennett, R. W., & Greenspan, S. L. (Eds.). (1994). *Applied Speech Technology.* Boca Raton, FL: CRC Press.

Tiffany, W. R. (1959). Nonrandom sources of variation in vowel quality. *Journal of Speech and Hearing Research, 2,* 305–317.

Tillman, T., & Carhart, R. (1966). An expanded test for speech discrimination utilizing CNC monosyllabic words (Northwestern University Auditory Test No. 6). Technical Report SAM-TR-66-55, USAF School of Aerospace Medicine, Aerospace Medical Division (AFSC), Brooks AFB, Texas.

Titze, I. R. (1988). The physics of small amplitude oscillation of the vocal folds. *Journal of the Acoustical Society of America, 83,* 1536–1552.

Titze, I. R. (1994). *Principles of Voice Production.* Englewood Cliffs, NJ: Prentice Hall (also available from Allyn & Bacon, Boston).

Titze, I. R. (1995). Motor and sensory components of a feedback-control model of fundamental frequency.

In F. Bell-Berti & L. Raphael (Eds.), *Producing Speech: Contemporary Issues* (pp. 309–320). Woodbury, NJ: AIP Press.

Titze, I. R., & Durham, P. L. (1987). Passive mechanisms influencing fundamental frequency control. In T. Baer, C. Sasaki, & K. S. Harris (Eds.), *Laryngeal Function in Phonation and Respiration* (pp. 304–319). San Diego: College-Hill (now Singular).

Titze, I. R., Mapes, S., & Story, B. (1994). Acoustics of the high tenor voice. *Journal of the Acoustical Society of America, 95,* 1133–1142.

Titze, I. R., & Talkin, D. (1979). A theoretical study of the effects of various laryngeal configurations on the acoustics of phonation. *Journal of the Acoustical Society of America, 66,* 60–74.

Trehub, S. E. (1976). The discrimination of foreign speech contrasts by infants and adults. *Child Development, 47,* 466–472.

Truby, H. (1959). Acoustico-cineradiographic analysis considerations with special reference to certain consonantal complexes. *Acta Radiol. (suppl. 182).*

Tuller, B., & Kelso, J. A. S. (1984). The timing of articulatory gestures: Evidence for relational invariants. *Journal of the Acoustical Society of America, 76,* 1030–1036.

Tuller, B., & Kelso, J. A. S. (1990). Phase transitions in speech production and their perceptual consequences. In M. Jeannerod (Ed.), *Attention and Performance XIII: Motor Representation and Control* (pp. 429–452). Hillsdale, NJ: Erlbaum.

Turner, C., & Robb, M. (1987). Audibility and recognition of stop consonants in normal and hearing-impaired subjects. *Journal of the Acoustical Society of America, 81,* 1566–1573.

Turner, C., Souza, P., & Forget, L. (1995). Use of temporal envelope cues in speech recognition by normal and hearing-impaired listeners. *Journal of the Acoustical Society of America, 97,* 2568–2578.

Umeda, N. (1975). Vowel duration in American English. *Journal of the Acoustical Society of America, 58,* 434–445.

Umeda, N. (1977). Consonant duration in American English. *Journal of the Acoustical Society of America, 61,* 846–858.

Van de Grift Turek, S., Dorman, M., & Franks, J. (1980). Identification of synthetic /bdg/ by hearing-impaired listeners under monotic and dichotic formant presentation. *Journal of the Acoustical Society of America, 67,* 1013–1040.

Vanderslice, R. (1967). Larynx vs. lungs: Cricothyrometer data refuting some recent claims concerning intonation and archetypality. *Work. Pap. Phonet., 7*, 67–79. Phonetics Laboratory, University of California at Los Angeles.

van Son, N., Bosman, A., Lamore, P., & Smoorenburg, G. (1993). The perception of complex harmonic patterns by profoundly hearing-impaired listeners. *Audiology, 32*, 308–327.

Van Tasell, D. (1981). Auditory perception of speech. In J. Davis & E. Hardick (Eds.), *Rehabilitative Audiology for Children and Adults*. New York: Wiley.

Van Tasell, D. (1993). Hearing loss, speech, and hearing aids. *Journal of Speech and Hearing Research, 36*, 228–244.

Verbrugge, R. R., & Shankweiler, D. (1977). Prosodic information for vowel identity. *Status Report on Speech Research, SR-51-52*, 27–35. (Haskins Laboratories).

Verdolini-Marston, K., Titze, I. R., & Druker, D. G. (1990). Changes in threshold phonation pressure with induced conditions of hydration. *Journal of Voice, 4*, 142–151.

Vihman, M. M. (1996). *Phonological Development: The Origins of Language in the Child*. Cambridge, MA: Blackwell.

Volaitis, L. E., & Miller, J. L. (1992). Phonetic prototypes: Influence of place of articulation and speaking rate on the internal structure of voicing categories. *Journal of the Acoustical Society of America, 92*, 723–735.

Watson, C. S., & Kewley-Port, D. (1989). Computer-based speech training (CBST): Current status and prospects for the future. In N. McGarr (Ed.), *Research on the Use of Sensory Aids for Hearing-Impaired Persons, Volta Review, 91*, 29–45.

Watson, C. S., Reed, D., Kewley-Port, D., & Maki, D. (1989). The Indiana Speech Training Aid (ISTRA) I: Comparisons between human and computer-based evaluation of speech quality. *Journal of Speech and Hearing Research, 32*, 245–251.

Werker, J. F. (1994). Cross-language speech perception: Developmental change does not involve loss. In J. C. Goodman & H. C. Nusbaum (Eds.), *The Development of Speech Perception: The Transition from Speech Sounds to Spoken Words* (pp. 93–120). Cambridge, MA: MIT Press.

Werker, J. F., Gilbert, J. V. H., Humphrey, K., & Tees, R. C. (1981). Developmental aspects of cross-language speech perception. *Child Development, 52*, 349–355.

Werker, J. F., & Logan, J. S. (1985). Cross-language evidence for three factors in speech perception. *Perception and Psychophysics, 37*, 35–44.

Werker, J. F., & Pegg, J. E. (1992). Infant speech perception and phonological acquisition. In C. A. Ferguson, L. Menn, & C. Stoel-Gammon (Eds.), *Phonological Development: Models, Research, Implications* (pp. 285–311). Timonium, MD: York.

Werker, J. F., & Tees, R. C. (1984). Phonemic and phonetic factors in adult cross-language speech perception. *Journal of the Acoustical Society of America, 75*, 1866–1878.

Westbury, J. R. (1983). Enlargement of the supraglottal cavity and its relation to stop consonant voicing. *Journal of the Acoustical Society of America, 73*, 1322–1336.

Whalen, D. H., & Liberman, A. L. (1987). Speech perception takes precedence over nonspeech perception. *Science, 237*, 169–171.

White, G. M., & Neely, R. B. (1976). Speech recognition experiments with linear prediction, bandpass filtering, and dynamic programming. *IEEE Transactions on Acoustics, Speech, and Signal Processing, 24*, 183–187.

Wickelgren, W. A. (1969). Context-sensitive coding, associative memory, and serial order in (speech) behavior. *Psychological Review, 76*, 1–15.

Wilhelms-Tricarico, R. (1995). Physiological modeling of speech production: Methods for modeling soft-tissue articulators. *Journal of the Acoustical Society of America, 97*, 3085–3098.

Zeng, F., & Turner, C. (1990). Recognition of voiceless fricatives for normal and hearing-impaired subjects. *Journal of Speech and Hearing Research, 33*, 440–449.

Zue, V. W. (1976). Acoustic characteristics of stop consonants: A controlled study. Dissertation submitted at the Massachusetts Institute of Technology.

Zue, V. W. (1985). The use of speech knowledge in automatic speech recognition. *Proceedings IEEE 73*, 1602–1615.

INDEX